CELLULAR AND MOLECULAR MECHANISMS OF DRUGS OF ABUSE AND NEUROTOXICITY

Cocaine, GHB, and Substituted Amphetamines

ANNALS OF THE NEW YORK ACADEMY OF SCIENCES
Volume 1074

CELLULAR AND MOLECULAR MECHANISMS OF DRUGS OF ABUSE AND NEUROTOXICITY

Cocaine, GHB, and Substituted Amphetamines

Edited by Syed F. Ali and Francesco Fornai

Published by Blackwell Publishing on behalf of the New York Academy of Sciences
Boston, Massachusetts
2006

Library of Congress Cataloging-in-Publication Data

Cellular and molecular mechanisms of drugs of abuse and neurotoxicity: cocaine, GHB, and substituted amphetamines / edited by Syed Ali, and Francesco Fornai

p. cm. – (Annals of the New York Academy of Sciences, ISSN 0077-8923 ; v. 1369)

Includes bibliographical references.

ISBN-13: 978-1-57331-629-3 (alk. paper)

ISBN-10: 1-57331-629-6 (alk. paper)

1. Drugs of abuse. 2. Neurotoxicology. 3. Amphetamines. 4. Cocaine. 5. Gamma-hydroxybutyrate. I. Ali, Sayed. II. Fornai, F. (Francesco) III. Itzhak, Y. (Yossef) IV. New York Academy of Sciences. V. Series.

[DNLM: 1. Cocaine–metabolism. 2. Amphetamines–adverse effects. 3. Amphetamines–metabolism. 4. Cocaine–adverse effects. 5. Neuro-toxicity Syndromes. 6. Street Drugs–pharmacokinetics. W1 AN626YL v.1369 2006 / QV 113 C393 2006]

RM316.C45 2006
615'.78–dc22

2006018863

The *Annals of the New York Academy of Sciences* (ISSN: 0077-8923 [print]; ISSN: 1749-6632 [online]) is published 28 times a year on behalf of the New York Academy of Sciences by Blackwell Publishing, with offices located at 350 Main Street, Malden, Massachusetts 02148 USA, PO Box 1354, Garsington Road, Oxford OX4 2DQ UK, and PO Box 378 Carlton South, 3053 Victoria Australia.

Information for subscribers: Subscription prices for 2006 are: Premium Institutional: \$3850.00 (US) and £2139.00 (Europe and Rest of World).
Customers in the UK should add VAT at 5%. Customers in the EU should also add VAT at 5% or provide a VAT registration number or evidence of entitlement to exemption. Customers in Canada should add 7% GST or provide evidence of entitlement to exemption. The Premium Institutional price also includes online access to full-text articles from 1997 to present, where available. For other pricing options or more information about online access to Blackwell Publishing journals, including access information and terms and conditions, please visit www.blackwellpublishing.com/nyas.

Membership information: Members may order copies of the *Annals* volumes directly from the Academy by visiting www.nyas.org/annals, emailing membership@nyas.org, faxing 212-888-2894, or calling 800-843-6927 (US only), or +1 212 838 0230, ext. 345 (International). For more information on becoming a member of the New York Academy of Sciences, please visit www.nyas.org/membership.

Journal Customer Services: For ordering information, claims, and any inquiry concerning your institutional subscription, please contact your nearest office:
UK: Email: customerservices@blackwellpublishing.com; Tel: +44 (0) 1865 778315; Fax +44 (0) 1865 471775
US: Email: customerservices@blackwellpublishing.com; Tel: +1 781 388 8599 or 1 800 835 6770 (Toll free in the USA); Fax: +1 781 388 8232
Asia: Email: customerservices@blackwellpublishing.com; Tel: +65 6511 8000; Fax: +61 3 8359 1120
Members: Claims and inquiries on member orders should be directed to the Academy at email: membership@nyas.org or Tel: +1 212 838 0230 (International) or 800-843-6927 (US only).

Printed in the USA.
Printed on acid-free paper.

Mailing: The *Annals of the New York Academy of Sciences* are mailed Standard Rate. **Postmaster:** Send all address changes to *Annals of the New York Academy of Sciences*, Blackwell Publishing, Inc., Journals Subscription Department, 350 Main Street, Malden, MA 01248-5020. Mailing to rest of world by DHL Smart and Global Mail.

Annals are available to subscribers online at the New York Academy of Sciences and also at Blackwell Synergy. Visit www.annalsnyas.org or www.blackwell-synergy.com to search the articles and register for table of contents e-mail alerts. Access to full text and PDF downloads of *Annals* articles are available to nonmembers and subscribers on a pay-per-view basis at www.annalsnyas.org.

The paper used in this publication meets the minimum requirements of the National Standard for Information Sciences Permanence of Paper for Printed Library Materials, ANSI Z39.48_1984.

ISSN: 0077-8923 (print); 1749-6632 (online)
ISBN-10: 1-57331-629-6 (paper); ISBN-13: 978-1-57331-629-3 (paper)

A catalogue record for this title is available from the British Library.

Digitization of the Annals of the New York Academy of Sciences:

An agreement has recently been reached between Blackwell Publishing and the New York Academy of Sciences to digitize the entire run of the Annals of the New York Academy of Sciences back to volume one, issue one.

The back files, which have been defined as all of those issues published before 1997, will be sold to libraries as part of Blackwell Publishing's Legacy Sales Program and hosted on the Blackwell Synergy website.

Copyright of all material will remain with the rights holder. Contributors: Please contact Blackwell Publishing if you do not wish an article or picture from the Annals of the New York Academy of Sciences to be included in this digitization project.

ANNALS OF THE NEW YORK ACADEMY OF SCIENCES

Volume 1074
August 2006

CELLULAR AND MOLECULAR MECHANISMS OF DRUGS OF ABUSE AND NEUROTOXICITY
Cocaine, GHB, and Substituted Amphetamines

Editors

SYED F. ALI AND FRANCESCO FORNAI

This volume is the result of a meeting entitled **Cellular and Molecular Mechanisms of Drugs of Abuse and Neurotoxicity: Cocaine, GHB and Substituted Amphetamines**, and held on August 16-19, 2005 on Isola di San Servolo, Venice, Italy.

CONTENTS

Part II. Methamphetamine Neurotoxicity

Part III. METH: Oxidative Stress, Neurodegeneration, and Neuroprotection

Part IV. METH and MPTP: Similarities and Differences

Part V. MDMA and Other Substituted Amphetamines

Part VI. Cocaine

Part VII. Heroine, Morphine, and Opiates

Part VIII. Nicotine and Marijuana

Part IX. GHB

Part X. Perinatal Exposure and Postnatal Outcome: Cocaine and Substituted Amphetamines

Financial assistance was received from:

- International Society for Neurochemistry
- Neuromed Pozzilli (IS)
- National Center for Toxicological Research, Food and Drug Administration, USA
- Venice International University
- Under the patronage of "Regione Veneto" and "Provincia di Venezia"

Preface

This volume contains reviewed versions of papers presented at the satellite meeting of the International Society for Neurochemistry Meeting and European Society for Neurochemistry. The satellite meeting entitled Cellular and Molecular Mechanisms of Drugs of Abuse and Neurotoxicity: Cocaine, GHB, and Substituted Amphetamines was held on Isola di San Servolo, August 16–19, 2005 at Venice International University, Venice, Italy. The overall atmosphere of the meeting, location, and especially the surroundings were just magnificent. Over 125 participants from 19 different countries attended the meeting. Because of the relatively small number of participants, each was able to enjoy the scientific exchange in a very relaxing and informal atmosphere.

The major goal of the conference was to understand the cellular and molecular mechanisms of drugs of abuse, such as cocaine, substituted amphetamines (D-amphetamine, methamphetamine, and MDMA), marijuana, nicotine, GHB, and organic solvents. Separate sessions were devoted to the underlying mechanisms of drug addiction such as genes and drugs of abuse; methamphetamine neurotoxicity; oxidative stress, neurotoxicity, neurodegeneration and neuroprotection; METH and MPTP neurotoxicity: similarities and differences; cocaine; MDMA and methylphenidate; heroine, morphine and opiates; nicotine, cannabinoids, CNS acting drugs and fMRI; influence of nutrition in drugs of abuse; GHB, GBL, 1,4-BD and solvents.

Several scientists presented clinical and basic studies aimed at understanding neurotoxic and addictive effects of drugs of abuse as well as developing new strategies to treat drug addiction. Although a tremendous body of data has been gathered on the molecular genetics of abused drugs, the molecular mechanisms responsible for the toxicity induced by exposure to these drugs remain to be fully elucidated. During the meeting there was constantly an informal atmosphere that allowed establishing connections and potential collaborations. This occurred particularly during the poster session, which was extremely productive. At the end of the conference, there was a panel discussion and open forum, which made the overall summary of the conference and future recommendation. The conference achieved its main goal, which was to bring together clinical and basic scientists in a multinational/multidisciplinary forum to exchange ideas and data related to this expanding field of research.

We express our gratitude to the organizations and the government agencies that supported this meeting. All papers included in this issue were reviewed by at least one referee, and we want to thank them for their valuable time and

Ann. N.Y. Acad. Sci. 1074: xv–xvi (2006). © 2006 New York Academy of Sciences.
doi: 10.1196/annals.1369.067

efforts. We also thank Blackwell Publishing and the staff of the *Annals of the New York Academy of Sciences* for their efficient processing of the manuscripts. Last, but not least, we want to thank many of our colleagues who helped us in the organization of this satellite meeting. The next ISN/ASN sponsored satellite meeting dealing with the same topic will be held on August 14–17, 2007, at the Princess Hotel in Belize City, Belize.

—**Syed F. Ali**
—**Francesco Fornai**

Opposite Regulation of Cocaine-Induced Intracellular Signaling and Gene Expression by Dopamine D1 and D3 Receptors

JIANHUA ZHANG[a] AND MING XU[b]

[a]*Department of Pathology, University of Alabama at Birmingham, Birmingham, Alabama 35294, USA*

[b]*Department of Cell Biology, Neurobiology and Anatomy, University of Cincinnati Medical Center, Cincinnati, Ohio 45267, USA*

ABSTRACT: Repeated exposure to cocaine induces persistent neuroadaptations that involve alterations in cellular signaling and gene expression mediated by dopamine (DA) receptors in the brain. Both dopamine D1 and D3 receptors mediate cocaine-induced behaviors and they are also coexpressed in the same neurons in the nucleus accumbens (NAc) and caudoputamen (CPu). We have investigated whether these two receptors coordinately regulate intracellular signaling and gene expression after acute and repeated cocaine administration. We found that extracellular signal-regulated kinase (ERK) activation and c-fos induction in the CPu following an acute cocaine administration is mediated by the D1 receptor and inhibited by the D3 receptor. ERK activation is necessary for acute cocaine-induced expression of fos family genes that include c-fos, fosB, and fra2. Furthermore, potential target genes of cAMP response element-binding (CREB) protein and/or AP-1 transcription complex, including dynorphin, neogenin, and synaptotagmin VII, are also oppositely regulated by D1 and D3 receptors after repeated cocaine injections. Lastly, such regulation requires proper ERK activation. These results suggest that D1 and D3 receptors oppositely regulate target gene expression by regulating ERK activation after cocaine administration.

KEYWORDS: cocaine; dopamine receptors; signal transduction; mitogen-activated protein kinases; c-fos; gene expression

Address for correspondence: Ming Xu, Ph.D., Department of Anesthesia and Critical Care, The University of Chicago, Chicago, IL 60637. Voice: 773-834-7937; fax: 773-702-4791.
e-mail: mxu@dacc.uchicago.edu

Ann. N.Y. Acad. Sci. 1074: 1–12 (2006). © 2006 New York Academy of Sciences.
doi: 10.1196/annals.1369.001

INTRODUCTION

A major feature of drug addiction is that it involves long-lasting neuroadaptations in the brain.[1–5] The brain dopamine (DA) system that projects to the nucleus accumbens (NAc), caudoputamen (CPu), and other forebrain structures is a primary neural substrate for mediating persistent changes induced by abused drugs.[6] There are two families of DA receptors identified so far.[7] The D1-family (D1 and D5) receptors activate adenylyl cyclases, while the D2-family receptors (D2, D3, and D4) inhibit adenylyl cyclases. The D1 receptor is abundantly expressed in the brain, including the NAc and CPu[7] whereas the D3 receptor is mostly expressed in the ventral striatum, a region where D1 receptor also exists.[7,8] We and others have previously used D1 and D3 mutant mice to demonstrate that these two receptors are involved in mediating both locomotor-stimulating and rewarding effects of psychostimulants.[9–17]

Signaling pathways and gene expression changes associated with different DA receptors are thought to play key roles in mediating drug-induced neuroadaptations in the brain. Cocaine induces the phosphorylation of cAMP response element-binding (CREB) protein and expression of immediate early genes (IEG) including c-fos and ΔfosB primarily in D1 receptor-producing neurons in both the NAc and CPu.[18–22] The induction of CREB and ΔfosB has been shown to oppositely modulate the rewarding behavioral effects of cocaine[23–25] and gene expression.[26] D3 receptors also regulate cocaine-induced gene expression changes.[16]

The mitogen-activated protein kinase (MAPK) pathways may mediate the behavioral effects of drugs of abuse. MAPKs are critical for cells to respond to environmental changes.[27,28] Extracellular signal-regulated kinases (ERKs), c-Jun N-terminal kinases (JNKs), and p38 are the three major groups of MAPKs in mammals.[27,28] Upon activation, MAPKs translocate into the cell nucleus and activate transcription factors, such as c-fos and CREB.[29] These kinases are activated by different stimuli through independent signaling pathways that mediate a variety of neuronal functions, including synaptic plasticity and learning and memory.[27–30] Exposure to drugs of abuse, such as cocaine and morphine, can also induce MAPK activation in the DA system and such activation may contribute to the development of drug-induced persistent changes in the brain.[31–34]

DA D1 and D3 receptors are coexpressed in neurons in the NAc and CPu.[8,35–37] D1 and D3 receptors can exert opposite effects in the brain. For example, we previously found that D1 and D3 receptor mutant mice exhibit attenuated and enhanced locomotor activity, respectively, compared to wild-type mice after acute cocaine administration.[10,14] Moreover, D1 and D3 receptors exhibit opposite regulation on c-fos expression in the islands of Calleja.[8,37] Although D1 receptors have been implicated in mediating acute cocaine-induced ERK activation,[32] whether D1 and D3 receptors coordinately regulate MAPK signaling and gene expression after cocaine administration remains largely unknown. We have investigated this issue. Our results suggest that D1 and D3 receptors exert opposite regulation on target gene expression by influencing ERK activation and c-fos induction after acute and chronic cocaine treatment.

MATERIALS AND METHODS

For details of D1 and D3 receptor mutant mouse models, signaling studies, and statistical analyses, see Zhang *et al.*[38] and references therein.

RESULTS

Acute Cocaine-Induced ERK Activation in the CPu is Mediated by D1 Receptors and Inhibited by D3 Receptors

Cocaine induces ERK activation in the striatum.[32] To investigate the role of D1 and D3 receptors in acute cocaine-induced MAPK activation, we evaluated how these two receptors are involved in ERK activation after acute cocaine injections using extracts from the CPu from D1 and D3 receptor mutant mice and wild-type littermates at different time points after acute cocaine injections. Western blot analyses showed that cocaine produced a similar time course in ERK phosphorylation in wild-type and D3 receptor mutant mice with a maximal effect at 20 min after the cocaine injection compared with that in saline-treated control mice.[38] Noticeably, the degree of ERK activation is 1.5-fold higher in the CPu in D3 receptor mutant mice than in wild-type mice 20 min after the cocaine injection, indicating that ERK activation is enhanced in D3 receptor mutant than in wild-type mice.[38] In contrast to that in wild-type and D3 receptor mutant mice, ERK activation is abolished in D1 receptor mutant mice.[38] Basal ERK phosphorylation is similar in the three groups of mice.[38] These results indicate that D1 and D3 receptors mediate opposite regulation in acute cocaine-induced ERK activation in the CPu.

Coordinated Actions of D1- and D2-Family Receptors at the Level of ERK Activation in the CPu are Modulated by D3 Receptors

We previously found that the D3 receptor mutation causes enhanced locomotor responses to a combined stimulation by D1- and D2-class agonists.[14] To investigate the molecular basis of D3 receptor modulation of D1- and D2-family receptor function, we determined how D3 receptors modulate ERK activation in response to D1- and D2-class receptor costimulation. We administered D1, D3 receptor mutant and wild-type mice with a D1-class agonist SKF81297, a D2-class agonist PD128907, or both. SKF81297 induced identical ERK phosphorylation in D3 receptor mutant and wild-type mice, but failed to do so in D1 receptor mutant mice.[38] Similarly, PD128907 induced equal levels of ERK activation in wild-type and D3 receptor mutant mice but not in D1 receptor mutant mice.[38] When the two agonists were administered together, ERK phosphorylation was also increased.[38] Similar to that after acute cocaine injections, there was a higher ERK activation in D3 receptor mutant mice than in wild type when the two agonists were coadministered.[38] This result indicates that during coactivation of D1- and D2-family receptors, stimulation of D3 receptors suppresses ERK activation.

ERK is Activated in D1 Receptor-Producing Neurons in the Striatum by Acute Cocaine Administration

We next determined whether cocaine-induced ERK activation occurs primarily in DA D1 receptor-expressing neurons by analyzing the distribution of phospho-ERK and dynorphin in the striatum using double immunostaining. We used brain sections prepared 20 min after the injection because at this time point cocaine induces maximal ERK activation. We found that phospho-ERK immunofluorescent signals mostly co-localize with those for dynorphin in the cytoplasm in the NAc and CPu.[38] This result indicates that ERK is activated in many but not all dynorphin-positive neurons in wild-type mice and suggests that the activation of ERK is mostly in D1 receptor-expressing neurons in the striatum.

Acute Cocaine Administration Does not Obviously Induce P38 and JNK Activation in the CPu

We next investigated whether cocaine-induced MAPK activation is specific for ERK. We performed Western blot analyses of p38 and JNK activation using antiphospho-p38 and antiphospho-JNK antibodies that recognize only the activated forms of p38 and JNK. We found no obvious p38 or JNK activation in the CPu in D1, D3 receptor mutant and wild-type mice within 2 h of the acute cocaine injection.[38] Furthermore, basal phosphorylation of p38 and JNK was similar in the three groups of mice.[38] These results indicate that D1 and D3 receptors do not obviously modulate p38 and JNK activation by acute cocaine treatment.

D1 and D3 Receptors Oppositely Regulate c-Fos Induction by Acute Cocaine Administration via Opposite Regulation of ERK Activation

Acute cocaine injections induce c-fos expression and ERK has been implicated in the c-fos induction process.[21,32] We analyzed whether the opposite regulation of D1 and D3 receptors on ERK activation extends into c-fos induction by acute cocaine injections. c-fos was not induced in the CPu in D1 receptor mutant mice compared to that in wild-type mice following a cocaine injection.[38] In contrast, there was a 1.7-fold increase in c-fos levels in the CPu in D3 receptor mutant mice compared to that in wild-type mice after cocaine injections.[38] Basal c-fos levels were similar in the CPu in the three groups of mice.[38] These results suggest that D1 and D3 receptors oppositely regulate c-fos induction in the CPu by acute cocaine injections.

To determine whether ERK activation is involved in the opposite regulation of c-fos induction by D1 and D3 receptors, we treated D3 receptor mutant and wild-type mice with a MEK-selective inhibitor SL327 before acute cocaine injections. SL327 inhibited acute cocaine-induced c-fos expression in the CPu in both groups of mice.[38] We previously showed that D1 receptors mediate fosB and fra2 induction by acute cocaine administration.[22] Noticeably, SL327 also attenuated the induction of fosB and fra2 in the CPu in wild-type and D3 receptor mutant mice.[38] These results suggest that the induction of several fos family proteins via DA receptors by acute cocaine treatment depends on the ERK signaling pathway.

D1 and D3 Receptors Also Oppositely Regulate Gene Expression After Chronic Cocaine Treatment

We previously showed that the D1 receptor mediates gene expression in the NAc and CPu upon repeated exposure to cocaine.[22] To investigate coregulation of gene expression by D1 and D3 receptors after chronic cocaine administration, we performed a systematic microarray analysis. We found that a number of potential cocaine-responsive genes in D1 and D3 receptor mutant mice showed opposite expression patterns compared to wild-type mice after repeated exposure to cocaine.[38,39] These genes included those encoding dynorphin, neogenin, and synaptotagmin VII.[38] We further investigated their differential expression in the striatum in D1 and D3 receptor mutant mice after repeated cocaine injections.

Immunohistostaining showed that the expression of dynorphin was decreased in the CPu and NAc in D1 receptor mutant mice, while increased in the CPu and NAc in D3 receptor mutant mice compared to those in wild-type mice, respectively, after chronic cocaine treatment.[38] Dynorphin levels remained similar in D1, D3 receptor mutant and wild-type mice in the cortex.[38] Western blot analysis showed that neogenin expression was decreased in both the NAc and CPu in wild-type mice by repeated cocaine injections.[38] In contrast, neogenin expression was less reduced in D3 receptor mutant mice and further decreased in D1 receptor mutant mice compared to that in wild-type mice, respectively.[38] Synaptotagmin VII was induced by repeated cocaine injections in both the NAc and CPu in wild-type mice.[38] Moreover, there was no obvious induction in synaptotagmin VII expression in D1 receptor mutant mice and an increase in synaptotagmin VII expression in D3 receptor mutant mice, respectively, compared to that in wild-type mice in both the NAc and CPu after repeated cocaine administration.[38] These results suggest that D1 and D3 receptors oppositely regulate the expression of certain target genes, including those encoding dynorphin, neogenin, and synaptotagmin VII, in the NAc and CPu after repeated cocaine injections.

The Opposite Regulation of Gene Expression by D1 and D3 Receptors After Chronic Cocaine Injections Requires ERK Activation

To determine whether neogenin and synaptotagmin VII expression requires the ERK signaling pathway, we performed Western blotting experiments using extracts prepared from both chronic cocaine-treated and SL327- and cocaine-treated wild-type mice. We found that, parallel to those found in D1 receptor mutant mice, inhibition of ERK activation further reduced neogenin and synaptotagmin VII expression in the NAc and CPu after repeated cocaine injections.[38] DNA sequence comparisons indicate that there are AP-1- and CREB-binding sites in the promotor regions of the genes encoding dynorphin, neogenin, and synaptotagmin VII.[38] Together, these findings indicate that the opposite regulation of expression of these genes by D1 and D3 receptors depends on ERK activation and may be mediated by the AP-1 transcription complexes, CREB, or both.

DISCUSSION

Repeated cocaine administration elicits persistent changes in the brain that likely involve gene expression changes mediated by DA receptors. D1 and D3 receptors are both expressed in the NAc and CPu that are known to be brain areas important for the development of drug-induced neuroadaptations. A large percentage of D3 receptor-producing neurons also coexpresses D1 receptors.[8,35–37] Moreover, coexisting D1 and D3 receptors mediate opposite responses.[8,9,14,37] The present study shows that D1 and D3 receptors exhibit opposite regulation of gene expression by oppositely regulating ERK activation after cocaine treatment.

Opposite Regulation in ERK Activation and c-Fos Induction in the CPu by D1 and D3 Receptors After Acute Cocaine Administration

MAPK activation has been implicated in mediating the rewarding effects of abused drugs. Acute cocaine injections activate ERK in the striatum.[32] Blockade of ERK activation abolishes the rewarding effects of cocaine.[32] Repeated cocaine treatment leads to a sustained ERK activation in the ventral tegmental area.[31] We now find that acute cocaine administration produces a time-dependent increase in ERK phosphorylation in the CPu in wild-type mice. Noticeably, ERK activation by acute cocaine injections is enhanced in the CPu in D3 receptor mutant mice yet abolished in the CPu in D1 receptor mutant mice, respectively, compared to that in wild-type mice. These findings suggest that D1 and D3 receptors exert opposite influence in ERK activation after acute exposure to cocaine. Moreover, cocaine-induced MAPK activation is limited to ERK and does not include p38 or JNK.

We also found that c-fos induction is abolished in the CPu in D1 receptor mutant mice while enhanced in the CPu in D3 receptor mutant mice, respectively, compared to that in the wild-type mice after acute cocaine injections. Moreover, inhibiting ERK activity reduces acute cocaine-induced fos family gene expression, including those encoding c-fos, fosB, and fra2. These results indicate that D1 and D3 receptors oppositely regulate cocaine-induced c-fos expression, and this regulation requires the ERK signaling pathway.

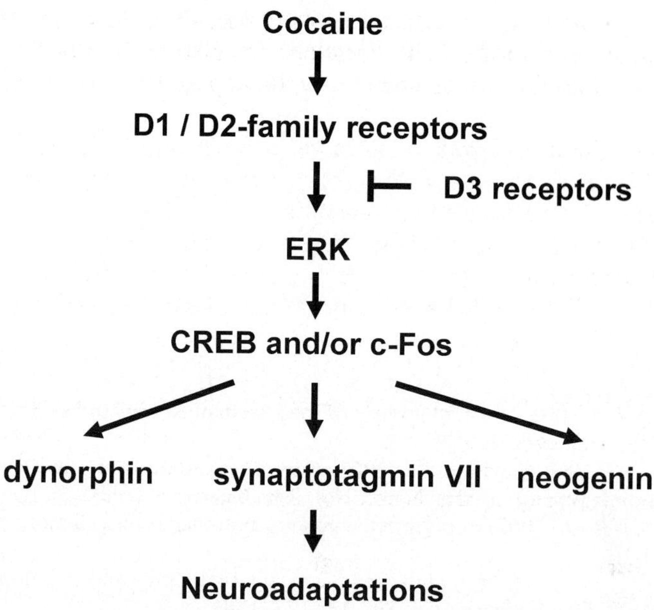

FIGURE 1. A model for D1 and D3 receptors in regulating ERK activation and gene expression after cocaine administration. Cocaine can induce ERK activation by stimulating D1- and D2-family receptors. Activated ERK, in turn, regulates c-fos and CREB and target gene expression. These gene expression changes may contribute to aspects of cocaine-induced persistent neuroadaptations. D3 receptors inhibit ERK activation and gene expression induced by combined stimulation of D1- and D2-class receptors.

Together, these results support a molecular model in which D3 receptors inhibit ERK activation and gene expression induced by costimulation of D1- and D2-family receptors (FIG. 1). Cocaine can activate ERK signaling by stimulating both D1- and D2-family receptors. Activated ERK induces CREB phosphorylation and c-fos expression that further regulate target gene expression, including that for dynorphin, synaptotagmin VII, and neogenin. Changes in the expression of these genes may contribute to different aspects of cocaine-induced long-term neuroadaptations. Since a large percentage of D1 and D3 receptors is coexpressed in the NAc and CPu, the inhibitory actions of D3 receptors may occur primarily in D1 receptor-expressing neurons.

ACKNOWLEDGMENTS

We thank Drs. L. Zhang, D. Lou, H. Jiao., D. Zhang, X. Wang, and Y. Xia for contributing to this work, and the Microarray Core at the Children's Hospital Research Foundation in Cincinnati for microarray hybridization and data scanning, and Drs. Y. Tang and F. Sharp for advice on microarray result analysis. J.Z is supported by the Epilepsy Foundation of America. M.X. is supported by NIDA (DA13786 and DA14644) and by the Epilepsy Foundation of America.

REFERENCES

1. Koob, G.F., P.P. Sanna & F.E. Bloom. 1998. Neuroscience of addiction. Neuron **21:** 467–476.
2. White, F.J. & P.W. Kalivas. 1998. Neuroadaptations involved in amphetamine and cocaine addiction. Drug Alcohol Depend. **51:** 141–153.
3. Nestler, E.J. 2001. Molecular basis of long-term plasticity underlying addiction. Nat. Rev. Neurosci. **2:** 119–128.
4. Hyman, S.E. & R.C. Malenka. 2001. Addiction and the brain: the neurobiology of compulsion and its persistence. Nat. Rev. Neurosci. **2:** 695–703.
5. Laakso, A. *et al.* 2002. Experimental genetic approaches to addiction. Neuron **36:** 213–228.
6. Koob, G.F. 1992. Drugs of abuse: anatomy, pharmacology and function of reward pathways. Trends Pharmacol. Sci. **13:** 177–184.
7. Missale, C. *et al.* 1998. Dopamine receptors: from structure to function. Physiol. Rev. **78:** 189–225.
8. Schwartz, J.C. *et al.* 1998. Functional implications of multiple dopamine receptor subtypes: the D1/D3 receptor coexistence. Brain Res. Brain Res. Rev. **26:** 236–242.
9. Xu, M. *et al.* 1994. Dopamine D1 receptor mutant mice are deficient in striatal expression of dynorphin and in dopamine-mediated behavioral responses. Cell **79:** 729–742.
10. Xu, M. *et al.* 1994. Elimination of cocaine-induced hyperactivity and dopamine-mediated neurophysiological effects in dopamine D1 receptor mutant mice. Cell **79:** 945–955.
11. Drago, J. *et al.* 1994. Altered striatal function in a mutant mouse lacking D1A dopamine receptors. Proc. Natl. Acad. Sci. USA **91:** 12564–12568.
12. Accili, D. *et al.* 1996. A targeted mutation of the D3 dopamine receptor gene is associated with hyperactivity in mice. Proc. Natl. Acad. Sci. USA **93:** 1945–1949.
13. Drago, J. *et al.* 1996. D1 dopamine receptor-deficient mouse: cocaine-induced regulation of immediate-early gene and substance P expression in the striatum. Neuroscience **74:** 813–823.
14. Xu, M. *et al.* 1997. Dopamine D3 receptor mutant mice exhibit increased behavioral sensitivity to concurrent stimulation of D1 and D2 receptors. Neuron **19:** 837–848.
15. Xu, M. *et al.* 2000. Behavioral responses to cocaine and amphetamine in D1 dopamine receptor mutant mice. Brain Res. **852:** 198–207.
16. Carta, A.R., C.R. Gerfen & H. Steiner. 2000. Cocaine effects on gene regulation in the striatum and behavior: increased sensitivity in D3 dopamine receptor-deficient mice. Neuroreport **11:** 2395–2399.

17. CAINE, S.B. *et al.* 2002. Decreased cocaine self-administration in dopamine D-1 receptor knockout mice. Drug Alcohol Depend. **66:** S25.
18. GRAYBIEL, A.M., R. MORATALLA & H.A. ROBERTSON. 1990. Amphetamine and cocaine induce drug-specific activation of the c-*fos* gene in striosome-matrix compartments and limbic subdivisions of the striatum. Proc. Natl. Acad. Sci. USA **87:** 6912–6916.
19. HOPE, B.T. *et al.* 1994. Induction of a long-lasting AP-1 complex composed of altered Fos-like proteins in brain by chronic cocaine and other chronic treatments. Neuron **13:** 1235–1244.
20. KONRADI, C. *et al.* 1994. Amphetamine regulates gene expression in rat striatum via transcription factor CREB. J. Neurosci. **14:** 5623–5634.
21. MORATALLA, R. *et al.* 1996. Cellular responses to psychomotor stimulant and neuroleptic drugs are abnormal in mice lacking the D1 dopamine receptor. Proc. Natl. Acad. Sci. USA **93:** 14928–14933.
22. ZHANG, D. *et al.* 2002. The dopamine D1 receptor is a critical mediator for cocaine-induced gene expression. J. Neurochem. **82:** 1453–1464.
23. CARLEZON, W.A. JR. *et al.* 1998. Regulation of cocaine reward by CREB. Science **282:** 2272–2275.
24. KELZ, M.B. *et al.* 1999. Expression of the transcription factor deltaFosB in the brain controls sensitivity to cocaine. Nature **401:** 272–276.
25. COLBY, C.R. *et al.* 2003. Striatal cell type-specific overexpression of DeltaFosB enhances incentive for cocaine. J. Neurosci. **23:** 2488–2493.
26. MCCLUNG, C.A. & E.J. NESTLER. 2003. Regulation of gene expression and cocaine reward by CREB and DeltaFosB. Nat. Neurosci. **6:** 1208–1215.
27. SCHAEFFER, H.J. & M.J. WEBER. 1999. Mitogen-activated protein kinases: specific messages from ubiquitous messengers. Mol. Cell. Biol. **19:** 2435–2444.
28. DAVIS, R.J. 2000. Signal transduction by the JNK group of MAP kinases. Cell **103:** 239–252.
29. ADAMS, J.P. & J.D. SWEATT. 2002. Molecular psychology: roles for the ERK MAP kinase cascade in memory. Annu. Rev. Pharmacol. Toxicol. **42:** 135–163.
30. MOROZOV, A. *et al.* 2003. Rap1 couples cAMP signaling to a distinct pool of p42/44MAPK regulating excitability, synaptic plasticity, learning, and memory. Neuron **39:** 309–325.
31. BERHOW, M.T., N. HIROI & E.J. NESTLER. 1996. Regulation of ERK (extracellular signal regulated kinase), part of the neurotrophin signal transduction cascade, in the rat mesolimbic dopamine system by chronic exposure to morphine or cocaine. J. Neurosci. **16:** 4707–4715.
32. VALJENT, E. *et al.* 2000. Involvement of the extracellular signal-regulated kinase cascade for cocaine-rewarding properties. J. Neurosci. **20:** 8701–8709.
33. CHOE, E.S. *et al.* 2002. Amphetamine increases phosphorylation of extracellular signal-regulated kinase and transcription factors in the rat striatum via group I metabotropic glutamate receptors. Neuropsychopharm. **27:** 565–575.
34. MAZZUCCHELLI, C. *et al.* 2002. Knockout of ERK1 MAP kinase enhances synaptic plasticity in the striatum and facilitates striatal-mediated learning and memory. Neuron **34:** 807–820.
35. SURMEIER, D.J., W.J. SONG & Z. YAN. 1996. Coordinated expression of dopamine receptors in neostriatal medium spiny neurons. J. Neurosci. **16:** 6579–6591.
36. LE MOINE, C. & B. BLOCH. 1996. Expression of the D3 dopamine receptor in peptidergic neurons of the nucleus accumbens: comparison with the D1 and D2 dopamine receptors. Neuroscience **73:** 131–143.

37. RIDRAY, S. *et al.* 1998. Coexpression of dopamine D1 and D3 receptors in islands of Calleja and shell of nucleus accumbens of the rat: opposite and synergistic functional interactions. Eur. J. Neurosci. **10:** 1676–1686.
38. ZHANG, L. *et al.* 2004. Cocaine-induced intracellular signaling and gene expression are oppositely regulated by the dopamine D1 and D3 receptors. J. Neurosci. **24:** 3344–3354.
39. ZHANG, D. *et al.* 2005. Gene expression changes induced by repeated cocaine administration through the dopamine D1 receptors. Neuropsychopharmacology **30:** 1443–1454.
40. VOSSLER, M.R. *et al.* 1997. cAMP activates MAP kinase and Elk-1 through a B-Raf- and Rap1-dependent pathway. Cell **89:** 73–82.
41. ROBERSON, E.D. *et al.* 1999. The mitogen-activated protein kinase cascade couples PKA and PKC to cAMP response element binding protein phosphorylation in area CA1 of hippocampus. J. Neurosci. **19:** 4337–4348.
42. WILLUHN, I., W. SUN & H. STEINER. 2003. Topography of cocaine-induced gene regulation in the rat striatum: relationship to cortical inputs and role of behavioural context. Eur. J. Neurosci. **17:** 1053–1066.
43. FAGERGREN, P. *et al.* 2003. Temporal upregulation of prodynorphin mRNA in the primate striatum after cocaine self-administration. Eur. J. Neurosci. **17:** 2212–2218.
44. COLLINS-HICOK, J. *et al.* 1994. Induction of the rat prodynorphin gene through Gs-coupled receptors may involve phosphorylation-dependent derepression and activation. Mol. Cell. Biol. **14:** 2837–2848.
45. COLE, R.L. *et al.* 1995. Neuronal adaptation to amphetamine and dopamine: molecular mechanisms of prodynorphin gene regulation in rat striatum. Neuron **14:** 813–823.
46. TESSIER-LAVIGNE, M. & C.S. GOODMAN. 1996. The molecular biology of axon guidance. Science **274:** 1123–1133.
47. ROBINSON, T.E. & B. KOLB. 1999. Alterations in the morphology of dendrites and dendritic spines in the nucleus accumbens and prefrontal cortex following repeated treatment with amphetamine or cocaine. Eur. J. Neurosci. **11:** 1598–1604.
48. ROBINSON, T.E. *et al.* 2002. Widespread but regionally specific effects of experimenter- versus self-administered morphine on dendritic spines in the nucleus accumbens, hippocampus, and neocortex of adult rats. Synapse **46:** 271–279.
49. SUDHOF, T.C. 2002. Synaptotagmins: why so many? J. Biol. Chem. **77**: 7629–7632.
50. CHAPMAN, E.R. 2002. Synaptotagmin: a Ca(2+) sensor that triggers exocytosis? Nat. Rev. Mol. Cell. Biol. **3:** 498–508.
51. SUGITA, S. *et al.* 2002. Synaptotagmins form a hierarchy of exocytotic Ca(2+) sensors with distinct Ca(2+) affinities. EMBO J. **21:** 270–280.
52. LIN, R.C. & R.H. SCHELLER. 2000. Mechanisms of synaptic vesicle exocytosis. Annu. Rev. Cell. Dev. Biol. **16:** 19–49.

Serial Analysis of Gene Expression in the Rat Striatum Following Methamphetamine Administration

NING SHENG CAI,[a] MICHAEL T. MCCOY,[a] BRUCE LADENHEIM,[a] JOHNALYN LYLES,[a] SYED F. ALI,[b] AND JEAN LUD CADET[a]

[a]*Molecular Neuropsychiatry Branch, National Institute on Drug Abuse-Intramural Research Program, Baltimore, Maryland 21224, USA*

[b]*Neurochemistry Laboratory, Division of Neurotoxicology, FDA/NCTR, Jefferson, Arkansas 72079, USA*

ABSTRACT: Methamphetamine (METH), a highly addictive drug, can cause degeneration of monoaminergic terminals and neuronal apoptosis in the mammalian brain. In the present article, we have used serial analysis of gene expression (SAGE) to investigate patterns of gene expression in the striata of rats that were given a neurotoxic dose of the drug. SAGE libraries were generated from animals treated with either saline or METH (40 mg/kg) and sacrificed 2 h later. A total of 315 transcripts were differentially expressed between the two libraries ($P < 0.05$), with 179 (56%) being upregulated and 136 (44%) being downregulated by the METH injection. Of these, CAATT enhancer-binding protein homologous protein (CHOP)/GADD153 (growth arrest- and DNA damage-inducible gene 153) was found to be upregulated by about threefold. Analysis of the expression of genes downstream of CHOP (DOCs) revealed significant METH-induced increases in their expression. Because DOC1 is an analog of carbonic anhydrase (CA) which is involved in the interconversion between carbon dioxide and the bicarbonate ion, we also measured the effects of METH on the expression of several CAs. These were significantly upregulated by METH in a time-dependent fashion. These results indicate that METH toxicity is mediated, in part, by drug-induced perturbations of physiological processes that are dependent on normal pH and CO_2 homeostasis.

KEYWORDS: METH; SAGE; neurotoxicity; CHOP; carbonic anhydrase

Methamphetamine (METH, CRANK, Speed) is a highly addictive drug that has replaced cocaine at the illicit drug of choice in some communities throughout the United States and the world.[1,2] METH is abused because it causes euphoria,

Address for correspondence: Jean Lud Cadet, M.D., Molecular Neuropsychiatry Branch, National Institute on Drug Abuse, National Institute of Health, 5500 Nathan Shock Drive, Baltimore, MD 21224. Voice: 410-550-2953; fax: 410-550-2745.
e-mail: jcadet@intra.nida.nih.gov

Ann. N.Y. Acad. Sci. 1074: 13–30 (2006). © 2006 New York Academy of Sciences.
doi: 10.1196/annals.1369.002

increased sense of well-being, and augmented sexual responses in the user.[2–4] However, at higher doses, it can cause motor dyskinesias, paranoid reactions, or acute psychotic reactions.[2,4] Prolonged use of large doses (up to several grams) of the drug can cause chronic neuropsychiatric syndromes including symptom complexes reminiscent of paranoid schizophrenia or mania.[1,2] METH abusers can also suffer from neuropsychological impairments.[5] Postmortem studies in humans have demonstrated significant decreases in the levels of dopamine (DA) and its metabolites in the brains of these patients [6] and exacerbation of neuronal death in the brains of HIV-infected patients.[7]

Studies of METH toxicity in rodent models have provided evidence that the drug can indeed cause marked depletion of DA and serotonin (5-HT) in the brain [8–11] (see Ref. 12 for a recent review). Evidence has also accumulated that METH can cause neuronal apoptosis both *in vitro* [12–15] and *in vivo*.[16–19] METH-induced neuronal apoptosis occurs via the activation of multiple cell death programs.[19] In our continuing attempts to try to identify molecular pathways that might be involved in METH-induced neurodegeneration, we have used serial analysis of gene expression (SAGE)[20] to investigate transcriptional responses in the rat striatum after a single injection of a neurotoxic dose of the drug.[19,21] Results from these investigations suggest that METH might cause some of its toxic effects through the disturbance of metabolic exchanges in the brain via CAATT enhancer-binding protein homologous protein (CHOP)-mediated upregulation of a novel form of carbonic anhydrase (CA)VI,[22] a member of a class of proteins that are involved in the catalysis of the hydration of carbon dioxide to form bicarbonate anions.[23]

MATERIALS AND METHODS

Animals and Drug Treatment

Sprague-Dawley rats (Charles River Lab, Raleigh, NC), weighing 230–280 g, received a single injection of METH (40 mg/kg)[19,21] or saline via intraperitoneal route. All animal-use procedures were according to the NIH guide for the Care and use of Laboratory Animals and were approved by the local Animal Care Committee. The rats were sacrificed 2 h after METH treatment for the SAGE analysis. Other rats were sacrificed at various time points for polymerase chain reaction (PCR) and Western blot analyses. After removal of the whole brain, the striatum was isolated and processed for RNA isolation.

RNA Isolation

Total RNA was isolated from striatum using TRIzol (Invitrogen, Carlsbad, CA) and according to the manufacturer's protocol. Approximately 10 mg of total RNA were used for the SAGE procedure.

Construction of SAGE Library

SAGE libraries were built using Invitrogen I- SAGE kit (Invitrogen) that is based on the technique developed by Velculescu *et al.*[20] Briefly, the mRNA (10 μg) was converted to cDNA using a biotinylated (T) 18 primer and Superscript II RNase H2 Reverse Transcriptase. The cDNA was converted to double-stranded cDNA and digested with *Nla*III as the anchoring enzyme; and cDNA fragments were captured using streptavidin-coated magnetic beads. After ligation of linkers to the *Nla*III-compatible sticky ends, the cDNA fragments were digested with the tagging enzyme *Bsm*FI (site present in linkers), thus generating 10 bp (base pairs) SAGE cDNA tags attached to the linkers. After blunting of the linker-cDNA products, dimerization, and PCR amplification (25 cycles) using primers directed against linker sequences, the linkers were excised by *Nla*III digestion. The released ditag was purified from the excised linkers by polyacrylamide gel electrophoresis and ligated to long multimers of ditags separated by *Nla*III sites. After size separation by polyacrylamide gel electrophoresis, the 400- to 800-bp fraction was excised from gel, purified, and cloned into the *Sph*I site of pZero-1 (Invitrogen). Transfection of one-fifth of this ligation mixture into 50-μL One Shot TOP10 Electrocomp *Escherichia coli* via electroporation yielded about 1600 colonies. The colonies were screened for inserts via PCR utilizing M13F and M13R as primers. The positive clones were sent to sequence.

Sequencing of SAGE Library

Sequence analysis was performed on 10 μL of insert PCR product, using the ABI Prism BigDye Terminator Cycle Sequencing Ready Reaction Kit and ABI Prism 3100 Genetic Analyzer (Applied Bio Systems Forster City, CA).

SAGE Data Analysis

SAGE libraries were analyzed using the SAGE2000 software that obtained from The Johns Hopkins University (Baltimore, MD, USA; http://www.sagenet.org). SAGE Transcripts were identified by comparison of the tags in the database with the NCBI tag to SAGEmap rat database dated August 21, 2004 (SAGEmap, http://www.ncbi.nlm.nih.gov/SAGE).

Functional Classes of Genes

Using the Database for Annotation Visualization and Integrated Discovery (DAVID), an online gene classification tool (available at http://david.niaid.nih.gov/David) the significantly altered known genes were classified.

TABLE 1. Summary of SAGE libraries

	Saline		METH	
	Tags	%	Tags	%
Known genes	5651	51	5746	51
ESTs	1928	18	2058	18
Unmatched transcripts	3435	31	3398	31
Total	11014	100	11202	100

Quantitative Real-Time RT-PCR Analysis

Rat striatum total RNA was extracted with an RNeasy Mini kit (Qiagen, Valenciá, CA), and 1 μg of total RNA was converted to cDNA using Advantage reverse transciption (RT) for PCR kit with oligo dT primer (BD Biosciences, San Jose, CA). PCR was performed with the LightCycler FastStart DNA Master SYBR Green I kit (Roche Applied Science Indianapolis, IN) as described in the manufacturer's protocol. Real-time detection of the emission intensity of SYBR green was performed using the LightCycler thermal cycler system (Roche Applied Science).

Western Blot Analyses

Western blot analysis was carried out with the striatum dissected from four METH- and saline-treated rats. Samples from four rats were pooled to form one group. The pooled striatum was homogenized in RIPA lysis buffer (Santa Cruz Biotechnology, Inc., Santa Cruz, CA) with a sonicator and maintained the temperature at 4°C throughout all procedures. The homogenates were transfered to microcentrifuge tubes, centrifuged at 10,000g for 10 min at 4°C. The supernatant were removed and centrifuged again. The supernatant fluid is the total tissue lysate. Electrophoresis and transfer of protein were according to standard protocols. Membrane blocking, primary and secondary antibody incubation, and chemiluminescence's reaction were carried out according to the protocol described by Santa Cruz Biotechnology. Monoclonal CHOP/GADD153 (growth arrest- and DNA damage-inducible gene 153) and tubulin antibody were purchased from Santa Cruz Biotechnology, Inc.

TABLE 2. METH-induced transcriptional changes in the rat striatum

	Up-regulated		Down-regulated		total	
classification	Transcripts	%	Transcripts	%	Transcripts	%
Known genes	139	77.7	84	61.8	223	70.8
ESTs	30	16.8	24	17.6	54	17.1
MRTs	10	5.6	28	20.6	38	12.1
Total	179	100	136	100	315	100

RESULTS

Generation of SAGE Data

In order to examine gene expression patterns in the rat striatum after METH, rats were given a single injection of a toxic dose of METH (40 mg/kg). A total of 22,000 tags were generated from the striata of saline-treated whereas 23,585 tags were generated from METH-injected rats. These data can be accessed at NCBI SAGEmap (accession number: GSM29627, GSM29626). These tags represent 8999 and 9121 unique transcripts, respectively. The unique tags were compared to the rat SAGEmap database prepared by NCBI.[24] TABLE 1 shows that these unique tags consisted of known genes (51%), expressed sequence tags (ESTs) (18%), and novel transcripts (31%) in both libraries. The frequency distribution of SAGE tags was also similar between the two libraries, with the vast majority of the tags (98%) being encountered 10 times or less and with relatively few tags having a frequency greater than 20 (2%). Thus, the two libraries are comparable in terms of the complexity of gene expression.

METH Administration Causes Significant Changes in Gene Expression in the Rat Striatum

Gene expression patterns in the two SAGE libraries were further compared statistically using SAGE2000[20] in order to assess the effects of the METH injections. There were 315 tags that were differentially expressed in the two libraries. Of these, 179 (56%) were upregulated and 136 (44%) were downregulated by METH (TABLE 2). A search of UniGene revealed that 223 of these were known genes, 54 were ESTs, whereas 38 were unmatched tags that we labeled METH-regulated tags (MRTs). The fold changes of METH induced upregulated and downregulated genes are shown in TABLES 3 and 4, respectively. TABLES 5 and 6 show all the ESTs that were differentially affected by METH. Several of the known genes have previously been reported to be affected by METH.[25–28] These include nerve-growth factor inducible gene B (NGFI-B or *Nor 77*),[18,19,25,27] heat shock proteins,[25,29,30] several ribosomal proteins,[31] and CHOP.[19] Most of the identified genes have not previously been reported to be affected by this drug.

In order to provide functional classification of the known genes that were affected by METH, we used the DAVID. FIGURES 1A and 1B show that the upregulated and downregulated genes belong to several functional categories, with a larger percentage belonging to genes whose products participate in the regulation of cell growth and/or maintenance, in protein metabolism and biosynthesis. Interestingly, many of these genes have yet to be classified.

TABLE 3. METH-induced upregulation of 50 known genes in the rat striatum

Tag	Saline	METH	Fold	*P* values	SYMBOL	Gene names	UniGene
ATTCACCTTG	0	8	>8	0.00	LOC246270	estrous-specific protein, 250 kDa	Rn. 92563
CAGTTGGGTT	0	6 >	6	0.02	Hnrpa1	heterogeneous nuclear ribonucleoprotein A1	Rn. 25771
TCCCTGTACA	0	6 >	6	0.02	Grifin	galectin-related interfiber protein	Rn. 26894
GCTGGAACTT	0	6	> 6	0.02	Lfg	lifeguard	Rn. 44942
GCCAAAAAAA	0	6	> 6	0.02	Klct	kinesin light chain KLCt	Rn. 64504
AAACCCACAC	0	6	> 6	0.02	Gad1	Glutamate decarboxylase 1 (brain)	Rn. 91245
CGCTGGACTC	0	5 >	5	0.04	Pmpcb	mitochondrial processing peptidase beta	Rn. 841
CCCATAATCC	0	5 >	5	0.04	SC2	synaptic glycoprotein SC2	Rn. 3380
CTTTTGAGTT	0	5 >	5	0.04	Vcp	valosin-containing protein	Rn. 3820
CCTTTTCCTT	0	5 >	5	0.04	Gdi1	GDP-dissociation inhibitor 1	Rn. 4000
CTTAAGGATC	0	5 >	5	0.04	Rda288	hypothetical RNA-binding protein RDA288	Rn. 7674
TTTGTTAAAA	0	5 >	5	0.04	Rtp801	HIF-1-responsive RTP801	Rn. 9775
TAGCTGAAAA	0	5 >	5	0.04	Nr4a1	immediate early gene transcription factor NGFI-B	Rn. 10000
GGAGATACCT	0	5 >	5	0.04	Nell2	nel-like 2 homolog (chicken)	Rn. 11567
GAGCAGGAGC	0	5 >	5	0.04	Hdac5	histone deacetylase 5	Rn. 18452
GACATTGGAC	0	5 >	5	0.04	Hpcl2	2-hydroxyphytanoyl-CoA lyase	Rn. 21425
GAGGACCCCC	0	5	> 5	0.04	Ptprd	protein tyrosine phosphatase, receptor type, D	Rn. 91202
GCCCTGGGTT	2	22	11.00	0.00	Pts	6-pyruvoyl-tetrahydropterin synthase	Rn. 87164
TAAAGCTGTT	1	11	11.00	0.00	LOC81816	ubiquitin-conjugating enzyme	Rn. 3530
TGCCCACCCG	1	10	10.00	0.01	Baiap2	brain-specific angiogenesis inhibitor 1-associated prote	Rn. 13017
ATGAAATCAA	2	19	9.50	0.00	Ndufa5	NADH dehydrogenase (ubiquinone) 1 alpha subcomple	Rn. 40171
TGTACTTGAA	2	17	8.50	0.00	Atp1a2	ATPase, Na+K+ transporting, alpha 2	Rn. 1042
TAACAGTTGC	1	7	7.00	0.04	Canx	calnexin	Rn. 1762
TCACTAAAGC	1	7	7.00	0.04	Glns	glutamine synthetase 1	Rn. 2204
GAGGCTTTGC	1	7	7.00	0.04	Hsp86	heat shock protein 86	Rn. 3277
GCTGACGCTC	1	7	7.00	0.04	Ube2d2	ubiquitin-conjugating enzyme E2D 2	Rn. 7390
TACCCTCACA	3	16	5.33	0.00	Rpl6	ribosomal protein L6	Rn. 2660
CTTTGATCGC	2	10	5.00	0.02	Ppp3ca	protein phosphatase 3, catalytic subunit, alpha isoform	Rn. 6866

Continued.

TABLE 3. ***Continued***

Tag	Saline	METH	Fold	*P* values	SYMBOL	Gene names	UniGene
CCTGTGGGTC	2	10	5.00	0.02	1G5	vesicle-associated calmodulin-binding protein	Rn. 9958
GTAATTAGAG	2	9	4.50	0.04	Glns	glutamine synthetase 1	Rn. 2204
CAAAAAAAAA	2	9	4.50	0.04	Tlk2	tousled-like kinase 2	Rn. 59536
GAATAATAAA	8	35	4.38	0.00	Hspa8	heat shock protein 8	Rn. 3672
TGTTCCAGAT	3	13	4.33	0.01	Calb1	calbindin 1	Rn. 3908
CCCTGAGCGG	5	20	4.00	0.00	Apoc4	apolipoprotein C-IV	Rn. 33157
CCCTGAGCGG	5	20	4.00	0.00	Tf	Transferrin	Rn. 91296
AGAGCAGGCC	3	12	4.00	0.03	Sirt6	sirtuin silent mating type information regulation 2 homo	Rn. 2109
TGTATAAAAA	3	12	4.00	0.03	TBB1	beta-tubulin T beta15	Rn. 37849
GTAAGCAAAA	16	63	3.94	0.00	Loc192255	polyubiquitin	Rn. 1253
GAATGACCTG	6	23	3.83	0.00	Rpl13a	ribosomal protein L13A	Rn. 92211
GAAAAAAAAA	3	11	3.67	0.04	LOC246307	asparaginase-like sperm autoantigen	Rn. 22774
TGCTAAGAAT	7	22	3.14	0.01	Ppp1cc	Protein phosphatase 1, catalytic subunit, gamma isofor	Rn. 1495
ACAAAAGCAC	5	15	3.00	0.03	Plp	proteolipid protein	Rn. 4550
CTGAGGAGGG	5	15	3.00	0.03	Ddit3	DNA-damage inducible transcript 3	Rn. 11183
CACATCTGGT	11	29	2.64	0.01	Hspa5	heat shock 70kD protein 5	Rn. 11088
TATGACTTAA	8	20	2.50	0.03	Rac1	ras-related C3 botulinum toxin substrate 1 (rho family, s	Rn. 980
GTGCTTTCAA	8	19	2.38	0.04	Cdh22	cadherin 22	Rn. 11397
CCGTGGGTGA	11	24	2.18	0.03	Rps23	ribosomal protein S23	Rn. 2139
ACCAACGAAA	12	26	2.17	0.03	Stmn4	stathmin-like 4	Rn. 5658
TGGAAATGAC	19	40	2.11	0.01	Col1a1	collagen, type 1, alpha 1	Rn. 2953
TGGAAATGAC	19	40	2.11	0.01	Bcat1	branched chain aminotransferase 1, cytosolic	Rn. 8273
GGAAGGTGGC	15	30	2.00	0.03	Apod	apolipoprotein D	Rn. 11339
ATAGCTTTCT	17	32	1.88	0.04	App	Amyloid beta (A4) precursor protein	Rn. 2104
GCTGGCAGCC	16	30	1.88	0.05	Ppp1ca	Protein phosphatase type 1 alpha, catalytic subunit	Rn. 2024
CTGAAACAGT	29	50	1.72	0.02	Penk-rs	preproenkephalin, related sequence	Rn. 10015
ACGTCTCAAA	37	62	1.68	0.02	Tuba1	alpha-tubulin	Rn. 54749

TABLE 4. METH-induced down-regulation of 25 known genes in the rat striatum

Tags	Saline	METH	Fold	*P* value	SYMBOL	GENENAME	UniGene
ATAGCAGCAC	9	0	> 9	0.001	Cox5b	cytochrome c oxidase subunit Vb	Rn. 6686
TTGGAACAAT	9	0	> 9	0.001	Ins2	insulin 2	Rn. 989
ACTCCTGTCC	8	0	> 8	0.003	Trhr	Thyrotropin releasing hormone receptor	Rn. 9962
CCAGGACAGT	6	0	> 6	0.013	Slc4a3	solute carrier family 4, member 3	Rn. 87739
CGACAGTCGA	6	0	> 6	0.013	Sv2b	synaptic vesicle glycoprotein 2 b	Rn. 9940
CTGCACTCCA	6	0	> 6	0.013	Sqstm1	sequestosome 1	Rn. 3432
GTGACCCTTA	6	0	> 6	0.013	Tyro3	TYRO3 protein tyrosine kinase 3	Rn. 8883
AGATGTGTTC	5	0	> 5	0.027	Tpm1	tropomyosin 1, alpha	Rn. 87540
GTCTCATCTC	5	0	> 5	0.027	Dlgh1	discs, large homolog 1 (Drosophila)	Rn. 89331
TTACACACCC	5	0	> 5	0.027	Rasd2	RASD family, member 2	Rn. 34097
CAATTGATAT	8	1	8.00	0.015	Tde1l	tumor differentially expressed 1, like	Rn. 2078
CAGGGCAGTT	8	1	8.00	0.015	Rab2	RAB2, member RAS oncogene family	Rn. 44916
CGACCAGCAG	8	1	8.00	0.015	Vdac2	voltage-dependent anion channel 2	Rn. 3343
GACTTGACAC	8	1	8.00	0.015	Scd2	stearoyl-Coenzyme A desaturase 2	Rn. 83595
CATTTGGTTG	7	1	7.00	0.028	Scp2	Sterol carrier protein 2, liver	Rn. 31887
CTGATCCCCA	7	1	7.00	0.028	Lamp1	Lysosomal-associated membrane protein 1 (120 k	Rn. 40177
TCGGAGAAGA	7	1	7.00	0.028	Ptms	parathymosin	Rn. 3609
TGTGTGTGTG	7	1	7.00	0.028	Neu1	Neuraminidase 1	Rn. 36634
CAAGGTGACA	20	4	5.00	0.000	Rps2	ribosomal protein S2	Rn. 2115
TTCAGCTCGA	17	4	4.25	0.002	Rps7	ribosomal protein S7	Rn. 2050
AGGCAGACAG	45	12	3.75	0.000	Eef1a1	eukaryotic translation elongation factor 1 alpha 1	Rn. 965
CAGATCTTTG	12	4	3.00	0.029	Ubc	ubiquitin C	Rn. 3761
AGCGGGAGGT	17	6	2.83	0.012	Stmn3	stathmin-like 3	Rn. 14961
TGGGCCAGAA	17	6	2.83	0.012	Rgs9	regulator of G protein signaling 9	Rn. 10903
GTGTGGCACA	18	7	2.57	0.015	Rps13	ribosomal protein S13	Rn. 4609
TTGGCTGCCC	26	11	2.36	0.006	Rps14	ribosomal protein S14	Rn. 36102

Continued.

TABLE 4. ***Continued***

Tags	Saline	METH	Fold	*P* value	SYMBOL	GENENAME	UniGene
GCCTCCAAGG	35	16	2.19	0.003	Gapd	Glyceraldehyde-3-phosphate dehydrogenase	Rn. 91450
GTGGGTGTGT	15	7	2.14	0.050	Rps15	ribosomal protein S15	Rn. 3391
GAGCGTTTTG	28	14	2.00	0.014	Ppia	Peptidylprolyl isomerase A (cyclophilin A)	Rn. 1463
AGAGCGAAGT	22	11	2.00	0.027	Rpl41	ribosomal protein L41	Rn. 2833
TCTGACCTGC	29	15	1.93	0.013	S100b	S100 calcium-binding protein, beta (neural)	Rn. 8937
GCTCTGATAT	21	11	1.91	0.038	Dbi	diazepam-binding inhibitor	Rn. 3285
CCAATGGTCC	50	29	1.72	0.005	Cst3	cystatin C	Rn. 956
TCTTCGTGAC	32	19	1.68	0.025	Sip30	SNAP25-interacting protein 30	Rn. 7624
CACAGCGTTG	79	47	1.68	0.001	Mobp	myelin-associated oligodendrocytic basic protein	Rn. 91185
TGGATCCTGA	34	21	1.62	0.030	Hbb	hemoglobin beta chain complex	Rn. 36966
TCAGGCTGCC	88	55	1.60	0.001	Fth1	ferritin, heavy polypeptide 1	Rn. 54447
CTAGTCTTTG	98	79	1.24	0.038	Rps29	Ribosomal protein S29	Rn. 34942

TABLE 5. List of ESTs up-regulated by METH

Tags	Saline	METH	Fold	*P* values	UniGene
TTCAAATCAC	0	11	> 11	0.0008	Rn. 3523
GACCCCTCAA	0	8	> 8	0.0048	Rn. 17175
ACTAACTGTG	0	7	> 7	0.0094	Rn. 7745
CTGATCCCCT	0	6	> 6	0.0207	Rn. 2058
ACAAAGGTTA	0	6	> 6	0.0207	Rn. 2517
AACAAAATTA	0	6	> 6	0.0207	Rn. 26543
TACCTGCTTG	0	5	> 5	0.0358	Rn. 15380
GTTATTTCTG	0	5	> 5	0.0358	Rn. 15120
TTTCCAAAGT	0	5	> 5	0.0358	Rn. 8068
TGAAGCAGAC	0	5	> 5	0.0358	Rn. 7031
TTTGCTCTTT	0	5	> 5	0.0358	Rn. 3816
TTCAACCTCA	0	5	> 5	0.0358	Rn. 13829
TCCTTTACAC	0	5	> 5	0.0358	Rn. 18949
GCTGGCCTCA	0	5	> 5	0.0358	Rn. 1342
TTAAATAAAT	0	5	> 5	0.0358	Rn. 8214
ATGGCTAATC	0	5	> 5	0.0358	Rn. 51070
GGTAAACACA	0	5	> 5	0.0358	Rn. 96446
TTAAATAAAT	0	5	> 5	0.0358	Rn. 102
TTGATCCTAC	0	5	> 5	0.0358	Rn. 8739
GCTGAACAGC	1	10	10.00	0.0081	Rn. 3027
AGGAGAAAGG	1	9	9.00	0.0149	Rn. 2547
CAGAGCTTTA	1	8	8.00	0.0253	Rn. 1620
TTGCAGGAAC	1	8	8.00	0.0253	Rn. 37874
ACACAGAAAT	1	8	8.00	0.0253	Rn. 1921
TATCCAAACA	1	8	8.00	0.0253	Rn. 3655
TGAGATACTC	1	8	8.00	0.0253	Rn. 7692
GCATAAGTTG	1	7	7.00	0.0430	Rn. 14632
GGGCAGTCCT	1	7	7.00	0.0430	Rn. 18327
TCAAAATGTC	1	7	7.00	0.0430	Rn. 2188
TTGAAATCAA	2	12	6.00	0.0089	Rn. 86600
GTATTTGCAA	4	22	5.50	0.0005	Rn. 12600
TGGAAATGGA	2	9	4.50	0.0426	Rn. 12944
CAAAAAAAAA	2	9	4.50	0.0426	Rn. 4133
CAAAAAAAAA	2	9	4.50	0.0426	Rn. 15873
CAAAAAAAAA	2	9	4.50	0.0426	Rn. 11543
AACTGTGTCG	2	9	4.50	0.0426	Rn. 35146
CAAAAAAAAA	2	9	4.50	0.0426	Rn. 7325
CAAAAAAAAA	2	9	4.50	0.0426	Rn. 12135
CAAAAAAAAA	2	9	4.50	0.0426	Rn. 86164
TGACTATTAA	5	22	4.40	0.0014	Rn. 94842
TGACTATTAA	5	22	4.40	0.0014	Rn. 2510
GTATGTGGAT	3	13	4.33	0.0141	Rn. 3135
TGTATAAAAA	3	12	4.00	0.0276	Rn. 83199
TACAAAATGC	4	16	4.00	0.0090	Rn. 17573
GAATGACCTG	6	23	3.83	0.0020	Rn. 6005
GTAAAAAAAA	4	15	3.75	0.0151	Rn. 44283
GTGGTTCACA	3	11	3.67	0.0391	Rn. 45309
GGGGGCCAGA	3	11	3.67	0.0391	Rn. 66301

Continued.

TABLE 5. *Continued*

Tags	Saline	METH	Fold	*P* values	UniGene
CTAAGTAAAG	3	11	3.67	0.0391	Rn. 66290
TATTACTTGT	4	14	3.50	0.0230	Rn. 24009
CAAGAGGCAC	5	16	3.20	0.0198	Rn. 1048
CAGAGTCGCT	6	18	3.00	0.0175	Rn. 7401
GGGGTCAGGC	5	14	2.80	0.0471	Rn. 17092
AGCAAAAGCC	9	25	2.78	0.0078	Rn. 7755
TTGGTCAAAC	8	21	2.63	0.0185	Rn. 13756
GATGTGGCTG	7	18	2.57	0.0321	Rn. 42155
CGCTGGTTCC	8	20	2.50	0.0270	Rn. 14687
GTGACTCACA	8	19	2.38	0.0407	Rn. 40372
GTGACTCACA	8	19	2.38	0.0407	Rn. 20356
GTGACTCACA	8	19	2.38	0.0407	Rn. 42802
GCCTTCCAAT	14	33	2.36	0.0090	Rn. 2437
ATAGCTTTCT	17	32	1.88	0.0418	Rn. 3856
TCCAATAAAG	39	73	1.87	0.0025	Rn. 973
TCCAATAAAG	39	73	1.87	0.0025	Rn. 36609
ATAACACATA	716	1015	1.42	0.0000	Rn. 94572

GADD153/CHOP and DOCs are Induced by METH Administration

Because CHOP, also known as GADD153 or DNA-damage inducible transcript 3,[32] is involved in cellular responses to stress,[32,33] we chose to further investigate the changes observed in its expression. Toward that end, we used RT-PCR to perform time- and dose-dependent experiments to analyze the effects of METH on CHOP expression in the rat striatum. FIGURE 2 shows that METH does indeed cause dose- (FIG. 2 A) and time-dependent (FIG. 2 B) changes in CHOP mRNA. A nontoxic dose of METH (10 mg/kg) did not cause any changes in CHOP expression whereas two toxic doses (20 and 40 mg/kg) of METH[21] caused two- to fourfold increases of METH at 2 h after the single METH injection. Assessment of the time course (FIG. 2 B) of the effects of the drug revealed that METH (40 mg/kg) caused increases in CHOP mRNA expression which started at 1 h after the drug injection, reached a maximum at 4 h, and then returned to normal. Western blot analysis also revealed significant increases in CHOP protein (FIG. 2 C).

CHOP is also a transcription factor which can regulate the expression of target genes some of which have been identified.[34] These have been labeled genes downstream of CHOP (DOCs) and include DOC 1, DOC4, and DOC6.[34] Because we wanted to know if the METH-induced changes in CHOP expression were mirrored by changes in the DOCs, we measured their expression and found that DOC mRNAs were significantly induced by the METH injection (FIG. 3). Because DOC1 is a novel form of CAVI[22] which belongs to a class of enzymes that catalyze the reversible hydration of CO_2 to form HCO_3^- and protons,[23] we also investigated the levels of striatal mRNAs for three CAs (CAVI, XII, and CAXIV) that are known to be located in the brain. These

TABLE 6. List of ESTs down-regulated by METH

Tags	Saline	METH	Fold	*P* values	UniGene
GCCAACGATC	7	0	> 7	0.0062	Rn. 27771
GCTTTCTTAC	6	0	> 7	0.0126	Rn. 95021
TCCGCAGTCA	6	0	> 7	0.0126	Rn. 50
ACCAAGATCT	5	0	> 7	0.0266	Rn. 98183
GTCTGACATA	5	0	> 7	0.0266	Rn. 22424
TAAGATTCTT	7	0	> 7	0.0062	Rn. 8614
AGAGGTGGTT	5	0	> 7	0.0266	Rn. 5135
TGACCAAGTG	5	0	> 7	0.0266	Rn. 17784
ATAATAGTTG	6	0	> 7	0.0126	Rn. 82736
GCTGCCCTCC	63	0	> 7	0.0000	Rn. 7037
GAGATCAGTT	8	0	> 7	0.0030	Rn. 78670
TAAGATTCTT	7	0	> 7	0.0062	Rn. 12355
CCTGCCCGTG	5	0	> 7	0.0266	Rn. 8286
GGAGGGGAAG	9	1	9.00	0.0077	Rn. 22772
GCCGTTCTTA	25	3	8.33	0.0000	Rn. 48996
CGCTGGGATG	8	1	8.00	0.0152	Rn. 8526
CTTTGCAATG	8	1	8.00	0.0152	Rn. 1298
TCACATCCAA	8	1	8.00	0.0152	Rn. 12600
TGTGTGTGTG	7	1	7.00	0.0284	Rn. 2463
TGTGTGTGTG	7	1	7.00	0.0284	Rn. 15881
AGGAGGACTT	7	1	7.00	0.0284	Rn. 22543
CAAGGTGACA	20	4	5.00	0.0005	Rn. 33237
CGCAAGGCCC	110	24	4.58	0.0000	Rn. 48153
GTAGAAGGAG	9	2	4.50	0.0243	Rn. 7347
GTTCAGCAAA	9	2	4.50	0.0243	Rn. 17168
CATTGGATAC	9	2	4.50	0.0243	Rn. 14920
TGCAGGCGAC	8	2	4.00	0.0408	Rn. 15712
GGGCACAGGA	8	2	4.00	0.0408	Rn. 7680
GTTCTCTGGC	8	2	4.00	0.0408	Rn. 5998
GTGTGTGGTG	8	2	4.00	0.0408	Rn. 3222
GTGTGTGGTG	8	2	4.00	0.0408	Rn. 65040
CCGCCCAAAG	12	4	3.00	0.0291	Rn. 28396
ACATCATAGA	12	4	3.00	0.0291	Rn. 397
TATGTCAGTA	16	7	2.29	0.0331	Rn. 18036
GTCCTATGAG	16	7	2.29	0.0331	Rn. 3678
GCCTCCAAGG	35	16	2.19	0.0028	Rn. 17312
GTGGGTGTGT	15	7	2.14	0.0498	Rn. 92852
GTGGGTGTGT	15	7	2.14	0.0498	Rn. 97783
GGAGGGGGAG	41	23	1.78	0.0081	Rn. 31467
TCGGGAGAGT	48	28	1.71	0.0076	Rn. 3254

isoforms of CA showed significant increases in their expression patterns, with increases beginning at 2 h and lasting a few hours after the METH treatment in the cases of CAVI and XIV (FIG. 4).

DISCUSSION

METH abuse is causing a major public health disaster throughout the world because of the many medical and neurological problems associated with its

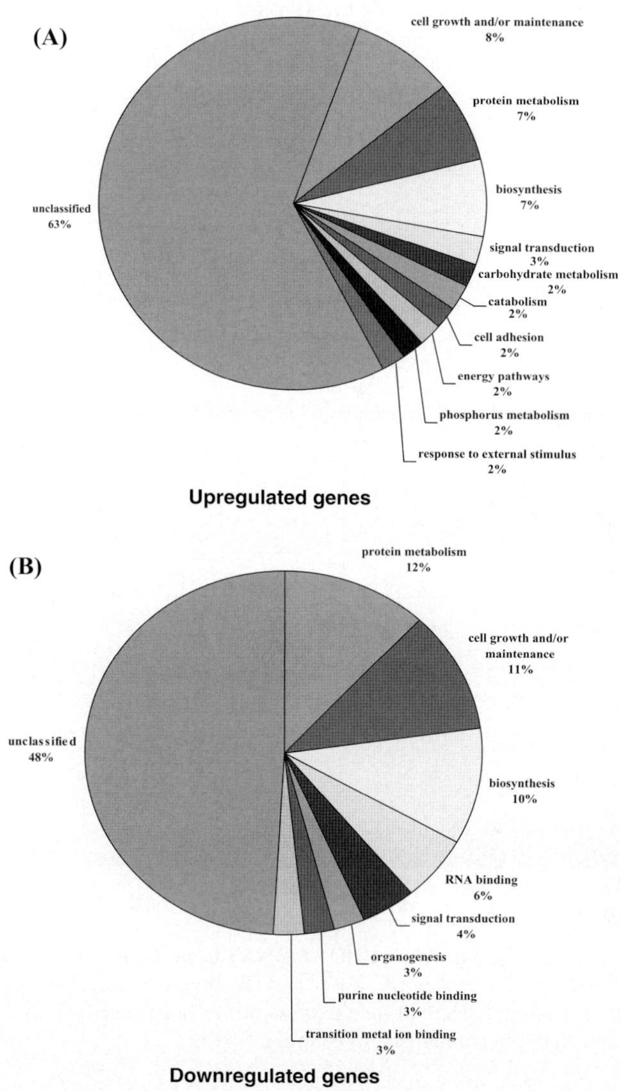

FIGURE 1. Functional classification of METH-induced upregulated (**A**) and downregulated (**B**) using the DAVID program. These genes belong to several functional categories, with a larger percentage belonging to genes whose products participate in the regulation of cell growth and/or maintenance, in protein metabolism and biosynthesis.

use. Some of these problems are due to the increasing larger doses of the drug that METH abusers have to take in order to maintain its euphoric effects.[35] These doses are known to cause long-term neurotoxic and neurodegenerative changes in animal models[36] and in humans.[5,37] Efforts to identify mechanisms that might be involved in METH-induced neurodegenerative effects have led

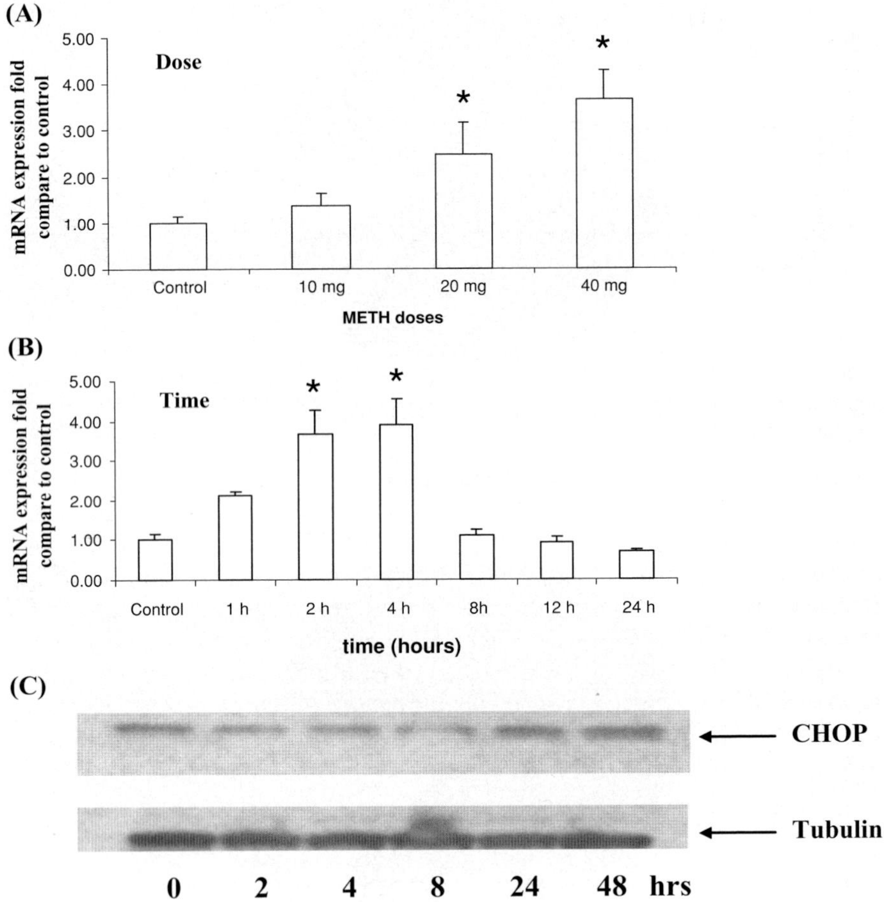

FIGURE 2. Effects of METH on CHOP mRNA (**A** and **B**) and protein (**C**) expression in the rat striatum. METH caused (**A**) dose- and (**B**) time-dependent increases in CHOP mRNA in the rat striatum. CHOP protein expression was also significantly increases after METH (**C**). $^*P < 0.05$, in comparison to controls.

to the conclusion that METH toxicity is dependent on cross-talks between several toxic mechanisms.[4,18,19,25,29,38,39] In the present study, we opted to use the unbiased SAGE technique[20] in an attempt to provide a comprehensive and quantitative analysis of the effects of METH on the rat striatal transcriptome. We reasoned that this approach might allow us to discover novel genes and/or pathways that have yet to be identified as culprits in the METH neurotoxicity cascade.

Indeed, this comprehensive approach allowed us to identify several known genes and novel tags that were affected by METH. These belong to several functional classes including cell growth and/or maintenance, protein metabolism,

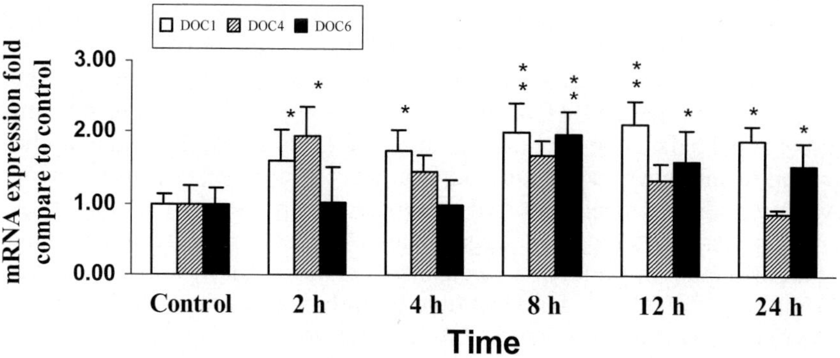

FIGURE 3. Effects of METH on DOC expression. DOC 1, DOC4, and DOC 6 showed significant METH-induced increases in their expression. $^*P < 0.05$; $^{**}P < 0.01$, in comparison with controls.

signal transduction, as well as classes of genes that are involved in regulating cellular responses to various stresses. Of the latter, we chose to further investigate the expression of CHOP/GADD153 which showed significant increases in a dose- and time-dependent fashion after a single METH injection. Because CHOP is a transcription factor that is involved in the regulation of the recently identified DOCs, we use quantitative PCR and showed that the DOCs were significantly upregulated by METH. In addition, because DOC1 is a novel form of CAVI,[40] we also measured the expression of three CAs because of the possibility that they might also be impacted by the METH injection. Our test of this idea revealed that there was indeed METH-induced upregulation of these

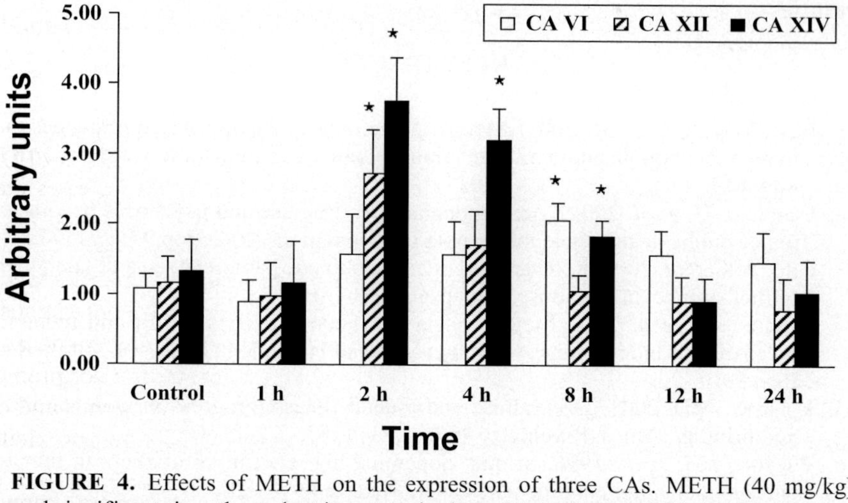

FIGURE 4. Effects of METH on the expression of three CAs. METH (40 mg/kg) caused significant time-dependent increases in three CA isoforms of CA (CAVI, XII, and CAXIV), with increases beginning at 2 h and lasting a few hours after the METH treatment in the cases of CAVI and XIV. $^*P < 0.05$, in comparison with controls.

CAs in the rat brain and suggests that METH might cause a general perturbation in acid–base balance in the brain because CAs are zinc metalloenzymes that catalyze the reversible hydration of CO_2 to form HCO_3^- and protons.[23] These METH-induced changes in CA might be in response to METH-induced perturbations of pH balance in the brain because METH is a weak base that has been reported to inhibit intracellular acidification.[41] Moreover, because increased CA expression has been reported to protect against stress-induced apoptosis,[42,43] it is not farfetched to suggest that CA induction in the present model might participate in protective mechanisms that serve to restore homeostasis subsequent to METH-mediated anionic perturbations in the rodent brain.

In conclusion, we have used SAGE to characterize the global transcription response of the rat striatum to an acute METH administration. Our observations suggest that METH toxicity is associated with significant perturbations of acid–base balance in the brain. When taken together with previous data indicating significant cross-talks between various toxic mechanisms after the administration of this drug, the present findings support the notion that METH-induced neurodegenerative effects are consequent to its multifaceted effects in the mammalian central nervous system. The identification and further characterization of the transcripts described here should provide potential new targets for the prevention and treatment of METH toxicity.

ACKNOWLEDGMENTS

We would like to give thanks to Dr. Patrice J. Morin, Dr. Lin Zhang, and Dr. Tugba Onal Suzek for their helpful advice with establishment of SAGE libraries.

REFERENCES

1. MATSUMOTO, T. *et al.* 2002. Methamphetamine in Japan: the consequences of methamphetamine abuse as a function of route of administration. Addiction **97:** 809–817.
2. FARRELL, M. *et al.* 2002. Methamphetamine: drug use and psychoses becomes a major public health issue in the Asia Pacific region. Addiction **97:** 771–772.
3. CHO, A.K. *et al.* 2001. Relevance of pharmacokinetic parameters in animal models of methamphetamine abuse. Synapse **39:** 161–166.
4. DAVIDSON, C. *et al.* 2001. Methamphetamine neurotoxicity: necrotic and apoptotic mechanisms and relevance to human abuse and treatment. Brain Res. Brain Res. Rev. **36:** 1–22.
5. VOLKOW, N.D. 2001. Drug abuse and mental illness: progress in understanding comorbidity. Am. J. Psychiatry **158:** 1181–1183.
6. WILSON, J.M. *et al.* 1996. Striatal dopamine nerve terminal markers in human, chronic methamphetamine users. Nat. Med. **2:** 699–703.
7. LANGFORD, D. *et al.* 2003. Patterns of selective neuronal damage in methamphetamine-user AIDS patients. J. Acquir. Immune. Defic. Syndr. **34:** 467–474.

8. CAPPON, G.D., C. PU & C.V. VORHEES. 2000. Time-course of methamphetamine-induced neurotoxicity in rat caudateputamen after single-dose treatment. Brain Res. **863:** 106–111.
9. CARMELIET, P. *et al.* 1998. Role of HIF-1alpha in hypoxia-mediated apoptosis, cell proliferation and tumour angiogenesis. Nature **394:** 485–490.
10. HOTCHKISS, A.J., M.E. MORGAN & J.W. GIBB. 1979. The long-term effects of multiple doses of methamphetamine on neostriatal tryptophan hydroxylase, tyrosine hydroxylase, choline acetyltransferase and glutamate decarboxylase activities. Life Sci. **25:** 1373–1378.
11. HOTCHKISS, A. & J.W. GIBB. 1980. Blockade of methamphetamine-induced depression of tyrosine hydroxylase by GABA transaminase inhibitors. Eur. J. Pharmacol. **66:** 201–205.
12. CADET, J. *et al.* 1997. Effects of UV and visible radiation on DNA-final base damage. Biol. Chem. **378:** 1275–1286.
13. DENG, X. *et al.* 2001. Methamphetamine causes widespread apoptosis in the mouse brain: evidence from using an improved TUNEL histochemical method. Brain Res. Mol. Brain Res. **93:** 64–69.
14. STUMM, G. *et al.* 1999. Amphetamines induce apoptosis and regulation of bcl-x splice variants in neocortical neurons. FASEB J. **13:** 1065–1072.
15. YAMAMOTO, Y. *et al.* 2002. Methamphetamine induces apoptosis in seminiferous tubules in male mice testis. Toxicol. Appl. Pharmacol. **178:** 155–160.
16. DENG, X. & J.L. CADET. 1999. Methamphetamine administration causes overexpression of nNOS in the mouse striatum. Brain Res. **851:** 254–257.
17. DENG, X. & J.L. CADET. 2000. Methamphetamine-induced apoptosis is attenuated in the striata of copper-zinc superoxide dismutase transgenic mice. Brain Res. Mol. Brain Res. **83:** 121–124.
18. JAYANTHI, S. *et al.* 2004. Methamphetamine induces neuronal apoptosis via cross-talks between endoplasmic reticulum and mitochondria-dependent death cascades. FASEB J. **18:** 238–251.
19. JAYANTHI, S. *et al.* 2005. Calcineurin/NFAT-induced up-regulation of the Fas ligand/Fas death pathway is involved in methamphetamine-induced neuronal apoptosis. Proc. Natl. Acad. Sci. USA **102:** 868–873.
20. VELCULESCU, V.E. *et al.* 1995. Serial analysis of gene expression. Science **270:** 484–487.
21. FUKUMURA, M. *et al.* 1998. A single dose model of methamphetamine-induced neurotoxicity in rats: effects on neostriatal monoamines and glial fibrillary acidic protein. Brain Res. **806:** 1–7.
22. SOK, J. *et al.* 1999. CHOP-dependent stress-inducible expression of a novel form of carbonic anhydrase VI. Mol. Cell Biol. **19:** 495–504.
23. PASTOREKOVA, S. *et al.* 2004. Carbonic anhydrases: current state of the art, therapeutic applications and future prospects. J. Enzyme Inhib. Med. Chem. **19:** 199–229.
24. LASH, A.E. *et al.* 2000. SAGEmap: a public gene expression resource. Genome Res. **10:** 1051–1060.
25. CADET, J.L. *et al.* 2001. Temporal profiling of methamphetamine-induced changes in gene expression in the mouse brain: evidence from cDNA array. Synapse **41:** 40–48.
26. THOMAS, D.M. *et al.* 2004. Identification of differentially regulated transcripts in mouse striatum following methamphetamine treatment—an oligonucleotide microarray approach. J. Neurochem. **88:** 380–393.

27. BACKMAN, C. & M. MORALES. 2002. Acute methamphetamine administration up-regulates NGFI-B mRNA expression in the striatum: co-localization with c-Fos immunoreactivity. Synapse **44:** 158–165.
28. ISHIGAMI, A. *et al.* 2003. The application of immunohistochemical findings in the diagnosis in methamphetamine-related death—two forensic autopsy cases. J. Med. Invest. **50:** 112–116.
29. CADET, J.L., M.T. MCCOY & B. LADENHEIM. 2002. Distinct gene expression signatures in the striata of wild-type and heterozygous c-fos knockout mice following methamphetamine administration: evidence from cDNA array analyses. Synapse **44:** 211–226.
30. KUPERMAN, D.I. *et al.* 1997. Methamphetamine-induced hyperthermia in mice: examination of dopamine depletion and heat-shock protein induction. Brain Res. **771:** 221–227.
31. NOAILLES, P.A. *et al.* 2003. Methamphetamine-induced gene expression profiles in the striatum of male rat pups exposed to the drug in utero. Brain Res. Dev. Brain Res. **147:** 153–162.
32. CHEN, Q. *et al.* 1992. Activation of the growth arrest and DNA damage-inducible gene gadd 153 by nephrotoxic cysteine conjugates and dithiothreitol. J. Biol. Chem. **267:** 8207–8212.
33. CARLSON, S.G. *et al.* 1993. Regulation of the C/EBP-related gene gadd153 by glucose deprivation. Mol. Cell Biol. **13:** 4736–4744.
34. WANG, X.Z. *et al.* 1998. Identification of novel stress-induced genes downstream of chop. EMBO J. **17:** 3619–3630.
35. CHO, A.K. & W.P. MELEGA. 2002. Patterns of methamphetamine abuse and their consequences. J. Addict. Dis. **21:** 21–34.
36. CADET, J.L., S. JAYANTHI & X. DENG. 2003. Speed kills: cellular and molecular bases of methamphetamine-induced nerve terminal degeneration and neuronal apoptosis. FASEB J. **17:** 1775–1788.
37. WILSON, J.M. *et al.* 1996. Differential changes in neurochemical markers of striatal dopamine nerve terminals in idiopathic Parkinson's disease. Neurology **47:** 718–726.
38. FROST, D.O. & J.L. CADET. 2000. Effects of methamphetamine-induced neurotoxicity on the development of neural circuitry: a hypothesis. Brain Res. Brain Res. Rev. **34:** 103–118.
39. ITZHAK, Y. *et al.* 2004. Long-lasting behavioral sensitization to psychostimulants following p-chloroamphetamine-induced neurotoxicity in mice. Neuropharmacology **46:** 74–84.
40. KURODA, M. *et al.* 1999. Induction of a secreted protein by the myxoid liposarcoma oncogene. Proc. Natl. Acad. Sci. USA **96:** 5025–5030.
41. SULZER, D. & S. RAYPORT. 1990. Amphetamine and other psychostimulants reduce pH gradients in midbrain dopaminergic neurons and chromaffin granules: a mechanism of action. Neuron **5:** 797–808.
42. RAISANEN, S.R. *et al.* 1999. Carbonic anhydrase III protects cells from hydrogen peroxide-induced apoptosis. FASEB J. **13:** 513–522.
43. POTTER, C. & A.L. HARRIS. 2004. Hypoxia inducible carbonic anhydrase IX, marker of tumour hypoxia, survival pathway and therapy target. Cell Cycle **3:** 164–167.

Dopamine Quinones Activate Microglia and Induce a Neurotoxic Gene Expression Profile

Relationship to Methamphetamine-Induced Nerve Ending Damage

DONALD M. KUHN, DINA M. FRANCESCUTTI-VERBEEM, AND DAVID M. THOMAS

Department of Psychiatry and Behavioral Neurosciences, Wayne State University School of Medicine and John D. Dingell VA Medical Center, Detroit, Michigan 48201, USA

ABSTRACT: Methamphetamine (METH) intoxication leads to persistent damage of dopamine (DA) nerve endings of the striatum. Recently, we and others have suggested that the neurotoxicity associated with METH is mediated by extensive microglial activation. DA itself has been shown to play an obligatory role in METH neurotoxicity, possibly through the formation of quinone species. We show presently that DA-quinones (DAQ) cause a time-dependent activation of cultured microglial cells. Microarray analysis of the effects of DAQ on microglial gene expression revealed that 101 genes were significantly changed in expression, with 73 genes increasing and 28 genes decreasing in expression. Among those genes differentially regulated by DAQ were those often associated with neurotoxic conditions including inflammation, cytokines, chemokines, and prostaglandins. In addition, microglial genes associated with a neuronally protective phenotype were among those that were downregulated by DAQ. These results implicate DAQ as one species that could cause early activation of microglial cells in METH intoxication, manifested as an alteration in the expression of a broad biomarker panel of genes. These results also link oxidative stress, chemical alterations in DA to its quinone, and microglial activation as part of a cascade of glial–neuronal crosstalk that can amplify METH-induced neurotoxicity.

KEYWORDS: dopamine quinone; methamphetamine; microglia; microarray analysis

Address for correspondence: Donald M. Kuhn, Ph.D., John D. Dingell VA Medical Center, Research & Development Service (11R), 4646 John R, Detroit, MI 48201. Voice: 313-576-4457; fax: 313-576-4466.

e-mail: donald.kuhn@wayne.edu

Ann. N.Y. Acad. Sci. 1074: 31–41 (2006). © 2006 New York Academy of Sciences.
doi: 10.1196/annals.1369.003

INTRODUCTION AND BACKGROUND

Methamphetamine (METH) is a member of the amphetamine family of drugs. METH abuse has reached alarming proportions leading numerous federal agencies including NIDA, ONDCP, and the DEA to liken it to an epidemic. In fact, the UN Office on Drugs and Crime reported that use of amphetamines, including METH and 3, 4-methyenedioxy methamphetamine (MDMA), has eclipsed that of cocaine and heroin on a global scale. The medical, legal, and societal problems associated with any rampant drug of abuse are compounded in the case of the amphetamines because many members of this pharmacological class cause persistent neuronal damage.[1] The consequences of METH abuse are manifested as persistent depletions of DA, inhibition of tyrosine hydroxylase, inactivation of the DA transporter (DAT), reduction in function of the vesicle monoamine transporter (VMAT), degeneration of fine, unmyelinated axons, and possibly apoptosis.[2–4] As a neurotransmitter, DA plays an essential role in numerous physiological, neuronal, and behavioral processes. A persistent reduction in DA neuronal function resulting from chronic METH abuse[5,6] could be expressed ultimately in the form of comorbid psychiatric or neurological diseases.

The mechanisms by which METH damages the DA neuronal system are not understood. Space constraints prohibit an exhaustive coverage of METH toxicity, and numerous excellent review articles have described the role of oxidative stress as a primary mediator of METH toxicity.[2,7–10] The neurotoxicity associated with METH involves DA and indicates that drug-induced toxicity is reduced when brain DA levels are lowered.[11–15] It is also known that reactive oxygen species and reactive nitrogen species, produced in response to METH intoxication, can react with DA to form the DA-quinone (DAQ). The rationale linking DAQ to METH neurotoxicity specifically, and to damage in DA neurons in general, is compelling. METH toxicity is accompanied by a significant increase in brain levels of DAQ.[16,17] In addition, the DA neurotoxicity of MPTP has also been linked to DAQ,[18] and the ability of DAQ to modify the same proteins (i.e., DAT, TH, TPH) that are modified *in vivo* by METH has been documented extensively.[19–22]

Bowyer *et al.*[23] were perhaps the first investigators to note that METH caused microglial activation. Since this interesting and important observation, evidence documenting microglial involvement in amphetamine neurotoxicity has grown considerably.[24–33] Assuming that microglia participate in the process of METH-induced nerve ending damage, the stimuli that provoke their activation is not understood. In light of evidence linking DAQ to METH neurotoxicity, and considering the ability of DAQ to promote redox cycling and oxidative stress, we hypothesized that DAQ could cause microglial activation. The present studies were designed to elucidate the gene expression profile induced by DAQ in mouse microglial cells.

MATERIALS AND METHODS

Microglial Cell Culture and Activation

Murine microglia BV-2 cells were grown in Dulbecco's Modified Eagle's Medium containing high glucose supplemented with 5% fetal calf serum, 1 mM sodium pyruvate, and 100 U/mL penicillin/streptomycin. Cultures were maintained at 37°C with 5% CO_2 in a humidified incubator. BV-2 cells were activated in serum-free media by DAQ (100 μM) prepared as previously described.[19] Activating conditions for DAQ were optimized through dose- and time-response analyses by measuring increases in expression of cyclooxygenase-2 (Cox-2) and c-fos protein within cells and increased secretion of tumor necrosis factor-α, glutamate, and prostaglandin E_2 into the culture media (data not shown). BV-2 cells were seeded at a density of 5×10^5 cells/well in a 6-well plate and allowed to adhere to substrate overnight. Cells were treated with activating conditions for 6 h after which media was removed and cells were washed three times with phosphate buffered saline, harvested into Trizol, and then stored at −80°C. Untreated cells were similarly washed and harvested. Three independent replicates of each experiment were carried out, resulting in three independent microarray chips for each activating condition and controls (12 total arrays).

RNA Isolation, Microarray Analysis, and Bioinformatics

RNA was extracted from frozen cells, purified using RNeasy Kits according to the manufacturer's instructions, treated with DNase I, and quantified by spectrophotometry. Synthesis of cDNA, production of labeled cRNA, microarray analysis, and bioinformatics were performed essentially as described previously by our lab.[31] Three independent replicates of all microglial activating conditions were analyzed by microarray analysis to protect against the potential variability associated with this technology.[34]

Statistical Analyses

All data were evaluated statistically in GeneSpring® (Agilent Technologies Palo Alto, CA, USA). Normalized gene expression values were subjected to an unpaired *t*-test using Bonferroni's multiple testing correction. For all tests, the significance level was set at $P < 0.05$.

RESULTS AND DISCUSSION

Treatment of cultured BV-2 cells with DAQ resulted in a dose- and time-dependent activation of the microglia, as evidenced by increased expression

TABLE 1. Genes upregulated at least 2.8-fold by DAQ

GenBank No.	Common name	Description
NM_009647	Ak4	DNA segment, Chr 4, ERATO Doi 298, expressed
AK016474	Apg12l	Autophagy 12-like (S. cerevisiae)
NM_013863	Bag3	Bcl2-associated athanogene 3
AF032460	Bcl2l11	BCL2-like 11 (apoptosis facilitator)
NM_016916	Blcap	Bladder cancer-associated protein homolog (human)
NM_009760	Bnip3	BCL2/adenovirus E1B 19kDa-interacting protein 1, NIP3
AV284384	Capza1	Capping protein (actin filament) muscle Z-line, alpha 1
NM_025821	Carhsp1	Calcium-regulated heat stable protein 1
AJ318863	Ccrl2	Chemokine (C-C motif) receptor-like 2
AK007630	Cdkn1a	Cyclin-dependent kinase inhibitor 1A (P21)
AW554231	Cldn12	Claudin 12
NM_021274	Cxcl10	Chemokine (C-X-C motif) ligand 10
BB049138	D7Ertd458e	DNA segment, Chr 7, ERATO Doi 458, expressed
NM_013760	Dnajb9	DnaJ (Hsp40) homolog, subfamily B, member 9
AF282255	Dscr1	Down syndrome critical region homolog 1 (human)
AF260717	Dscr1	Down syndrome critical region homolog 1 (human)
L07264	Dtr	Diphtheria toxin receptor
NM_013642	Dusp1	Dual specificity phosphatase 1
NM_130447	Dusp16	Dual specificity phosphatase 16
BC005486	Ets2	E26 avian leukemia oncogene 2, 3′ domain
AV026617	Fos	FBJ osteosarcoma-related oncogene
W07885	Foxo3	Forkhead box O3
BB795235	Fzd5	Frizzled homolog 5 (Drosophila)
AF180518	Gabarapl1	GABA-A receptor-associated protein-like 1
AK010420	Gadd45b	Growth arrest and DNA-damage-inducible 45 beta
NM_008102	Gch1	GTP cyclohydrolase 1
NM_011819	Gdf15	Growth differentiation factor 15
BB142123	Gpr44	G protein-coupled receptor 44
NM_025293	Gtlf3a	Gene trap locus F3a
AK008756	Hig1	Hypoxia-induced gene 1
M12573	Hspa1a	Heat shock protein 1A
NM_008321	Idb3	Inhibitor of DNA binding 3
NM_010500	Ier5	Immediate early response 5
BC026605	Jmjd1a	Jumonji domain containing 1A
U20344	Klf4	Kruppel-like factor 4 (gut)
AK004719	Mdm2	Transformed mouse 3T3 cell double minute 2
AK004987	Mkks	McKusick–Kaufman syndrome protein
NM_010807	Mlp	MARCKS-like protein
BM729431	Mrps6	Mitochondrial ribosomal protein S6
NM_008654	Myd116	Myeloid differentiation primary response gene 116
NM_019750	Nat6	N-acetyltransferase 6
AF323918	Ndel1	Nuclear distribution gene E-like homolog 1 (A. nidulans)
AV248273	Nfe2l2	Nuclear factor, erythroid derived 2, like 2
NM_010907	Nfkbia	Nuclear factor of kappa light chain gene enhancer, alpha
BM210600	Npn3	Neoplastic progression 3
BC011325	Npn3	Neoplastic progression 3
BB237825	Osm	Oncostatin M

(continued)

TABLE 1. ***(Continued)***

GenBank No.	Common name	Description
NM_009344	Phlda1	Pleckstrin homology-like domain, family A, member 1
BM234765	Plk2	Polo-like kinase 2 (Drosophila)
BI410130	Pnrc1	Proline-rich nuclear receptor coactivator 1
NM_134084	Ppif	Peptidylprolyl isomerase F (cyclophilin F)
NM_011171	Procr	Protein C receptor, endothelial
NM_019983	Rabgef1	RAB guanine nucleotide exchange factor (GEF) 1
BB280137	Rabgef1	RAB guanine nucleotide exchange factor (GEF) 1
BB757103	Rassf1	Ras association (RalGDS/AF-6) domain family 1
NM_015811	Rgs1	Regulator of G-protein signaling 1
BC018275	Rhob	Ras homolog gene family, member B
BB507557	Rora	RAR-related orphan receptor alpha
NM_008871	Serpine1	Serine (or cystine) proteinase inhibitor, clade E, member 1
AF366401	Sertad1	SERTA domain containing 1
NM_009174	Siah2	Seven in absentia 2
NM_011990	Slc7a11	Solute carrier family 7 (cationic amino acid transporter)
BC025091	Soat1	Sterol O-acyltransferase 1
M59378	Tnfrsf1b	Tumor necrosis factor receptor superfamily, member 1b
NM_009404	Tnfsf9	Tumor necrosis factor (ligand) superfamily, member 9
AK016482	Tollip	Toll-interacting protein
BB740529	Treml4	Triggering receptor expressed on myeloid cells-like 4
AV132698	Ubap1	Ubiquitin-associated protein 1
U50279	Vegfa	Vascular endothelial growth factor A
AA124553	Za20d2	Zinc finger, A20 domain containing 2
BC027135	Zfp295	Zinc finger protein 295
NM_023322	Zfp99	Zinc finger protein 99

NOTE: Changes in gene expression for all listed genes were statistically significant ($P < 0.05$). In some cases, genes are listed more than once if they have more than one GenBank No.

of intracellular Cox-2 and c-fos protein, and through increased secretion into the cell culture media of tumor necrosis factor-α, glutamate, and prostaglandin E_2 (data not shown). Each of these effects has been used previously to document microglial activation after provocation of cells by various stimuli. As the initial step in characterizing the molecular pathways through which DAQ leads to microglial activation, we subjected DAQ-activated BV-2 cells to microarray analysis using Affymetrix microarray chips. Cells were exposed to 100 μM DAQ and harvested after 6 h of treatment. It was observed that DAQ had a profound effect on microglial gene expression. The Affymetrix Mouse Genome 430 2.0 Array used presently contains 45,101 probe sets, representing more than 39,000 transcripts and variants of more than 34,000 genes. Of these, 15,802 probe sets were consistently called "present" or "marginal" in untreated BV-2 cells. These probe sets were culled further by removing expressed sequence tags, hypothetical proteins, cDNA clones, and GenBank number-only entries, yielding a list of 9882 annotated genes. This list of genes in untreated

BV-2 cells is a fair representation of the resting microglial transcriptome. More than 1195 annotated microglial genes were differentially regulated by DAQ using a factor of at least 2.8-fold increased or decreased to define a change in expression. This number was reduced to 914 when the genes were filtered additionally on the GeneSpring analytical tool of "confidence" to remove genes with unreliable signal values from gene chip processing. When the entire gene list was subjected to analysis using an unpaired *t*-test with Bonferroni's multiple testing correction (in GeneSpring), DAQ significantly ($P < 0.05$) changed the expression of 101 genes, with 73 increased in expression and 28 decreased in expression. The apparent reduction in the number of genes whose expression was changed significantly (i.e., 101) from those changed by a factor of 2.8-fold or more (i.e., 914) is deceiving. The statistical tests embedded in GeneSpring are very stringent and include multiple testing corrections. It is perhaps more relevant, from a biological perspective, to consider fold-change as a primary indicator, and then place these differentially regulated genes within relevant biological and molecular pathways (see TABLES 1–3 below). In consideration of space constraints, only those microglial genes whose expression was changed to a statistically significant extent are included in the following tables. The larger lists of genes differentially regulated by DAQ are available as Excel files and will be provided upon request to interested readers by email.

Genes whose expression was increased by 2.8-fold or greater by DAQ were stratified according to gene ontology and the results included a broad array of genes from most biological processes and molecular functions. In particular, genes with signal transduction activity, to include cytokines, growth factors, and receptor binding were well represented. Included in this classification of molecular function genes were genes that participate in central nervous system (CNS) inflammation, such as chemokine (C-X-C motif) ligand 10, chemokine (C-C motif) receptor-like 2, and the tumor necrosis factor receptor 1b superfamily. A number of heat shock protein genes, nitric oxide synthase (inducible), and Cox-2, each of which has been linked previously to METH-induced neurotoxicity, were also upregulated. It was also noted that GTP cyclohydrolase 1, the rate-limiting enzyme in the biosynthesis of tetrahydrobiopterin, the essential cofactor for the inducible form of nitric oxide synthase, was also increased in expression. The solute carrier gene Slc7a11 encodes the cystine–glutamate antiporter, the protein transporter through which microglia secrete glutamate. Increases in Slc7a11 expression could contribute to the glutamate excitotoxicity previously associated with METH neurotoxicity.[35] A list of genes increased in expression by a factor of 2.8-fold to a statistically significant extent is presented in TABLE 1.

Genes whose expression was decreased by DAQ also spanned most categories of molecular function and biological processes as specified by the Gene Ontology analytical software. It was interesting that caveolin 2, a gene involved in cellular endocytosis was decreased in expression, suggesting that the ability of microglia to clear cellular debris could be compromised. The purinergic

TABLE 2. Genes downregulated at least 2.8-fold by DAQ

GenBank No.	Common name	Description
BQ174638	Ank2	Ankyrin 2, brain
BM245154	Apc	Adenomatosis polyposis coli
BM246535	Arhgap15	Rho GTPase-activating protein 15
NM_007496	Atbf1	AT motif-binding factor 1
NM_016900	Cav2	Caveolin 2
NM_009847	Cd2ap	CD2-associated protein
BB201368	Evi2a	Ecotropic viral integration site 2a
AK018078	Gnaq	Guanine nucleotide-binding protein, alpha q polypeptide
NM_018748	Golga4	Golgi autoantigen, golgin subfamily a, 4
AV377824	Gpr21	G protein-coupled receptor 21
NM_008413	Jak2	Janus kinase 2
NM_010612	Kdr	Kinase insert domain protein receptor
NM_008535	Lyl1	Lymphoblastomic leukemia
AV297525	Mll3	Myeloid/lymphoid or mixed-lineage leukemia 3
NM_010881	Ncoa1	Nuclear receptor coactivator 1
BM230024	Nin	Ninein
NM_008845	Pip5k2a	Phosphatidylinositol-4-phosphate 5-kinase, type II, alpha
AV317262	Plxnc1	Plexin C1
NM_133249	Ppargc1b	Peroxisome proliferative activated receptor, gamma
BB523906	Prkcbp1	Protein kinase C-binding protein 1
AV232438	Pten	Phosphatase and tensin homolog
AV316937	Sgol2	Shugoshin-like 2 (S. pombe)
BB828008	Snx13	Sorting nexin 13
BB732892	Top2b	Topoisomerase (DNA) II beta
BM214109	Tpr	Translocated promoter region
AV295157	Vps35	Vacuolar protein sorting 35
AK012075	Wdfy3	WD repeat and FYVE domain containing 3
AW987152	Zfp217	Zinc finger protein 217

NOTE: Changes in gene expression for all listed genes were statistically significant ($P < 0.05$).

receptor P2X was also decreased in expression and is of interest because this receptor is present on microglia where it is thought to mediate neuroprotective functions of these cells. It was also of interest that toll-like receptor 4, the receptor through which lipopolysaccharide causes microglial activation was diminished in expression. Sestrin 1, which participates in establishing cellular antioxidant firewalls, was also decreased in expression, creating the possibility that oxidative functions of microglia could exceed antioxidant defenses and contribute to an imbalance in favor of oxidative stress. A list of genes decreased in expression by a factor of 2.8-fold to a statistically significant extent is presented in TABLE 2.

Finally, we compared those microglial genes whose expression was changed 2.8-fold or greater by DAQ to striatal genes whose expression was changed to a similar extent after *in vivo* METH treatment of mice.[31] The results are presented

TABLE 3. Genes changed in expression in response to DAQ (BV-2 cells) or METH (*in vivo*)

GenBank No.	Common name	Description
Upregulated		
NM_013863	Bag3	Bcl2-associated athanogene 3
U50712	Ccl12	Chemokine (C-C motif) ligand 12
AK007630	Cdkn1a	Cyclin-dependent kinase inhibitor 1A (P21)
NM_013498	Crem	cAMP responsive element modulator
M12573	Hspa1a	Heat shock protein 1A
BC003727	Il1a	Interleukin 1 alpha
M57525	Il1rn	Interleukin 1 receptor antagonist
NM_007707	Socs3	Suppressor of cytokine signaling 3
Downregulated		
BM250919	Dlg7	Discs, large homolog 7 (Drosophila)
NM_009027	Rasgrf2	RAS protein-specific guanine nucleotide-releasing factor 2

NOTE: All genes were changed in expression by a factor of 2.8-fold or greater.

in TABLE 3. Obviously, the striatal genes changed in expression by METH cannot be linked directly to microglial cells. Similarly, the microglial genes changed in expression by DAQ cannot be linked directly to METH because it is not known if alterations in striatal DAQ content plays a role in the *in vivo* activation of microglia seen after a neurotoxic regimen of METH. Nevertheless, this list of genes is quite interesting and includes several cytokine-related factors (e.g., chemokine ligand 12, interleukin 1 alpha, interleukin 1 receptor antagonist, and suppressor of cytokine signaling 3) and heat shock protein 1A. The involvement of cytokines[36] and heat shock proteins[37] in METH neurotoxicity has been documented and, when considered with the present results, suggests that microglia could represent a common factor linking these factors to METH.

The use of large format microarrays to characterize the response of the CNS to METH has provided very interesting clues to the molecular pathways used by this stimulant drug of abuse to cause neurotoxicity. The present demonstration that DAQ can invoke changes in expression of a rather large number of microglial genes effectively complements the work of Le *et al.*,[38] who showed that DAQ-modified cell membranes can cause microglial activation. Taken together, the profile of microglial genes whose expression was altered by DAQ indicates enhanced expression of genes that contribute to inflammatory processes, cell and membrane damage, and cytokine production. At the same time, reductions in expression of "neuronally protective" receptors on microglia would limit chemotactic and anti-inflammatory capability, and act in concert with those upregulated microglial genes that mediate inflammatory effects to amplify neuronal damage. The present results also link oxidative stress, chemical alterations in DA to its quinone, and microglial activation as

that fluoxetine inhibits the function of G protein activated inwardly rectifying K^+ (GIRK) channel in Xenopus oocyte. Recently Fumagalli *et al.*[3] found that chronic fluoxetine administration inhibits extracellular signal-regulated kinase 1/2 phosphorylation in rat brain.

For 15 years, we have studied the structure and function of 14-3-3 protein by analyses of gene structure.[4] On the other hand, we have examined the gene expression in the brain by using DNA microarray method. Recently we have published two papers about the pharmacological effects of phencyclidine and clozapine on the gene expression in the mouse brain.[5,6] In the present article, we attempted to apply the DNA microarray method for studies on chronic administration of fluoxetine into mouse and to compare the data on these mice with those in control mice.

MATERIALS AND METHODS

Animals

We used male mice weighting about 40 g from local breeder (Charles River Laboratories, Yokohama, Japan). The care and use of the animals were carried out following the principles of the Laboratory Animal Care and approved by the Animal Care Committee of the Niigata University School of Medicine. The animals were allowed free access to food and water.

Drugs

Fluoxetine (Prozac), a product of Sigma Chemical (St. Louis, MO), was dissolved in dimethyl sulfoxid (DMSO).

Injection Program

Fluoxetine was administered to the mice as follows. In the chronic experiments, fluoxetine (0.4 mg/0.1 mL) was injected intraperitoneally into mice (40 g) once a day for 20 days. About 20 h after last injection, mice were decapitated and the brains were isolated. DMSO was injected into the control mice.

Hybridization Analysis

Total RNA was prepared from the mouse cerebral cortical tissues by using Isogen according to the procedures of Nippon Gene (Toyama, Japan).[7] cDNA was synthesized from this RNA by the conventional reverse-transcription procedure and labeled by [α-^{32}P]dATP. Clontech Atlas Mouse 1.2 Array membrane was hybridized using the expression hybridization solution containing

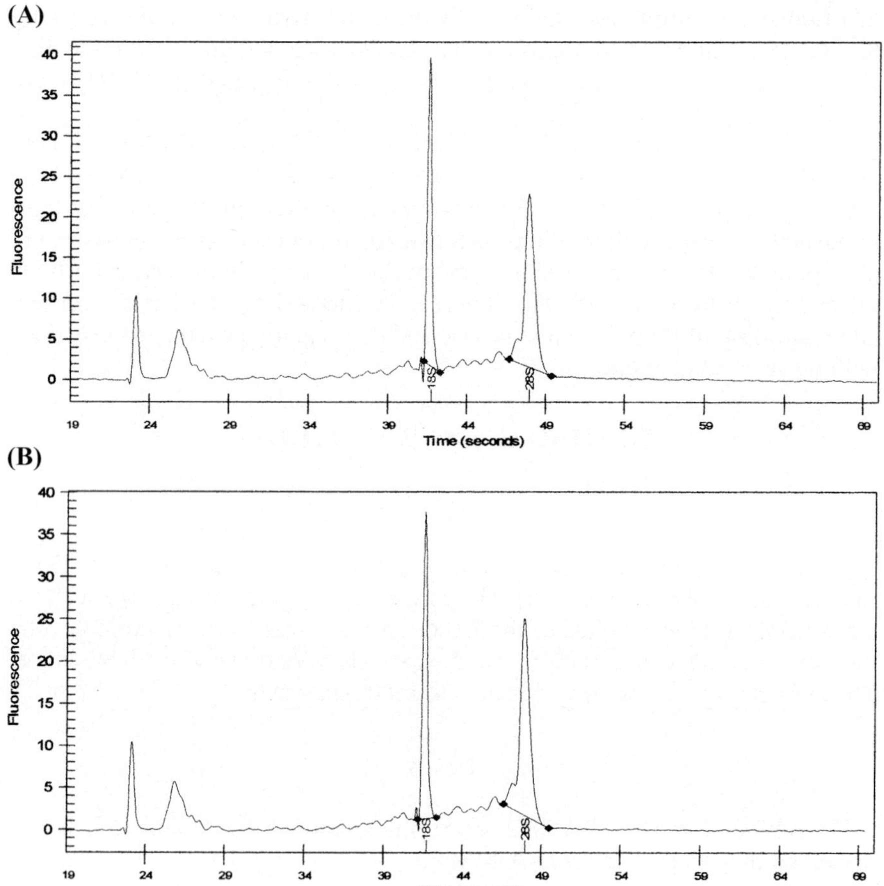

FIGURE 1. The electrophoretic patterns of total RNAs from the control and fluoxetine-injected mouse brains. (**A**) Control RNA, (**B**) RNA from fluoxetine-injected mouse brain.

[^{32}P]-labeled cDNA probe overnight at 68°C as described in detail in Atlas cDNA Expression Arrays, a user manual published by Clontech Laboratories (Shinjuku, Tokyo).[8] The hybridized Atlas Mouse 1.2 Array membrane was washed, and the hybridization pattern was analyzed by autoradiography and quantified by phosphorimaging.

RESULTS

DNA microarray technology was introduced to the analysis of gene expression several years ago. This technology has been described in detail in recent manuals, such as DNA Microarrays, A Molecular Cloning Manual, which was

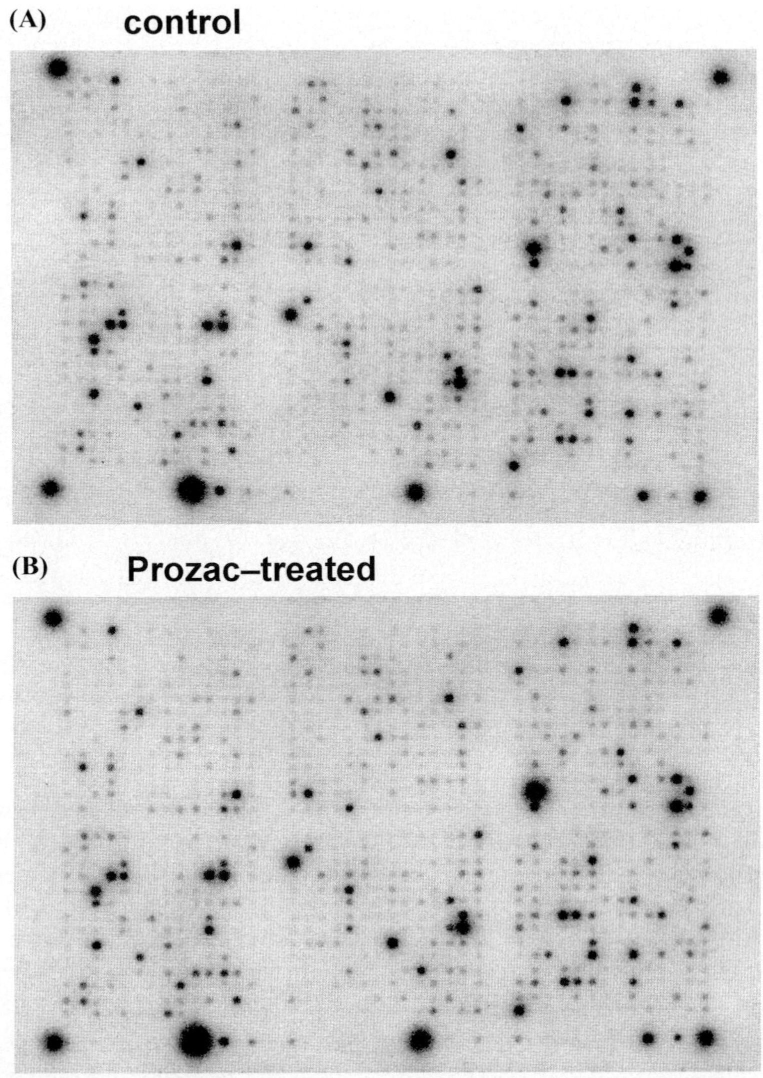

FIGURE 2. The hybridized arrays to Clontech's Atlas Mouse 1.2 Array Membrane. (**A**) Control mouse, (**B**) the fluoxetine-injected mouse.

published by the Cold Spring Harbor Laboratory Press, NY.[9] In the Materials and Methods section of the present article, this technology is briefly summarized.

In the first step of this experiment, we isolated total RNA from the brains of the control and fluoxetine-injected mice by using Isogen. The electrophoretic patterns of total RNAs from the control and drug-treated mouse brains were

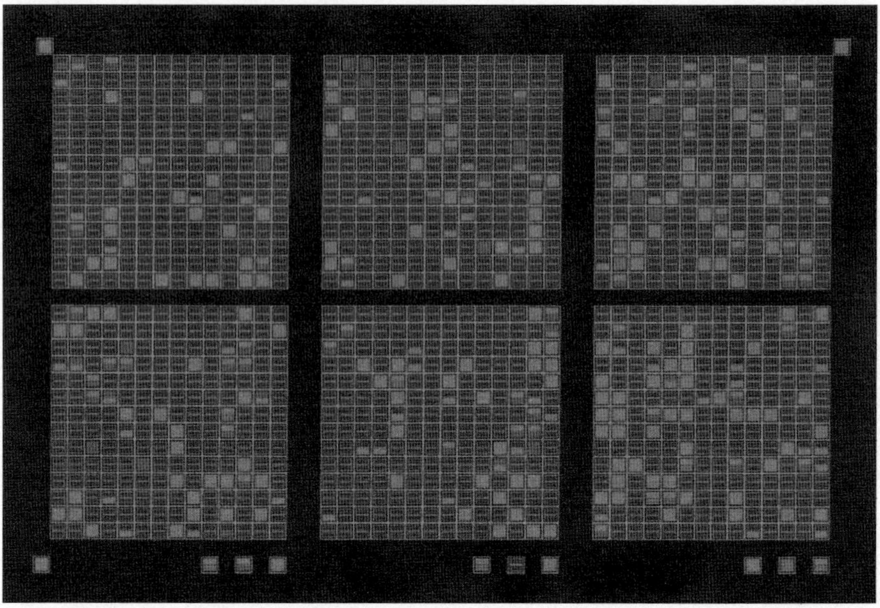

FIGURE 3. The analyses of the results of the differential expression in the control and fluoxetine-treated mice using Atlas Array Image Software. The upregulation of the spot signal in the fluoxetine-treated mouse is shown as red and the downregulation is shown as blue.

examined. These findings indicated that these RNAs were not degradated as shown in FIGURES 1 A and 1 B. cDNA probes were prepared from total RNA by the conventional reverse-transcription procedure using Atlas gene-specific primer mixture. Then the probes were hybridized to Clontech's Atlas Mouse 1.2 Array membrane overnight. The hybridized arrays were washed and then scanned using an image scanner. The data of these experiments are shown in FIGURE 2. FIGURE 2 A shows the data from the control mouse, and FIGURE 2 B shows the data from the fluouxetine-injected mouse. FIGURE 2 B did not appear to show any difference in comparison with FIGURE 2 A, although some spot signals in FIGURE 2 B appear to be upregulated.

FIGURE 3 shows the analyses of the results of the differential expression in the control (A) and drug-treated animals (B) using Atlas Array Image Software.[10] In FIGURE 3, the upregulation of the spot signal in the fluoxetine-treated mouse (B) is shown as red, and the downregulation is shown as blue. The number of the downregulated spot signals is very many, although the number of the upregulated spot signals is a little. The color image shown in FIGURE 3 is also shown in black and white in FIGURE 4. All data from FIGURES 1, 2, 3, and 4 are summarized in 40 tables. Particularly TABLE 1 shows the existence of very many downregulated spot signals in the fluoxetine-treated mouse. The data

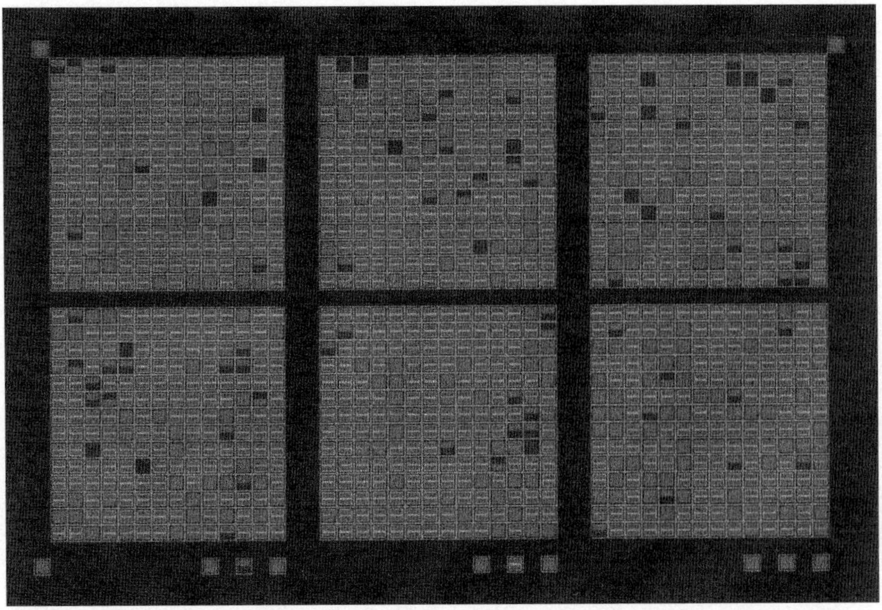

FIGURE 4. The analyses of the results in FIGURE 3 in black and white.

in these figures and tables show that the spot intensity of cholecystockinin,[11] prostaglandin D2 synthase,[12] S-100 protein,[13] and 14-3-3 protein[4] largely decreased in the fluoxetine-treated mouse brain and the spot intensity of 45 kDa Ca-binding protein precurser,[14] γ-aminobutyric acid (GABA) receptor,[15] and neurfilament L protein[16] increased a little.

DISCUSSION

In our previous papers, we reported gene expression profiles in the brains from phencyclidine-treated mouse and clozapine-treated mouse by using a DNA microarray method.[5,6] As we described in the discussion of the previous paper,[6] it is still doubtful whether the selection of 1176 spots in Atlas Mouse 1.2 Array is suitable for the study of gene expression in the brain. Potier *et al.*[17] used DNA microarray method in order to study gene expression in the knockout mouse and Ngai[18] also used DNA microarray method to study gene expression in selected model systems, including the developing cerebellum, olfactory bulb, and cortical neurons of the mouse.

As it was reported in the introduction of this article, fluoxetine inhibits serotonin uptake, serotonin receptor activity, muscle and neuronal acetylcholine receptors, GIRK, and extracellular signal-regulated kinase 1/2 phosphorylation in brain. In our present article, we found that the number of the downregulated

TABLE 1. Spot intensity of spot signals in the control and the fluoxetine-treated mice

		Spot Intensity				RATIO			
#	Coordinate	Control	Prozac-treated	Ratio	Difference	UP	DOWN	Gene	GenBank #
1	A01a	13	5	Down	−8			? BRAIN-SPECIFIC POLYPEPTIDE PEP-19 (BRAIN-SPECIFIC ANTIGEN PCP-4)	X17320
2	A10i	18	9	0.50	−9		2.0	? EARLY GROWTH RESPONSE PROTEIN 2 (EGR-2) (KROX-20 PROTEIN)	X06746
3	A13d	33	18	0.55	−15		1.8	Hematopoietically expressed homeobox protein (HHEX); proline-rich homeodomain-containing transcription factor (PRHX)	Z21524
4	A13g	22	13	0.59	−9		1.7	LIM domain-binding protein 1 (LDB1); nuclear LIM interactor (NLI) + LIM homeobox protein cofactor 2 (CLIM2)	U69270; U70375 + U89488
5	B02a	35	19	0.54	−16		1.8	Brain factor 1 (Hfhbf1)	U36760
6	B03a	19	10	0.53	−9		1.9	? Epidermal growth factor receptor kinase substrate EPS8	L21671
7	B03b	22	11	0.50	−11		2.0	Erf; Ets-related transcription factor	U58533
8	B05f	36	13	0.36	−23		2.8	Atonal protein homolog 2 (ATOH2; ATH2); helix-loop-helix protein MATH2; NEX1	D29678
9	B10l	16	8	0.50	−8		2.0	? Cdk5; cyclin-dependent kinase 5	U29086
10	B12f	176	93	0.53	−83		1.9	Prothymosin alpha (PTMA)	X56135
11	C02m	557	1197	2.15	640	2.1		TRANSTHYRETIN PRECURSOR (PREALBUMIN) (TBPA) (TTR) (ATTR)	D89076

Continued

TABLE 1. ***Continued***

#	Coordinate	Spot Intensity		Ratio	Difference	RATIO		Gene	GenBank #
		Control	Prozac-treated			UP	DOWN		
12	C03i	29	11	0.38	−18		2.6	Neurofibromatosis 1	X54924
13	C04b	216	120	0.56	−96		1.8	Thyroid hormone receptor alpha 1 (THRA); MR1A1; c-erbA alpha	X51983
14	C04d	31	12	0.39	−19		2.6	Transcription factor AP-1; c-jun proto-oncogene; AH119	J04115
15	C04j	44	26	0.59	−18		1.7	Jund	J05205
16	C09b	215	120	0.56	−95		1.8	HSP86; heat shock 86-kDa protein	M36830
17	C10b	53	17	0.32	−36		3.1	Oxidative stress-induced protein mRNA	U40930
18	C11c	19	10	0.53	−9		1.9	? CCHB3; calcium channel (voltage-gated; dihydropyridine-sensitive; L-type) beta-3 subunit)	U20372
19	D03i	158	90	0.57	−68		1.8	Clusterin precursor (CLU); clustrin; apolipoprotein J (APOJ); sulfated glycoprotein 2 (SGP2; MSGP2)	L08235
20	D05c	51	27	0.53	−24		1.9	Basic fibroblast growth factor receptor 1 precursor (BFGF-R; FGFR1); MFR; FLG	M28998
21	D06j	71	40	0.56	−31		1.8	Cholecystokinin	X59520
22	D11n	15	2	Down	−13			Prepro-orexin	AF041242
23	E13i	38	18	0.47	−20		2.1	Transducin beta-2 subunit	U34960
24	G45	19	36	1.89	17	1.9		45-kDa calcium-binding protein precursor (CAB45); stromal cell-derived factor 4 (SDF4)	U45977

NOTE: ? = Weak signal (low trust).

spot signals is very many in the fluoxetine-injected mouse, although the number of the upregulated spot signals is a little. These experimental results may be related with the many inhibitory effects of fluoxetine as described above. According to the studies of Miledi *et al.*,[1] Kobayashi *et al.*,[2] and Fumagalli *et al.*,[3] fluoxetine inhibits the function of acetylcholine receptor, GIRK, and extracellular signal-regulated kinase 1/2 phosphorylation in brain. Fluoxetine is an antidepressant drug, but it may have the considerably strong inhibitory effect on the gene expression in the mouse brain.

CONCLUSION

In order to examine the effects of fluoxetine on the gene expression in the mouse brain, we have used the DNA microarray methods. As the results of these experiments, we found the downregulation of many spot signals in the fluoxetine-treated mice, for example, cholecystokinin and prostaglandin D2 synthase.

REFERENCES

1. GARCIA-COLUNGA, J., J.N. ANAD & R. MILEDI. 1997. Blockage of muscle and neuronal nicotinic acetylcholine receptors by fluoxetin (Prozac). Proc. Natl. Acad. Sci. USA **94:** 2041–2044.
2. KOBAYASHI, T., K. IKEDA & T. KUMANISHI. 1998. Effect of clozapine on the δ- and κ-opioid receptors and G-protein activated K^+ (GIRK) channel expressed in Xenopus oocytes. Br. J. Pharmacol. **123:** 421–426.
3. FUMAGALLI, F., R. MOLTENI, F. CALABRESC, *et al.* 2005. Chronic fluoxetine administration inhibits extracellular signal-regulated kinase 1/2 phosphorylation in rat brain. J. Neurochem. **93:** 1551–1560.
4. TAKAHASHI, Y. 2003. The 14-3-3 proteins; gene, gene expression and function. Neurochem. Res. **28:** 1265–1273.
5. TOYOOKA, K., M. USUI, K. WASHIYAMA, *et al.* 2002. Gene expression profiles in the brain from phencyclidine-treated mouse by using DNA microarray. Ann. N. Y. Acad. Sci. **965:** 10–20.
6. TAKAHASHI, Y., T. KUMANISHI & S. HAYASHI. 2004. Using a DNA microarray method to examine gene expression in brain from clozapine-injected mice. Ann. N. Y. Acad. Sci. **1025:** 561–569.
7. NIPPON GENE COMPANY. 1999. Isogen, In Manual, 349–358.
8. CLONTECH COMPANY. 1999. Atlas cDNA Expression Arrays. User Manual, 1–43.
9. BOWTELL, D.R. & J. SAMBROOK. 2003. DNA Microarrays; A Molecular Cloning Manual, Cold Spring Harbor Laboratory Press. Cold Spring Harbor, New York.
10. CLONTECH COMPANY. 1999. Atlas Array Image Software. User Manual.
11. KUWANO, R., K. ARAKI, H. USUI, *et al.* 1984. Molecular cloning and nucleotide sequence of cDNA coding for rat brain cholecystokinin precursor. J. Biochem. **96:** 923–926.

12. SAMUELSSON, B. 1985. Leucotriens and related compounds. *In* Advances in Prostaglandin, Thromboxane and Leukotriene Research, Vol. 15. O. Hayaishi & S. Yamamoto, Eds.: 1–9. Raven Press. New York.
13. ZOMZELY-NEURATH, C.E. 1982. The nervous system-specific protein S-100. *In* Handbook of Neurochemistry, Vol. 5. A. Lajtha, Ed.: 65–100. Plenum Publishing Corporation. New York.
14. TAKAHASHI, Y., T. YAMAKUNI, H. USUI, *et al.* 1989. The studies on cerebellar Ca-binding protein, spot35 protein by cDNA and gene cloning techniques. *In* Calcium Protein Signaling. H. Hidaka, Ed.: 257–262. Plenum Publishing Corporation. New York.
15. HIROUCHI, M., R. KUWANO, T. KATAGIRI, *et al.* 1989. Nucleotide and deduced amino acid sequences of $GABA_A$ receptor α-subunit from human brain. Neurochem. Internat. **15:** 33–38.
16. TAKAHASHI, S., T. IWANAGA, Y. TAKAHASHI, *et al.* 1984. Neuron-specific enolase, neurofilament protein and S-100 protein in the olfactory mucosa of human fetuses. Cell Tissue Res. **238:** 231–234.
17. POTIER, M.-C., N. GOLFIER, GIEBELIN, *et al.* 2001. Differential gene expression in brain from knock-out mice using DNA microarrays. J. Neurochem. **78**(Suppl. 1): 110.
18. NGAI, J. 2001. Gene expression profiling in the nervous system. J. Neurochem. **78**(Suppl. 1): 110.

Short-Term Effects of Adolescent Methylphenidate Exposure on Brain Striatal Gene Expression and Sexual/Endocrine Parameters in Male Rats

WALTER ADRIANI,[a] DAMIANA LEO,[b] MARIA GUARINO,[c] ALESSIA NATOLI,[c] EMMA DI CONSIGLIO,[d] GIOVANNA DE ANGELIS,[d] ELSA TRAINA,[c] EMANUELA TESTAI,[d] CARLA PERRONE-CAPANO,[b] AND GIOVANNI LAVIOLA[a]

[a]*Department of Cell Biology & Neurosciences, Behavioural Neuroscience Section, Istituto Superiore di Sanità, I-00161 Roma, Italy*

[b]*Institute of Genetics and Biophysics "A. Buzzati Traverso," CNR, Napoli I-80131, Italy*

[c]*Department of Drug Research and Evaluation, Istituto Superiore di Sanità, Roma I-00161, Italy*

[d]*Department of Environment and Primary Prevention, Istituto Superiore di Sanità, Roma I-00161, Italy*

ABSTRACT: Exposure to methylphenidate (MPH) during adolescence is the elective therapy for attention deficit/hyperactivity disorder (ADHD) children, but raises major concerns for public health, due to possibly persistent neurobehavioral changes. Rats (30- to 44-days old) were administered MPH (2 mg/kg, i.p once daily) or saline (SAL). At the end of the treatment we collected plasma, testicular, liver, and brain (striatum) samples. The testes and liver were used to evaluate conventional reproductive and metabolic endpoints. Testes of MPH-exposed rats weighed more and contained an increased quantity of sperm, whereas testicular levels of testosterone (TST) were markedly decreased. The MPH treatment exerted an inductive effect on enzymatic activity of TST hydroxylases, resulting in increased hepatic TST catabolism. These findings suggest that subchronic MPH exposure in adolescent rats could have a trophic action on testis growth and a negative impact on TST metabolism. We have analyzed striatal gene expression profiles as a consequence of MPH exposure during adolescence, using microarray technology.pagebreak More than 700 genes were upregulated in the striatum

Address for correspondence: W. Adriani, Department of Cell Biology & Neurosciences, Behavioural Neuroscience Section, Istituto Superiore di Sanità, viale Regina Elena 299, I-00161 Roma, Italy. Voice: +39-06-4990-2105; fax: +39-06-495-7821.
e-mail: adriani@iss.it

Ann. N.Y. Acad. Sci. 1074: 52–73 (2006). © 2006 New York Academy of Sciences.
doi: 10.1196/annals.1369.005

of MPH-treated rats (foldchange >1.5). A first group of genes were apparently involved in migration of immature neural/glial cells and/or growth of novel axons. These genes include matrix proteases (ADAM-1, MMP14), their inhibitors (TIMP-2, TIMP-3), the hyaluronan-mediated motility receptor (RHAMM), and growth factors (transforming growth factor-β3 [TGF-β3] and fibroblast growth factor 14 [FGF14]). A second group of genes were suggestive of active axonal myelination. These genes mediate survival of immature cells after contact with newly produced axonal matrix (laminin B1, collagens, integrin alpha 6) and stabilization of myelinating glia-axon contacts (RAB13, contactins 3 and 4). A third group indicated the appearance and/or upregulation of mature processes. The latter included genes for : K+ channels (TASK-1, TASK-5), intercellular junctions (connexin30), neurotransmitter receptors (adrenergic alpha 1B, kainate 2, serotonin 7, GABA-A), as well as major proteins responsible for their transport and/or anchoring (Homer 1, MAGUK MPP3, Shank2). All these genes were possibly involved in synaptic plasticity, namely the formation, maturation, and stabilization of new neural connections within the striatum. MPH treatment seems to potentiate synaptic plasticity, which is an age-dependent developmental phenomenon that adolescent rats are very likely to show, compared to adults. Our observations suggest that adolescent MPH exposure causes only transient changes in reproductive and hormonal parameters, and a more enduring enhancement of neurobehavioral plasticity.

KEYWORDS: puberty; testosterone; myelination; neurotransmission; genomic approach

INTRODUCTION

Attention deficit/hyperactivity disorder (ADHD), a common chronic neurobehavioral disease of childhood, is viewed as an executive dysfunction, according to the dominant model. However, alternative accounts present ADHD as a motivational dysfunction, characterized by attempts to escape or avoid delay, and arising from altered reward processes in fronto-striatal circuits.[1,2] Methylphenidate (MPH) is a psychostimulant currently prescribed to children diagnosed with ADHD, actually representing the elective therapy ("Ritalin"). MPH interacts with the same brain pathways activated by drugs of abuse, producing striatal dopamine (DA) overflow similarly to cocaine. [3] Hence, exposure to MPH during adolescence has raised major concerns for public health, due to possible adverse long-term effects.[4]

Studies in rodents are useful to define molecular and behavioral responses to MPH. Recent reports in rats showed that exposure to MPH during adolescence caused behavioral changes enduring into adulthood, including enhanced psychomotor responses to cocaine and increased cocaine self-administration,[5] reduced rewarding power, and increased sensitivity to the aversive effects of cocaine,[6] as well as depressive-like effects in the forced-swim test.[7] Furthermore, adult animals treated with MPH during adolescence are less responsive to natural rewards, showing increased stressful and anxiety-like behaviors,[8] and lower levels of impulsivity.[9]

Molecular evidence suggests that repeated psychostimulant exposure causes stable changes in gene expression and persistent alterations in dendritic morphology within the mesocorticolimbic DA system, the main pathway of the brain reward circuitry.[10] Similar plastic changes in reward-related circuits might also occur after repeated MPH, especially with adolescent exposure.[4] Recent reports showed increased *dynorphin* expression in the dorsal striatum at the end of the adolescent treatment [11] and increased *CREB* expression within the nucleus accumbens (NAc) shell at adulthood.[6] Acute exposure to MPH is known to alter the expression of c-fos and substance P preferentially in the dorsal striatum.[12] However, the whole molecular consequences of chronic exposure to MPH during critical periods of development are poorly understood.[4] Our work was aimed to identify the short-term effects of subchronic treatment with MPH during adolescence. To study gene expression changes, we have used microarray technology, to simultaneously screen the expression of more than 15,000 transcripts in the rat striatum.

As for potential side effects of MPH treatment, there may be room for a major concern as well. Indeed, as prepubertal individuals are repeatedly treated with a psychostimulant drug, adverse effects on gonadic maturation and physical growth may be expected. Generally, no major adverse effects of Ritalin treatment are reported in rats.[13] However, little is known about actual MPH effects on gonadal and hormonal parameters, because only few works are available.[14] So far, there are no studies in humans on the possible effects of MPH on reproduction, and the reproductive toxicity data from experimental animal studies are considered insufficient to draw conclusions.[15] A slight reduction in sperm motility, a dose-related decrease of absolute epididymis and testis weight, and an increase of the relative testis weight, were found in pubertal mice fed with diets containing MPH at high concentrations.[16]

Relatively more efforts have been made to study effects of prolonged psychostimulant exposure on reproductive and hormonal parameters. Recent results clearly demonstrate that repeated psychostimulant administration can sensitize and thus increase the natural motivation for sex behavior.[17] This effect was explained in terms of direct drug effects on mesolimbic reward system. However, peripheral effects on puberty onset and maturation of gonads were not taken into account. In general, differently from the case of Ritalin, a psychostimulant-related suppression of growth and sexual maturation is classically reported.[18] Accordingly, repeated psychostimulant administration overtly decreases plasma levels of androgen hormones in rats.[19]

It should be underlined that MPH and other psychostimulants are classically reported to decrease prolactin.[20] In the male rats, increasing titers of prolactin are involved in testicular development during puberty onset. Prolactin may also facilitate the action of other sex hormones on maturation of male gonads.[21] Thus, a retardation in puberty-related physiological parameters, and/or an altered metabolism of sex hormones, may be expected as a consequence of subchronic MPH treatment. For this reason, conventional reproductive (testicular) and metabolic (hepatic) endpoints have been evaluated. This was aimed to identify the possible short-term and long-lasting effects on spermatogenesis, gonadal growth, and testosterone (TST) metabolism, induced by the administration of MPH in adolescent rats.

Experimental Approach

Three groups of adolescent male rats were administered MPH (2 mg/kg, intraperitoned [i.p]) or saline (SAL). A first group was injected only once (on postnatal day [PND] 44), and sacrificed 2 h after injection. This group was aimed at investigating *acute* MPH effect during adolescence. A second group was treated for 14 days (PND 30–44, once daily), and sacrificed 2 h after the last treatment injection. This group was aimed at investigating *short-term* subchronic effects of MPH during adolescence. A third group was treated for 14 days (PND 30–44, once daily), and sacrificed 2 months after the last injection. This group was aimed at investigating *long-term* subchronic effects of MPH exposure during adolescence. In all three groups, trunk-blood samples were collected immediately after sacrifice, for detection of hormonal parameters. After sacrifice, all animals were quickly dissected, testes and liver being collected. The reproductive (testicular) endpoints included absolute and relative testis weight, sperm head count number (per testis and per gram of testis), and the intratesticular TST levels (per testis and per gram of testis). The metabolic (hepatic) endpoints included TST hydroxylase activity and aromatase (CYP19) activity assays. Brain striatum samples were also quickly collected, for assessment of gene expression using the whole-genome approach.

Male Reproductive (Testicular) Endpoints

Testes were removed and weighed. The right testes were decapsuled, homogenized, and sonicated. A 0.2-mL aliquot of the testicular sample was diluted 1:10 with deionized H_2O and evaluated for sperm head number, according to Meistrich.[22] To evaluate testicular TST, the residual homogenates were extracted three times with diethylether, evaporated to dryness under N_2 flow and appropriately diluted in physiological SAL solution containing dimethylsulphoxide (in accordance with the detection range of the hormone). The concentration of TST was determined by immuno-enzymatic test (ELISA assay). Data were analyzed using a one-way ANOVA, with pretreatment (MPH versus SAL) as a within-litter factor.

TABLE 1. Reproductive parameters from rats treated with MPH (2 mg/kg) or SAL during adolescence for 14 days and sacrificed 2 h after the last injection (short-term subchronic effect)

Parameter	SAL pre-exposed	MPH pre-exposed
Body weight (g)	196.0 ± 4.8	195.2 ± 5.0
testes weight (g)	1.038 ± 0.019	1.114 ± 0.020*
Testis/body weight ratio (× 1000)	5.30 ± 0.11	5.72 ± 0.11*
Total sperm/testis (million)	61.02 ± 4.82	73.58 ± 2.61*
Total sperm/testis, weight standardized	59.50 ± 4.47	67.03 ± 3.70
TST/ testis (ng)	72.17 ± 4.42	52.30 ± 9.39
TST/testis, weight standardized	70.16 ± 3.26	46.72 ± 7.32*

*$P < 0.05$ when compared to SAL pre-exposed.

It is clearly evident from tables that all effects were seen only as a short-term response to subchronic MPH (TABLE 1). It is interesting to note that acute MPH produced no effects (TABLE 2), indicating that a repeated treatment is needed for adaptive changes to occur. Moreover, MPH effects were no longer evident as a long-term effect (TABLE 3), indicating that MPH-induced changes were not long lasting and recovered over time.

As for the profile of short-term effects, reproductive endpoints were clearly affected by MPH exposure. The weight of testes was increased by drug treatment, being 8% higher in MPH than in SAL rats. Because whole-body weight was unaffected, the testis/body weight ratio was also increased around 8%. These findings suggest a trophic action of MPH exposure on testis growth. The total quantity of sperm was increased by 20% in MPH-treated rats. However, when standardized for the weight of testes, we found only a nonsignificant

TABLE 2. Reproductive parameters from rats treated with MPH (2 mg/kg) or SAL during adolescence only for 1 day and sacrificed 2 h after the injection (acute effect)

Parameter	SAL pre-exposed	MPH pre-exposed
Body weight (g)	155.6 ± 2.4	155.4 ± 3.5
testes weight (g)	1.031 ± 0.030	1.027 ± 0.031
Testis/body weight ratio (× 1000)	6.53 ± 0.14	6.60 ± 0.20
Total sperm/testis (million)	54.90 ± 9.92	67.66 ± 4.84
Total sperm/testis, weight standardized	54.59 ± 10.79	66.55 ± 2.37
TST/testis (ng)	48.99 ± 7.72	58.88 ± 16.39
TST/testis, weight standardized	47.38 ± 6.56	57.16 ± 14.65

NOTE: No significant effects of acute MPH during adolescence were found.

TABLE 3. Reproductive parameters from rats treated with MPH (2 mg/kg) or SAL during adolescence for 14 days and sacrificed 2 months after the last injection (long-term subchronic effects)

Parameter	SAL pre-exposed	MPH pre-exposed
Body weight (g)	349.0 ± 6.6	359.9 ± 11.3
testes weight (g)	1.676 ± 0.058	1.643 ± 0.069
Testis/body weight ratio (× 1000)	4.82 ± 0.28	4.60 ± 0.28
Total sperm/testis (million)	183.9 ± 11.8	188.2 ± 7.8
Total sperm/testis, weight standardized	107.8 ± 3.8	109.3 ± 2.7

NOTE: No long-term effects of subchronic MPH during adolescence were found.

tendency toward an increase of sperm. Production of sperm per gram of testis seems to be unaffected. As a whole, the increase in quantity of sperm follows the increase in testicular dimensions, rather than be due to a truly increased production rate.

Finally, the concentration of TST within the testes was clearly diminished by drug treatment. Indeed, a 40% decrease was evident in MPH-treated rats, compared to controls. This finding is consistent with literature on psychostimulants, reporting decreased plasma levels of androgen hormones in the rat.[19] However, this effect was only transient, and is likely to represent an adaptive physiological response to the drug treatment. Noteworthy, no differences in TST titers were found in adult rats, suggesting a full recovery from transient endocrine alterations experienced during the adolescent period.

These findings suggest that subchronic MPH exposure in adolescent rats could have a trophic action on testis growth and a negative impact on the production of testicular TST. More information, about the possible impairment of the Sertoli and Leydig cell function and/or about a possible disruption of the hypothalamic-pituitary-testicular axis, is obviously needed. This would allow to clarify if the observed effects are due to a direct action of MPH on the testicular cells or conversely to a centrally mediated effect. However, the role of hepatic TST metabolism has been investigated in the present work (see below).

However, as far as long-term effects are concerned, there were no longer detectable differences once the animals became adults. Thus, according to clinical and preclinical[13] evidence, we can conclude that MPH exposure during adolescence does not produce any enduring alteration on the function of male sexual organs. Moreover, differently from what is observed with other psychostimulant drugs, body weight was never affected. This observation may perhaps be used to reassure parents of ADHD children, confirming that Ritalin treatment is devoid of major adverse consequences on general growth patterns.

Metabolic (Hepatic) Endpoints

Hepatic microsomes were prepared as previously described.[23] The protein content was determined using bovine serum albumin as standard.[24] The activity of TST hydroxylase in the microsomal samples was determined by the method described elsewhere[25] with minor modifications. The enzymatic activity was measured under the linear range of reaction time, substrate, and protein concentrations. The assay was performed by 10 min incubation (37°C) of 1 mg/mL hepatic microsomal protein with 1 mM TST, 2 mM G6P, 2 U/mL G6PDH, and 1 mM NADP in buffer (50 mM Tris, 1 mM EDTA [pH 7.4]). The incubation was stopped by the addition of dichloromethane. Corticosterone as internal standard (IS) was then added. Blanks were carried out using standard incubation mixture without NADP. TST, its metabolites, and IS were extracted and then detected by high-performance liquid chromatography (HPLC).

CYP19 activity in liver microsomes was measured by a tritiated-water formation assay as previously described.[26] Microsomal samples (0.4 mg/mL) were incubated with 4 mM G6P, 2 U/mL G6PDH, 143.5 μM unlabeled-Δ^4, and 1.2 μCi/mL [1β-^{3}H]-Δ^4. The reaction was started by the addition of 0.5 mM NADP and carried out for 80 min (37°C). Blanks were carried out using standard incubation mixture without NADP. The reaction was stopped by the addition of chloroform and deionized water. Samples were then extracted and the radiolabeled steroids were removed by the addition of a suspension of charcoal-dextran coated. The release of tritiated water was measured using scintillation counter LS6500 Beckman liquid.

Data were analyzed using one-way ANOVA followed by Bonferroni's test. Our results indicate that liver weights and liver/body weight ratios were unaffected by MPH treatment. No differences in the hepatic microsomal protein content between control and acutely/subchronically MPH-treated rats were observed (not shown). CYP19 is a member of the CYP family that catalyses the aromatization of TST into estrogens (i.e., estradiol). CYP19 activity was measured, to evaluate its role in maintaining steroid hormones homeostasis. Preliminary results show that, in rat hepatic microsomes, no significant alterations of CYP19 activity were evident after either acute or subchronic treatment with MPH, compared to controls (see TABLE 4).

In the liver, different cytochrome P450 isoenzymes (CYPs) can monohydroxylate TST at several positions, or dehydrogenate to produce androstenedione. The effect of MPH on the rate of the regio- and stereo-selective TST metabolism was studied by measuring, in hepatic microsomes, TST 6α, 7α, 6β, 16α, 16β, 2β hydroxylase-specific activities (producing the corresponding hydroxylated TST metabolites) and dehydrogenase-specific activity (producing androstenedione). Our data show that MPH treatment caused a statistically significant increase of the formation rate of all TST metabolites, with the exception of androstenedione (FIG. 1). The inductive effect resulted in an increase of TST catabolism, ranging from 1.1- to 1.8-fold, without a close correlation

TABLE 4. CYP19 activity levels in hepatic microsomal samples from adolescent rats, treated with MPH (2 mg/kg) or SAL only once (acute group) or for 14 days (subchronic group), and sacrificed 2 h after the last injection

Treatment group	CYP19 activity (nmol/mg prot min)
SAL acute	2.21 ± 0.38
MPH acute	2.76 ± 0.46
SAL sub-chronic	1.41 ± 0.10
MPH sub-chronic	1.56 ± 0.62

Data are expressed as nmol/mg prot min and represent the mean ± SD of samples run in duplicate on three different microsomal preparations. No effects of either acute or subchronic MPH administration were found.

with any specific CYP-mediated activity. When we compared the inductive effect due to either acute or subchronic treatment with MPH, no significant differences were observed.

As a whole, the MPH exposure resulted in increased hepatic TST catabolism and reduced testicular TST levels. These two findings seem to support each other and are in good agreement with literature, reporting decreased androgen

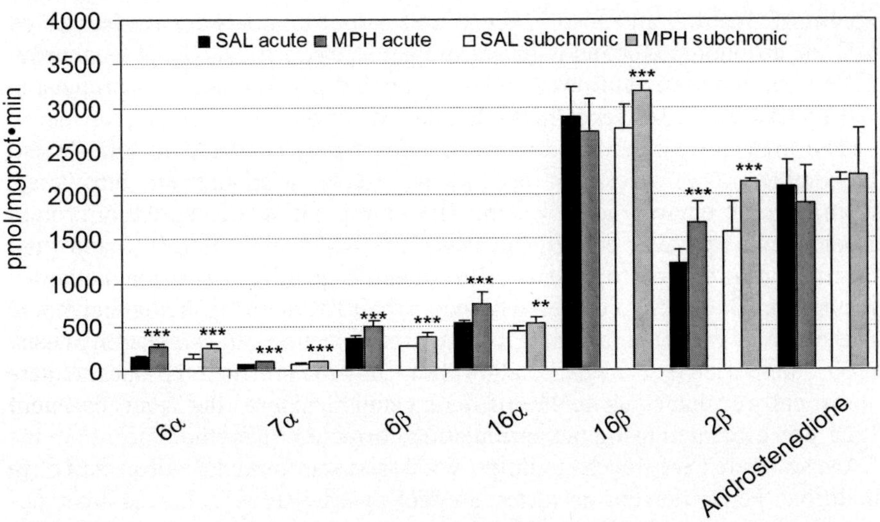

FIGURE 1. Rate of TST catabolism by hepatic microsomal samples from adolescent rats, treated with MPH (2 mg/kg) or SAL only once (acute group) or for 14 days (subchronic group), and sacrificed 2 h after the last injection. Closed and open bars represent results on control animals with SAL injection(s), while stripped and dotted bars represent results on animals with the MPH treatment, respectively. Each set of four bars represents the levels of a single TST metabolite (as indicated in the abscissa). Data are expressed as pmol/mg prot min and represent the mean ± SD of samples run in duplicate on three different microsomal preparations.*** $P \leq 0.001$; ** $P \leq 0.01$.

hormones after psychostimulants in rats.[19] and after MPH in mice.[16] This set of data is thus consistent with our initial hypothesis of a disruption in male hormonal endpoints. Conversely, contrary to our initial expectations, MPH treatment during adolescence in rats seemed to produce a transient acceleration of testis maturation, which may well be taken as an index of a precocious puberty onset. This set of data suggests an opposite trend, compared to our initial hypothesis of a retardation in reproductive endpoints.

Genome-Wide Expression Profiling in Brain Striatum

Brain striatal samples, from the "short-term sub-chronic" group, were used for the expression profiling approach. Samples from the "acute" and the "long-term sub-chronic" groups were used for reverse transciption polymerase chain reaction (RT-PCR) validation, namely to assess if selected genes, showing changes in the microarray data set, were also showing changes in the other two conditions. These results have been reported elsewhere.[9] For the microarray technique, total RNA was isolated using a combination of Tri Reagent (Sigma-Aldrich, Milan, Italy) and RNeasy Kit (Qiagen, Milan, Italy). Samples were treated with DNase (RNase-free DNase set, Qiagen) when still bound to Qiagen columns. Quantity and absorbance at 260/280 of total RNA was assessed by UV spectrophotometer and with agarose gel electrophoresis. Double-stranded cDNA was synthesized from total RNA, labeled with biotin and hybridized to Affimetrix Rat 230A GeneChips. Detailed Methods are described elsewhere.[9]

The images were analyzed with the Affy (freely available at: http://www.bioconductor.org) package for the R (freely available at: http://cran.r-project.org) environment system. The extrapolation of expression values from the images was carried out using the RMA algorithm.[27,28] and their normalization was performed using the quantile-quantile regression method.[29] In addition, data were prefiltered based on their fitting to the theoretical model of the Li and Wong algorithm.[30,31] and on the detection call calculation of each probe, supported by the MAS-5 algorithm. Only the prefiltered probesets were statistically evaluated using three different statistical tests: the False Discovery Rate was evaluated using the permutation corrected *t*-test implemented in the SAM software (SAM website [http://www-stat.stanford.edu/~tibs/SAM]). In addition, the Bonferroni-corrected Student's *t*-test was run.

Only the genes common to all the three statistical filters, having a False Discovery Rate median value equal to 0 and P values <0.01 were considered as candidate genes and used for the clustering analysis. Hierarchical clustering of the samples was applied considering the whole prefiltered probesets, and the significant probesets were used to evaluate the quality of replicates and the coherence of the data set. Moreover, the significant genes were divided in classes of expression profile with the k-means clustering method. Functional-clustering analysis was also performed in order to link the significant genes

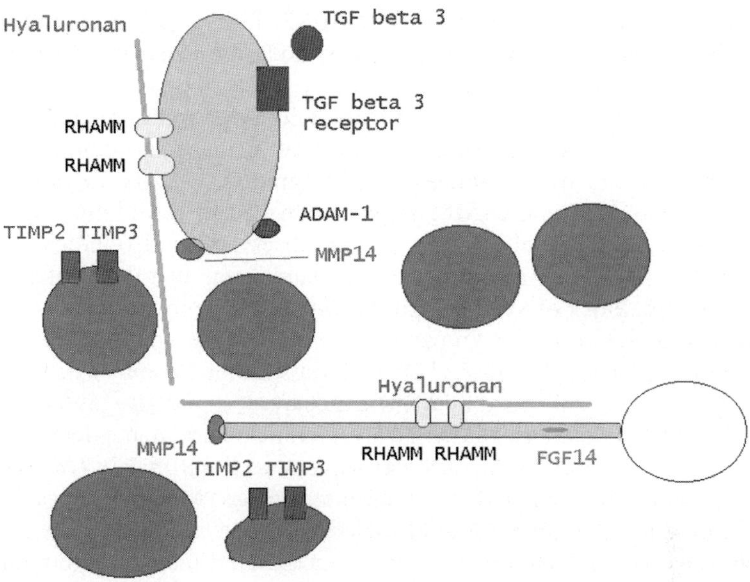

FIGURE 2. Migration of glial precursors and/or growth of novel axons (in light gray) inside the striatum, in the presence of the resident cells (in dark gray), which are untouched structural elements. All shown proteins, known to contribute to this developmental process, were upregulated by MPH exposure.

to the Gene Ontology database annotations. A Fisher test was applied on each functional family overrepresented, using 0.05 as cutoff.

More than 700 genes were upregulated in MPH-treated rats (fold-change$>$1.5). Among these genes, several families of genes were represented.[9] Only some selected genes will be discussed here, whose functions are known and hence a role in MPH-treated rats can be extrapolated. These genes will permit us to speculate about processes occurring within the brain striatum as an adaptation to subchronic MPH exposure. Hypotheses will be formulated about migration of immature glial/neural precursors, growth and myelination of novel axonal projections, reorganization of intercellular communication, through rearrangement of electric signaling and dendritic spines. The profile of effects which involves the function of synapses, their plasticity, and their neurotransmission, are described elsewhere.[9]

Migration of Glial/Neural Cells and Novel Axonal Projections

A first group of genes were apparently involved in migration of immature neural/glial cells and/or growth of novel axons (FIG. 2). These genes include the hyaluronan-mediated motility receptor (RHAMM), matrix proteases

(ADAM-1, MMP14), their inhibitors (TIMP-2, TIMP-3), and growth factors (transforming growth factor-β3 [TGF-β3] and fibroblast growth factor 14 [FGF14]).

The protein RHAMM (namely, "receptor for hyaluronan-mediated motility") is a member of the hyaladherin family of hyaluronan-binding proteins. RHAMM has a key role in adhesion and migration, via interactions of cells with hyaluronan.[32] The RHAMM receptor plays a role in cell motility within the nervous system as well. Recent *in vitro* observations also indicate the involvement of RHAMM in neurite motility, suggesting that this protein might be an important index of axon outgrowth *in situ*.[33] We provide a first evidence that the expression of genes, known to be involved in axon growth, is significantly increased in rats following MPH administration. We may hence propose that axon growth is enhanced by MPH exposure.

Matrix metalloproteinases (MMPs) are a family of zinc-dependent endopeptidases, which are able to degrade various extracellular matrix (ECM) components, for instance, ADAM-1 ("A Disintegrin And Metalloprotease") is an integrin-binding, membrane-bound metalloprotease. Its role in the nervous system is poorly understood.[34] Another upregulated membrane-bound metalloproteinase, called MMP-14, is better characterized. In a recent study, the expression of MMP-14 was demonstrated in human brain tumors of various types. There was strong evidence suggesting that MMP-14 is produced at the leading edge of the invading glia cells.[35,36] In physiological nontumor situations, MMP-14 may play a key role, allowing migration of newly produced glial cells through the existing structures. This functional process may hence be enhanced by MPH administration.

As MMPs degrade the components of the ECM, the most significant determinant of proteolytic events in tissue remodeling is the actual balance between MMPs and their inhibitors, called tissue inhibitors of metalloproteinases (TIMPs).[37] Information about production site of TIMPs is available from brain lesions studies. In adult rat cortex, TIMP-2 and TIMP-3 are found in astrocytes of deep cortex and in the underlying white matter.[38] TIMP production is particularly strong, especially in those structures that are more inhibitory for axon regeneration. Taken together, this set of genes are suggesting active brain remodeling, consisting of axons that are growing and glial cells that are migrating. Indeed, existing structures appear to protect themselves during this process. Again, MPH administration possibly enhances brain plasticity in adolescent brains.

A group of DA-related neurotrophins is also upregulated. FGF14 is known to be expressed in the developing and adult central nervous system (CNS). FGF14-deficient mice have reduced responses to DA agonists.[39] Functions of FGF14 include neuronal signaling and axonal trafficking. Strikingly, the FGF14 protein appears to be transported into neuronal processes of the basal ganglia.[39] Our data, suggesting increased neurotransmission in the striatum of MPH-exposed rats, are consistent with the mechanisms of action of MPH, that

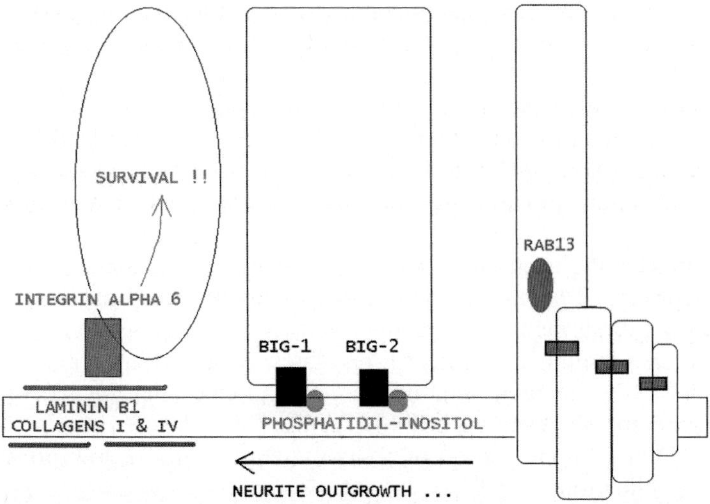

FIGURE 3. Myelination of a newly growing axon. The glia-axon contact is a cue for survival of the glial cell (left). The myelination process then requires stabilization of the contact (middle), and wrapping of the axon by the repeated folding of the glial cell (right). All shown proteins, known to play a key role in these three steps, were upregulated by MPH exposure.

is believed to block the DA transporter, thus increasing the DA concentration in the target areas of the DAergic system.[3]

TGF-β is a product of astroglial cells, with a well-established trophic action on DAergic neurons. TGF-β is required for both induction and survival of ventral-midbrain DAergic neurons. Consistently, neutralization of TGF-β completely abolishes the production of DAergic neurons *in vitro*.[40] Also, TGF-β is possibly required for mediating the survival of cortical and striatal neurons, grown in the presence of glial cells.[41] Together, these results identify the TGF-β as an essential mediator for the induction and maintenance of midbrain DAergic projections.

More specifically, TGF-β3 is known to be expressed in adult human astrocytes, where it may play a role in glioblast differentiation and guidance of neuroblast migration.[42] TGF-β3 also causes a reduction of connexin43 mRNA (see below) in cortical and striatal astroglial cells.[43] The finding of an upregulation for TGF-β3 and its receptor is a consistent with a working hypothesis of active brain remodeling.

Myelination of Axons after Glial Contact

A second group of genes were suggestive of active axonal myelination (FIG. 3). These genes mediate survival of immature myelinating cells after contact with newly produced axonal matrix (laminin B1, collagen alpha1(IV), integrin alpha 6), and subsequent stabilization of myelinating glia-axon contacts (PI4KII, contactins 3 and 4). In this frame, it is well known that myelin sheaths of the CNS are produced by the oligodendrocytes. Noteworthy, a key turning point in the destiny of immature oligodendrocytes is whether or not they eventually contact an axon. Newly formed oligodendrocytes that fail to contact axons undergo apoptosis. Conversely, oligodendrocytes will survive and produce mature myelin only following contact with their target axons.

In particular, the survival signal origins from an interaction between the laminins produced by the axons and their integrin receptors expressed on oligodendrocyte surface. Specifically, when myelin-forming oligodendrocytes contact axonal laminins, an integrin-regulated switch in survival signaling is activated.[44–46] It has been demonstrated that alpha6 integrin is actually the laminin receptor which enhances the survival of oligodendrocytes.[44–46] Hence, the MPH-induced upregulation of alpha6 integrin could be interpreted as an index of myelination.

On the other hand, laminin B1 and collagen alpha 1(IV) are specific components of nonsynaptic ECM surrounding the axon, being not abundant near synapses.[47] The increased expression of B1 laminin and type IV collagen may thus indicate that axonal growth is occurring.[48] Moreover, laminin B1 upregulation is also reported within myelinating cells following axonal contact.[49] Hence, the MPH-induced upregulation of B1 laminin and collagen alpha1(IV) is also consistent with the hypothesis of MPH-induced enhanced myelination.

The process of myelination in the rat CNS consists of an initial phase of wrapping, when a tight junction develops between the joining tips of the oligodendrocytic process.[50] The myelinated axon is not homogeneous across its length, but the succession of Ranvier nodes and myelinated traits identifies two distinct regions. The nodal traits, where action potentials occur, are rich in Na(+) and K(+) channels. Conversely, paranodal traits are wrapped by myelinating oligodendrocytes and are characterized by contactin proteins.[51] In particular, specialized adhesion sites are found between the axon and myelinating glial cells. These sites, flanking the Ranvier nodes, are called axoglial paranodal junctions.[52] The paranodal junctions express on the axonal membrane contactins, a family of glycosylphosphatidylinositol-anchored proteins. Contactins mediate neuron-glial contacts and organize axonal subdomains at the node of Ranvier of myelinated fibers.[53] Two genes for contactins, namely BIG-1 and BIG-2, were upregulated in our microarray data.

BIG-1 (alias contactin3) and BIG-2 (alias contactin4) are members of the immunoglobulin (Ig) superfamily, with six Ig-like domains, four fibronectin type III-like repeats, and a glycosyl phosphatidylinositol-anchoring domain. The expression of BIG-1 and BIG-2 mRNA is restricted to specific subsets of neurons.[54,55] Recombinant BIG-1 and BIG-2 proteins have a neurite outgrowth-promoting activity, suggesting that both may be involved in the formation and maintenance of specific networks in the brain.[54,55] The finding of upregulation

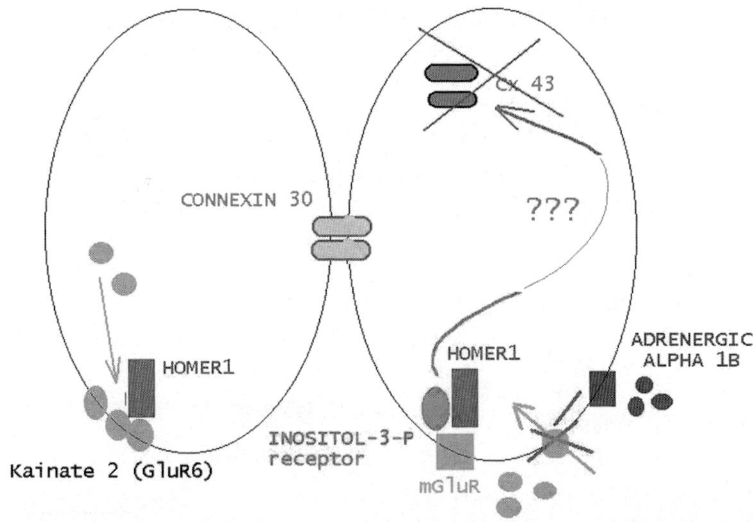

FIGURE 4. Intercellular communication between two adjacent glial cells. The metabolites spread from cell to cell via the gap junctions. The expression of protein connexin30 was upregulated by MPH exposure, whereas the more classical protein connexin43 (cx43) may be hypothesized to be functionally deactivated.

of both BIG-1 and BIG-2 in MPH-treated rats suggests that outgrowth and myelination of axons is actually occurring.

Because contactins are ultimately anchored to the cell membrane via a phosphatidyl inositol, a further evidence for this hypothesis would be provided by the finding of the upregulation in genes related to phosphatidyl-inositol metabolism. Interestingly, the Phosphatidyl-Inositol-4-Kinase type II (PI4KII) was upregulated. This gene family was recently characterized[56]: PI4KII is concentrated at synapses and in the region of the Golgi complex in neuronal perikarya, and plays a critical role in the cycle of phosphoinositide synthesis and hydrolysis.[56]

Intercellular Communication, Electric Signaling, Dendritic Spines

A third group of upregulated genes are known to be involved in intercellular connection and in synapting signaling (FIG. 4 and 5), thus indicating a global remodeling of striatal communication pathways. These genes encode for intercellular gap junctions (connexin30), electric channels (TASK-1, TASK-5), neurotransmitter receptors (adrenergic alpha-1B, kainate 2, serotonin 7, GABA-A), as well as major proteins responsible for their transport and/or anchoring (Homer-1, MAGUK MPP3, Shank2). All these genes were involved in synaptic plasticity, namely the formation, maturation, and stabilization of new neural connections within the striatum.[9]

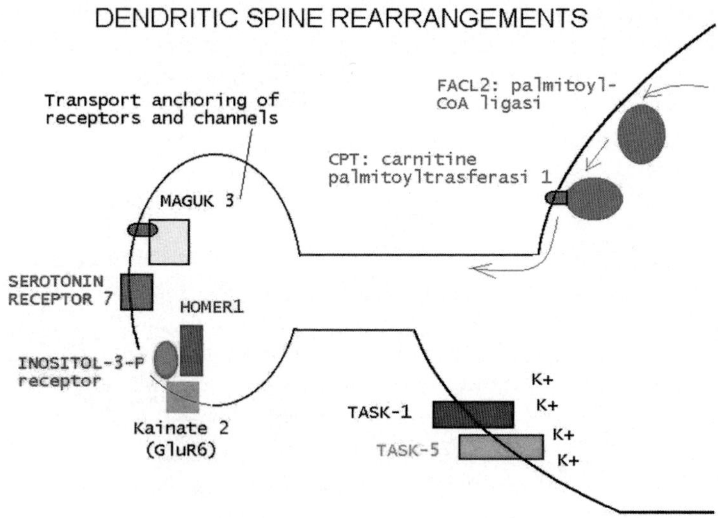

FIGURE 5. Schematic representation of a dendritic spine in a neural cell. All shown proteins, known to form the architecture of dendritic spines, were upregulated by MPH exposure.

Intercellular Communication

In glia, metabolic signals are transferred within the cytoplasm of adjacent cells via gap junctions. Indeed, these functional pores allow spreading of cytoplasmic metabolites from one cell to another. The major and ubiquitous gap-junction protein is connexin43, but astrocytes also produce a second protein called connexin30. It is localized in astrocytes, at gap junctions with another astrocyte or with an oligodendrocyte.[57,58] Thus, connexin30 is expressed by in gray but not white matter, and emerges relatively late during brain maturation.[57] In particular, expression of connexin30 increases during the first 3 weeks after birth and reaches its maximum at 4 weeks,[59] namely during adolescence. This late onset of connexin30 expression suggests that it may have a role in communication among mature astrocytes.

The intriguing aspect of this protein is that it seems to influence behavioral parameters. Recent work in connexin30-/- mice has shown reduced exploratory activity in the open field and object exploration task, and anxiogenic behavior in the open field.[60] Conversely, inactivation of connexin43 in astrocytes produces an increase of exploratory activity and an anxiolytic-like effect.[61] Such data highlight the importance of gap-junction signaling in behavioral processes, suggesting that connexins can alter the behavioral reactivity to novel environments. In this light, psychoactive drugs may produce their behavioral effects not only via a classical modulation of neurotransmission, but also through changes in connexin30 expression. We hypothesize that MPH exposure might lead to increased expression of connexin30 together with a decreased expression of connexin43 (see FIG. 4). Intriguingly, the finding of an upregulation of connexin30 in MPH-treated rats from the present study may be a cue, suggesting that connexins may represent important but yet unknown factors, certainly deserving further investigation.

Electric Signaling

TASK-1 and TASK-5 belong to a new family of potassium channels, which has been recently identified. These channels have two pore domains in tandem and four transmembrane segments, and are active as dimers. These channels are widespread in both excitable and nonexcitable cells. Their currents are quasi-instantaneous, noninactivating, insensitive to classic K(+) channel blockers, and active at all membrane potentials.[62] These channels have been designated as background K(+) channels, setting the resting membrane potential in many cell types. TASK-1 immunoreactivity is prominently found in cerebellum, somatic motoneurons,[63] and in hippocampal astrocytes.[64]

A recent study revealed that TASK-1 are most strongly expressed in many neurons likely to be cholinergic, noradrenergic, or serotonergic.[65] In contrast, TASK-5 expression is predominantly associated with the central auditory pathway. Interestingly, TASK-5 channels may play a role in the transmission of temporal information in the auditory system.[65] These two observations may help to define an hypothesis regarding the striata of MPH-treated rats, where an upregulation of both TASK-1 and TASK-5 was found. Specifically, these two channel proteins may be respectively involved either in striatal serotonergic functions or in processing temporal information. Intriguingly, these two possibilities are not mutually exclusive, because one of the roles for striatal serotonin pathways is actually to subserve an integrated perception about "timing" of reward delivery.[66] Again, microarray data may have delivered a cue toward an important but yet unknown factor, deserving further investigation.

Dendritic Spines

The number of neurotransmitter receptors in the postsynaptic membrane and their functional coupling to intracellular signaling cascades are important determinants of synaptic strength and hence potential markers of plasticity. Normal dendritic spines have a rather constant structure, where certain specific proteins are always present (see FIG. 5). These proteins are: (*a*) glutamate ionotropic receptors (GluRs); (*b*) at least one associated protein of the MAGUK (membrane-associated guanylate kinase) family; and (*c*) Homer, which interacts with inositol-3-phosphate receptors (IP3Rs).[67] We found that genes belonging to all these three specific classes were upregulated in MPH-treated rats, a finding that may suggest the formation of novel dendritic spines. Indeed, among many upregulated genes, we found: (*a*) the kainate 2 subunit of

GluRs (Grik2); (*b*) the "membrane protein, palmitoylated 3" (MPP3), that is the member 3 of the MAGUK p55 subfamily; and (*c*) Homer-1a and the inositol 1,4,5-triphosphate receptor 2 (Itpr2). There is hence a nice correspondence between actual findings and changes expected based on available literature. Interestingly, overexpression of Homer-1a is known to enhance α-amino-3-hydroxy-5-methyl-4-isoxazol propionate (AMPA)/kainate receptor function by increasing synaptic clustering of these receptors.[68] Moreover, all Homer proteins physically link inositol 1,4,5-triphosphate receptors in the subsynaptic endoplasmic reticulum,[69] thus providing a link to intracellular signaling cascades. Again, from these considerations, the formation of novel dendritic spines, or enhanced functional activity of the existing ones, might be suggested. These two processes would respectively indicate structural versus functional plasticity of striatal connections. Intriguingly, such dendritic-spine rearrangement may possibly occur due to novel outgrowing axons reaching their target.

Members of the MAGUK protein family have emerged as central organizers of multicomponent signaling complexes. The MAGUKs use multiple domains to cluster ion channels and receptors, and play a fundamental role in the transport and anchoring of these specific proteins toward synapses and cellular junctions.[70] Genes of this family interact with adhesion molecules and cytosolic signaling proteins, and play a major role in the formation, maintenance, and plasticity of glutamatergic synapses.[71] The specific MAGUK protein which was upregulated in our rats, namely MPP3, is palmitoylated. This fact implies that the protein palmitoylation process could also be upregulated, to account for increased MPP3 synthesis. Two genes actually confirm this picture: Palmitoyl-CoA ligase (FACL2), which converts free palmitoyl acid into palmitoyl-CoA,[72] and carnitine palmitoyltransferase (CPT), which may be important for phospholipid and triglyceride fatty acid turnover in neurons.[73]

CONCLUSION

This article, focusing about consequences of MPH exposure during adolescence, considered various parameters, ranging from gonadal maturation to hepatic metabolism up to brain (striatal) gene expression. We have shown a disruption in male hormonal endpoints, both in terms of gonadal TST levels and hepatic TST catabolism. However, an opposite trend emerges for reproductive endpoints, consisting of a transient increase in testicular growth and spermatogenesis, and perhaps suggesting precocious puberty onset. We wish to underline that all these effects were only transient (being evident at short term) and not enduring (being absent at long term).

As for the brain, subchronic MPH treatment seems to potentiate the expression of specific genes, which activity is indicative of neural and synaptic plasticity. Enhanced remodeling of brain (striatal) architecture and connectivity is specifically proposed. This is a developmental (i.e., age-dependent) phenomenon that control adolescent rats are also very likely to show, when compared to adults. Our observations suggest that adolescent MPH exposure may cause fundamental structural and functional changes in reward-related striatal circuits. These might in turn account for the positive modulatory action of MPH on altered behavioral processing, shown by animal models of ADHD.

In summary, adolescent MPH exposure may have some transient side effects on hormonal and reproductive parameters, but centrally mediated "therapeutic" effects on behavioral plasticity[74] are still enduring when animals get into adulthood.

ACKNOWLEDGMENTS

This study was supported by joint NIH-ISS Project, Ministry of Health, Italy, and by Dipartimento Nazionale Antidroga, Pres. Cons. Min., Italy (to GL). We wish to thank Giovanni Dominici for expert technical help.

REFERENCES

1. SAGVOLDEN, T. & J.A. SERGEANT. 1998. Attention deficit/hyperactivity disorder—from brain dysfunction to behavior. Behav. Brain Res. **94:** 1–10.
2. SONUGA-BARKE, E.J. 2003. The dual pathway model of AD/HD: an elaboration of neuro-developmental characteristics. Neurosci. Biobehav. Rev. **27:** 593–604.
3. SWANSON, J.M. & N.D. VOLKOW. 2002. Pharmacokinetic and pharmacodynamic properties of stimulants: implications for the design of new treatments for ADHD. Behav. Brain Res. **130:** 73–78.
4. CARLEZON, W.A. JR. & C. KONRADI. 2004. Understanding the neurobiological consequences of early exposure to psychotropic drugs: linking behavior with molecules. Neuropharmacology **47:** 47–60.
5. BRANDON, C.L., M. MARINELLI, L.K. BAKER & F.J. WHITE. 2001. Enhanced reactivity and vulnerability to cocaine following methylphenidate treatment in adolescent rats. Neuropsychopharmacology **25:** 651–661.
6. ANDERSEN, S.L., A. ARVANITOGIANNIS, A.M. PLIAKAS, *et al.* 2002. Altered responsiveness to cocaine in rats exposed to methylphenidate during development. Nat. Neurosci. **5:** 13–14.
7. CARLEZON, W.A. JR. S.D. MAGUE & S.L. ANDERSEN. 2003. Enduring behavioral effects of early exposure to methylphenidate in rats. Biol. Psychiatry **54:** 1330–1337.
8. BOLANOS, C.A., M. BARROT, O. BERTON, *et al.* 2003. Methylphenidate treatment during pre- and periadolescence alters behavioral responses to emotional stimuli at adulthood. Biol. Psychiatry **54:** 1317–1329.
9. ADRIANI, W., D. LEO, D. GRECO, *et al.* 2005. Methylphenidate administration to adolescent rats determines short- and long-term changes on reward-related behavior and striatal gene expression. Neuropsychopharmacology Nov 23; [Epub ahead of print].
10. NESTLER, E.J. 2004. Molecular mechanisms of drug addiction. Neuropharmacology **47:** 24–32.

11. Brandon, C.L. & H. Steiner. 2003. Repeated methylphenidate treatment in adolescent rats alters gene regulation in the striatum. Eur. J. Neurosci. **18:** 1584–1592.
12. Yano, M. & H. Steiner. 2004. Topography of methylphenidate (Ritalin)-induced gene regulation in the striatum: differential effects on c-Fos, substance P and opioid peptides. Neuropsychopharmacology **22:** 1–15.
13. Pizzi, W.J., E.C. Rodc, J.E. Barnhart. 1987. Differential effects of methylphenidate on the grouth of neonatal and adolescent rats. Neurotoxicol. Teratol. **9:** 107–111.
14. Greelcy, G.H. Jr, J.S. Kizer. 1980. The effects of chronic methylphenidate treatment on the groth and endocrine function in the developing rat. J. Pharmacol. Exp. Ther. **215:** 545–551.
15. NIH. 2005. NTP-CERHR Monograph on the potential Human Reproductive and Developmental Effects of Methylphenidate. Publication No. 05–4473.
16. Morrissey, R.E., B.A. Schwetz, J.C. Lamb, *et al.* 1988. Evaluation of rodent sperm, vaginal cytology and reproductive organ weight data from National Toxicology Program 13-week studies. Fundam. Appl. Toxicol. **11:** 343–358.
17. Fiorino, DF & Phillips AG. 1999. Facilitation of sexual behavior in male rats following d-amphetamine-induced behavioral sensitization. Psychopharmacology **142:** 200–208.
18. Lurie S & O' Quinn A. 1991. Neuroendocrine responses to methylphenidate and d-amphetamine: applications to attention-deficit disorder. J. Neuropsychiatry Clin Neurosci. **3:** 41–50.
19. Budziszewska B, Jaworska-Feil L & Lason W. 1996. The effect of repeated amphetamine and coaine administration on adrenal, gonadal and thyroid hormone levels in the rat plasma. Exp. Clin. Endocrinol. Diabetes **104:** 334–338.
20. Muller E.E., Locatelli V, Cella S, *et al.* 1983. Prolactin-lowering and releasing drugs. Mechanisms of action and therapeutic applications. Drugs **25:** 399–432.
21. Becu-Villalobos D, Lacau-Mengido IM, Diaz-Torga G.S., *et al.* 1992. Ontogenic studies of the neural control of adenohypophyseal hormones in the rat. IL Prolactin. Cell. Mol. Neurobiol. **12:** 1–19.
22. Meistrich, M.L. 1989. Evaluation of reproductive toxicity by testicular sperm head counts. J. Am. Coll. Toxicol. **8:** 551–566.
23. Testai, E. & L. Vittozzi. 1986. Biochemical alterations elicited in rat liver microsomes by oxidation and reduction products of chloroform metabolism. Chem. Biol. Interact. **59:** 157–171.
24. Oyama, V.I. & H. Eagle. 1956. Measurement of cell growth in tissue culture with a phenol reagent (folin-ciocalteau). Proc. Soc. Exp. Biol. Med. **91:** 305–307.
25. Sanwald, P., E.A. Blankson, B.D. Dulery, *et al.* 1995. Isocratic high-performance liquid chromatographic method for the separation of testosterone metabolites. J. Chromatogr. B **672:** 207–385.
26. You, L., M. Sar, E. Bartolucci, *et al.* 2001. Induction of hepatic aromatase by p,p'-DDE in adult male rats. Mol. Cell. Endocrinol. **178:** 207–214.
27. Irizarry RA, Hobbs B, Collin F, *et al.* 2003. Exploration, normalization, and summaries of high density oligonucleotide array probe level data. *Biostatistics*. **4:** 249–264.
28. Irizarry, RA, Bolstad BM, Collin F. *et al.* 2003. Summaries of Affymetrix GeneChip probe level data. *Nucleic Acids Res*. **15:** c15.
29. Bolstad, BM, Irizarry RA, Astrand M, *et al.* 2003. A comparison of normalization methods for high density oligonucleotide array data based on variance and bias. *Bioinformatics* **22:** 185–193.

30. LI C. & W.H. WONG. 2001. Model-based analysis of oligonucleotide arrays: expression index computation and outlier detection. Proc Natl Acad Sci. USA **98:** 31–36.
31. LI C. & W.H. WONG. 2001. Model-based analysis of oligonucleotide array: model validation, design issues and standard error application. Genome Biol. **2:** 32.1–32.11.
32. LYNN, B.D., X. LI, P.A. CATTINI, *et al.* 2001. Identification of sequence, protein isoforms, and distribution of the hyaluronan-binding protein RHAMM in adult and developing rat brain. J. Comp. Neurol. **439:** 315–330.
33. NAGY, J.I., M.L. PRICE, W.A. STAINES, *et al.* 1998. The hyaluronan receptor RHAMM in noradrenergic fibers contributes to axon growth capacity of locus coeruleus neurons in an intraocular transplant model. Neuroscience **86:** 241–255.
34. GERST, J.L., A.K. RAINA, I. PIRIM, *et al.* 2000. Altered cell-matrix associated ADAM proteins in Alzheimer disease. J. Neurosci. Res. **59:** 680–684.
35. ROOPRAI, H.K., T. VANMETER, G.J. RUCKLIDGE, *et al.* 1998. Comparative analysis of matrix metalloproteinases by immunocytochemistry, immunohistochemistry and zymography in human primary brain tumours. Int. J. Oncol. **13:** 1153–1157.
36. BELIEN, A.T., P.A. PAGANETTI & M.E. SCHWAB. 1999. Membrane-type 1 matrix metalloprotease (MT1-MMP) enables invasive migration of glioma cells in central nervous system white matter. J. Cell Biol. **144:** 373–384.
37. VAILLANT, C., M. DIDIER-BAZES, A. HUTTER, *et al.* 1999. Spatiotemporal expression patterns of metalloproteinases and their inhibitors in the postnatal developing rat cerebellum. J. Neurosci. **19:** 4994–5004.
38. MUIR, E.M., K.H. ADCOCK, D.A. MORGENSTERN, *et al.* 2002. Matrix metalloproteases and their inhibitors are produced by overlapping populations of activated astrocytes. Brain Res. Mol. Brain Res. **100:** 103–117.
39. WANG, Q., M.E. BARDGETT, M. WONG, *et al.* 2002. Ataxia and paroxysmal dyskinesia in mice lacking axonally transported FGF14. Neuron **35:** 25–38.
40. FARKAS, L.M., N. DUNKER, E. ROUSSA, *et al.* 2003. Transforming growth factor-beta(s) are essential for the development of midbrain dopaminergic neurons in vitro and in vivo. J. Neurosci. **23:** 5178–5186.
41. KRIEGLSTEIN, K., B. REUSS, D. MAYSINGER & K. UNSICKER. 1998. Short communication: transforming growth factor-beta mediates the neurotrophic effect of fibroblast growth factor on midbrain dopaminergic neurons. Eur. J. Neurosci. **10:** 2746–2750.
42. JOHNSON, M.D., M.T. JENNINGS, L.I. GOLD & H.L. MOSES. 1993. Transforming growth factor-beta in neural embryogenesis and neoplasia. Hum. Pathol. **24:** 457–462.
43. REUSS, B., R. DERMIETZEL & K. UNSICKER. 1998. Fibroblast growth factor 2 (FGF-2) differentially regulates connexin (cx) 43 expression and function in astroglial cells from distinct brain regions. Glia **22:** 19–30.
44. FROST, E.E., P.C. BUTTERY, R. MILNER & C. FRENCH-CONSTANT. 1999. Integrins mediate a neuronal survival signal for oligodendrocytes. Curr. Biol. **9:** 1251–1254.
45. COLOGNATO, H., W. BARON, V. AVELLANA-ADALID, *et al.* 2002. CNS integrins switch growth factor signalling to promote target-dependent survival. Nat. Cell Biol. **4:** 833–841.
46. DECKER, L. & C. FRENCH-CONSTANT. 2004. Lipid rafts and integrin activation regulate oligodendrocyte survival. J. Neurosci. **24:** 3816–3825.

47. SANES, J.R., E. ENGVALL, R. BUTKOWSKI & D.D. HUNTER. 1990. Molecular heterogeneity of basal laminae: isoforms of laminin and collagen IV at the neuromuscular junction and elsewhere. J. Cell Biol. **111:** 1685–1699.
48. SIIRONEN, J., M. SANDBERG, V. VUORINEN & M. ROYTTA. 1992. Laminin B1 and collagen type IV gene expression in transected peripheral nerve: reinnervation compared to denervation. J. Neurochem. **59:** 2184–2192.
49. DOYU, M., G. SOBUE, E. KEN, *et al.* 1993. Laminin chains gene expression in transected and regenerating nerves: regulation by axonal signals. J. Neurochem. **60:** 543–551.
50. DERMIETZEL, R. & H. KROCZEK. 1980. Interlamellar tight junctions of central myelin. I. Developmental mechanisms during myelogenesis. Cell Tissue Res. **213:** 81–94.
51. MATHIS, C., N. DENISENKO-NEHRBASS, J.A. GIRAULT & E. BORRELLI. 2001. Essential role of oligodendrocytes in the formation and maintenance of central nervous system nodal regions. Development **128:** 4881–4890.
52. DENISENKO-NEHRBASS, N., C. FAIVRE-SARRAILH, L. GOUTEBROZE & J.A. GIRAULT. 2002. A molecular view on paranodal junctions of myelinated fibers. J. Physiol. Paris **96:** 99–103.
53. FALK, J., C. BONNON, J.A. GIRAULT & C. FAIVRE-SARRAILH. 2002. F3/contactin, a neuronal cell adhesion molecule implicated in axogenesis and myelination. Biol. Cell. **94:** 327–334.
54. YOSHIHARA, Y., M. KAWASAKI, A. TANI, *et al.* 1994. BIG-1: a new TAG-1/F3-related member of the immunoglobulin superfamily with neurite outgrowth-promoting activity. Neuron **13:** 415–426.
55. YOSHIHARA, Y., M. KAWASAKI, A. TAMADA, *et al.* 1995. Overlapping and differential expression of BIG-2, BIG-1, TAG-1, and F3: four members of an axon-associated cell adhesion molecule subgroup of the immunoglobulin superfamily. J. Neurobiol. **28:** 51–69.
56. GUO, J., M.R. WENK, L. PELLEGRINI, *et al.* 2003. Phosphatidylinositol 4-kinase type IIalpha is responsible for the phosphatidylinositol 4-kinase activity associated with synaptic vesicles. Proc. Natl. Acad. Sci. USA **100:** 3995–4000.
57. NAGY, J.I., D. PATEL, P.A. OCHALSKI & G.L. STELMACK. 1999. Connexin30 in rodent, cat and human brain: selective expression in gray matter astrocytes, co-localization with connexin43 at gap junctions and late developmental appearance. Neuroscience **88:** 447–468.
58. RASH, J.E., T. YASUMURA, F.E. DUDEK & J.I. NAGY. 2001. Cell-specific expression of connexins and evidence of restricted gap junctional coupling between glial cells and between neurons. J. Neurosci. **21:** 1983–2000.
59. KUNZELMANN, P., W. SCHRODER, O. TRAUB, *et al.* 1999. Late onset and increasing expression of the gap junction protein connexin30 in adult murine brain and long-term cultured astrocytes. Glia **25:** 111–119.
60. DERE, E., M.A. DE SOUZA-SILVA, C. FRISCH, *et al.* 2003. Connexin30-deficient mice show increased emotionality and decreased rearing activity in the open-field along with neurochemical changes. Eur. J. Neurosci. **18:** 629–638.
61. FRISCH, C., M. THEIS, M.A. DE SOUZA-SILVA, *et al.* 2003. Mice with astrocyte-directed inactivation of connexin43 exhibit increased exploratory behaviour, impaired motor capacities, and changes in brain acetylcholine levels. Eur. J. Neurosci. **18:** 2313–2318.

62. LESAGE, F. & M. LAZDUNSKI. 2000. Molecular and functional properties of two-pore-domain potassium channels. Am. J. Physiol. Renal Physiol. **279:** F793–F801.
63. TALLEY, E.M., G. SOLORZANO, Q. LEI, *et al.* 2001. Cns distribution of members of the two-pore-domain (KCNK) potassium channel family. J. Neurosci. **21:** 7491–7505.
64. KINDLER, C.H., C. PIETRUCK, C.S. YOST, *et al.* 2000. Localization of the tandem pore domain K+ channel TASK-1 in the rat central nervous system. Mol. Brain Res. **80:** 99–108.
65. KARSCHIN, C., E. WISCHMEYER, R. PREISIG-MULLER, *et al.* 2001. Expression pattern in brain of TASK-1, TASK-3, and a tandem pore domain K(+) channel subunit, TASK-5, associated with the central auditory nervous system. Mol. Cell Neurosci. **18:** 632–648.
66. CARDINAL, R.N., C.A. WINSTANLEY, T.W. ROBBINS & B.J. EVERITT. 2004. Limbic corticostriatal systems and delayed reinforcement. Ann. N. Y. Acad. Sci. **1021:** 33–50.
67. PETRALIA, R.S., Y.X. WANG, N. SANS, *et al.* 2001. Glutamate receptor targeting in the postsynaptic spine involves mechanisms that are independent of myosin Va. Eur .J. Neurosci. **13:** 1722–1732.
68. HENNOU, S., A. KATO, E.M. SCHNEIDER, *et al.* 2003. Homer-1a/Vesl-1S enhances hippocampal synaptic transmission. Eur. J. Neurosci. **18:** 811–819.
69. THOMAS, U. 2002. Modulation of synaptic signalling complexes by Homer proteins. J. Neurochem. **81:** 407–413.
70. FANNING, A.S. & J.M. ANDERSON. 1999. Protein modules as organizers of membrane structure. Curr. Opin. Cell Biol. **11:** 432–439.
71. MONTGOMERY, J.M., P.L. ZAMORANO & C.C. GARNER. 2004. MAGUKs in synapse assembly and function: an emerging view. Cell Mol. Life Sci. **61:** 911–929.
72. CAO, Y., K.J. MURPHY, T.M. MCINTYRE, *et al.* 2000. Expression of fatty acid-CoA ligase 4 during development and in brain. FEBS Lett. **467:** 263–267.
73. ARDUINI, A., N. DENISOVA, A. VIRMANI, *et al.* 1994. Evidence for the involvement of carnitine-dependent long-chain acyltransferases in neuronal triglyceride and phospholipid fatty acid turnover. J. Neurochem. **62:** 1530–1538.
74. ADRIANI, W. & G. LAVIOLA. 2004. Windows of vulnerability to psychopathology and therapeutic strategy in the adolescent rodent model. Behav. Pharmacol. **15:** 341–352.

Effects of L-Carnitine Pretreatment in Methamphetamine and 3-Nitropropionic Acid-Induced Neurotoxicity

ZBIGNIEW K. BINIENDA,[a] BEATA D. PRZYBYLA,[a]
BONNIE L. ROBINSON,[a] NADIA SALEM,[b] ASHRAF VIRMANI,[c]
ANTONINO AMATO,[b] AND SYED F. ALI[a]

[a]*Division of Neurotoxicology, National Center for Toxicological Research, Food and Drug Administration, Jefferson, Arkansas 72079, USA*

[b]*Sigma-tau Research, Inc., Gaithersburg, Maryland 20877, USA*

[c]*Research and Development, Sigma-tau HealthScience, Pomezia 00040, Italy*

ABSTRACT: Adult, male Sprague-Dawley rats were injected with 3-nitropropionic acid (3-NPA) at 30 mg/kg or methamphetamine (METH) at 20 mg/kg alone or following pretreatment with L-cartnitine (LC) at 100 mg/kg. Rectal temperature was measured before and 4 h following treatment. Animals were sacrificed at 4 h posttreatment. Monoamine neurotransmitters, dopamine (DA) and serotonin (5-HT), and their metabolites were analyzed in the striatum using high-performance liquid chromatography method coupled with electrochemical detection (HPLC/ED). Transcripts of several genes related to DA metabolism were quantified using real time reverse transciption polymerase chain reaction (RT-PCR). Core temperature decreased significantly after 3-NPA acid and increased in METH-treated rats ($P < 0.05$). Temperature change at 4 h exhibited a significant LC effect for 3-NPA, preventing hypothermia ($P < 0.05$) and no effect for METH. Concentration of DA and 5-HT, and their metabolites, 3,4-dihydroxyphenylacetic acid (DOPAC), homovanillic acid (HVA), and 5-hydroxyindoleacetic acid (5-HIAA), increased significantly in 3-NPA and decreased in METH-treated rats. An increase in DOPAC/DA turnover and serotonin observed after 3-NPA was abolished in LC-/3-NPA-treated rats. In both 3-NPA- and METH-treated rats, LC prevented an increase in DA receptor D_1 gene expression. It appears that carnitine effect preventing hypothermia after 3-NPA treatments may be related not only to its mitochondriotropic actions but also to inhibitory effect on the DA and 5-HT systems activated after the exposure to 3-NPA. The same effect observed at the transcriptional level, at least for the DA receptor D_1, may account for protection against METH toxicity.

KEYWORDS: methamphetamine; 3-nitropropionic acid; carnitine; mitochondria; striatum; neuroprotection

Address for correspondence: Dr. Zbigniew K. Binienda, Division of Neurotoxicology, HFT-132, FDA/NCTR, Jefferson, AR 72079–9502. Voice: 870-543-7920; fax: 870-543-7745.
e-mail: zbinienda@nctr.fda.gov

**Ann. N.Y. Acad. Sci. 1074: 74–83 (2006). © 2006 New York Academy of Sciences.
doi: 10.1196/annals.1369.006**

INTRODUCTION

The systemic administration of d-methamphetamine (METH) leads to rapid dopamine (DA) release and hyperthermia followed by a depletion of DA and serotonin (5-HT), as well as the DA and 5-HT transporters DAT, vesicular monoamine transporter-2 (VMAT-2), and serotonin transporter (SERT). The monoamine synthesizing enzymes, tyrosine hydroxylase (TH) and tryptophan hydroxylase (TPH) are also depleted by METH administration.[1–6]

Reports indicate involvement of DA receptors in METH-evoked neurotoxicity. It has been shown that METH-induced monoamine depletions were attenuated by selective DA receptor inhibition.[7–9] Pretreatment with DA receptor D_1 and D_2 antagonists in rats exposed to METH also resulted in attenuation of DAT increasing activity induced by METH.[10] It has been reported that METH-induced energy impairment plays a role in METH neurotoxicity in the striatum. DA depletion induced by exposure to METH was associated with a rapid decrease in striatal adenosine 5′-triphosphate (ATP) level.[11] Mitochondrial energy enhancement via nicotinamide pretreatment attenuated the reductions of striatal DA and ATP contents.[12]

Mitochondrial energy disruption is a frequently observed effect of neurotoxicants, including inhibitors of mitochondrial electron transport chain such as MPTP (as MPP^+; complex I), 3-nitropropionic acid (3-NPA; complex II), antimycin A (complex III), and cyanide (complex IV). We focused on 3-NPA, an environmental toxicant, irreversible inhibitor of succinate dehydrogenase (SDH), a component of mitochondrial complex II.[13] 3-NPA is a toxicant produced in moldy crops (sugarcane, peanuts, etc.) in amount sufficient to cause severe neuromuscular disorders (dystonia) when consumed by humans.[14] Similarly to METH, the acute exposure to 3-NPA leads to a loss of ATP content[15] and dopaminergic activation,[16] however, in contrary to METH-induced hyperthermia, 3-NPA administration is accompanied by hypothermia.[17]

The aim of our article was to assess monoamine activation and relate it to temperature changes observed in these two different experimental conditions. The reverse transciption polymerase chain reaction (RT-PCR) was used subsequently to evaluate changes in gene expression at the transcription level during 3-NPA and METH exposures. A pretreatment with L-carnitine (LC), an enhancer of mitochondrial metabolism,[18] was applied to test the neuroprotective effect of LC against both neurotoxicants on the cellular level.

MATERIAL AND METHODS

Compounds

3-NPA, LC, and (+)-METH hydrochloride were purchased from Sigma-Aldrich (St. Louis, MO). 3-NPA was dissolved in 0.1 M phosphate buffer (pH 7.4). LC and METH were dissolved in Plasma-Lyte A, an electrolyte solution (pH 7.4) before injections took place.

Animals, Treatments, and Temperature Monitoring

Adult, male Sprague-Dawley rats from the FDA/NCTR breeding colony (Jefferson, AR) were used. Animals were kept under controlled environmental conditions (temperature 22°C, relative humidity 45–55%, 12-h light/dark cycle) and housed individually with food and water supplied *ad libitum*. Animal care and use procedures were followed along the guidelines of the Association for Assessment and Accreditation of Laboratory Animal Care International (AAALAC) and approved by the Institutional Animal Care and Use Committee (IACUC). Rats were injected with 3-NPA subcutaneously (s.c.) at 30 mg/kg or METH intraperitoneally (i.p.) at 20 mg/kg alone or dosed with LC i.p. at 100 mg/kg 30 min prior to 3-NPA and METH treatment. Rectal temperature was monitored before injections and before sacrifice using a Fluke 714 Thermocouple Calibrator (Fluke, Co., Everett, WA).

Neurochemical Measurements

Animals were sacrificed 4 h posttreatment by decapitation. The corpora striata were dissected onto ice, immediately frozen in liquid nitrogen, and stored at –80°C. The concentration of DA and 5-HT, and their metabolites, 3,4-dihydroxyphenylacetic acid (DOPAC) and 5-hydroxyindoleacetic acid (5-HIAA), were analyzed in the striatum using HPLC/ED method.[19] Data were analyzed using a one-way analysis of variance (ANOVA) followed by multiple comparisons of treated groups versus the control (Holm–Sidak method) with the significance set at $P < 0.05$ (Sigma Stat).

RT-PCR

Total RNA was isolated from one striatum using Tri Reagent (Molecular Research Center, Cincinatti, OH) and Rneasy Kit (Qiagen, Valencia, CA). Samples were treated with DNase (RNase-free DNase set, Qiagen) when still bound to Qiagen columns. The integrity and purity of RNA was determined with the RNA 6000 LabChip kit and Agilent 2100 Bioanalyzer (Agilent Technologies, Wilmington, DE). The cDNA was prepared using Scipt (Bio-Rad Laboratories, Inc., Hercules, CA). The SYBR Green PCR assays were performed on cDNA samples using iQ SYBR Green Supermix (BioRad). A standard curve was prepared for each target gene and for the endogenous reference (18S ribosomal RNA). An ANOVA was used for data analysis. The differences between treated and control animals were considered significant when $P \leq 0.05$.

RESULTS AND DISCUSSION

The alterations in core temperature after 3-NPA and METH are illustrated in FIGURE 1. Although, temperature change at 4 h posttreatment exhibited a significant LC effect for 3-NPA, preventing hypothermia ($P < 0.05$), there was no significant LC effect for METH, not preventing hyperthermia ($P = 0.72$). Similar effect of LC preventing brain temperature drop following 3-NPA injection was observed when the intracranial temperature was continuously monitored directly via implanted probes.[20] The inhibition of SDH and oxidative phosphorylation by 3-NPA leads to a metabolic condition that resembles ischemia/hypoxia where the oxidation of lipids as well as carbohydrates is compromised. In the brain, the exposure to 3-NPA is accompanied by a near 50% ATP loss in different regions within first hour posttreatment.[14] A decrease of core temperature may reflect the acute condition of mitochon-

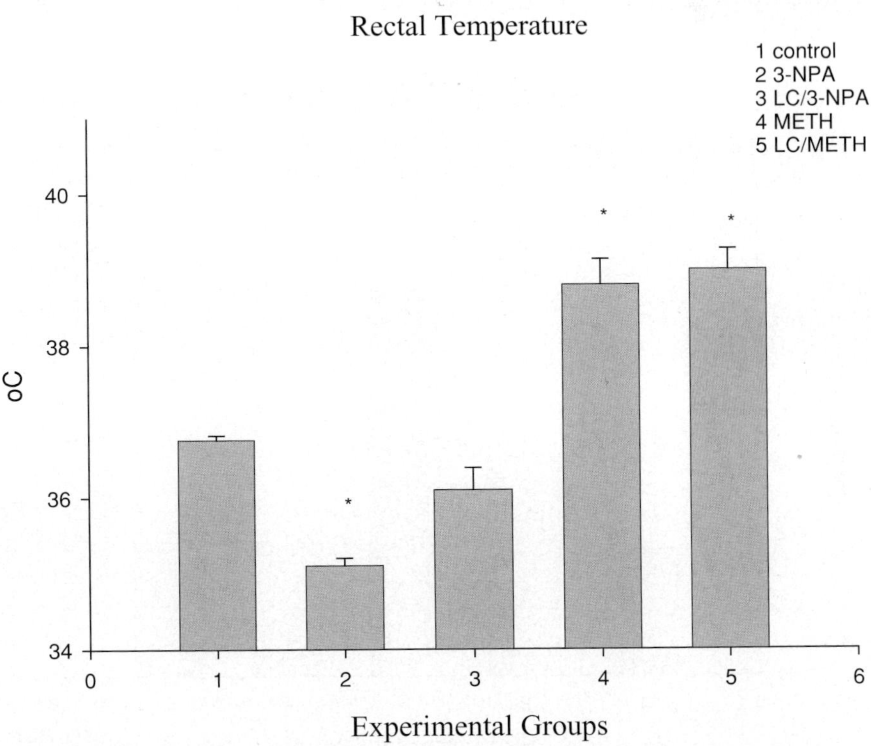

FIGURE 1. The effects of 3-NPA and METH administration alone and after pretreatment with LC on the core temperature within 4 h of exposure. Mean ± SEM. * $P < 0.05$ different from control at time 0.

TABLE 1. Concentration of DA, 5-HT and their metabolites HVA, DOPAC, and 5-HIAA in the striatum of rats treated with 3-NPA, METH alone, or after LC pretreatment.

Neurotransmitter Treatment	DA	5-HT	HVA	DOPAC	5-HIAA
Control (saline)	601.3 ± 18.1	78.8 ± 5.1	52.1 ± 1.7	108.3 ± 5.9	38.1 ± 4.5
3-NPA	674.1 ± 2.0*	127.6 ± 8.3*	98.8 ± 5.6*	370.2 ± 13.2*	70.0 ± 5.2*
LC/3-NPA	675.6 ± 26.9	87.1 ± 17.5	79.3 ± 11.0*	216.5 ± 43.4*	49.0 ± 7.7
METH	518.5 ± 40.6	38.4 ± 3.8*	45.4 ± 5.5	98.5 ± 7.7	22.8 ± 1.3*
LC/METH	554.1 ± 50.9	47.1 ± 9.7*	76.1 ± 14.3	108.6 ± 19.5	25.9 ± 3.6*

Mean ± SEM. $n = 5$ rats/group. * $P < 0.05$

drial dysfunction. Whereas LC enhances mitochondrial lipid β-oxidation in all cells, the exogenous LC in the brain has a high potential to promote energy production by reducing excessive acetyl-CoA accumulation during mitochondrial dysfunction induced by 3-NPA that blocks key enzymes of carbohydrate

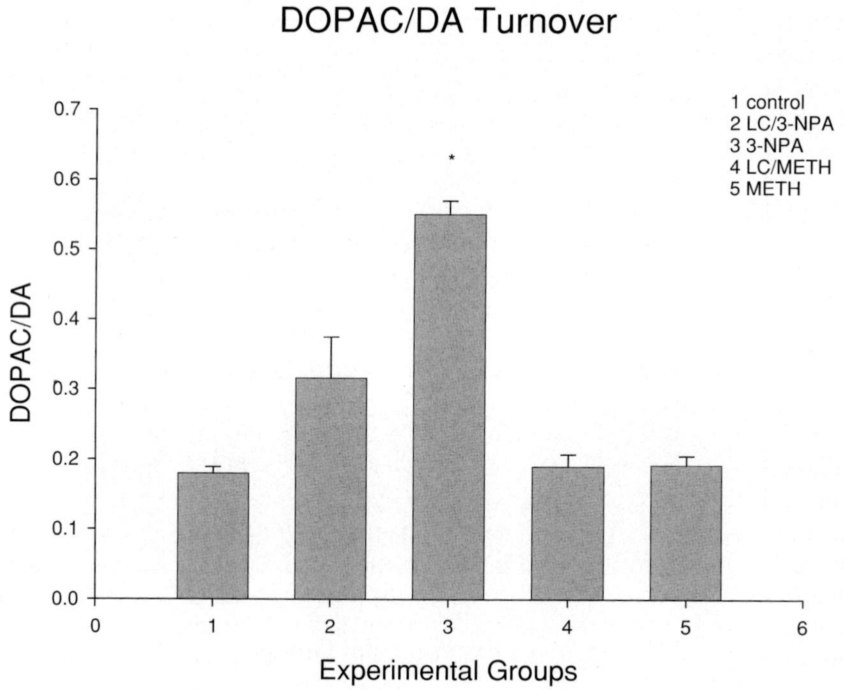

FIGURE 2. DOPAC/DA turnover index in rats treated with 3-NPA and METH alone or after pretreatment with LC. Mean ± SEM. * $P < 0.05$.

TABLE 2. Primer sequences for six rat genes used in RT-PCR analysis

GenBank	Gene name*	Primer 5′-3′
NM_012546	D1	GCAAATCCGGCGCATC
	Drd1a	GGTCTGGCAATTCTTGGCA
NM_012547	D2	CCAAAGATGCAGCGGCC
	Drd2	GTGTGCTCGACCACTGAGCTAG
NM_012740	TH	CCATGAGCTGTTGGGACATG
	Th	CCTGGGGAGAACTGGGGCAA
NM_013198	MAOB	TGACCCAGTATGGAAGGGTTCT
	Maob	TGAAGCTGTCTCGGTGCCT
NM_013031	VMAT2	GCTGCGGGACAGCCG
	Slc18a2	AGCAGCGCAAGGAACACG
X62145	(18 S)	TTSGAACGTCTGCCCTATCAA
		ATGGTAGGCACGGCGACTA

*Current Rat Genome Database names reported in italics.

metabolism.[21] On the other hand, the ATP loss after the exposure to METH is not as dramatic as with the 3-NPA and is observed in the striatum but not in other brain regions.[11] Therefore, potential hypothermic effect of the ATP loss on the core temperature would be much lower. In contrary, direct or indirect action of many factors including monoamines, thyroid hormones, uncoupling proteins (UCP-3), and mediators of inflammatory responses (interleukins, cytokines) leads to a phenomenon of hyperthermia observed after METH treatment.[9,20–23]

Thermoregulation is achieved by convergence of temperature-sensitive information by the spinal cord, brain stem, and hypothalamus. It is generally accepted that the hypothalamus is the highest integrator and coordinator of the thermal information. Among many neurotransmitters and neuromodulators, DA and 5-HT appear to have a prominent role in thermoregulation by the hypothalamus.[24] In our study, concentrations of DA, 5-HT, and their metabolites increased significantly in 3-NPA and decreased in METH-treated rats (TABLE 1). Activation of the serotonergic system results in the increased heat loss and reduced heat production.[24] The hypothermic effect has been also achieved by injections of DA into the caudate nucleus or DA agonist, apomorphin, into the substantia nigra.[25] The administration of DA receptor D_1 and D_2 antagonists was shown to attenuate hyperthermia induced by METH injections as well as to prevent monoamine depletions following METH treatment.[9] In the present study, the increase in 5-HT and DOPAC/DA turnover observed in the striatum after 3-NPA injection was prevented by carnitine pretreatment; however, carnitine did not affect monoamine concentration in METH-treated rats (FIG. 2).

Preliminary results of the gene expression (TABLE 2) obtained after RT-PCR in the present study, indicate an activation of genes encoding for the DA receptor D_1 in both treatments that was alleviated by carnitine (FIGS. 3 and 4).

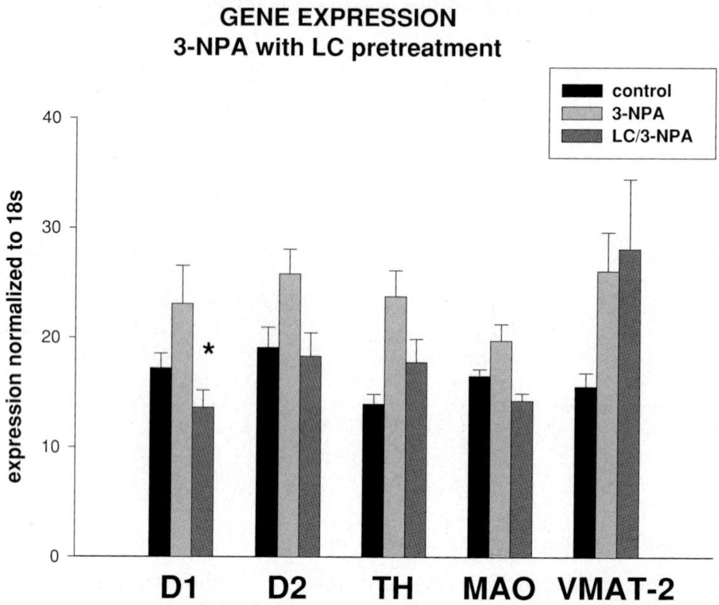

FIGURE 3. Expression of genes encoding of DA receptors D1 and D2, TH, monoamine oxidase-B (MAO), VMAT-2 in rats treated with 3-NPA alone or after pretreatment with LC. Mean ± SEM. * $P \leq 0.05$ when compared with control.

Although an increase in gene expression in the 3-NPA rats has not reached the statistical significance, it was nearly two-fold higher in METH-treated animals than in control ($P < 0.05$). The increase in expression of TH gene following METH exposure remained significantly different from control despite LC pretreatment. Similarly, a reduction in expression of VMAT gene was not changed by LC pretreatment. It has been shown that pretreatment with DA receptor D_1 and D_2 antagonists in rats exposed to METH prevented the increase in DAT activity induced by METH.[10] It appears that carnitine might exert inhibitory effect on DA receptor D_1 formation that may be relevant to neuroprotection against both 3-NPA and METH.

CONCLUSIONS

It appears that the effect of carnitine in the prevention of hypothermia after 3-NPA treatments may be related not only to its mitochondriotropic actions but also to inhibitory effect on the DA and 5-HT systems activated after the exposure to 3-NPA. The same effect observed at the transcriptional level, at least for the DA receptor D_1, may account for protection against METH toxicity. Temperature changes, especially hypothermia following 3-NPA exposure,

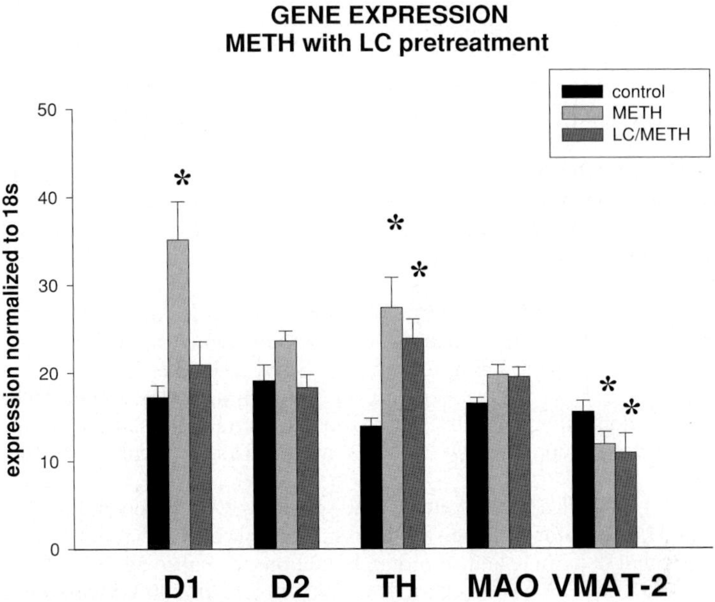

FIGURE 4. Expression of genes encoding of DA receptors D1 and D2, TH, MAO, and VMAT-2 in rats treated with METH alone or after pretreatment with LC. Mean ± SEM. * $P \leq 0.05$ when compared with control.

appears to reflect alterations in monoamine neurotransmitter systems additive to alterations in cellular energy metabolism.

ACKNOWLEDGMENT

The authors express their gratitude to Janice L. Summage, Brigitte DeCoursey, and Karen D. Cannon for an excellent technical support in this study.

The views presented in this article do not necessarily reflect those of the Food and Drug Administration.

REFERENCES

1. Fukumura, M., G.D. Cappon, H.W. Broening, *et al.* 1998. Methamphetamine-induced dopamine and serotonin reductions in neostriatum are not gender-specific in rats with comparable hyperthermic responses. Neurotoxicol. Teratol. **20:** 441–448.
2. Ali, S.F., G.D. Newport, R.R. Holson, *et al.* 1994. Low environmental temperatures or pharmacologic agents that produce hypothermia decrease methamphetamine neurotoxicity in mice. Brain Res. **658:** 33–38.

3. FLECKENSTEIN, A.E., R.R. METZGER, D.G. WILKINS, *et al.* 1997. Rapid and reversible effects of methamphetamine on dopamine transporters. J. Pharmacol. Exp. Ther. **382:** 45–49.
4. KOKOSHKA, J.M., R.R. METZGER, D.G. WILKINS, *et al.* 1998. Methamphetamine treatment rapidly inhibits serotonin, but not glutamate transporters in rat brain. **799:** 78–83.
5. RAU, K.S., E. BIRDSALL, J.E. HANSON, *et al.* 2005. Bupropion increases striatal vesicular monoamine transport. Neuropharmacology. **49:** 820–830.
6. O'CALLAGHAN, J.P. & D.B. MILLER. 1994. Neurotoxicity profiles of substituted amphetamines in the C57BL/6J mouse. J. Pharmacol. Exp. Ther. **270:** 741–751.
7. SONSALLA, P.K., J.W. GIBB & G.R. HANSON. 1986. Roles of D_1 and D_2 dopamine receptor subtypes in mediating the methamphetamine-induced changes in monoamine systems. J. Pharmacol. Exp. Ther. **238:** 932–937.
8. O'DELL, S.J., F.B. WEIHMULLER & J.F. MARSHAL. 1993. Methamphetamine-induced dopamine overflow and injury to striatal dopamine terminals: attenuation by dopamine D_1 and D_2 antagonists. J. Neurochem. **60:** 1792–1799.
9. BROENING, H.W., L.L. MORFORD & C.V. VORHEES. 2005. Interactions of dopamine D_1 and D_2 receptor antagonists with d-methamphetamine-induced hyperthermia and striatal dopamine and serotonin reductions. Synapse **56:** 84–93.
10. METZGER, R.R., H.M. HAUGHLEY, D.G. WILKINS, *et al.* 2000. Methamphetamine-induced rapid decrease in dopamine transporter function: role of dopamine and hyperthermia. J. Pharmacol. Exp. Ther. **295:** 1077–1085.
11. CHAN, P., D.A. DI MONTE, J.-J. LUO, *et al.* 1994. Rapid ATP loss caused by methamphetamine in the mouse striatum: relationship between energy impairment and dopaminergic neurotoxicity. J. Neurochem. **62:** 2484–2487.
12. HUANG, N.K., F.J. WAN, C.J. TSENG, *et al.* 1997. Nicotinamide attenuates methamphetamine-induced striatal dopamine depletion in rats. Neuroreport **27:** 1883–1885.
13. ALSTON, T.A., L. MELA & H.J. BRIGHT. 1977. 3-Nitropropionate, the toxic substance of Indigofera, is a suicide inactivator of succinate dehydrogenase. Proc. Natl. Acad. Sci. USA **74:** 3767–3771.
14. MING, L. 1995. Moldy sugarcane poisoning—a case report with a brief review. Clin. Toxicol. **33:** 363–367.
15. BROUILLET, E., B.G. JENKINS, B.T. HYMAN, *et al.* 1993. Age-dependent vulnerability of the striatum to the mitochondrial toxin 3-nitropropionic acid. J. Neurochem. **60:** 356–359.
16. NISHINO, H., M. KUMAZAKI, A. FUKUDA, *et al.* 1997. Acute 3-nitropropionic acid intoxication induces striatal astrocytic cell death and dysfunction of the blood-brain barrier: involvement of dopamine toxicity. Neurosci. Res. **27:** 343–355.
17. NONY, P.A., A.C. SCALLET, R.L. ROUNTREE, *et al.* 1999. 3-Nitropropionic acid (3-NPA) produces hypothermia and inhibits histochemical labelling of succinate dehydrogenase (SDH) in rat brain. Metab. Brain Dis. **14:** 83–94.
18. BINIENDA, Z. & A. VIRMANI. 2003. The mitochondriotropic effects of L-carnitine and its esters in the central nervous system. Curr. Top. Med. Chem. **3:** 275–282.
19. IMAM, S.Z. & S.F. ALI. 2001. Aging increases the susceptibility to methamphetamine-induced dopaminergic neurotoxicity in rats: correlation with peroxynitrite production and hyperthermia. J. Neurochem. **78:** 1–10.

20. BINIENDA, Z. 2003. Neuroprotective effects of L-carnitine in induced mitochondrial dysfunction. Ann. N. Y. Acad. Sci. **993:** 289–295.
21. DI LISA, F. 2002. Biochemical and pharmacological relevance of carnitine. Rivista Italiana di Nutrizione Parenterale ed Enterale **20:** 1–10.
22. SPRAGUE, J.E., N.M. MALLET, D.E. RUSYNIAK, *et al.* 2004. UCP3 and thyroid hormone involvement in methamphetamine-induced hyperthermia. Biochem. Pharmacol. **68:** 1339–1343.
23. CADET, J.L., S. JAYANTHI, M.T. MCCOY, *et al.* 2001. Temporal profiling of methamphetamine-induced changes in gene expression in the mouse brain: evidence from cDNA array. Synapse **41:** 40–48.
24. BRUCK, K. & E. ZEISBERGER. 1990. Adaptive changes in thermoregulation and their neuropharmacological basis. *In* Thermoregulation: Physiology and Biochemistry. E. Schonbaum & P. Lomax, Eds.: 255–307. Pergamon Press, New York, NY.
25. BROWN, S.J., C.V. GISOLFI & F. MORA. 1982. Temperature regulation and dopaminergic system in the brain: does the substantia nigra play a role? Brain Res. **234:** 275–286.

Convergent Roles of α-Synuclein, DA Metabolism, and the Ubiquitin-Proteasome System in Nigrostriatal Toxicity

FRANCESCO FORNAI,[a,b] GLORIA LAZZERI,[a]
ADOLFO BANDETTINI DI POGGIO,[a] PAOLA SOLDANI,[a]
ANTONIO DE BLASI,[b] FERDINANDO NICOLETTI,[b,c]
STEFANO RUGGIERI,[b,c] AND ANTONIO PAPARELLI[a]

[a]*Department of Human Morphology and Applied Biology, University of Pisa, 56126 Pisa, Italy*

[b]*Laboratory of Neurobiology of Movement Disorders I.R.C.C.S., I.N.M. Neuromed, 86077 Pozzilli, Isernia, Italy*

[c]*University of Rome "La Sapienza," 01185 Rome, Italy*

ABSTRACT: Recent studies disclosed the relevance of specific molecules for the onset of Parkinson's disease (PD) and for the composition of neuronal inclusions. The scenario which is now emerging leads to identify a potential common pathway named the ubiquitin-proteasome (UP) system. In line with this, striatal or systemic inhibiton of the UP system causes experimental Parkinsonism characterized by the formation of neuronal inclusions. 1-Methyl-4-phenyl-1,2,3,6-tetrahydropyridine (MPTP), which is also a complex I inhibitor, has been used for decades to produce experimental Parkinsonism with no evidence for neuronal inclusions in rodents. This leaves open the question whether neuronal inclusions need an alternative mechanism or the inhibition of complex I needs to be carried out continuously to build up inclusions. In the present article, we administered continuously MPTP. In these experimental conditions we compared the neurological consequence of intermittent versus continuous MPTP. In both cases we observed a severe dopamine (DA) denervation and cell loss. However, when MPTP was delivered continuously, spared DA nigral neurons develop ubiquitin, parkin, and α-synuclein positive inclusions, which are not detectable after intermittent dosing. The onset of Parkinsonism is associated with inhibition of the UP system. We compared these results with those obtained with amphetamine derivative *in vivo* and *in vitro* in which occurrence of neuronal inclusions was associated with inhibition of the UP system and we evaluated the role of DA metabolism in inducing these effects.

Address for correspondence: Francesco Fornai, M.D., Department of Human Morphology and Applied Biology, University of Pisa, Via Roma, 55, I-56126 Pisa, Italy. Voice: +39-50-2218610; fax: +39-50-2218606.
e-mail: f.fornai@med.unipi.it

Ann. N.Y. Acad. Sci. 1074: 84–89 (2006).
doi: 10.1196/annals.1369.007

KEYWORDS: Parkin-levels; Parkinsonism; methamphetamine (METH); neurodegeneration; striatum nervous systems

INTRODUCTION

Parkinson's disease (PD) is a neurodegenerative disorder which affects dopaminergic neurons of the substantia nigra and noradrenergic neurons of locus coeruleus. The classic subcellular alterations which can be observed in the spared catecholamine neurons in these brain areas consist of neuronal inclusions named Lewy bodies (LB).[1] These inclusions occur also in cholinergic cells[2] and appear as structures made up of a hyaline core and a pale peripheral halo,[3,4] which, at an ultrastructural level corresponds to filamentous material forming fibrillary elements characterized by the presence of the protein α-synuclein. Moreover, LB can be found in the telencephalon (amygdala, frontotemporal isocortex, and the caudate putamen basal ganglia),[5] where they are smaller and variously shaped.[6]

The definition of LB follows specific immunohistochemical markers because they contain ubiquitin,[7] α-synuclein,[8] parkin,[9] synphillin-1,[10] torsin A,[11] cyclins,[12] and cytoskeletal proteins.[13] A number of proteins found in LB are part of a multienzymatic pathway named the ubiquitin-proteasome (UP) system.

Whereas reproducing striatal DA denervation and nigral cell loss is a routine procedure going on for decades in PD research, the modeling of neuronal inclusions was not possible until recently. In fact, during the last few years, increased knowledge on inherited Parkinsonism led to focus on specific proteins which occur in neuronal inclusions and belong to the UP system. In-depth analysis of these proteins led to disclose a potential biochemical cascade which might be responsible for the pathogenesis of both inherited and sporadic forms of PD. In line with this, the pharmacological manipulation of the UP system led to modeling PD in a way, which apart from reproducing striatal DA denervation and nigral and locus coeruleus cell loss, extended to reproduce neuronal inclusions and to disclose the role of DA metabolism in this process. Similarly, following a reversed approach an altered DA metabolism achieved via administration of amphetamine derivatives produces an inhibition of the UP system, as shown in the present manuscript (FIG. 1), which leads to the occurrence of neuronal inclusions.[14,15]

THE PROTEASOME SYSTEM IN EXPERIMENTAL PARKINSONISM

The presence of ubiquitinated proteins within neuronal inclusions is one of the hallmarks of neurodegeneration. These inclusions contain various

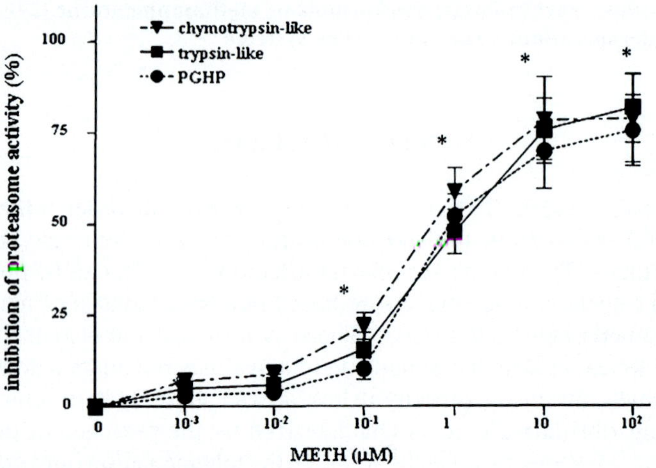

FIGURE 1. Methamphetamine produces proteasome inhibition. Dose-dependent effects of methamphetamine on the three main enzymatic activities of the proteasome in PC12 cell cultures.

components of the UP pathway, which operates as an intracellular protein-clearing system.[16,17] The UP system consists of a multienzymatic pathway placed mainly in the endoplasmic reticulum which becomes activated during oxidative stress which works to process misfolded protein. By using electron microscopy, we found neuronal inclusion induced by proteasome inhibitors (lactacystin/epoxomycin) or amphetamine derivatives[14,15,18] appearing at first as multilamellar whorls and further developing as nonmembrane limited bodies, real inclusions featuring an electrondense core. These inclusions accumulate dose dependently and require doses of UP inhibitors/amphetamines lower than what is necessary to induce cell death. This suggests that only a moderate dysfunction of the UP system determines the onset of inclusions, whereas increasing the dosage leads to cell death.

MILD AND PROLONGED- VS. STRONG AND SHORT-ACTING NEUROTOXICITY

Sporadic administration of the mitochondrial toxin 1 methyl-4-phenyl-1,2,3,6-tetrahydropyridine (MPTP) at relative high doses damages dopaminergic neurons but does not produce inclusions. Recently, we compared the effects of sporadic MPTP injections with continuous MPTP administration using an osmotic minipump.[19] We found that both MPTP exposures cause severe striatal dopamine (DA) depletion, and nigral cell loss, but only continuous MPTP exposure leads to typical progressive behavioral changes and triggers formation of nigral inclusions immunoreactive for ubiquitin and α-synuclein. Moreover, only continuous MPTP infusions leads to inhibition of the UP system which was long-lasting.[19] Interestingly, in this recent publication we found that the presence of α-synuclein was critical in order to bridge the biochemical effects of the neurotoxin with proteasome inhibition.[19]

A specific point, that deserves a special emphasis concerns the selectivity of the damage following widespread proteasome inhibition either it is achieved directly with enzyme inhibitors, or indirectly with mitochondrial neurotoxins. In fact, only a few neuronal systems are affected in degenerative disorders and this selectivity is preserved when a dysfunction of the UP system takes place. In keeping with PD, this apply to the selective vulnerability of the DA system and its tendency to spontaneous degeneration. In a similar way, the high sensititvity of DA neurons (axon terminals) to methamphetamine which causes proteasome inhibition deserves a specific analysis.

THE CONTRIBUTION OF DA METABOLISM

The role of DA and DA metabolites can be demonstrated by the neuroprotection induced by transient depletion of nigrostriatal DA or enhanced neurotoxicity induced by DA-increasing drugs. This apply both to methamphetamine- and proteasome inhibitors-induced neuronal inclusions.[14,15] In fact we found that both can be suppressed following administration of the tyrosine hydroxylase (TH) inhibitor, αMpT. Blocking DA synthesis with αMpT partially prevents inclusions formation unless DA synthesis is restored by the adding L-3,4,-dihydroxyphenyl alanine (L-DOPA). This can be achieved also in chromaffin cell cultures by blocking the conversion of DA to norepinephrine (NE). The role of DA might be related to the spontaneous oxidation of DA into DA-quinones; in fact, the blockade of oxidative deamination using the nonselective monoamine-oxidase inhibitor pargyline worsens neurotoxicity as does L-DOPA administration. This lends substance to a recent hypothesis on the occurrence of toxic adducts between DA-quinones and α-synuclein as a critical biochemical step in PD.[20,21] In keeping with this, DA neurons are selectively vulnerable to various neurotoxins which increase cytosolic DA content. This is the case of methamphetamine,[22] malonate,[23] or the absence of vesicular DA transporter especially when joined with normal expression of membrane DA transporter.[24–27] There is a growing body of evidence which focuses on free cytosolic DA as a critical agent for DA-containing neurons. In summary *in vivo* and *in vitro* data joined together indicate that DA-containing cells are vulnerable. This specific vulnerability is bound to the presence of high levels of DA in their cytosol.[27,28]

ACKNOWLEDGMENTS

Pfizer Italia s.r.l. is gratefully acknowledged for supporting part of these studies.

REFERENCES

1. Forno, L.S. *et al.* 1986. Locus ceruleus lesions and eosinophilic inclusions in MPTP-treated monkeys. Ann. Neurol. **20:** 449–455.
2. Pollanen, M.S., D.W. Dickson & C.B. Bergeron. 1993. Pathology and biology of the Lewy body. J. Neuropathol. Exp. Neurol. **52:** 183–191.
3. Ohama, E. & F. Ikuta. 1976. Parkinson's disease: distribution of Lewy bodies and monoamine neuron system. Acta Neuropathol. **34:** 311–319.
4. Zweig, R.M. *et al.* 1989. The pedunculopontine nucleus in Parkinson's disease. Ann. Neurol. **26:** 41.
5. Okazaki, H. *et al.* 1961. Diffuse intracytoplasmic ganglionic inclusions (Lewy type) associated with progressive dementia and quadriparesis in flexion. J. Neuropathol. Exp. Neurol. **20:** 237–244.
6. Duffy, P.E. *et al.* 1967. Cholinesterase in adult and ambryonic hypothalamus. A combined cytochemical alectron microscopic study. Arch. Neurol. **16:** 385–403.
7. Lennox, G. *et al.* 1989. Anti-ubiquitin immunocytochemisrty is more sensitive than conventional techniques in the detection of diffuse Lewy body disease. J. Neurol. Neurosurg. Psychiatry **52:** 67–71.
8. Spillantini, M.G. *et al.* 1997. α-Synuclein in Lewy bodies. Nature **388:** 839–840.
9. Schlossmacher, M.G. *et al.* 2002. Parkin localizes to the Lewy bodies of Parkinson disease and dementia with Lewy bodies. Am. J. Pathol. **160:** 1655–1667.
10. Lee, G. *et al.* 2004. Casein kinase II-mediated phosphorylation regulates alpha-synuclein/synphilin-1 interaction and inclusion body formation. J. Biol. Chem. **279:** 6834–6839.
11. Sharma, N. *et al.* 2001. A close association of torsinA and alpha-synuclein in Lewy bodies: a fluorescence resonance energy transfer study. Am. J. Pathol. **159:** 339–344.
12. Lee, S.S. *et al.* 2003. Cell cycle aberrations by alpha-synuclein over-expression and cyclin B immunoreactivity in Lewy bodies. Neurobiol. Aging **24:** 687–696.
13. Ross, C.A. & M.A. Poirier. 2004. Protein aggregation and neurodegenerative disease. Nat. Med. **10:**S10–S17.
14. Fornai, F. *et al.* 2004a. Methamphetamine produces neuronal inclusions in the nigrostriatal system and in PC12 cells. J. Neurochem. **88:** 114–123.
15. Fornai, F. *et al.* 2003. Fine structure and biochemical mechanisms underlying nigrostriatal inclusions and cell death after proteasome inhibition. J. Neurosci. **23:** 8955–8966.
16. Bence, N.F. *et al.* 2001. Impairment of the ubiquitin-proteasome system by protein aggregation. Science **292:** 552–555.
17. Chung, K.K. *et al.* 2001. The role of the ubiquitin-proteasomal pathway in Parkinson's disease and other neurodegenerative disorders. Trends Neurosci. **24:** S7–S14.
18. Fornai, F. *et al.* 2004. DNA damage and ubiquitinated neuronal inclusions in the substantia nigra and striatum ao mice following MDMA (ecstasy). Psychopharmacology **173:** 353–363.
19. Fornai, F. *et al.* 2005. Parkinson-like syndrome induced by continuous MPTP infusion: convergent roles of the ubiquitin-proteasome system and alpha-synuclein. Proc. Natl. Acad. Sci. USA **102:** 3413–3418.
20. Conway, K.A. *et al.* 2001. Kinetic stabilization of the alpha-synuclein protofibril by a dopamine alpha-synuclein adduct. Science **294:** 1257–1258.

21. SULZER, D. 2001. Alpha-synuclein and cytosolic dopamine: stabilizing a bad situation. Nat. Med. **7:** 1280–1282.
22. SCHMITH, C.J. *et al.* 1985. Role of dopamine in the neurotoxic effects of metamphetamine. J. Pharmacol. Exp. Ther. **233:** 539–544.
23. MOY, L.Y. *et al.* 2000. Role for dopamine in malonate-induced damage in vivo in striatum and in vitro in mesencephalic cultures. J. Neurochem. **74:** 1656–1665.
24. GAINETDINOV, R.R. *et al.* 1998. Increased MPTP neurotoxicity in vesicular monoamine transporter 2 heterozygote knock-out mice. J. Neurochem. **70:** 1973–1978.
25. JONES, S.R. *et al.* 1998. Mechanism of amphetamine action revealed in mice lacking the dopamine transporter. J. Neurosci. **18:** 1979–1986.
26. FUMAGALLI, F. *et al.* 1999. Increased metamphetamine neurotoxicity in heterozygous vesicular monoamine transporter 2 knock-out mice. J. Neurosci. **19:** 2424–2431.
27. MILLER, G.W. *et al.* 1999. Dopamine transporter and neuronal injury. Trends Pharmacol. Sci. **20:** 424–429.
28. SPEIDEL, D. *et al.* 2005. CAPS1 regulates catecholamine loading of large dense-core vesicles. Neuron **46:** 75–88.

Association Study of the Dihydropyrimidinase-Related Protein 2 Gene and Methamphetamine Psychosis

H. UJIKE,[a,b] A. SAKAI,[c] K. NAKATA,[d] Y. TANAKA,[a] T. KODAKA,[a] Y. OKAHISA,[a] M. HARANO,[b,e] T. INADA,[b,f] M. YAMADA,[b,g] T. KOMIYAMA,[b,h] T. HORI,[b,h] Y. SEKINE,[b,i] N. IWATA,[b,j] I. SORA,[b,k] M. IYO,[b,l] N. OZAKI,[b,m] AND S. KURODA[a]

[a]*Department of Neuropsychiatry, Okayama University Graduate School of Medicine, Dentistry and Pharmaceutical Sciences, Okayama 700-8558, Japan*

[b]*JGIDA (Japanese Genetics Initiative for Drug Abuse)*

[c]*Kasaoka Hospital, Kasaoka 714-0022, Japan*

[d]*Kinoko Espoir Hospital, Kasaoka 714-0071, Japan*

[e]*Department of Neuropsychiatry, Kurume University School of Medicine, Kurume, Japan*

[f]*Department of Psychiatry, Teikyo University School of Medicine, Ichihara Hospital, Ichihara, Japan*

[g]*Department of Psychogeriatrics, National Institute of Mental Health, National Center of Neurology and Psychiatry, Kodaira, Japan*

[h]*Division of Psychiatry, National Center Hospital for Mental, Nervous and Muscular Disorders, National Center of Neurology and Psychiatry, Kodaira, Japan*

[i]*Department of Psychiatry and Neurology, Hamamatsu University School of Medicine, Hamamatsu, Japan*

[j]*Department of Psychiatry, Fujita Health University School of Medicine, Toyoake, Japan*

[k]*Department of Psychobiology, Tohoku University Graduate School of Medicine, Sendai, Japan*

[l]*Department of Psychiatry, Graduate School of Medicine, Chiba University, Chiba, Japan*

[m]*Department of Psychiatry, Nagoya University Graduate School of Medicine, Nagoya, Japan*

Address for correspondence: Hiroshi Ujike, M.D., Ph.D., Department of Neuropsychiatry, Okayama University Graduate School of Medicine, Dentistry and Pharmaceutical Sciences, 2-5-1 Shikata-cho, Okayama 700-8558, Japan. Voice: +81-86-235-7242; fax: +81-86-235-7246.
e-mail: hujike@cc.okayama-u.ac.jp

Ann. N.Y. Acad. Sci. 1074: 90–96 (2006).
doi: 10.1196/annals.1369.008

ABSTRACT: Dihydropyrimidinase-related protein 2 (DRP-2 or DPYSL-2)mediates the intracellular response to collapsin, a repulsive extracellular guidance cue or axonal outgrowth. DRP-2 is also referred to as collapsin response mediator protein 2 (CRMP-2). We have previously demonstrated that the DRP-2 gene is associated with susceptibility to schizophrenia, but not to bipolar disorders. In addition, a genetic association was observed with paranoid-type schizophrenia, but not with hebephrenic-type schizophrenia. It has been well documented that repeated abuse of methamphetamine (METH) for a long period frequently produces psychotic symptoms, such as auditory hallucinations and delusions that are hardly distinguishable from those of paranoid-type schizophrenia. Therefore, we hypothesized that a certain genetic variant of the DRP-2 gene may affect individual vulnerability to the development of METH-induced psychosis. We examined the genetic association by a case–control method. The polymorphism *2236T>C in the 3′ untranslated region of the DRP-2 gene, which has been shown to be a negative genetic risk factor for paranoid-type schizophrenia, was analyzed in 198 patients with METH psychosis and 221 corresponding healthy controls in a Japanese population. No significant association of the DRP-2 gene with METH psychosis was found. Neither did we find an association with the clinical phenotype of METH psychosis, such as the age of first consumption of METH, latency to development of psychosis after METH abuse, prognosis of psychosis after detoxification from METH use, complication of spontaneous relapse of psychosis without reconsumption of the drug, or multisubstance abuse status. These findings indicate that a genetic variant of the DRP-2 gene may not affect the risk of METH psychosis or any clinical phenotype of the disorder.

KEYWORDS: substance abuse; dihydropyrimidinase-related protein 2; collapsin response mediator protein 2; association study; methamphetamine psychosis; Japanese population

INTRODUCTION

Dihydropyrimidinase-related protein 2 (DRP-2, OMIM *602463), which also has been independently identified as CRMP-2 (collapsin response mediator protein 2), TOAD-64, Ulip2 UNC-33, or DPYSL-2 (dihydropyrimidinase-like 2), is a homolog of human dihydropyrimidinase.[1] DRP-2 is highly expressed in the brain, especially during prenatal development, and is crucial for axonal outgrowth and determination of the fate of the axon and dendrites, possibly by promoting neurite elongation and branching via microtubule assembly.[2–5] DRP-2 activity is regulated by phosphorylation. Glycogen synthase kinase-3β phosphorylates DRP-2, an inactive form, and induces neuronal polarity.[6]In contrast, neurotrophin-3 increases nonphosphorylated DRP-2, an active form, probably via activation of PI3 kinase and Akt, and induces axon outgrowth.[6]

The neurodevelopmental disturbance hypothesis is now widely accepted as one of the promising hypotheses for the etiology of schizophrenia. Because dysfunction of DRP-2 may induce aberrant axon/neurite and brain wiring during development of the brain, DRP-2 is a candidate molecule for the pathogenesis of schizophrenia. Johnston-Wilson *et al.*[7] revealed that DRP-2 protein is significantly decreased in the frontal cortex of schizophrenics. We have examined the genetic association between the DRP-2 gene and endogenous psychoses at five single nucleotide polymorphisms (SNPs) and found that the *2236T>C SNP, located in the 3′ untranslated region, was strongly associated with susceptibility to schizophrenia but not to bipolar disorders in a Japanese population[8,9] Our finding was recently replicated by Hong *et al.*[10] in Caucasian schizophrenics. A genetic association with DRP-2 was more prominently observed in the paranoid type than the hebephrenic type of schizophrenia. It has been well documented that repeated abuse of methamphetamine (METH) frequently produces psychotic symptoms, such as delusions and auditory hallucinations that are quite similar to those observed in patients with paranoid-type schizophrenia.[11] In the clinical course, once METH psychosis has developed, patients show frequent relapses with or without reconsumption of METH and gradual progression of severity, which has been called a sensitization phenomenon.[12] Such longitudinal characteristics are also common in a subgroup of patients with paranoid-type schizophrenia. Based on the striking resemblance of psychiatric symptoms and disease processes between the paranoid type of schizophrenia and METH psychosis, we hypothesized that DRP-2 may be involved in the etiology or development of not only endogenous psychosis but also substance-induced psychosis. Therefore, we examined the genetic association of the *2236T>C SNP of the DRP-2 gene with METH-induced psychosis in a Japanese population.

METHODS

Subjects

The subjects comprised 167 unrelated patients with METH-induced psychosis disorder (136 male and 31 female, 36.2 ± 11.8 years [average ± SD]) and 221 unrelated healthy controls (171 male and 50 female, 36.6 ± 10.6 years) matched for age, gender, and geographical origin. The patients met F15.5 of the ICD-10-DCR criteria and were outpatients or inpatients of psychiatric hospitals of the JGIDA. The controls were mostly medical staff members who had no past or family history of drug dependence or psychotic disorders. All subjects were Japanese. This study was initiated after receiving the approval of the ethical committee of each participating institution of the JGIDA. Written informed consent was obtained from all participants.

Clinical Phenotypes

The patients with METH psychosis were divided into two subgroups according to the following clinical phenotypes: age at first METH consumption, duration of METH use before onset of psychosis, prognosis of psychosis after detoxification from METH and therapy (transient type versus prolonged type), and presence or absence of spontaneous relapse without METH reconsumption. The rationales of why we focused on these clinical features were described previously.[13] In dividing the subgroups, the median values were adopted as the cutoff point.

Genotyping and Statistics

Peripheral blood was obtained from the subjects, and the genomic DNA was extracted from peripheral leukocytes using a standard procedure. Genotyping of the *2236T>C SNP of the DRP-2 gene was performed by the PCR–RFLP method as previously reported. The presence of Hardy–Weinberg equilibrium was tested using a χ^2 goodness-of-fit test. Comparisons of allele and genotype frequencies were carried out using the χ^2 test for 2×2 and 2×3 contingency tables.

RESULTS

The genotype distribution was not significantly different from that expected according to the Hardy–Weinberg equilibrium in any group or in any subgroup. The genotype distribution and allele frequency of the *2236T>C SNP of the DRP-2 gene of patients with METH psychosis and controls are shown in TABLE 1. No significant difference was observed in either allele or genotype frequency between the two groups (allele: $\chi^2 = 0.0623$, $df = 1$, $P = 0.84$; genotype: $\chi^2 = 0.216$, $df = 2$, $P = 0.90$).

To further investigate the roles of the DRP-2 gene in the pathophysiology of psychosis, we examined its association with several clinical phenotypes of METH psychosis, such as the age at first consumption of METH, latency to

TABLE 1. Genotype and allele frequencies of *2236T>C SNP of DRP-2 gene in patients with METH psychosis and healthy controls

		Genotype				Allele		
*2236T > C	N	TT	TC	CC	*P*	T	C	*P*
Control	221	70.1%	27.1%	2.7%		83.7%	16.3%	
METH psychosis	164	70.7%	27.4%	1.8%	0.90	84.5%	15.5%	0.84

TABLE 2. Effects of DRP-2 gene on clinical phenotypes of METH psychosis

		Genotype				Allele		
Subgroups of METH psychosis	N	TT	TC	CC	*P*	T	C	*P*
Age of first consumption of METH								
<20 year	96	70.8%	27.1%	2.1%	0.98	84.4%	15.6%	0.91
≥20 year	103	69.9%	28.2%	1.9%		84.0%	16.0%	
Latency to onset of psychosis after METH abuse								
<3 year	76	72.4%	26.3%	1.3%	0.57	85.5%	14.5%	0.29
≥3 year	82	64.6%	32.9%	2.4%		81.1%	18.9%	
Prognosis of psychosis								
Transient	91	69.2%	29.7%	1.1%	0.52	84.1%	15.9%	0.88
Prolonged	67	73.1%	23.9%	3.0%		85.1%	14.9%	
Spontaneous relapse of psychosis without METH reconsumption								
+	71	67.6%	29.6%	2.8%	0.63	82.4%	17.6%	0.41
−	95	72.6%	26.3%	1.1%		85.8%	14.2%	
Multiple substance abuse status								
−	59	71.2%	25.4%	3.4%	0.71	83.9%	16.1%	0.51
mild	62	66.1%	32.3%	1.6%		82.3%	17.7%	
heavy	71	76.1%	22.5%	1.4%		87.3%	12.7%	

Prognosis of METH psychosis: *Transient type*, psychotic symptoms improved within 1 month after detoxification from METH along with initiation of therapy with neuroleptics; *Prolonged type*, psychotic symptoms continued for more than 1 month even after detoxification from METH along with initiation of therapy with neuroleptics.

Multiple substance abuse status: *Mild*, abuse of METH and substances that are relatively easy to acquire in Japan, such as toluene, hypnotics, and antitussive agents; *Heavy*, abuse of METH and substances relatively difficult to acquire in Japan, such as cannabinoids, morphine, and cocaine.

onset of psychosis after abuse, prognosis of psychosis after therapy, spontaneous relapse even without reconsumption of METH, and multiple substance abuse status, which show individual variation and may in part be regulated genetically. However, there was no significant association of the gene with any clinical phenotype of METH psychosis (TABLE 2).

DISCUSSION

The present study found that the DRP-2 gene was not associated with susceptibility to METH psychosis. Neither was the DRP-2 gene associated with any clinical phenotype of METH psychosis, such as latency to onset of psychosis after METH abuse, prognosis after therapy, or spontaneous relapse of psychosis without reconsumption of METH. It is unlikely that dysfunction of DRP-2 is involved in METH psychosis. Previously, we reported that the DRP-2 gene was associated with schizophrenia of the paranoid type.[8] Schizophrenia of the paranoid type and METH psychosis show striking similarity in clinical symptoms and course, which may imply shared mechanisms underlying the two different psychoses.[11,12] However, a genetic variant of DRP-2 may be a specific factor in the etiology of schizophrenia rather than a factor in the development of psychotic symptoms. In contrast, we have reported that the Akt1 gene shared a genetic risk for both endogenous and substance-induced psychosis,[14,15] and that the cannabinoid receptor type 1 (CNR1)[16,17] and dopamine transporter-1[13] genes were specific factors for METH psychosis.

Significant associations of the DRP-2 gene with schizophrenia have been proven in two different populations, Japanese[8] and Caucasian.[10] The C allele of the *2236T>C SNP of the DRP-2 gene was a negative risk factor for Japanese schizophrenics, but it was a positive risk factor for Caucasian schizophrenics. This inconsistency may result from a population difference. Alternatively, it is possible that different alleles or haplotypes of the same gene may affect the susceptibility to schizophrenia in different populations. Accordingly, SNPs other than *2236T>C may be associated with METH psychosis. Further analyses using additional SNPs covering the entire DRP-2 gene are necessary to demonstrate a relationship between the DRP-2 gene and METH psychosis.

ACKNOWLEDGMENT

This work was partly supported by the Zikei Institute of Psychiatry (Okayama, Japan) and Grants-in-Aid from the Japanese Ministry of Health, Labor and Welfare.

REFERENCES

1. Hamajima, N., K. Matsuda, S. Sakata, *et al.* 1996. A novel gene family defined by human dihydropyrimidinase and three related proteins with differential tissue distribution. Gene **180:** 157–163.
2. Byk, T., T. Dobransky, C. Cifuentes-Diaz, *et al.* 1996. Identification and molecular characterization of unc-33-like phosphoprotein (Ulip), a putative mammalian homolog of the axonal guidance-associated unc-33 gene product. J. Neurosci. **16:** 688–701.
3. Goshima, Y., F. Nakamura, P. Strittmatter, *et al.* 1995. Collapsin-induced growth cone collapse mediated by an intracellular protein related to UNC-33. Nature **376:** 509–514.
4. Minturn, J.E., H.J.L. Fryer, D.H. Geschwind, *et al.* 1995. TOAD-64, a gene expressed early in neuronal differentiation in the rat, is related to unc-33, a *C. elegans* gene involved in axon outgrowth. J. Neurosci. **15:** 6757–6766.
5. Inagaki, N., K. Chihara, N. Arimura, *et al.* 2001. CRMP-2 induces axons in cultured hippocampal neurons. Nat. Neurosci. **4:** 781–782.
6. Yoshimura, T., Y. Kawano, N. Arimura, *et al.* 2005. GSK-3beta regulates phosphorylation of CRMP-2 and neuronal polarity. Cell **120:** 137–149.
7. Johnston-Wilson, N.L., C.D. Sims, J.P. Hofmann, *et al.* 2000. Disease-specific alterations in frontal cortex brain proteins in schizophrenia, bipolar disorder, and major depressive disorder. Mol. Psychiatry **5:** 142–149.

8. NAKATA, K., H. UJIKE, A. SAKAI, *et al.* 2003. The human dihydropyrimidinase-related protein 2 gene on chromosome 8p21 is associated with paranoid-type schizophrenia. Biol. Psychiatry **53:** 571–576.
9. NAKATA, K., H. UJIKE, Y. TANAKA, *et al.* 2003. No association between the dihydropyrimidinase-related protein 2 (DRP-2) gene and bipolar disorder in humans. Neurosci. Lett. **349:** 171–174.
10. HONG, L.E., I. WONODI, M.T. AVILA, *et al.* 2005. Dihydropyrimidinase-related protein 2 (DRP-2) gene and association to deficit and nondeficit schizophrenia. Am. J. Med. Genet. B. Neuropsychiatr. Genet. **136:** 8–11.
11. UJIKE, H. & M. SATO. 2004. Clinical features of sensitization to methamphetamine observed in patients with methamphetamine dependence and psychosis. Ann. N. Y. Acad. Sci. **1025:** 279–287.
12. UJIKE, H. 2002. Stimulant-induced psychosis and schizophrenia: the role of sensitization. Curr. Psychiatry Report **4:** 177–184.
13. UJIKE, H., M. HARANO, T. INADA, *et al.* 2003. Nine- or fewer repeat alleles in VNTR polymorphism of the dopamine transporter gene is a strong risk factor for prolonged methamphetamine psychosis. Pharmacogenomics J. **3:** 242–247.
14. IKEDA, M., N. IWATA, T. SUZUKI, *et al.* 2005. Positive association of AKT1 haplotype to Japanese methamphetamine use disorder. Int. J. Neuropsychopharmacol. **28:** 1–5.
15. IKEDA, M., N. IWATA, T. SUZUKI, *et al.* 2004. Association of AKT1 with schizophrenia confirmed in a Japanese population. Biol. Psychiatry **56:** 698–700.
16. UJIKE, H., M. TAKAKI, K. NAKATA, *et al.* 2002. CNR1, central cannabinoid receptor gene, associated with susceptibility to hebephrenic schizophrenia. Mol. Psychiatry **7**: 515–518.
17. UJIKE, H. & Y. MORITA. 2004. New perspectives in the studies on endocannabinoid and cannabis: cannabinoid receptors and schizophrenia. J. Pharmacol. Sci. **96:** 376–381.

Repeated Methamphetamine Administration Alters Expression of the NMDA Receptor Channel ε2 Subunit and Kinesins in the Mouse Brain

HIDEKO YAMAMOTO,[a] KAZUHIDE IMAI,[b] ETSUKO KAMEGAYA,[a] YUKIO TAKAMATSU,[a] MASASHI IRAGO,[a] YOKO HAGINO,[a] SINYA KASAI,[a] KIYO SHIMADA,[b,c] TOSHIFUMI YAMAMOTO,[a,d] ICHIRO SORA,[a,e] HISASHI KOGA,[b,c] AND KAZUTAKA IKEDA[a]

[a]*Division of Psychobiology, Tokyo Institute of Psychiatry, Tokyo 156-8585, Japan*

[b]*Chiba Industry Advancement Center, Chiba, Japan*

[c]*Department of Genome Informatics, Laboratory for Genome Informatics, Kazusa DNA Research Institute, Japan*

[d]*Molecular Recognition, Yokohama City University, Yokohama, Japan*

[e]*Department of Psychobiology, Tohoku University, School of Medicine, Japan*

ABSTRACT: Repeated amphetamine administration results in behavioral sensitization. Behavioral sensitization related to abuse and/or relapse may be associated with stable changes in gene expression. To explore the participating genes, we examined the changes in gene expression levels 24 h or 21 days (long-term withdrawal period) after chronic methamphetamine (METH) treatment for 2 weeks. The expression of several genes related to glutamatergic neural transmission was altered, although changes in the corresponding protein expression were not always consistent with the results for mRNA expression. Of interest, in the frontal cortex of mice treated with METH for 2 weeks, protein expression levels of KIF17 and the N-methyl-D-asparate (NMDA) receptor channel ε2 subunit (NRε2) were concomitantly increased. The alteration in expression of these proteins, KIF17 and NRε2, might be a part of the molecular basis of the behavioral sensitization to METH.

KEYWORDS: methamphetamine; cDNA array; frontal cortex; kinesin; NMDA receptor

Address for correspondence: H. Yamamoto, Division of Psychobiology, Tokyo Institute of Psychiatry, Tokyo 156-8585, Japan. Voice: +81-3-3304-5701; fax: +81-3-3329-8035.
e-mail: yamahide@prit.go.jp

**Ann. N.Y. Acad. Sci. 1074: 97–103 (2006). © 2006 New York Academy of Sciences.
doi: 10.1196/annals.1369.009**

INTRODUCTION

The primary targets for drugs of abuse are the dopaminergic neurons that project from the ventral tegmental area of the midbrain to the nucleus accumbens (NAc). Moreover, glutamatergic afferents from medial prefrontal cortex (mPFC) to the NAc are thought to be crucial to the development of addictive behavior. Both cocaine and amphetamine have been reported to increase extracellular glutamate levels in the mPFC.[1,2] In addition, recent studies have suggested that glutamate transmission in the mPFC may be altered in sensitized animals,[3,4] the findings of which may be summarized as follows: (*a*) Neurons in the mPFC show an increased responsiveness to glutamate following repeated exposure to amphetamine. (*b*) Furthermore, K^+-stimulated glutamate efflux in the mPFC was enhanced in animals following repeated exposure to methamphetamine (METH).[4]

We have investigated changes in gene expression after chronic METH treatment by using a newly developed cDNA array system comprising mouse KIAA (mKIAA) cDNA clones and Western blotting.[5,6] KIAA clones were originally obtained from a human cDNA sequencing project in progress to accumulate protein-coding sequence (CDS) information on unidentifed human genes.[7] Already, more than 2000 human long cDNAs, systematically designated as KIAA plus a 4-digit number, have been newly identified and characterized. Mainly, KIAA clones are characterized by their long cDNAs (>4 kb) sequences encoding large proteins (>50 kDa) and by their source (brain). Therefore, this considerable population of KIAA clones reflects a large number of high-molecular-weight proteins expressed in the brain. Information regarding mKIAA genes has been released and is available in an online database (http://www.kazusa.or.jp/rouge/).

In the present study, using the cDNA array system, we examined the effects of repeated low-dose administration of METH that produces conditioned place preference in mice on gene expression levels in their brain. The low-dose of METH was chosen to eliminate toxicity-related genes, such as heat shock proteins. To confirm the obtained cDNA array data, we performed Western blot analyses and verified the protein expression changes.

MATERIALS AND METHODS

Materials

Antibodies specific for kinesin family member (KIF) 17, NRε2, and GLT-1 were purchased from Sigma-Aldrich, Inc. (St. Louis, MO). The antibodies for KIF17b and KIF5C were raised against recombinant proteins corresponding to amino acids 3069–3767 mapping to the amino terminus of mKIAA1405

(KIF17b) and to amino acids 2864–3109 mapping to the amino terminus of mKIAA0531 (KIF5C), respectively.

Tissue Preparation From Mice Chronically Treated With METH

The experimental procedures and housing conditions were approved by our Institutional Animal Care and Use Committee, and all animals were cared for and treated humanely in accordance with our institutional guidelines on animal experimentation. All mice were housed 5–6 to a cage with free access to food and water in animal room maintained on a 12-h light/dark cycle (lights on at 08:00 h). Ten-week-old male C57BL/6J mice received saline or METH injection (2 mg/kg, i.p.) for 14 days once a day between 13:00 and 15:00 h and were sacrified 24 h or 2 weeks after the last injection. After decapitation, the frontal cortex or hippocampus from 20 mice per treatment group were quickly dissected on ice, and immediately frozen at $-80°C$. These dissected tissues from 20 mice per treatment group were pooled and used for the cDNA array experiment. For SDS-PAGE/Western blotting analysis, the tissues from 6–10 mice per treatment group were pooled and used.

Microarray Analysis: RNA Isolation, Probe Labeling, and Microarray Hybridization

Microarray analysis was conducted as previously described.[6] Briefly, total RNA was isolated from pooled tissues by using an RNeasy kit (Qiagen Inc., Valencia, CA). Then mRNA-enriched RNA (poly A^+ RNA) was isolated from the total RNA by using a Dinabeads mRNA Purification Kit (Dynal Biotech, Lake Success, NY). The quantity and quality of RNA were assessed by spectrophotometry and electrophoresis on denaturing agarose gels. Radiolabeled cDNA probes were prepared from 1.0 μg of heat-denatured (70°C, 10 min) poly A^+ RNA or 0.1 μg Tet1-PolyA^+ RNA in the presence of random nonamer, dATP, dTTP, dGTP, [^{33}P]dCTP, Superscript II reverse transcriptase, and RNase inhibitor at 43°C for 1 h. Subsequently, the RNA in the reaction mixture was decomposed by incubation with RNaseH and RNaseA at 37°C for 10 min. Labeled DNAs were purified with QIAquick PCR Purification Kit (Qiagen Inc.) and quantified by using a liquid scintillation counter.

Approximately 1700 mKIAA clones and 63 well-characterized non-mKIAA cDNAs were each blotted onto a nylon membrane. In brief, mKIAA cDNA plasmids were amplified using the TempliPhi DNA amplification kit (Amersham Bioscience Co., Piscataway, NJ) and then spotted onto a nylon Biodyne Plus membrane (Pall Corporation, East Hills, NY) attached to a slide glass using a GeneTac RA1 microarrayer (Genomic Solutions, Ann Arbor, MI).[8] To reduce the false-positive rate, we used three membranes per labeled DNA probes prepared from an mRNA sample. Array membranes were prehybridized for 1 h at 68°C in 0.4 mL of PerfectHyb (Toyobo Co., Ltd., Osaka, Japan) hybridization buffer for each membrane. Purified labeled DNA probes together with 50 μg mouse Cot-1 DNA, 2 μg polyA, and 1/100 (counts/counts of labeled DNAs) Tet1 were heat-denatured (100°C for 5 min). After prehybridization, the membranes were hybridized with the mixture of these labeled DNA probes overnight at 68°C in a 10-mL vial in a rotating hybridization oven. Membranes were washed at 68°C with 2 × SSC (150 mM NaCl and 15 mM sodium citrate)/1% SDS twice for 15 min and then at 68°C with 0.1 × SSC/1% SDS twice for 30 min each time. They were subsequently dried and exposed to an imaging plate for 2–3 days. Image acquisition and quantification were performed with a FLA-8000 (Fuji Photo Film, Inc., Tokyo, Japan). The calculation of the gene expression level and the statistical analysis of the data were performed according to the system provided by *phoretix* software (Nonlinear Dynamics Ltd., Newcastle upon Tyne, UK).

Western Blotting

The pooled tissues were homogenized in an ice-cold PBS buffer containing protease inhibitors. The samples (10 μg/lane) were resolved on a 5–20% gradient polyacrylamide-SDS gel, and proteins were electrotransferred onto polyvinylidene fluoride membranes by using a semi-dry blotter. Nonspecific sites were blocked with Blocking One solution (Nacarai Tesque, Inc., Kyoto, Japan), and incubated overnight at room temperature with primary antibodies (KIF17, 1:10,000 dilution; NRε2, 1:5,000 dilution) in Can Get SignalTM (Toyobo Co., Ltd., Osaka, Japan) or Tris-buffered saline containing 0.5% Tween-20 (TBS/TW) and 1/20 vol. of Blocking One solution, respectively. Next, the membranes were washed and incubated with peroxidase-labeled secondary antibody (1:50,000 dilution; Zymed Lab., Inc., South San Francisco, CA) for 1 h at room temperature. Finally, they were washed repeatedly with TBS/TW, incubated with SuperSignal^{TM} WestDura Extended Duration Substrate (Pierce Biotech., Inc., Rockford, IL) for 10 min, and exposed to Amersham ECL film.

The intensities of the immunoreactive bands were calculated by use of NIHimage software, and their sizes were compared with prestained molecular weight standards (New England Biolabs, Beverly, MA).

RESULTS AND DISCUSSION

We examined the changes in gene expression levels 24 h or 21 days (long-term withdrawal period) after chronic METH (2 mg/kg, i.p.) treatment for 2 weeks. METH-induced changes (more than 30%) in gene expression were found in 228 clones in the hippocampus and in 37 clones in the frontal cortex 24 h after chronic METH administration. After long-term withdrawal, stable changes remained in 10 (131 when oppositely directed changes were included)

TABLE 1. mRNA expression analysis by use of mouse cDNA arrays

	Frontal cortex		Hippocampus	
	(% of saline control)			
Glutamate transporters/receptors/kinesins	METH	Withdraw	METH	Withdraw
EAAC1	97	113	95	88
GLAST	98	96	89	102
GLT-1	101	87	71	82
mGluR1	90	107	86	139
mGluR5	93	86	95	78
NRε2	90	72	80	82
NRε3	100	87	127	121
NRε4	81	61	151	106
NRζ1	107	92	90	79
mKIAA0004 kinectin 1 (kinesin receptor)	94	114	94	124
mKIAA1448 kinesin family member 1B	112	91	84	100
mKIAA0591 kinesin family member 1B	108	94	94	74
mKIAA0591 kinesin family member 1B	118	90	88	101
mKIAA0706 kinesin family member 1C	104	89	78	92
mKIAA0359 kinesin family member 3B	96	128	91	104
mKIAA0531 kinesin family member 5C	109	98	76	94
mKIAA0639 kinesin family member 13B	99	98	146	112
mKIAA1405 kinesin family member 17B	95	97	123	115
mKIAA1708 kinesin family member 21A	109	95	76	86
mKIAA1236 kinesin family member 26A	107	96	115	110

Each experimental datum is the average of eight determinations.

clones in the hippocampus, and 1 (111 with oppositely directed changes included) clones in the frontal cortex. In these comparisons, their gene expression profiles markedly differed.

In the CNS, GLT-1 and GLAST are expressed primarily in astrocytes, whereas EAAC1 is restricted to neurons.[9] Recent studies indicate that GLT-1 and GLAST play major roles in glutamate clearance in the forebrain under normal conditions and in preventing excitotoxic brain damage under pathological conditions.[10–12] No changes in the gene expression levels of 2 of these 3 glutamate transporter subtypes, GLAST and EAAC1, in response to chronic METH treatment were observed (TABLE 1), whereas the gene expression of GLT-1 in the hippocampus was slightly decreased. We performed Western blot analysis using anti-GLT-1-selective antiserum. However, the amount of GLT-1 protein was not changed in the hippocampus (97% of saline control for short- and 101% for long-term withdrawal).

Considering the finding that neurons in the mPFC show an increased responsiveness to glutamate following repeated exposure to amphetamine,[13] repeated exposure to amphetamine may cause neuronal adaptations of glutamate receptors. Gene expression profiles of ε2–ε4 subunits of the N-methyl-D-asparate (NMDA) receptor channel in the frontal cortex were

TABLE 2. Comparison of mRNA and protein expressions

% of saline control (average)		F. Cortex		Hippocampus	
Gene		Subchronic METH	METH + Withdrawal	Subchronic METH	METH + Withdrawal
KIF5C	cDNA array	109.3	97.9	76.1	94.3
	Western blot	116.6	119.3	105.2	94.3
KIF17b	cDNA array	94.6	96.8	122.8	114.6
KIF17	Western blot	124.7	91.5	102.1	88.0
KIF17b	Western blot			96.4	108.4
NR ε2	cDNA array	89.7	71.7	80.2	81.5
	Western blot	132.8	104.0	126.2	121.4

The data of cDNA array were extracted from data in TABLE 1.

The sequence of KIF17b is almost the same as that from 754 amino acid to 1038 amino acid (C-terminus region) of KIF17. Therefore, cDNA array including the KIF17b clone recognized the expression of KIF17 mRNA.

relatively decreased after long-term withdrawal (TABLE 1). By contrast, in the hippocampus, gene expression of these subunits did not change in the same direction. Of interest, in the frontal cortex of mice treated with METH for 2 weeks, protein expression levels of KIF17 and NRε2 subunit were concomitantly increased (TABLE 2).

NMDA receptor channels are transported in dendrites by KIF17.[14] KIF17, a plus-end-directed motor localized mainly in dendrites, co-localizes with the NRε2 subunits and moves from the cell body toward the postsynaptic region.[15] The alteration in expression of these proteins, KIF17 and NMDA receptor channel, might be involved in the increased responsiveness to glutamate after repeated METH treatment.

CONCLUSION

Glutamatergic sensitization has been implicated in the development of psychostimulant abuse; in particular, the PFC seems to play a critical role in mediating several important components of addictive behaviors. In the present study, we found concomitant increases in protein expressions of the NRε2 subunit and its carrier KIF17, suggesting that these proteins may be partly involved in sensitized glutamate transmission following repeated exposure to METH.

ACKNOWLEDGMENTS

We are grateful to Dr. Keiko Matsuoka for her helpful assistance. This work was supported by a research grant (17025054) from the MEXT of Japan, and by grants (H17-pharmaco-001, H16-iyaku-029, H15-kou-3-03) from the MHLW of Japan.

REFERENCES

1. Del Arco, A., R. Martinez & F. Mora. 1998. Amphetamine increases extracellular concentrations of glutamate in the prefrontal cortex of the awake rat: a microdialysis study. Neurochem. Res. **23:** 1153–1158.
2. Reid, M.S., K. Hsu, Jr. & S.P. Berger. 1997. Cocaine and amphetamine preferentially stimulate glutamate release in the limbic system: studies on the involvement of dopamine. Synapse **27:** 95–105.
3. Peterson, J.D., M.E. Wolf & F.J. White. 2000. Altered responsiveness of medial prefrontal cortex neurons to glutamate and dopamine after withdrawal from repeated amphetamine treatment. Synapse **36:** 342–344.
4. Stephans, S.E. & B.K. Yamamoto. 1995. Effect of repeated methamphetamine administrations on dopamine and glutamate efflux in rat prefrontal cortex. Brain Res. **700:** 99–106.
5. Yamamoto, H., K. Imai, Y. Takamatsu, *et al.* 2004. Changes in expression of the mouse homologues of KIAA genes after subchronic methamphetamine treatment. Ann. N. Y. Acad. Sci. **1025:** 92–101.
6. Yamamoto, H., K. Imai, Y. Takamatsu, *et al.* 2005. Methamphetamine modulation of gene expression in the brain: analysis using customized cDNA microarray system with the mouse homologues of KIAA genes. Brain Res. Mol. Brain Res. **137:** 40–46.
7. Nomura, N., N. Miyajima, T. Sazuka, *et al.* 1994. Prediction of the coding sequences of unidentified human genes. I. The coding sequences of 40 new genes (KIAA0001 - KIAA0040) deduced by analysis of randomly sampled cDNA clones from human immature myeloid cell line KG-1. (Suppl.), DNA Res. **1:** 47–56.
8. Yamakawa, H., S. Yokoyama, T. Hiran, *et al.* 2004. A simple and robust method for preparation of cDNA nylon microarrays. DNA Res. **11:** 353–360.
9. Rothstein, J.D., L. Martin, A.I. Levey, *et al.* 1994. Localization of neuronal and glial glutamate transporters. Neuron **13:** 713–725.
10. Rothstein, J.D., M. Dykes-Hoberg, C.A. Pardo, *et al.* 1996. Knockout of glutamate transporters reveals a major role for astroglial transport in excitotoxicity and clearance of glutamate. Neuron **16:** 675–686.
11. Tanaka, K., K. Watase, T. Manabe, *et al.* 1997. Epilepsy and exacerbation of brain injury in mice lacking the glutamate transporter GLT-1. Science **276:** 1699–1702.
12. Watase, K., K. Hashimoto, M. Kano, *et al.* 1998. Motor discoordination and increased susceptibility to cerebellar injury in GLAST mutant mice. Eur. J. Neurosci. **10:** 976–988.
13. Peterson, J.D., M.E. Wolf & F.J. White. 2000. Altered responsiveness of medial prefrontal cortex neurons to glutamate and dopamine after withdrawal from repeated amphetamine treatment. Synapse **36:** 342–344.
14. Setou, M., T. Nakagawa, D.H. Seog & N. Hirokawa. 2000. Kinesin superfamily motor protein KIF17 and mLin-10 in NMDA receptor-containing vesicle transport. Science **288:** 1796–1802.
15. Guillaud, L., M. Setou & N. Hirokawa. 2003. KIF17 dynamics and regulation of NR2B trafficking in hippocampal neurons. J. Neurosci. **23:** 131–140.

Genes and Gene Expression in the Brains of Human Alcoholics

PETER R. DODD,[a] S. TRACEY BUCKLEY,[b] ALLISON L. ECKERT,[a] PHILOMENA F. FOLEY,[a] AND DAVID J. INNES[a]

[a]*School of Molecular and Microbial Sciences, University of Queensland, Brisbane Q4072, Australia*

[b]*Perinatal Research Centre, Royal Brisbane and Women's Hospital, Brisbane 4072, Australia*

ABSTRACT: Chronic alcohol misuse by human subjects leads to neuronal loss in regions such as the superior frontal cortex (SFC). Propensity to alcoholism is associated with several genes. γ-Aminobutyric acid (GABA)$_A$ receptor expression differs between alcoholics and controls, whereas glutamate receptor differences are muted. We determined whether genotype differentiated the regional presentation of GABA$_A$ and glutamate-NMDA (*N*-methyl-D-aspartate) receptors in SFC. Autopsy tissue was obtained from alcoholics without comorbid disease, alcoholics with liver cirrhosis, and matched controls. *ADH1C*, *DRD2B*, *EAAT2*, and *APOE* genotypes modulated GABA$_A$-β subunit protein expression in SFC toward a less-effective form of the receptor. Most genotypes did not divide alcoholics and controls on glutamate-NMDA receptor pharmacology, although gender and cirrhosis did. Genotype may affect amino acid transmission locally to influence neuronal vulnerability.

KEYWORDS: pathogenesis; substance misuse and dependence; brain damase; phenotype; cerebral cortex; excitotoxicit

INTRODUCTION

Long-term alcohol misuse by human subjects can result in localized loss of neurons (by ~20%) in the superior frontal cortex (SFC).[1] Other cortical areas, including motor, show no significant differences in neuron number between alcoholics and controls. Reduced mean neuronal surface area and pruning of the dendritic arbor occur widely in alcoholic cortex, indicative of generalized neuronal shrinkage.[2]

Address for correspondence: Peter R. Dodd, Ph.D., School of Molecular and Microbial Science, University of Queensland, Brisbane 4072, Australia. fax: +61-7-3365-4699.
e-mail: p.dodd@uq.edu.au

**Ann. N.Y. Acad. Sci. 1074: 104–115 (2006). © 2006 New York Academy of Sciences.
doi: 10.1196/annals.1369.010**

These abnormalities could result from altered brain function: chronic alcohol ingestion might change neurotransmission. γ-Aminobutyric acid (GABA) is the most abundant inhibitory neurotransmitter in the brain.[3] It exerts its effects through three classes of GABA receptors, especially the $GABA_A$ site.[4] GABA neurotransmission maintains the inhibition: excitation balance through tonic regulation of the major excitatory central nervous system (CNS) transmitter, glutamate.[5] About 16–23% of synapses use GABA.[6] $GABA_A$ receptors, which are pentameric complexes, are the site of action of many drugs, including ethanol.[5] Complexes are formed from a number of subunit isoforms, which are classified α_{1-6}, β_{1-3}, γ_{1-3}, δ, ε, π, and θ. The most common complex in laboratory animals comprises the $\alpha_1\beta_2\gamma_2$ combination.[7–11] Recombinant studies have shown that variation in subunit composition confers differences in pharmacological properties and hence function.[12,13] Alcohol abuse could alter the subunit composition of the receptor in human subjects; alternatively, individuals predisposed to alcoholism may intrinsically possess different subunit profiles. We have shown that the SFC in alcoholics exhibits variant expression of $GABA_A$ receptor α-subunit gene transcripts,[14] suggesting that the $GABA_A$ site is involved in the actions of alcohol misuse. Others have reported alterations in the gene expression of a number of $GABA_A$ subunit genes.[15–17] It has proved more difficult to demonstrate consistent differences in the form and pharmacology of glutamate ionotropic receptors between human alcoholic and control brains, although such effects have been widely reported in animal models.

Alcoholism involves multiple gene-environment interactions.[18] Predisposition to alcohol misuse may be influenced by many genes.[19] A number of alcoholism-associated candidate genes have been identified. These include genes coding for alcohol-metabolizing enzymes, such as alcohol dehydrogenase (ADH) and aldehyde dehydrogenase (ALDH); and others coding for proteins that mediate neurotransmission, such as the dopamine D2 receptor (*DRD2*), various subunits of the $GABA_A$ receptor (e.g., the β_2-subunit gene *GABRB2*) and the glutamate-NMDA (*N*-methyl-D-aspartate) receptor (e.g., the NR2B subunit gene *GRIN2B*), the excitatory amino acid transporter #2 (EAAT2; the *SLC1A2* gene), and the serotonin (5-HT) transporter (the *SLC6A4* gene). None of these genes contributes more than a small proportion of alcoholism risk, and each may be associated with different aspects of the condition.

We studied interactions between alcoholism-associated genes and the expression of $GABA_A$ receptor β_1-, β_2-, and β_3-subunit isoform proteins. We also studied [^{3}H]MK801 binding to synaptic membranes as a measure of glutamate-NMDA receptor pharmacology. Samples of SFC and primary motor cortex (PMC) were obtained at autopsy from high-consumption alcoholics without other drug misuse, with and without comorbid cirrhosis of the liver, and from matched controls, using protocols we have developed and validated for the human brain.[20]

METHODS

Tissue

Cases and controls were of northern European origin and were subjected to autopsy with informed written consent from the coroner or the next of kin, under clearance from the University of Queensland Human Ethics Committee (HEC #H/09/Biochem/NHMRC/98 and H/212/BIOCHEM/00). Full macroscopic and microscopic postmortem examinations were performed and the cause of death determined. Pieces of cerebral cortex (1–5 cm^3) were dissected at the autopsy, immersed in ice-cold 0.32 M sucrose, slowly frozen, and stored at –80°C until analyzed. This procedure is optimal for the preservation of human brain samples.[21] The other hemisphere was fixed in formalin for pathological examination. For each case, information regarding general health, diet, alcohol intake, medication, and the presence of alcohol-related diseases such as cirrhosis of the liver, was available from medical records and postmortem reports. No subject used here had clinical or pathological evidence of neurological or psychiatric disease, including Wernicke–Korsakoff psychosis, prior to death. No patient was a polysubstance or intravenous drug user, and none was on prescribed neuroactive medication. Controls had consumed $<$20 g of ethanol per day or were teetotalers; alcoholics were defined by an intake of $>$80 g of ethanol per day throughout most of their adult life (over 30 years on average).

Membrane Preparation

Frozen samples from SFC and PMC were dissected frozen, thawed briefly in 0.32 M sucrose at 37°C, immediately transferred to 10 vols of ice-cold dH_2O, weighed, and dispersed using a motor-driven Teflon-glass homogenizer (Kimble/Kontes, Vineland, NJ). The homogenate was centrifuged at 1000 *g* for 5 min at 4°C. The supernatant was removed and dispensed into 100 μL aliquots and stored at −80°C. Protein concentrations were determined by the method of Lowry *et al.*[22]

Western Blotting

SDS-polyacrylamide gel electrophoresis was performed by standard methods.[23] Samples (5 μg) were diluted 1:1 (v/v) in 2 × sample buffer (2% SDS, 10% glycerol, 5% 2-mercaptoethanol, 62.5 mM Tris-HCl, pH 6.8) and boiled for 5 min. A molecular weight (MW) marker and a standard, prepared by pooling SFC and PMC samples from all cases, were included on every gel. A 10% separation gel with a 3% stacking gel were run at 200 V for ~45 min. Proteins were transferred to polyvinylidene fluoride (PVDF) and the membranes blocked in 5% Blotto overnight at 4°C. After incubation with the appropriate primary antibody (Santa Cruz Biotechnologies, Santa Cruz, CA) diluted 1/2000 in 1% Blotto in Tris-buffered saline with 0.1% v/v Tween-20 (TBST), the membranes were washed 3 × 10 min in TBST. Membranes were incubated with secondary antibody and washed. Bands were detected by chemiluminescence and quantified by densitometry against the standard curve. Care was taken that the intensity of the unknown bands fell between the values of the lowest and highest standards on every gel; samples were diluted and rerun to ensure this where necessary. Values were adjusted for the total protein concentration in each sample.

[^{3}H]MK801 Binding

Synaptic membranes were prepared and binding assays performed as previously described.[24] Incubations with a range of unlabeled MK801 concentrations were subjected to Satchard analysis by nonlinear methods to give K_D and B_{MAX} values. Incubations at a fixed MK801 concentration and varying concentrations of unlabeled glutamate were analyzed by fitting composite sigmoidal curves to give estimates of agonist affinity and efficacy.[24]

Genotyping

DNA was prepared from samples of brain tissue by phenol extraction.[25] Polymerase chain reaction (PCR)-based genotyping was carried out according to standard protocols using published primers. Details are presented elsewhere.[26]

Data Analysis

Normal probability plots showed that the values were log-normally distributed, and they were converted to natural logarithms before analysis. The data set was analyzed by ANOVA using Statistica (Statsoft Inc., Tulsa, OK). Genotype was included as a categorical variable, simplified by separating subjects that were homozygous for the disease-associated allele from all others.

RESULTS

We did not undertake a comprehensive analysis of genotype frequencies in our study populations. Such studies employ several hundred subjects or more, which is difficult to achieve in autopsy-tissue work. Rather, we relied on literature reports of genes associated with alcohol misuse, and sought to determine how possession of different genotypes affected the expression of

TABLE 1. *DRD2 Taq 1B* genotype[31] frequencies in alcoholics undifferentiated for comorbid liver cirrhosis

	Alcoholics	Controls	Total
DRD2-B1,B1	18	5	23
DRD2-B1,B2	22	20	42
DRD2-B2,B2	42	62	104
	82	87	169

NOTE: $\chi^2 = 11.151$; df = 3; $P = 0.004$.

key mediators of amino acid transmission at the molecular and pharmacological levels. We did, however, ask whether our subject pool conformed to the literature. Examples are shown in TABLES 1 and 2: for the dopamine receptor *DRD2* gene, 49% of alcoholics had at least one B1 allele, whereas only 29% of controls did; similarly for the $GABA_A$ receptor β_2 subunit *GABRB2* gene, 34% of alcoholics had one or more alleles with the T polymorphism, whereas only 9% of controls did. In the latter instance it may be seen that the frequency of the minor allele was too low to be fully informative, so analysis was confined to a comparison between subjects with and without at least one copy of the minor allele. In all other examples reported here, subjects homozygous for the disease-associated allele were separated from the others. In the case of the *ADH1C* gene, genotype frequency was affected by comorbid liver disease. Thus, genotype frequencies fell short of significance in a comparison between uncomplicated alcoholics and controls ($\chi^2 = 4.412$, df = 3, $n = 96$; $P = 0.11$), but they did differ significantly between cirrhotic alcoholics and controls ($\chi^2 = 6.147$, df = 3, $n = 102$; $P < 0.05$). This was not seen for any other genotype tested.

The effect of *DRD2B* genotype on $GABA_A$-β protein expression was assessed. In SFC, β_2 expression was highest in uncomplicated alcoholics homozygous for the B1 allele, whereas expression in controls was unaffected by *DRD2B* genotype (FIG. 1). No significant differences were seen in PMC. Controls and alcoholics showed very similar levels of β_3 expression for each *DRD2B* genotype in both cortical regions (not shown).

TABLE 2. *GABRB2* genotype[32] frequencies in alcoholics undifferentiated for comorbid liver cirrhosis

	Alcoholics	Controls	Total
GABRB2-C,C	70	100	170
GABRB2-C,T	16	10	26
GABRB2-T,T	5	0	5
	82	87	169

NOTE: $\chi^2 = 9.972$, df; = 3; $P = 0.007$.

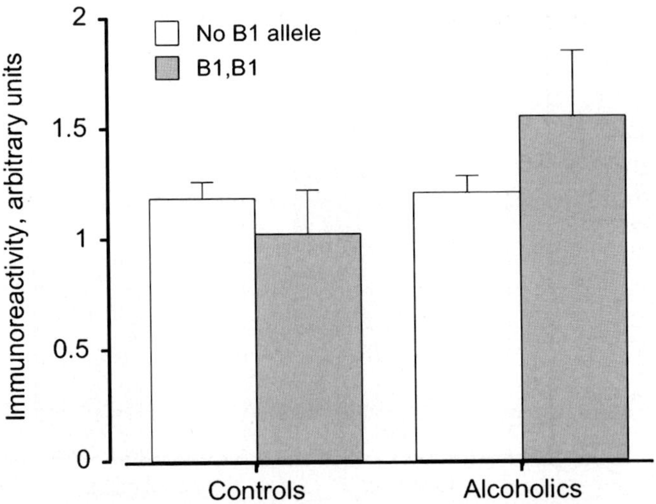

FIGURE 1. Interactions between genotype and alcoholism on the expression of the $GABA_A$ receptor β protein isoforms in SFC: *DRB2B* and β_2.

ADH1C genotype had differential effects on β_2 and β_3 expression. As FIGURE 2 shows, β_2 expression in SFC tended to be stronger in alcoholics homozygous for the γ2 allele, whereas the opposite pattern was observed with β_3 expression (FIG. 3). The net effect was to markedly alter the β_2:β_3 ratio in

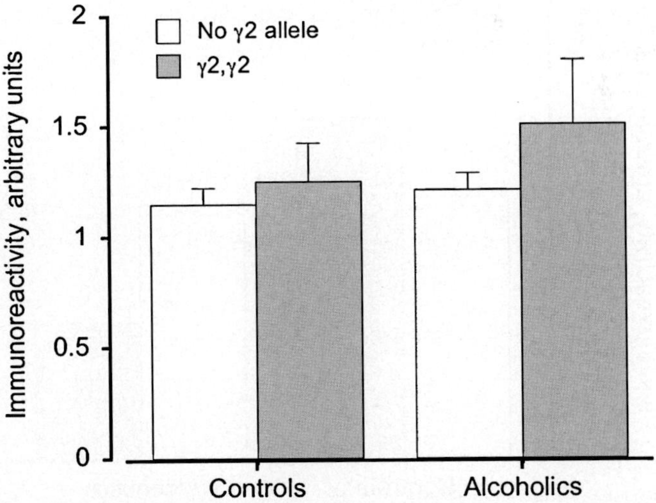

FIGURE 2. Interactions between genotype and alcoholism on the expression of the $GABA_A$ receptor β protein isoforms in SFC: *ADH1C* and β_2.

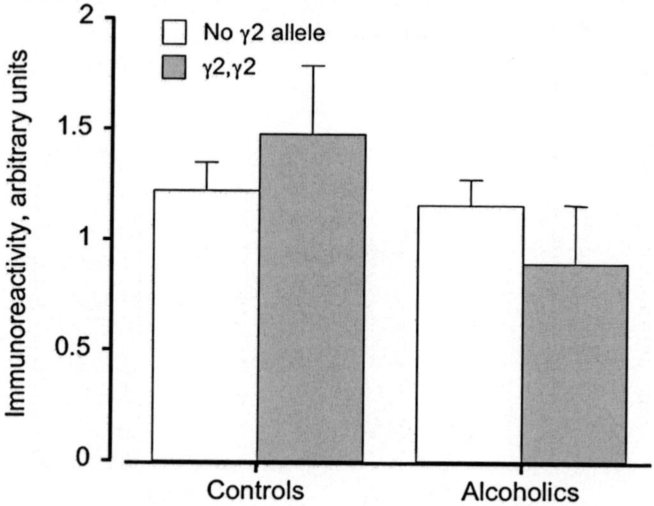

FIGURE 3. Interactions between genotype and alcoholism on the expression of the $GABA_A$ receptor β protein isoforms in SFC: *ADH1C* and β_3.

alcoholic SFC in alcoholics homozygous for the disease-associated allele. It may be seen that genotype had no effect on the expression of either isoform protein in controls (FIGS. 2 and 3).

The gene for the glutamate transporter EAAT2, *SLC1A2*, affected β_3 expression in uncomplicated alcoholics in a similar fashion to, but more strongly

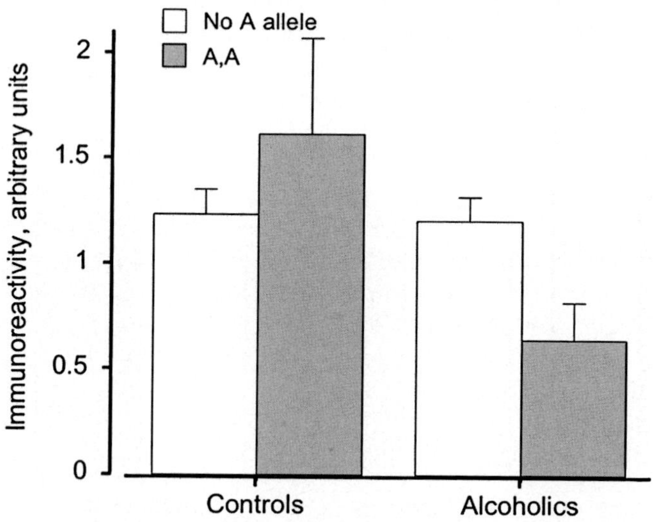

FIGURE 4. Interactions between genotype and alcoholism on the expression of the $GABA_A$ receptor β protein isoforms in SFC: *SLC1A2* and β_3.

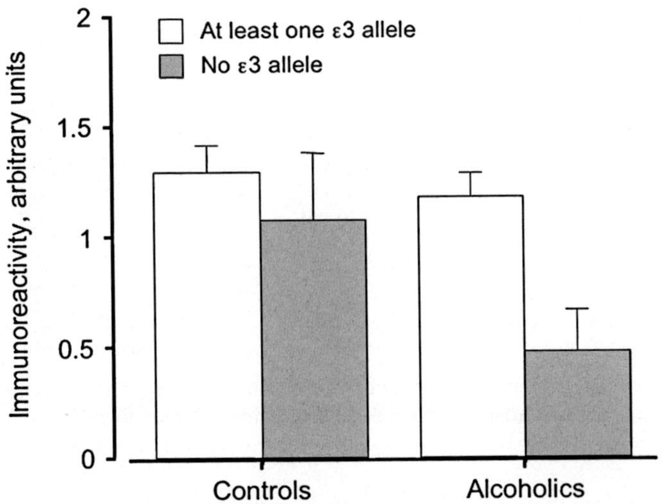

FIGURE 5. Interactions between genotype and alcoholism on the expression of the $GABA_A$ receptor β protein isoforms in SFC: *APOE* and β_3.

than, the *ADH1C* gene (FIG. 4). That is, controls homozygous for the minor allele showed stronger β_3 expression in SFC than controls with at least one major allele, whereas the reverse was true for alcoholics. There was little difference in β_3 expression between controls and alcoholics possessing at least one major allele (FIG. 4). However, this genotype showed no significant interaction with alcoholism for β_2 expression (not shown).

A related phenomenon was observed with *APOE* genotype (FIG. 5). There was reduced expression of β_3 protein selectively in subjects who did not possess at least one ϵ3 allele in alcoholic SFC. There was no significant difference in β_3 protein expression in PMC, and there was no significant alcoholism-related variation in regional β_2 protein expression.

The effects of gender and genotype on glutamate-NMDA receptor pharmacology were examined. It may be seen that females had receptors with a lower overall affinity for MK801 than males, a difference that was even more marked in SFC than in PMC (FIG. 6 A). However, receptor efficacy (the maximal extent to which glutamate enhances [^{3}H]MK801 binding) was lower in females than in males (FIG. 6 B). Female cirrhotic alcoholics selectively showed markedly higher NMDA receptor binding capacity, an index of receptor density, than either control females, female alcoholics without comorbid disease, or males with or without alcoholism or cirrhosis (FIG. 7). Pilot studies showed that NMDA-receptor-binding capacity was particularly high in female cirrhotic alcoholics with the disease-associated *GABRB2* allele (not shown) although case numbers were too small to view this result with confidence. Similarly, there was a statistically significant complex interaction between cirrhotic-alcoholic

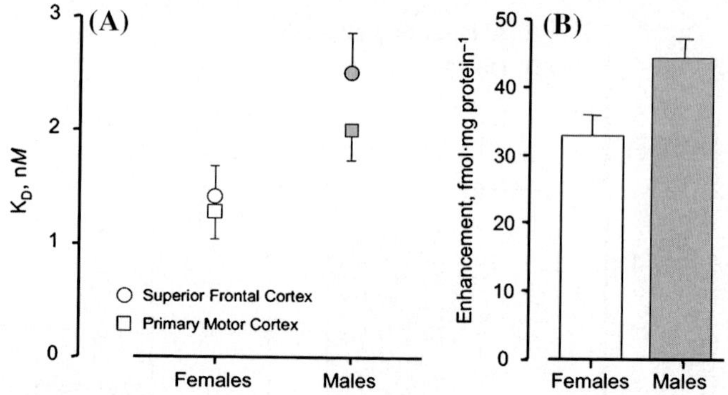

FIGURE 6. Interactions between gender and cortical area on glutamate-NMDA receptor affinity and efficacy. (**A**) affinity for MK801; (**B**) maximal glutamate-enhanced [^{3}H]MK801 binding, an index of agonist efficacy. Data were averaged across alcoholic and control subjects.

status, gender, and *SLC1A2* genotype (not shown), but again it must be cautioned that obtaining sufficient numbers of subjects for such a conclusion to be reliable is always going to be extremely difficult. No other genotype or gender interaction with alcoholism—with or without cirrhosis—was statistically significant for any other gene tested.

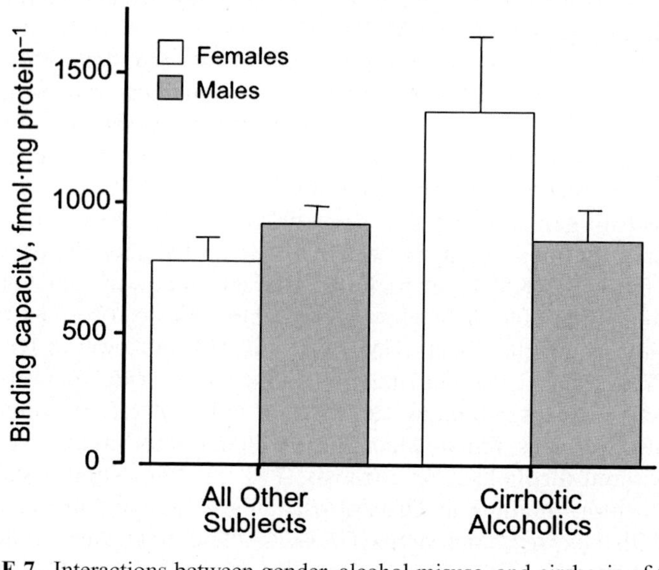

FIGURE 7. Interactions between gender, alcohol misuse, and cirrhosis of the liver on glutamate-NMDA-receptor-binding capacity. Data were averaged across SFC and PMC.

DISCUSSION

Discrete regions and cell populations in the brain are selectively vulnerable to the effects of alcohol. Recombinant studies have shown that variations in the subunit composition of the $GABA_A$ and glutamate-NMDA receptors can result in alterations in receptor efficacy, pharmacology, and functionality. Thus, long-term and excessive ingestion of alcohol may disrupt amino acid transmitter function. Alternatively, variant combinations of receptor subtypes might occur in subjects predisposed to the development of alcoholism. However, the findings presented here, showing significant interactions between a subject's genotype, alcoholism status, and expression of receptors frequently unrelated to the genotype under analysis, make the latter conclusion unlikely. It is more likely that subjects with particular genotypes would have exhibited more or less similar extents of expression of these receptor subunits in the absence of superimposed alcohol misuse. This is consistent with studies in laboratory animals, where alcohol administration changes protein expression in comparable ways. Of particular interest in this context are the studies of Devaud and colleagues, who have shown differential effects of alcohol administration on glutamate-NMDA receptor expression and pharmacology in male and female rats.[27]

There have been some animal studies on the effect of genetic make-up on gene expression, usually by assaying the transcripts or proteins encoded by the gene of interest. However, it is clear from studies in laboratory mice that knocking out a single gene can alter the expression of many hundreds of mRNA transcripts, most of which have no clear association with the knocked-out gene. Microarray analysis has been used to compare knockout strains that differ in their alcohol responsiveness, in order to find transcripts in common that might be involved in the response to alcohol.[28] The transcripts so identified derived from genes with range of chromosomal locations, often different from the locus of the knocked-out gene. Effect sizes in these studies are commonly less than twofold, typical for microarray studies in human brain.[29] Analogously, the only known "gene knockout" related to alcoholism in human subjects is the *ALDH2* gene (ALDH2-2,2 homozygotes have no ALDH activity); while the latter is protective against alcoholism, it is rarely found in Caucasians, the subjects in the present study. Nevertheless, different alleles of alcoholism-associated genes might affect the expression of a range of genes; the effect sizes might be smaller, or the range lesser in extent, than are found in knockout studies. The $GABA_A$ isoform protein data shown here probably benefited from a multiplier effect: in expression studies proteins commonly show larger effect sizes.[30]

Overall, two patterns of difference were seen between alcoholic subjects and controls that may have a bearing on pathogenesis. Alleles associated with alcoholism appeared to reduce β_3:β_2 ratios in the pathologically affected SFC. As recombinant studies have shown that $GABA_A$ receptors contain β_2 subunits are less efficacious at mediating chloride ion influx in response to any given concentration of applied GABA, this subunit switching would have the effect of attenuating $GABA_A$-mediated inhibition. Hence, $GABA_A$ receptors might *passively* mediate neuronal susceptibility in SFC in alcoholics without comorbid liver disease. In contrast, there were significant differences between the sexes in glutamate-NMDA receptor affinity, capacity and efficacy, most notably in female cirrhotic alcoholics. Thus, glutamate-NMDA sites may play an *active* part in SFC neuronal death in alcoholics with cirrhosis, with female cirrhotic alcoholic particularly at risk—especially if they inherit certain alcoholism-associated genes.

ACKNOWLEDGMENTS

We are grateful to the National Health and Medical Research Council and the Australian Associated Brewers. Human autopsy tissue was obtained from the NHMRC Brain Tissue Consortium.

REFERENCES

1. KRIL, J.J. *et al.* 1997. The cerebral cortex is damaged in chronic alcoholics. Neuroscience **79:** 983–998.
2. HARPER, C.G. & J.J. KRIL. 1990. Neuropathology of alcoholism. Alcohol Alcohol. **25:** 207–216.
3. OLSEN, R.W. & A.J. TOBIN. 1990. Molecular biology of $GABA_A$ receptors. FASEB J. **4:** 1469–1480.
4. LÜDDENS, H. & E.R. KORPI. 1995. Biological function of $GABA_A$/benzodiazepine receptor heterogeneity. J. Psychiatr. Res. **29:** 77–94.
5. ENNA, S.J. 1997. The GABA Receptors. Humana. Totowa, NJ.
6. HORNUNG, J.-P. & N. DE TRIBOLET. 1994. Distribution of GABA-containing neurons in human frontal cortex: a quantitative immunocytochemical study. Anat. Embryol. (Berl.) **189:** 139–145.
7. DAVIES, P.A. *et al.* 1997. Insensitivity to anaesthetic agents conferred by a class of $GABA_A$ receptor subunit. Nature **385:** 820–823.
8. HEDBLOM, E. & E.F. KIRKNESS. 1997. A novel class of $GABA_A$ receptor subunit in tissues of the reproductive system. J. Biol. Chem. **272:** 15346–15350.
9. JECHLINGER, M. *et al.* 1998. Subunit composition and quantitative importance of hetero-oligomeric receptors: $GABA_A$ receptors containing α_6 subunits. J. Neurosci. **18:** 2449–2457.
10. NEELANDS, T.R. *et al.* 1999. Spontaneous and γ-aminobutyric acid (GABA)-activated $GABA_A$ receptor channels formed by ϵ subunit-containing isoforms. Molec. Pharmacol. **55:** 168–178.
11. WHITING, P.J. 1999. The $GABA_A$ receptor gene family: new targets for therapeutic intervention. Neurochem. Int. **34:** 387–390.
12. YMER, S. *et al.* 1990. Structural and functional characterization of the γ_1 subunit of $GABA_A$/benzodiazepine receptors. EMBO J. **9:** 3261–3267.
13. SIGEL, E., R. BAUR & P. MALHERBE. 1993. Recombinant $GABA_A$ receptor function and ethanol. FEBS Lett. **324:** 140–142.

14. LEWOHL, J.M., D.I. CRANE & P.R. DODD. 1997. Expression of the α_1, α_2 and α_3 isoforms of the $GABA_A$ receptor in human alcoholic brain. Brain Res. **751:** 102–112.
15. MITSUYAMA, H. *et al.* 1998. $GABA_A$ receptor α_1, α_4, and β_3 subunit mRNA and protein expression in the frontal cortex of human alcoholics. Alcohol. Clin. Exp. Res. **22:** 815–822.
16. PARSIAN, A. & C.R. CLONINGER. 1997. Human $GABA_A$ receptor α_1 and α_3 subunit genes and alcoholism. Alcohol. Clin. Exp. Res. **21:** 430–433.
17. MHATRE, M.C. & M.K. TICKU. 1994. Chronic ethanol treatment upregulates the GABA receptor β subunit expression. Brain Res. Mol. Brain Res. **23:** 246–252.
18. SANDER, T. *et al.* 1999. Association analysis of sequence variants of $GABA_A$ α_6, β_2, and γ_2 gene cluster and alcohol dependence. Alcohol. Clin. Exp. Res. **23:** 427–431.
19. RADEL, M. & D. GOLDMAN. 2001. Pharmacogenetics of alcohol response and alcoholism: the interplay of genes and environmental factors in thresholds for alcoholism. Drug Metab. Dispos. **29:** 489–494.
20. HYND, M.R. *et al.* 2003. Biochemical and molecular studies using human autopsy brain tissue. J. Neurochem. **85:** 543–562.
21. DODD, P.R. *et al.* 1986. Optimization of freezing, storage, and thawing conditions for the preparation of metabolically active synaptosomes from frozen rat and human brain. Neurochem. Pathol. **4:** 177–198.
22. LOWRY, O.H. *et al.* 1951. Protein measurement with the Folin-phenol reagent. J. Biol. Chem. **193:** 265–275.
23. LAEMMLI, U.K. 1970. Cleavage of structural proteins during the assembly of the head of bacteriophage T4. Nature **227:** 680–685.
24. RAGNARSSON, L. *et al.* 2002. Spermine modulation of the glutamate-NMDA receptor is differentially responsive to conantokins in normal and Alzheimer disease human cerebral cortex. J. Neurochem. **81:** 765–779.
25. SAMBROOK, J., E.F. FRITSCH & T. MANIATIS. 1989. Extraction, purification, and analysis of messenger RNA from eukaryotic cells. *In* Molecular Cloning: a Laboratory Manual. C. Nolan, Ed.: 61–662. Cold Spring Harbor Press. Cold Spring Harbor, NY.
26. FOLEY, P.F. *et al.* 2004. Association studies of neurotransmitter gene polymorphisms in alcoholic Caucasians. Ann. N. Y. Acad. Sci. **1025:** 39–46.
27. DEVAUD, L.L., P. ALELE & C. RITU. 2003. Sex differences in the central nervous system actions of alcohol. Crit. Rev. Neurobiol. **15:** 41–59.
28. PONOMAREV, I. *et al.* 2004. Convergent analysis of cDNA and short oligomer microarrays, mouse null mutants and bioinformatics resources to study complex traits. Genes Brain Behav. **3:** 360–368.
29. LEWOHL, J.M. *et al.* 2000. Gene expression in human alcoholism: microarray analysis of frontal cortex. Alcohol. Clin. Exp. Res. **24:** 1873–1882.
30. GHAEMMAGHAMI, S. *et al.* 2003. Global analysis of protein expression in yeast. Nature **425:** 737–741.
31. CASTIGLIONE, C.M. *et al.* 1995. Evolution of haplotypes at the DRD2 locus. Amer. J. Hum. Genet. **57:** 1445–1456.
32. LOH, E.-W. *et al.* 1999. Association between variants at the $GABA_A\beta_2$, $GABA_A\alpha_6$ and $GABA_A\gamma_2$ gene cluster and alcohol dependence in a Scottish population. Mol. Psychiatry **4:** 539–544.

Association Study of the Tumor Necrosis Factor-α Gene and Its 1A Receptor Gene with Methamphetamine Dependence

A. NOMURA,[a,b,c] H. UJIKE,[a,b] Y. TANAKA,[a] M. KISHIMOTO,[a] K. OTANI,[a] Y. MORITA,[a] A. MORIO,[a] M. HARANO,[b,d] T. INADA,[b,e] M. YAMADA,[b,f] T. KOMIYAMA,[b,g] T. HORI,[b,g] Y. SEKINE,[b,h] N. IWATA,[b,i] I. SORA,[b,j] M. IYO,[b,k] N. OZAKI,[b,l] AND S. KURODA[a]

[a]*Department of Neuropsychiatry, Okayama University Graduate School of Medicine, Dentistry and Pharmaceutical Sciences, Okayama 700-8558, Japan*

[b]*Japanese Genetics Initiative for Drug Abuse (JGIDA), Japan*

[c]*Kasaoka Hospital, Kasaoka, Japan*

[d]*Department of Neuropsychiatry, Kurume University School of Medicine, Kurume, Japan*

[e]*Department of Psychiatry, Teikyo University School of Medicine, Ichihara Hospital, Ichihara, Japan*

[f]*Department of Psychogeriatrics, National Institute of Mental Health, National Center of Neurology and Psychiatry, Kodaira, Japan*

[g]*Division of Psychiatry, National Center Hospital for Mental, Nervous and Muscular Disorders, National Center of Neurology and Psychiatry, Tokyo, Japan*

[h]*Department of Psychiatry and Neurology, Hamamatsu University School of Medicine, Hamamatsu, Japan*

[i]*Department of Psychiatry, Fujita Health University School of Medicine, Nagoya, Japan*

[j]*Department of Psychobiology, Tohoku University Graduate School of Medicine, Sendai, Japan*

[k]*Department of Psychiatry, Graduate School of Medicine, Chiba University, Chiba, Japan*

[l]*Department of Psychiatry, Nagoya University Graduate School of Medicine, Nagoya, Japan*

Address for correspondence: Hiroshi Ujike, M.D., Ph.D., Department of Neuropsychiatry, Okayama University Graduate School of Medicine, Dentistry and Pharmaceutical Sciences, 2-5-1 Shikata-cho, Okayama 700-8558, Japan. Voice: +81-86-235-7242; fax: +81-86-235-7246.
e-mail: hujike@cc.okayama-u.ac.jp

Ann. N.Y. Acad. Sci. 1074: 116–124 (2006).
doi: 10.1196/annals.1369.011

ABSTRACT: Recent preclinical findings that repeated treatment with methamphetamine (METH) induced an increase in tumor necrosis factor-α (TNF-α) mRNA in some brain regions and that TNF-α blocked METH neurotoxicity and rewarding effects suggest TNF-α, a multifunctional pro-inflammatory cytokine, may be involved in METH dependence. We hypothesized that genetic polymorphisms of the TNF-α gene and its receptor genes may be associated with vulnerability to METH dependence. Genetic association of -308G>A and -857C>T in the promotor region of the TNF-α gene, and 36A>G in exon 1 of the TNF receptor 1A gene (TNFR-SF1A), were analyzed in patients with METH dependence ($n = 185$) and healthy controls ($n = 221$) in a Japanese population. No significant association of alleles or haplotypes of the TNF-α or TNFR-SF1A genes with METH dependence was found. Neither was any significant association of clinical phenotype with METH dependence found. These results suggest that genetic variations in the TNF-α gene and its receptor genes may not be involved in individual vulnerability to METH dependence.

KEYWORDS: tumor necrosis factor-α; substance dependence; case-control association study

INTRODUCTION

Substance dependence and substance-induced psychoses are serious problems worldwide.[1,2] In Japan, methamphetamine (METH) has been the most popular drug of abuse since World War II, and METH dependence and METH-related crimes are severe social problems.[3] On the other hand, genetic factors are important and relatively strong contributors to the risk for psychostimulant-use disorders. Intensive family, twin, and adoption studies have indicated that genetic factors substantially influence vulnerability to psychostimulant-use disorders.[4]

Tumor necrosis factor-α (TNF-α) is a pleiotropic pro-inflammatory cytokine that plays various roles in lipid metabolism, coagulation, insulin resistance, obesity, infections, and autoimmune conditions.[5] Cytokines and TNF-α may be involved in the development of dependence, brain damage, or substance-induced psychoses due to abuse of illegal drugs. Recently, it was found that repeated treatment with METH increased TNF-α mRNA and AP-1 binding in discrete regions of the mouse brain[6] and activated c-Jun and other members involved in the pathway leading to c-Jun activation,[7] and that TNF-α blocked METH neurotoxicity and reward.[8,9] These findings suggest that TNF-α plays protective roles in METH toxicity and dependence. To address possible roles of TNF-α systems in METH dependence, we performed a genetic association study of the TNF-α gene and its receptor 1A gene (TNFR-SF1A, also known as TNFR1 or TNFAR, OMIM *191190) in a population of Japanese patients with METH dependence.

METHODS

Subjects

Participants in this study included 185 unrelated patients with METH dependence (148 males and 37 females; mean age 36.8 ± 11.9 years) who were outpatients or inpatients of psychiatric hospitals of the Japanese Genetics Initiative for Drug Abuse (JGIDA). All participants were Japanese, born and living in limited regions of Japan. Diagnoses were made using the international statistical classification of the disease, revision 10, diagnostic criteria. Two trained psychiatrists assessed these diagnoses on the basis of all available information, including hospital records. Control subjects included 221 healthy age-, gender-, and region-matched volunteers (171 males and 50 females, mean age 36.3 ± 10.5 years), recruited primarily from the medical staff. Only unaffected subjects who had no known personal or family history of major psychiatric diseases, including alcoholism, were included in this study. The patients were divided into subgroups by clinical phenotype, multi-substance abuse status, and age at initial consumption of METH. This study was performed after obtaining approval from the ethics committees of each participating member institution of the JGIDA, and all subjects provided written informed consent for the use of their DNA samples for this research.

Genotyping

The genomic DNA was extracted from peripheral leukocytes using standard procedures. Genotyping of single nucleotide polymorphisms (SNPs), -308G>A and -857C>T of the TNF-α gene and 36A>G of the TNFR-SF1A

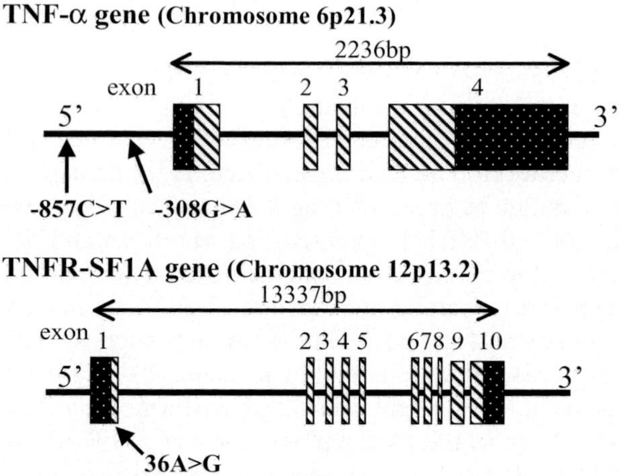

FIGURE 1. Motifs of the locus of SNPs.

gene (FIG. 1), was performed using polymerase chain reaction restriction fragment length polymorphism. Primers and restrictive enzymes recognizing polymorphisms were as follows: TNF-α-308G>A, 5′-agg caa tag gtt ttg agg gcc at-3′, 5′-tcc tcc ctg ctc cga ttc cg-3′, *Nco*I; TNF-α-857C>T, 5′-aag tcg agt atg ggg acc ccc cgt taa-3′, 5′-ccc cag tgt gtg gcc ata tct tct t-3′, *Hin*II; TNFR-SF1A 36A>G, 5′-tct ccc att ccc ctg cct cag c-3′, 5′-tgg gac cag gcc gtg atc tct atg c-3′, *BseN*I.

Statistical Analyses

Hardy–Weinberg equilibrium was tested using a χ^2 goodness-of-fit test. Linkage disequilibrium and haplotype analyses were performed using SNPAlyze software (Dynacom, Japan). To evaluate the statistical significance of differences in genotype distributions and allele frequencies between controls and patients and between clinical subgroups of patients, a χ^2 test was applied.

RESULTS

The genotype distributions of -308G>A and -857C>T of the TNF-α gene and 36A>G of the TNFR-SF1A gene were not significantly different from those expected according to Hardy–Weinberg equilibrium in any group or any subgroup. The genotype distributions and allele frequencies of the three SNPs of the patients with METH dependence and controls are shown in TABLE 1. No significant association of METH dependence was found with the -308G>A and -857C>T polymorphisms of the TNF-α gene (-308G>A, allele, χ^2 = 0.58, df = 1, P = 0.45; genotype, χ^2 = 0.59, df = 1, P = 0.44; -857C>T, allele, χ^2 = 2.44, df = 1, P = 0.12; genotype, χ^2 = 2.64, df = 2, P = 0.27), and 36A>G of the TNFR-SF1A gene (allele, χ^2 = 0.58, df = 1, P = 1.0; genotype, χ^2 = 0.54, df = 2, P = 0.76).

Two SNPs of the TNF-α, -308G>A and -857C>T, were located close to each other, and EM algorithm analysis using the SNPAlyze program showed they were in strong linkage disequilibrium (D' = 1.00 and r^2 = 0.0055). Haplotype analysis was performed on the two SNPs, and three haplotypes, AC, AT, and GC, at -308G>A and -857C>T loci were found (TABLE 2). Estimated frequencies of haplotypes of the TNF-α gene of patients with METH dependence and controls were not significantly different.

To further examine possible roles of TNF-α systems in the development of METH dependence and the etiology of its rewarding effects, clinical phenotypes of METH dependence, the age at first consumption of METH, and multi-substance abuse status were analyzed (TABLE 3). There were, however, no significant associations of SNPs of the TNF-α and TNFR-SF1A genes with either phenotype.

TABLE 1. Genotype and allele frequencies of polymorphisms -308G>A and -857C>T of the TNF-α gene, and 36A>G of the TNFR-SF1A gene in patients with METH dependence and controls

	Genotypes					Alleles			
TNF-α-308G>A	N	GG	GA	AA	*P*	N	G	A	*P*
Control (%)	214	207 (96.7)	7 (3.3)	0 (0.0)		428	421 (98.4)	7 (1.6)	
METH dependence (%)	184	175 (95.1)	9 (4.9)	0 (0.0)	0.44	368	359 (97.6)	9 (2.4)	0.45
TNF-α-857C>T	N	CC	CT	TT	*P*	N	C	T	*P*
Control (%)	219	134 (61.2)	68 (31.1)	17 (7.8)		438	336 (76.7)	102 (23.3)	
METH dependence (%)	183	123 (67.2)	52 (28.4)	8 (4.4)	0.27	366	298 (81.4)	68 (18.6)	0.12
TNFR-SF1A 36A>G	N	AA	AG	GG	*P*	N	A	G	*P*
Control (%)	216	151 (69.9)	59 (27.3)	6 (2.8)		432	361 (83.6)	71 (16.4)	
METH dependence (%)	179	131 (73.2)	44 (24.6)	4 (2.2)	0.76	366	306 (83.6)	60 (16.4)	1.00

TABLE 2. Case–control haplotype analysis at -308G>A and -857C>T loci of the TNF-α gene

Haplotype		Frequencies			
-308G>A	-857C>T	Control	METH	χ^2	*P*
G	C	0.75	0.79	1.53	0.22
G	T	0.23	0.19	2.43	0.12
A	C	0.017	0.025	0.65	0.42

Permutation *P* value = 0.32.

DISCUSSION

The two SNPs of the TNF-α examined in the present study, -308G>A and -857C>T, are located in the promoter region of the gene (FIG. 1), which implies that they are functional SNPs. The -308G>A polymorphism was found to be associated with the HLA-A1-B8-DR3-DQ2 haplotype and affected the affinity of factor binding.[10] Luciferase assay showed that -308A allele produced twofold greater transcription activity than the -308G allele.[11,12] Similarly, the -857C>T polymorphism was shown to be associated with HLA-DRB1*0405, and the -857T allele showed 1.7-fold greater transcription activity than the -857C allele.[13] TNF receptor 1A, like another subtype, 1B, is a cell-surface receptor molecule and transduces the TNF-α signal upon ligand binding. The extracellular domains of these receptors can also be shed by proteolytic cleavage and act as natural inhibitors of TNF-α activity. The 36A>G SNP of the TNFR-SF1A is located in exon 1 (FIG. 1) and is a nonfunctional silent mutation. However, it is the closest frequent exonic polymorphism to all the known TNF-associated periodic syndromes, dominantly inherited autoinflammatory disorder-associated mutations found on exons 2-4, which encode the TNFR-SF1A extracellular domain.[14,15] It is likely that 36A>G of the TNFR-SF1A gene is in linkage disequilibrium with unknown functional SNPs of the gene. Actually, significant associations of 36A>G of the TNFR-SF1A gene with anemia in rheumatoid arthritis[16] and familial rheumatoid arthritis[17] have been reported.

Nakajima *et al.*[9] showed that exogenously applied TNF-α suppressed METH-induced hyperlocomotion in mice. It also attenuated the rewarding response to METH in conditioned place-preference and drug discrimination tests and METH-induced dopaminergic neurotoxicity in mice. They also revealed that mice with targeted deletion of the TNF-α gene showed enhanced response to locomotor sensitization and the rewarding and neurotoxic effects of METH compared with wild-type mice. These neuroprotective roles of TNF-α against METH dependence and neurotoxicity resulted from activation of the plasmalemmal and vesicular dopamine transporters and inhibition the METH-induced increase of extracellular dopamine release. Therefore, the TNF-α

TABLE 3. Association of TNF-α and TNFR-SF1A genes with subgroups of METH dependence divided by clinical phenotype

	Genotypes					Alleles			
Multi-substance abuse status TNF-α-308G>A	N	GG	GA	AA	*P*	N	G	A	*P*
No (%)	58	55 (94.8)	3 (5.2)	0 (0.0)		116	113 (98.4)	3 (1.6)	
Yes (%)	132	125 (94.7)	7 (5.3)	0 (0.0)	1.00	264	257 (97.6)	7 (2.4)	1.00
TNF-α-857C>T	N	CC	CT	TT	*P*	N	C	T	*P*
No (%)	58	134 (61.2)	68 (31.1)	17 (7.8)		116	96 (82.8)	20 (17.2)	
Yes (%)	130	123 (67.2)	52 (28.4)	8 (4.4)	0.27	260	216 (83.1)	44 (16.9)	1.00
TNFR-SF1A 36A>G	N	AA	AG	GG	*P*	N	A	G	*P*
No (%)	56	41 (73.2)	14 (25.0)	1 (1.8)		112	96 (85.7)	16 (14.3)	
Yes (%)	128	91 (71.1)	34 (26.6)	3 (2.3)	0.94	256	216 (84.4)	40 (15.6)	0.75
Age at initial METH consumption TNF-α-308G>A	N	GG	GA	AA	*P*	N	G	A	*P*
20 years > (%)	95	90 (94.7)	5 (5.3)	0 (0.0)		190	185 (97.4)	5 (2.6)	
20 years ≤ (%)	99	94 (94.9)	5 (5.1)	0 (0.0)	1.00	198	193 (97.5)	5 (2.5)	1.00
TNF-α-857C>T	N	CC	CT	TT	*P*	N	C	T	*P*
20 > (%)	94	67 (71.3)	26 (27.7)	1 (1.1)		188	160 (85.1)	28 (14.9)	
20 ≤ (%)	99	64 (64.6)	28 (28.3)	7 (7.1)	0.11	198	156 (78.8)	42 (21.2)	0.11
TNFR-SF1A 36A>G	N	AA	AG	GG	*P*	N	A	G	*P*
20 > (%)	91	62 (68.1)	27 (29.7)	2 (2.2)		182	151 (83.0)	31 (17.0)	
20 ≤ (%)	99	76 (76.8)	21 (21.2)	2 (2.0)	0.30	198	173 (87.4)	25 (12.6)	0.23

system works as a negative feedback system to the METH effects on the brain. It is possible that individuals with a hyperfunctional -308A or -857T allele of the TNF-α gene may be resistant to METH reward or METH-induced sequlae, including psychosis. However, the present study showed no association of functional alleles of -308A or -857T of the TNF-α gene with susceptibility to METH dependence or any clinical phenotype of METH dependence. There was also no significant association of these SNPs with susceptibility to METH-induced psychosis and its prognosis (data not shown), nor was a significant association of the TNFR-SF1A gene with METH dependence found. Accordingly, our genetic study did not provide any evidence that supports negative feedback roles for the TNF-α system in METH-induced reward and neurotoxicity. However, our negative findings should be confirmed by further examination of additional SNPs covering the entire TNF-α and TNFR-SF1A genes in other populations.

ACKNOWLEDGMENTS

This study was partly supported by the Zikei Institute of Psychiatry (Okayama, Japan) and Grants-in-Aid from the Japanese Ministry of Health, Labor and Welfare.

REFERENCES

1. REHM, J., R. ROOM, W. VAN DEN BRINKT, *et al.* 2005. Problematic drug use and drug use disorders in EU countries and Norway: an overview of the epidemiology. Eur. Neuropsychopharmacol. **15:** 389–397.
2. ANGLIN, M.D., C. BURKE, B. PERROCHET, *et al.* 2000. History of the methamphetamine problem. J. Psychoactive Drugs **32:** 137–141.
3. UJIKE, H. & M. SATO. 2004. Clinical features of sensitization to methamphetamine observed in patients with methamphetamine dependence and psychosis. Ann. N. Y. Acad. Sci. **1025:** 279–287.
4. TSUANG, M.T., M.J. LYNONS, S.A. EISEN, *et al.* 1996. Genetic influences on DSM-III-R drug abuse and dependence: a study of 3,372 twin pairs. Am. J. Med. Genet. **67:** 473–477.
5. VASSALI, P. 1992. The pathophysiology of tumor necrosis factors. Annu. Rev. Immunol. **10:** 411–452.
6. FLORA, G., Y.W. LEE, A. NATH, *et al.* 2002. Methamphetamine-induced TNF-alpha gene expression and activation of AP-1 in discrete regions of mouse brain: potential role of reactive oxygen intermediates and lipid peroxidation. Neuromolecular Med. **2:** 71–85.
7. JAYANTHI, S., M.T. MCCOY, B. LADENHEIM, *et al.* 2002. Methamphetamine causes coordinate regulation of Src, Cas, Crk, and the Jun N-terminal kinase-Jun pathway. Mol. Pharmacol. **61:** 1124–1131.
8. YAMADA, K. & T. NABESHIMA. 2004. Pro- and anti-addictive neurotrophic factors and cytokines in psychostimulant addiction: mini-review. Ann. N. Y. Acad. Sci. **1025:** 198–204.

9. NAKAJIMA, A., K. YAMADA, T. NAGAI, *et al.* 2004. Role of tumor necrosis factor-alpha in methamphetamine-induced drug dependence and neurotoxicity. J. Neurosci. **24:** 2212–2225.
10. WILSON, A.G., N. DE VRIES, F. POCIOT, *et al.* 1993. An allelic polymorphism within the human tumor necrosis factor alpha promoter region is strongly associated with HLA A1, B8, and DR3 alleles. J. Exp. Med. **177:** 557–560.
11. KROEGER, K.M., K.S. CARVILLE & L.J. ABRAHAM. 1997. The -308 tumor necrosis factor-alpha promoter polymorphism effects transcription. Mol. Immunol. **34:** 391–399.
12. WILSON, A.G., G.W. DUFF, H.O. MCDEVITT, *et al.* 1997. Effects of a polymorphism in the human tumor necrosis factor promoter on transcriptional activation. Proc. Natl. Acad. Sci. USA **94:** 3195–3199.
13. HIGUCHI, T., N. SEKI, S. KAMIZONO, *et al.* 1998. Polymorphism of the 5′-flanking region of the human tumor necrosis factor (TNF)-alpha gene in Japanese. Tissue Antigens **51:** 605–612.
14. MCDERMOTT, M.F., I. AKSENTIJEVICH, J. GALON, *et al.* 1999. Germline mutations in the extracellular domains of the 55 kDa TNF receptor, TNFR1, define a family of dominantly inherited autoinflammatory syndromes. Cell **97:** 133–144.
15. AKSENTIJEVICH, I., J. GALON, M. SOARES, *et al.* 2001. The tumour necrosis factor receptor-associated periodic syndrome: new mutations in TNFR-SF1A, ancestral origins, genotype-phenotype studies, and evidence for further genetic heterogeneity of periodic fevers. Am. J. Hum. Genet. **269:** 301–314.
16. GLOSSOP, J.R., P.T. DAWES, A.B. HASSELL, *et al.* 2005. Anemia in rheumatoid arthritis: association with polymorphism in the tumor necrosis factor receptor I and II genes. J. Rheumatol. **32:** 1673–1678.
17. DIEUDE, P., J. OSORIO, E. PETIT-TEIXEIRA, *et al.* 2004. European Consortium on Rheumatoid Arthritis Families. A TNFR1 genotype with a protective role in familial rheumatoid arthritis. Arthritis Rheum. **50:** 413–419.

Longitudinal Clinical Course Following Pharmacological Treatment of Methamphetamine Psychosis Which Persists after Long-Term Abstinence

KAZUFUMI AKIYAMA

Department of Psychiatry, Dokkyo Medical University School of Medicine, Mibu, Tochigi 321-0293, Japan

ABSTRACT: The present article investigated clinical symptoms and their longitudinal clinical course following pharmacological treatment in 32 female incarcerated patients suffering from methamphetamine (METH) psychosis who were referred to psychiatric consultation. The length of METH-abuse periods of the patients ranged from 2 to 31 years. A total of 31 patients suffered from psychosis at abstinence after 5–31 months from the self-injection of METH. Nine of these 31 patients experienced episodes of psychotic relapse. The following symptoms were observed: auditory hallucination (29 cases), delusion of persecution (29 cases), thought broadcasting (24 cases), visual hallucination (22 cases), depressive mood (29 cases), and suicidal idea (22 cases). Patients exhibited symptoms of psychosis and depression, which persisted for more than several months despite commencement of administration of antipsychotics and antidepressants. There were significant correlations among length of periods required for improvement in total Brief Psychiatric Rating Scale (BPRS) scores, and BPRS subscale scores representing positive symptoms and depression/anxiety dimensions. Three groups of patients, according to severity of positive and depressive/anxiety symptoms, showed apparent differences in prognoses during pharmacological treatment. Average degree of extrapyramidal symptoms significantly correlated with average daily dose of antipsychotics and length-of-treatment period required for improvement in BPRS subscale scores representing positive symptom dimension. These results suggest that both psychotic and affective symptoms are involved in therapeutic response and prognosis of METH psychosis.

KEYWORDS: methamphetamine psychosis; persistent type; symptom dimensions; pharmacological treatment; differential prognoses; liability to extrapyramidal symptoms

Address for correspondence: Kazufumi Akiyama, M.D., Ph.D., Department of Psychiatry, Dokkyo Medical University School of Medicine, Kitakobayashi 880, Mibu, Tochigi 00-321-0293, Japan. Voice: +81-282-87-2153; fax: +81-282-86-5187.
e-mail: kazufuak@dokkyomed.ac.jp

Ann. N.Y. Acad. Sci. 1074: 125–134 (2006).
doi: 10.1196/annals.1369.012

INTRODUCTION

Methamphetamine (METH) is a major psychostimulant abused in Asian/Pacific countries, and Japan experienced two major epidemics in the past. The second epidemic did not subside completely, and many patients who began abusing METH during this epidemic have continued to abuse it. Thus, Japan is now facing its third epidemic since 1995.[1] Culminating evidence has indicated that chronic METH abuse gradually leads to the development of a psychotic state resembling paranoid schizophrenia.[2–5] Japanese investigators have noticed that long-term abuse of METH predisposes its users to psychosis that persists despite long-term abstinence.[1–5] Ujike and Sato[1] proposed that, according to the time course after abstinence, METH psychosis may well be classified into transient, prolonged, and persistent types. The transient type results from direct effect of METH *per se*, and rapidly desists upon urinary excretion of METH. With the prolonged type, psychotic state continues up to 1 month after abstinence. Finally, the persistent type represents the proportion of patients exhibiting psychotic states after long-term abstinence beyond 1 month. Japanese investigators have assumed that among the varied types of METH psychosis, the persistent type affects about 40% of the total patients suffering from METH psychosis.[1] Mikami *et al.*[6] reported that patients with the persistent type, who were severely disturbed and had high rate of family history of schizophrenia, exhibited notably poor exploratory eye movement, which served as a vulnerability marker of schizophrenia. Conversely, the other investigators have pointed out that persistent psychosis in METH abusers may be attributable to the presence of comorbid psychiatric disorders.[7,8] The present article investigated clinical symptoms and response to pharmacotherapy during longitudinal clinical course in 32 female patients with METH psychosis in Japan.

SUBJECTS AND METHODS

Women who were identified as guilty of offenses against the Stimulant Control Law, and incarcerated, were referred to psychiatric consultation. A total of 32 patients who suffered from psychotic state, such as auditory hallucination and delusion of persecution, were recruited from incarcerated patients requiring treatment, and those who had only slight or moderate symptom severity, such as anxiety or insomnia, were excluded. Patients who had a history of psychosis exhibiting a presence of schizophrenia prior to first METH use were also excluded. Observation under detention confirmed that eligible patients were kept abstinent since their last self-injection of METH. They underwent interviews in a routine clinical setting for assessment of current psychiatric symptoms and treatment response to pharmacotherapy.

Because use of METH is illegal in Japan, the subjects were informed that their legal status would not be affected by confession of METH abuse.

Their symptoms were measured using a 24-item Brief Psychiatric Rating Scale (BPRS) which allows ratings of 1 (absent) – 7 (extremely severe) for each symptom and the extraction of clusters forming symptom dimensions (positive, negative, manic, and depression/anxiety).[9,10] Thus, in the 24-item BPRS, positive symptoms comprise bizarre behavior, unusual thought content, disorganization, hallucination, and suspiciousness. Negative symptoms comprise blunted affect, motor retardation, emotional withdrawal, and self-neglect. Manic excitement comprises motor hyperactivity, elevated mood, excitement, distractibility, hostility, and grandiosity. Depression/anxiety comprises depression, anxiety, suicidality, and guilt. Interviews were repeated usually biweekly or bimonthly either until they were discharged or at most for 120 months (observation period).

Either haloperidol or risperidone was randomly administered to patients as a first-line antipsychotic. Administration doses were based on usual clinical practice. When extrapyramidal symptoms occurred, haloperidol was replaced by risperidone or perospirone. Similarly, risperidone was administered as a first-line antipsychotic, and when extrapyramidal symptoms occurred, it was replaced by quetiapine. The various antipsychotics doses were gauged based on the equivalent milligram dosage of haloperidol. That is, 1 mg of haloperidol was regarded as equivalent to either 0.5 mg of risperidone, 4 mg of perospirone, or 33 mg of quetiapine. Antidepressants and mood stabilizers were administered as they were needed. Either imipramine or fluvoxamine was administered as an antidepressant, both being regarded as equipotent.

Patients underwent brief neurological examination for occurrence of extrapyramidal symptoms such as tremor, dysarthria, rigidity, gait disturbance, and akathisia. Magnitude of extrapyramidal symptoms was defined by the cumulative numbers of occurring symptoms. Length-of-treatment period required for reduction of total BPRS scores and BPRS-subscale scores representing each symptom dimension was defined in terms of weeks, when cumulative rating of total BPRS scores and BPRS subscale scores were less than 32 and 10, respectively. However, when patients were discharged before such improvement was achieved, the weeks of discharge was regarded in this length. Correlation among magnitude of psychiatric symptoms, extrapyramidal symptoms, doses of therapeutic drugs, and length-of-treatment period required for symptom reduction were examined by using Spearman's correlation coefficient by rank.

RESULTS

Baseline data of the patients' profiles were depicted in FIGURE 1. Age at the first consultation ranged from the early 20s to the early 40s (FIG. 1 A). Duration from the last self-injection to the first consultation was several months due to detention (FIG. 1 B). A total of nine patients experienced episodes of spontaneous psychotic relapse during this abstinence period, for which psychotic state

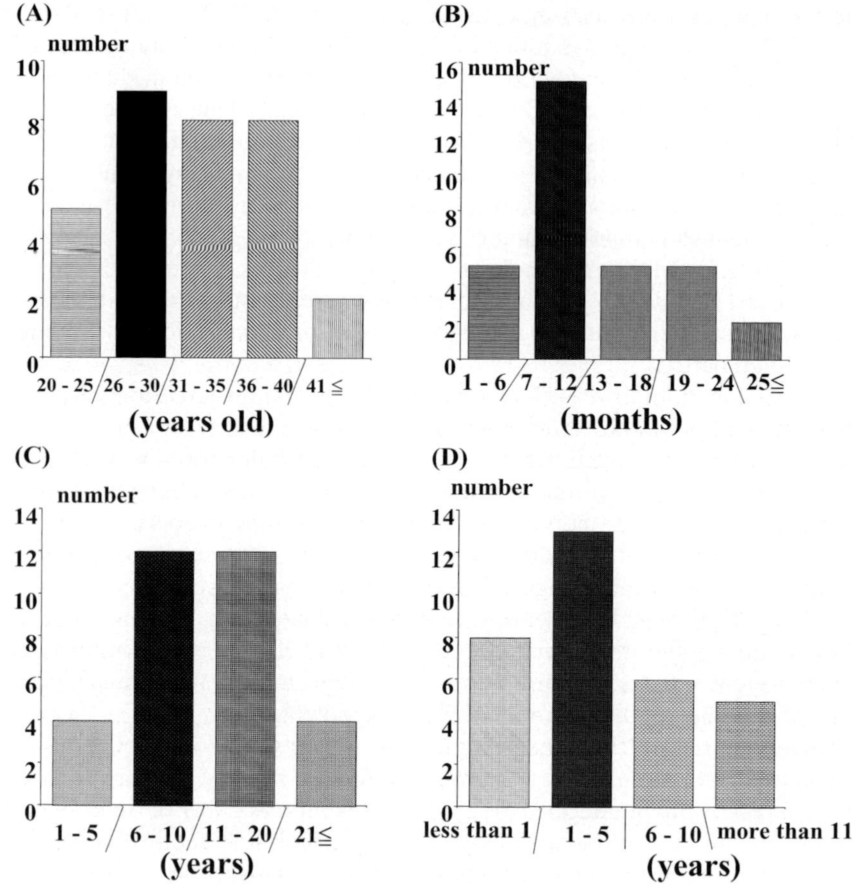

FIGURE 1. Baseline data of subjects' profiles.

initially subsided but subsequently recurred. Length of METH-abuse period ranged from 1 year to more than 20 years (FIG. 1 C). Latencies from beginning of METH abuse to emergence of an initial psychotic episode ranged from less than 1 year to more than 11 years (FIG. 1 D). Three patients had depressive episodes prior to their first METH use. Symptoms that were characteristic of schizophrenia and mood disorder were frequently observed (TABLE 1), those being auditory hallucination, delusion of persecution, thought broadcasting, visual hallucination, somatic hallucination, depressive mood, and suicidal idea. Cumulative ratings of BPRS subscale representing each symptom dimension were averaged throughout the observation period for an individual patient such that an averaged rating of one symptom dimension was plotted synchronously with other symptom dimension. FIGURE 2 shows significant positive correlations between positive symptom dimension and depression/anxiety symptom

TABLE 1. Symptoms observed at first consultation

Auditory hallucination (29/32 = 90.6 %)
Delusion of persecution (29/32 = 90.6 %)
Thought broadcasting (24/32 = 75%)
Visual hallucination (22/32 = 68.8%)
Somatic hallucination (13/32 = 40.6%)
Depressive mood (29/32 = 90.6 %)
Suicidal idea (22/32 = 68.8%)

dimension ($P = 0.003$). According to this correlation, the patients were arbitrarily classified into three groups who had low, moderate, and high ratings of combined positive symptom and depression/anxiety. FIGURE 3 shows the average of the cumulative ratings of total 24-item BPRS scores among patients belonging to the three different groups during the observation period. The three groups showed apparent differential prognostic courses during the observation period under pharmacological treatment. Unexpectedly, it took 5 months to ameliorate symptoms even in the low-rating group. Conversely, the high-rating group did not recover in spite of intensive pharmacological treatment.

Among the whole group of patients, there were significant correlations between length of periods required for improvement in total BPRS scores, and BPRS-subscale scores representing positive symptom and depression/anxiety dimensions (total versus positive symptom, $P < 0.0001$; total *versus*. depression/anxiety, $P < 0.0001$; positive symptom versus depression/anxiety $P < 0.0001$, data not shown). There was no significant correlation between these lengths of periods and duration of METH abuse (data not shown). Average degree of extrapyramidal symptoms significantly correlated with average daily dose of antipsychotics ($P = 0.0023$, FIG. 4) and length-of-treatment period required for improvement in BPRS-subscale scores representing positive symptom dimension ($P = 0.02$, FIG. 4). Haloperidol and risperidone were administered to 15 and 13 patients, respectively, as a first-line antipsychotic. All patients, receiving haloperidol as a first-line antipsychotic, exhibited extrapyramidal symptoms. Haloperidol administration was continued in only 1 patient, but replaced by risperidone and perospirone in 12 and 2 patients, respectively. A total of 8 patients receiving risperidone as a first-line antipsychotic exhibited extrapyramidal symptoms. Risperidone was thus replaced by quetiapine in the 8 patients. Quetiapine proved to relieve extrapyramidal symptoms, and resulted in favorable response in 4 cases. However, psychotic symptoms were exacerbated in 4 cases.

DISCUSSION

The cross-sectional features of METH psychosis which were revealed by the present study are in general agreement with previous reports.[2–5,7] Except

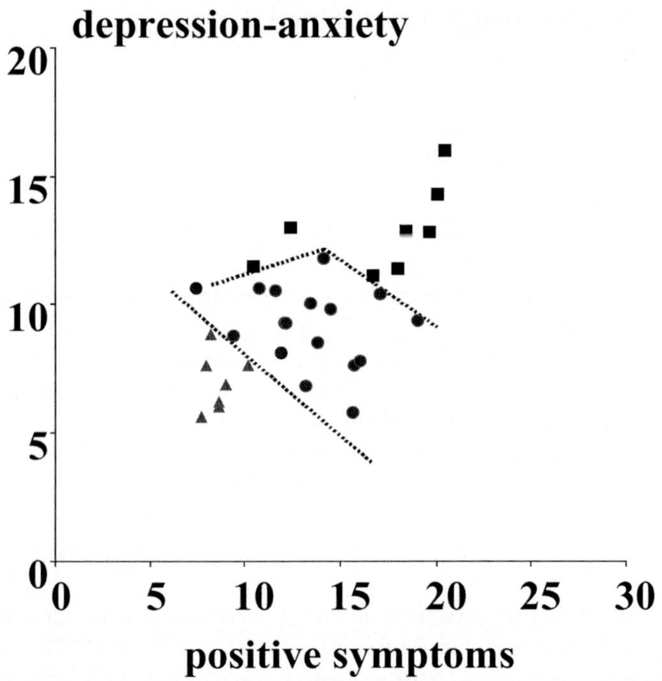

FIGURE 2. Correlation between rating of BPRS-subscale representing positive symptoms and depression/anxiety ($P = 0.003$ according to Spearman's correlation coefficient by rank). Each point represents average rating of positive symptoms and depression/anxiety in individual patients. Patients were classified into three groups according to severity (low▲, moderate ●, and high ■) of positive symptoms and depression/anxiety.

for one patient, the psychiatric symptoms had either continued for more than 1 month since the last self-injection or recurred following initial withdrawal during this abstinence period under detention. The subjects experiencing recurrence were regarded as having spontaneous relapse and were included in the persistent-type METH psychosis. It should be noted that the subjects in the present study do not represent a general population of METH abuse, including habitual users. Thus, the present study has a methodological limitation, in that only psychiatrically disturbed patients were examined, implying a possibility that their premorbid psychopathology might make them more prone to either craving psychostimulants or developing psychosis than the general population. Nonetheless, a prolonged period of METH abuse ranging from 1 year to more than 20 years in the persistent-type patients suggests that long-term abuse period significantly contributes to development of a refractory psychotic state, as was previously suggested.[7,11] With respect to a neuroimaging study using positron emission tomography, Sekine *et al.*[11] reported that a significant reduction in the dopamine transporter continued after METH abstinence up to

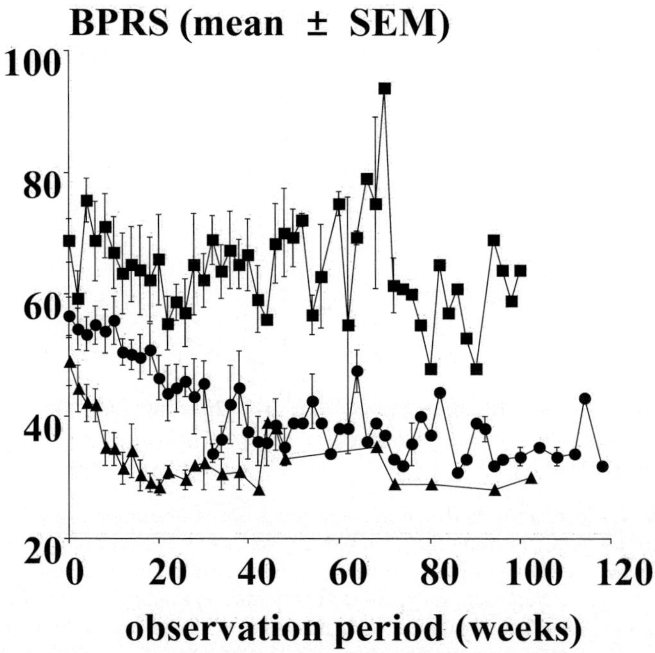

FIGURE 3. Three groups, which are labeled with ▲, ●, and ■ had low, moderate, and high ratings, respectively, of severity of combined positive symptoms and depression/anxiety.

20 months, and that such reduction was associated with longer abuse period. Alternatively, a proportion of persistent type of METH psychosis is underlain by enduring vulnerability. This assumption is supported by a psychophysiological study that shows persistent-type patients who were severely disturbed and had high rate of family history of schizophrenia exhibited poor exploratory eye movements as observed in schizophrenic subjects.[6]

Patients in the present study were also associated with negative symptoms and affective symptoms. Existence of negative symptoms in METH psychosis is compatible with a previous study which were preformed using BPRS[6] and a rating scale of two-factor dimensional model of METH psychosis.[12] Patients in the present study mimic schizophrenia paranoid type ($n = 26$), disorganized type ($n = 4$), or delusional disorder ($n = 1$) with ($n = 20$) or without ($n = 11$) concomitant mood disorder. A previous study examining patients incarcerated for METH abuse in Taiwan reported that the rates of major depression whose first episode occurred prior to first METH use was 7.6% and 3.8% in subjects with METH psychosis, and those without METH psychosis, respectively.[7] The same group of investigators reported that as many as 36% of the female, but not male, METH abusers exhibited suicidal behavior.[8] As many patients of the present study began METH abuse in their youth, it is unclear, except for three

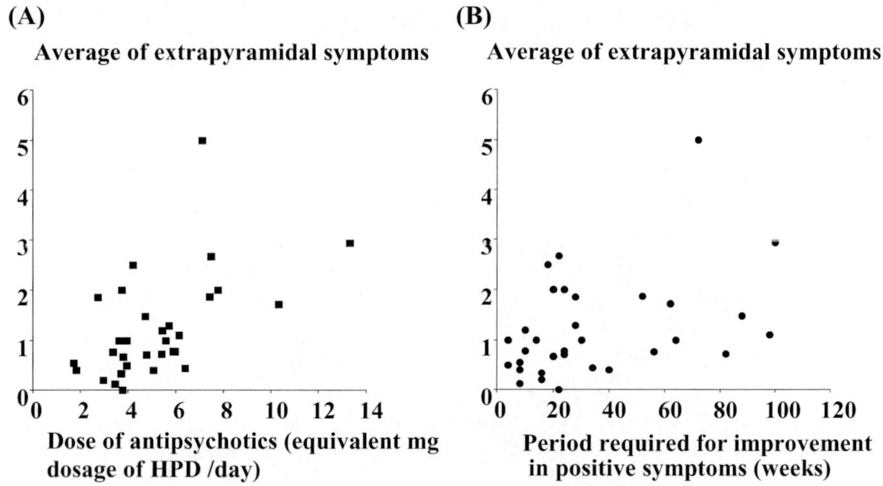

FIGURE 4. Correlation between average daily doses of antipsychotics and average degree of extrapyramidal symptoms [$P = 0.0023$, according to Spearman's correlation coefficient by rank, (**A**) and between length-of-treatment period required for improvement in BPRS-subscale scores representing positive symptoms and average degree of extrapyramidal symptoms [$P = 0.02$, according to Spearman's correlation coefficient by rank, (**B**)].

cases with previous mood episode, whether their affective symptoms reflect the presence of comorbid disorder or presence of a previously latent disorder. Practically, however, high rates of suicidal tendency commonly observed is consistent with the previous report from Taiwan[8] and warrants attention as it applies to suicide risk in the treatment of female patients with METH psychosis. According to diagnostic criteria of Diagnostic and Statistical Manual of Mental Disorders, fourth edition (DSM-IV) previous exposure to psychostimulant not only excludes diagnosis of schizophrenia, but also diagnosis of amphetamine psychosis is excluded if psychosis continues beyond 1 month of abstinence. Occurrence of a group of patients suffering from persistent psychosis may result from both premorbid vulnerability and long-term abuse, and this aspects requires further study.

Only a few studies examined longitudinal clinical course of patients with METH psychosis following pharmacological treatment.[5,13] Iwanami *et al.* [5] reported that psychotic symptoms continued for more than 3 months after commencement of treatment with antipsychotics in subjects representing 16% population of METH-abused inpatients in Tokyo Metropolitan Matsuzawa Hospital during a period between 1988 and 1991 in the second epidemic. Yeh *et al.*[13] reported that scores of delusion and hallucination in schedule for affective disorders and schizophrenia were improved after 6 months of admission, but did not mention the pharmacological treatment. Although the present study is hampered by small sample size, differential responses to pharmacotherapy is noteworthy. Based on two-dimensional distributions between positive and depression/anxiety symptoms, both of which were represented as an average rating during the observational period, three groups were arbitrarily differentiated based on their relative (low, intermediate, and high) magnitude of symptoms. It turned out that these three groups represented differential treatment response groups. Among all patients, there were significant correlations between length of periods required for improvement in total BPRS scores, and BPRS-subscale scores representing positive symptoms and depression/anxiety dimensions. This aspect implies a unique psychiatric clinical course in terms of psychosis intermingling with affective change, and suggests that affective as well as psychotic symptoms are targets for pharmacotherapy of METH psychosis. Also from the present study, it should be noted that extrapyramidal symptoms were liable to occur in patients with METH psychosis who were resistant to pharmacotherapy, suggesting that the use of second-generation antipsychotics are preferable as suggested in previous studies.[14,15]

The present study had several limitations which were retrospective and performed on a selected small number of patients, and did not use instruments allowing comprehensive assessment of premorbid schizoid/schizotypal personality trait.[7] Nevertheless, it reinforces a viewpoint that chronic abuse of METH leads to vulnerability to paranoid psychosis which resembles schizophrenia and at least partially coincides with affective symptoms. Occasionally, the symptoms persist after long-term abstinence, and are refractory to pharmacotherapeutical intervention.

REFERENCES

1. UJIKE, H. & M. SATO. 2004. Clinical features of sensitization to methamphetamine observed in patients with methamphetamine dependence and psychosis. Ann. N. Y. Acad. Sci. **1025:** 279–287.
2. SATO, M., C.-C. CHEN, K. AKIYAMA & S. OTSUKI. 1983. Acute exacerbation of paranoid psychotic state after long-term abstinence in patients with previous methamphetamine psychosis. Biol. Psychiatry **18:** 429–440.
3. SATO, M. 1992. Lasting vulnerability to psychosis in patients with previous methamphetamine psychosis. Ann. N. Y. Acad. Sci. **654:** 160–170.
4. KONUMA, K. 1994. Use and abuse of amphetamines in Japan. *In* Amphetamine and its Analogs, Psychopharmacology, Toxicology, and Abuse. A.K. Cho & D.S. Segal, Eds.: 415–435. Academic Press. San Diego, CA.
5. IWANAMI, A., A. SUGIYAMA, N. KUROKI, *et al.* 1994. Patients with methamphetamine psychosis admitted to a psychiatric hospital in Japan. A preliminary report. Acta Psychiatr. Scand. **89:** 428–432.
6. MIKAMI, T., N. NARUSE, Y. FUKURA, *et al.* 2003. Determining vulnerability to schizophrenia in methamphetamine psychosis using exploratory eye movements. Psychiatry Clin. Neurosci. **57:** 433–440.
7. CHEN, C.-K., S.-K. LIN, P.C. SHAM, *et al.* 2003. Premorbid characteristics and co-morbidity of methamphetamine users with and without psychosis. Psychol. Med. **33:** 1407–1414.

8. LIN, S.-K., D. BALL, C.-C. HSIANO, *et al.* 2004. Psychiatric comorbidity and gender differences of persons incarcerated for methamphetamine abuse in Taiwan. Psychiatry Clin. Neurosci.**58:** 206–212.
9. LUKOFF, D., K.H. NUECHTERLEIN & J. VENTURA. 1986. Manual for expanded brief psychiatric rating scale (BPRS). Schizophr. Bull. **12:** 594–602.
10. VENTURA, J., K.H. NUECHTERLEIN, K.L. SUBOTNIK, *et al.* 2000. Symptom dimensions in recent-onset schizophrenia and mania: a principal components analysis of the 24-item brief psychiatric rating scale. Psychiatry Res. **97:** 129–135.
11. SEKINE, Y., M. IYO, Y. OUCHI, *et al.* 2001. Methamphetamine-related psychiatric symptoms and reduced brain dopamine transporters studied with PET. Am. J. Psychiatry **158:** 1206–1214.
12. SRISURAPANONT, M., R. ALI, J. MARSDEN, *et al.* 2003. Psychotic symptoms in methamphetamine psychotic in-patients. Int. J. Neuropsychopharmacol. **6:** 347–352.
13. YEH, H.-S, Y.-C. LEE, H.-J. SUN & S.-R. WAN. 2001. Six months follow-up of patients with methamphetamine psychosis. Chin. Med. J. (Taipei) **64:** 388–394.
14. MIRSA, L. & L. KOFOED. 1997. Risperidone treatment of methamphetamine psychosis. Am. J. Psychiatry **154:** 1170.
15. MIRSA, L.K., L. KOFOED, J.R. OESTERHELD & G.A. RICHARDS. 2000. Olanzapine treatment of methamphetamine psychosis. J. Clin. Psychopharmacol. **20:** 393–394.

Distinct Mechanisms Mediating Methamphetamine-Induced Neuronal Apoptosis and Dopamine Terminal Damage Share the Neuropeptide Substance P in the Striatum of Mice

JUDY P.Q. ZHU, WENJING XU, AND JESUS A. ANGULO

Department of Biological Sciences, Hunter College of the City University of New York, New York 10021, USA

ABSTRACT: Methamphetamine (METH) is an addictive psychostimulant that induces damage to the dopamine terminals and the apoptosis of some neurons of the striatum. Our laboratory demonstrated using either a single bolus dose (30 mg/kg) or a binge (10 mg/kg 4× at 2-h intervals) of METH that pharmacological blockade of the substance P receptor (neurokinin-1) attenuates METH-induced damage to both the presynaptic dopamine terminals and the apoptosis of some neurons of the striatum. To determine the phenotype of striatal neuron ablated by METH, we combined TUNEL (Terminal Deoxyncleotidyl Transferase-Mediated dUTP Nick End Labeling) with immunofluorescence for selective markers of projection and interneurons. METH induces the loss of approximately 20% of the projection neurons. The cholinergic and γ-aminobutyric acid (GABA)-parvalbumin interneurons sustain losses of 30% and 50%, respectively. The somatostatin/neuropeptide Y (NPY)/nitric oxide synthase (NOS) interneurons are not impacted by METH. To investigate the mechanism by which substance P mediates METH-induced damage in this part of the brain, we ablated the striatal interneurons that express the neurokinin-1 receptor (NK-1R) with the selective neurotoxin substance P-SAP. Ablation of the NK-1R-expressing interneurons prevented METH-induced apoptosis in the striatum but was without effect on depletion of dopamine terminal markers. We propose that substance P mediates the apoptosis of some striatal neurons via the intrastriatal activation of nitric oxide synthesis. In contrast, substance P may mediate damage of the dopamine terminals via an extrastriatal mechanism involving the substantia nigra and cortical glutamate release.

KEYWORDS: striatum; methamphetamine; neurotoxicity; apoptosis; substance P; neurokinin-1 receptor

Address for correspondence: Dr. Jesus A. Angulo, Department of Biological Sciences, Hunter College, 695 Park Avenue, New York, NY 10021. Voice: 212-772-5232; fax: 212-772-5230.
e-mail: angulo@genectr.hunter.cuny.edu

Ann. N.Y. Acad. Sci. 1074: 135–148 (2006). © 2006 New York Academy of Sciences.
doi: 10.1196/annals.1369.013

INTRODUCTION

Methamphetamine (METH) use is rapidly increasing in the United States posing a health problem because this psychostimulant causes damage in the brain. Evidence of the neurotoxic effects of METH on dopamine neurons was reported by Kogan *et al.*[1] and Seiden *et al.*[2] METH also causes damage to serotonergic neurons.[3,4] Unequivocal demonstration of the neuronal damage induced by METH came from immunocytochemical studies[5,6] and the application of the silver stain.[7] METH has been shown to cause inhibition of the enzyme tyrosine hydroxylase (TH)[1] and inactivation[8] and oligomerization[9] of striatal dopamine transporters. In addition to the neurochemical and morphological damage inflicted on the dopaminergic and serotonergic terminals, METH induces neuronal cell loss. Exposure to METH causes the loss of some neurons in the striatum and the cortex of rodents.[10–12] The damaging effects of METH in the brain may be mediated in part by the excessive release of glutamate. For example, antagonists of the NMDA (*N*-methyl-D-aspartate) subtype of glutamate receptor protect from METH-induced neural damage.[13] The overflow of striatal dopamine elicited by METH and required for neural damage, can be attenuated by antagonists of the NMDA receptor.[14] METH induces the overflow of glutamate in the striatum[15] and agents that abrogate this increase also decrease METH-induced depletion of striatal dopamine content.[16]

The excessive overflow of dopamine induced by METH is detrimental to neurons because of the production of reactive oxygen species. METH has been implicated in the generation of superoxide radicals via the auto-oxidation of catecholamines.[17,18] The auto-oxidation of dopamine is associated with increased activity of neuronal nitric oxide synthase and elevated levels of nitric oxide.[19] Pharmacological inhibition of nitric oxide synthase or deletion of the gene for this enzyme in neurons protects the striatum from METH.[20,21] In the striatum, the neuronal nitric oxide synthase is co-localized with the neurokinin-1 receptor (NK-1R) in 95% of the somatostatin interneurons.[22] Because we have observed that pharmacological blockade of the NK-1R protects the striatum of mice from METH,[23,24] we investigated the role of this receptor by ablation of the NK-1R-expressing interneurons of the striatum with the selective neurotoxin [sar,[9] met(O_2)[11]] substance p-saporin (SSP-SAP). We also report on the phenotype of striatal neuron lost in the aftermath of METH.

MATERIALS AND METHODS

Animals

Ten-week-old male ICR mice (Taconic, Germantown, NY) were housed individually on a 12-h light/dark cycle with food and water available *ad libitum*. All animals were habituated for 2 weeks prior to commencement of intraperitoneal (i.p.) drug administration or intrastriatal microinjection. All procedures of animal use were performed according to the *National Institutes of Health Guide for the Care and Use of Laboratory Animals* and were approved by the Institutional Animal Care and Use Committee at Hunter College of the City University of New York.

Drug Preparation and Administration

METH (30 mg/kg of body weight) (Sigma, St. Louis, MO) was dissolved in phosphate-buffered saline (PBS), pH 7.6, and administered as a single i.p. injection to 10- or 13-week-old (3 weeks after intrastriatal microinjection) ICR mice (Taconic). The NK-1R antagonist, WIN 51,708 (Sigma/RBI, St. Louis), was dissolved in 45% 2-hydroxylpropyl-β-cyclodextrin (Sigma/RBI) and PBS (1:4) and administered i.p. 30 min prior to METH treatment. SAP (Advance Targeting Systems, San Diego, CA) and SSP-SAP (Advance Targeting Systems) were dissolved in PBS and administered by intrastriatal injection. After treatment, (24 h or 3 days post-METH; 3 weeks postintrastriatal microinjection) animals were either euthanized by decapitation or were first anesthetized with i.p. injections of ketamine/acepromazine (100 mg/kg, 3 mg/kg of body weight) and then perfused transcardially with 30 mL of PBS with heparin followed by 30 mL of 4% paraformaldehyde in PBS. Brains were then either dissected out and immediately placed on dry ice or postfixed in 4% paraformaldehyde in PBS overnight and cryoprotected in 30% sucrose in PBS at 4°C. Tissue was then frozen and stored at –80°C until use.

Autoradiographic Analysis of Dopamine Transporter

Fresh frozen 20 μm coronal sections were dried in a dessicator and then incubated in 0.073 nM [^{125}I]RTI-121- (2200 Ci/mmol; New England Nuclear, Boston, MA) buffered solution (137 mM NaCl, 2.7 mM KCl, 10.14 mM Na2HPO4, 1.76 mM KH2PO4, 10 mM NaI) for 1 h at room temperature. Nonspecific binding was determined using 10 uM GBR-12909 (Sigma). After incubation, sections were washed twice with chilled buffer for 20 min and then quickly rinsed with chilled distilled water. Slides were allowed to air-dry overnight and exposed on Hyperfilm MP (Amersham Pharmacia, Piscataway, NJ) together with a [^{125}I] microscale. Binding of [^{125}I]RTI-121 was quantified by densitometry with use of a computer-based NIH image analysis system.

TH Western Blot

Striatal tissue was dissected and homogenized with lysis buffer (50 mM Tris-HCL pH 7.4, 150 mM NaCl, 320 mM sucrose, 5 mM HEPES, 1 mM EDTA,

1 mM EGTA, 1 mM PMSF, 1 mM DTT, 1% Inhibitor Cocktail [1.04 mM AEBSF, 0.8 uM aprotinin, 0.02 mM leupeptin, 0.04 mM bestatin, 0.015 mM pepstatin A, 0.014 mM E-64 (Sigma)]). Homogenates were centrifuged at 800 *g* for 5 min at 4°C. Supernatants were further centrifuged at 3000 *g*, and supernatants were then used for Western blot analysis. After protein concentration was determined by the Bradford assay, samples were denatured in Laemmli sample buffer containing 20% β-mercaptoethanol for 10 min at 85°C. Samples were then subjected to 10% SDS-PAGE gel, and proteins were transferred onto PVDF membranes. Membranes were blocked with 5% nonfat dry milk and probed with mouse anti-TH (1:1000, Chemicon, Temecula, CA) overnight at 4°C with gentle rocking. Membranes were washed with TBS and incubated with HRP-conjugated goat anti-mouse (1:1000; Santa Cruz Biotech, Santa Cruz, CA) for 1 h at room temperature. After a wash with TBS, proteins were detected with the use of the SuperSignal West Pico Chemilumescent Substrate (Pierce, Rockford, IL) and apposed onto Hyperfilm ECL film (Amersham Biosciences Corporation, Piscataway, NJ). For internal standards, membranes were stripped and reprobed with mouse anti-β-actin (1:10,000; Sigma). Densitometry was performed using a computerized image analysis system with NIH software. The relative density of each band was normalized against that of β-actin.

Intrastriatal Microinjections

Mice were anesthetized with inhaled isoflurane (2.5% for induction, 2% for maintenance) and their heads were placed in a stererotaxic frame (Model 5000; David Kopf Instruments, Tujunga, CA). A hole was drilled on the skull and a 25 gauge 2 uL Hamilton microinjection syringe was lowered into the striatum. Distance of injection sites from bregma was determined using a mouse brain atlas[25]: anteroposterior +0.5 mm; mediolateral ±2.0 mm; dorsventral –2.5 mm. The microinjection needle was left in position for 5 min prior to drug injection of 1.0 μL PBS (pH 7.4), 1.0 μL (4 ng/μL) of SAP (Advance Targeting Systems), or 1.0 μL (4 ng/μL) SSP-SAP (Advance Targeting Systems). Drugs were injected over a 10-min (~0.1 μL/min) period and the needle was left in place for an additional 5 min before removal from the striatum.

TUNEL Histochemistry

The method is as previously described.[26] In brief, fresh frozen 20 μm coronal sections were taken between bregma 0.38 mm ± 0.1 mm and fixed in 4% paraformaldehyd (PFA) for 30 min. After PBS wash, sections were immersed in 0.4% Triton-X-100 in PBS for 5–10 min at 70°C. Sections were washed and TUNEL (Terminal Deoxyncleotidyl Transferase-Mediated dUTP Nick End

Labeling) reactions (Roche Applied Science, Indianapolis, IN) were applied directly onto sections and incubated for 1 h in a humidified chamber. After TUNEL staining, sections were counterstained with DAPI. Stained sections were washed in PBS and coverslipped with Vectashield (Vector Laboratories, Burlingame, CA). Images were taken using Molecular Dynamics CLSM Multiprobe 2001 scanning confocal system.

Double-Labeling: Immunocytochemistry of NK-1R and TH

Dual staining of the NK-1R and TH was processed on striatal 20 μm coronal sections from 3 weeks postintrastriatal surgery. Nonspecific-binding sites are blocked with a combination of 5% normal goat serum (Vector Laboratories) and 5% normal donkey serum (Chemicon) in 0.2% Triton X-100 in PBS for 1 h. Sections were then incubated with a mixture of rabbit anti-NK-1R (1:1000; Chemicon) with 2% normal goat serum and mouse anti-TH (1:200; Chemicon) with 2% normal donkey serum in 0.2% Triton-X-100 in PBS overnight at 4°C. After washing with PBS, sections are incubated with a mixture of fluorescein isothiocyanate (FITC)-conjugated donkey anti-rabbit (1:1000; Chemicon) with 2% normal goat serum and Cy3-conjugated goat anti-mouse (1:1000; Chemicon) with 2% normal donkey serum in 0.2% Triton-X-100 in PBS for 1 h. After washing with PBS, sections are mounted on glass slides and overlaid with a coverslip using Vectashield (Vector Laboratories). Sections were viewed with the Nikon Eclipse E400 epifluorescent microscope (Melville, NY) and photographed with a Hamamatsu digital camera C4742-95 (Bridgewater, NJ).

Double-Labeling: Immunocytochemistry of NK-1R and TUNEL Staining

Dual staining of the NK-1R and TUNEL staining were processed on striatal 20 μm coronal sections from 3 weeks postintrastriatal surgery. Sections were rinsed in PBS and then immersed in heated 0.4% Triton-X-100 in PBS for 5 min and immediately washed in PBS. Staining of NK-1R and TUNEL labeling were then processed as described above. Sections were viewed with the Nikon Eclipse E400 epifluorescent microscope and photographed with a Hamamatsu digital camera C4742-95.

Cell Counts and Quantification

Coronal sections were taken from bregma 0.38 ± 0.1 mm. TUNEL-positive cells were quantified from 20-μm-thick coronal sections in an area of 0.26 mm^2 for each region of interest in the caudate-putamen (CPu) (dorsal-medial [DM], dorsal-lateral [DL], ventral-medial [VM], and ventral-lateral [VL]).[26]

Statistical Analysis

Analysis was performed from mean ± SEM. Differences between groups were analyzed by ANOVA followed by *post hoc* comparison using Fisher's protected least significance test. The significance criterion is set at $P < 0.05$.

RESULTS

Pharmacological Blockade of the NK-1R Protects from METH

A bolus dose of METH (30 mg/kg, i.p.) induces significant loss of dopamine terminal markers: dopamine transporters (FIG. 1, receptor autoradiography) and TH (FIG. 2, Western blots) 3 days after the injection. To assess the role of the NK-1Rs in these depletions, we treated the mice 30 min before the METH bolus with a systemic injection of the nonpeptide NK-1R antagonist WIN-51,708 (5 mg/kg, i.p.). Pretreatment with WIN-51,708 dramatically attenuated METH-induced depletions of both striatal dopamine transporters and TH (FIGS. 1 and 2, respectively) and also inhibited the induction of glial fibrillary acidic protein by METH in the striatal astrocytes (data not shown). These results demonstrate that blocking the NK-1R attenuates the METH-induced toxicity of the dopamine terminals of the striatum.

We have assessed METH-induced striatal apoptosis by the TUNEL assay. Unlike toxicity of the dopamine terminals that reaches a peak at day 3 post-METH, striatal apoptosis reaches a peak at 24 h after a bolus injection of METH (30 mg/kg).[26] METH induces TUNEL staining in approximately 25% of the

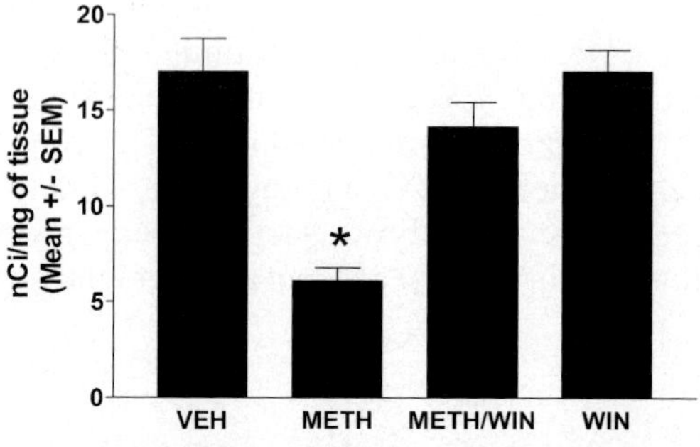

FIGURE 1. The NK-1R antagonist WIN-51,708 (WIN) prevents METH-induced reduction of striatal dopamine transporter sites at day 3 post- METH (autoradiographic study). The mice ($n = 6$) received one injection of METH (30 mg/kg, i.p.). A separate group received WIN (5 mg/kg, i.p.) 30 min prior to METH. Binding of [^{125}I]RTI-121 to striatal dopamine transporter sites was quantitated by image analysis of X ray autoradiograms. VEH, vehicle; SEM, standard error of the mean values. $^{*}P < 0.05$ (ANOVA).

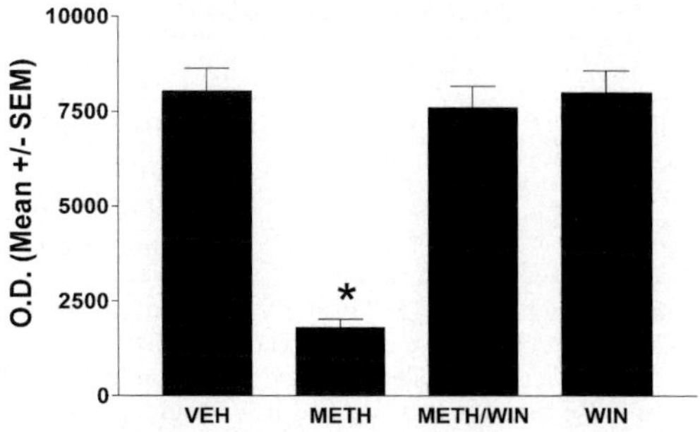

FIGURE 2. Pharmacological blockade of the NK-1Rs with WIN-51,708 (WIN, 5 mg/kg) prevents METH-induced reduction of TH in the striatum at day 3 post-METH (Western blot analysis). The mice were treated as described in the legend to FIGURE 1. SEM, standard error of the mean values. $^{*}P < 0.05$ (ANOVA).

striatal neurons (FIG. 3). Treatment with WIN-51,708 (5 mg/kg) 30 min before METH attenuated this striatal apoptosis (FIG. 3). We have found that 5 mg/kg of WIN-51,708 is the most effective dose to attenuate both METH-induced apoptosis and dopamine terminal toxicity (data not shown). To estimate the number of striatal neurons undergoing apoptosis, we combined TUNEL and NeuN (a neuronal specific marker) immunofluorescence. An overlay of the two chromophores demonstrates that nearly all TUNEL-positive cells are also positive for NeuN, indicating that METH induces apoptosis principally in the striatal neurons (*Neuroscience*, submitted). These results indicate that in addition to preventing dopamine terminal loss, blocking NK-1Rs significantly attenuates the apoptosis of some striatal neurons.

Because the striatum is composed of various kinds of neurons, to determine the phenotype of the neurons undergoing apoptosis, we combined TUNEL

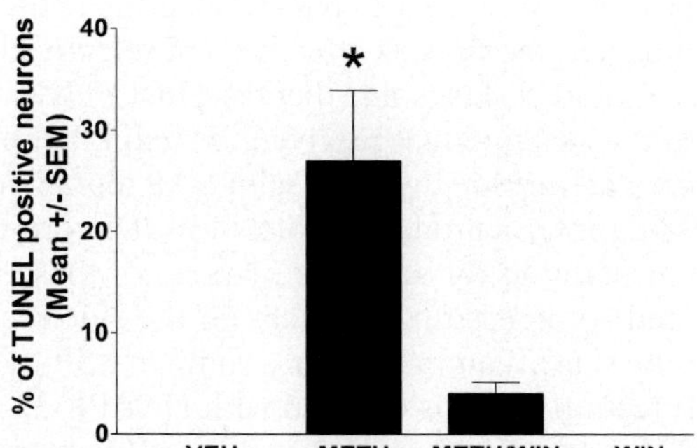

FIGURE 3. Pretreatment with WIN-51,708 (5 mg/kg, i.p.) attenuates METH-induced apoptosis in the striatum. METH was injected i.p. at a dose of 30 mg/kg. Apoptosis was assessed at 24 h post-METH by TUNEL. SEM, standard error of the mean values. $^{*}P <$ 0.05 compared to METH.

TABLE 1. Phenotype of striatal neurons killed by METH[a]

Type of Neuron	% of total	Marker	% ablated
Striatonigral/striatopallidal	90[a]	DARPP-32	20
Cholinergic	<2[b]	ChAT	30
GABA-parvalbumin	3-5[c]	Parvalbumin	50
Somatostatin/NOS/NPY	1-2[d]	Somatostatin	0

[a]The mice received one injection of METH (30 mg/kg, i.p.) and were sacrificed 24 h after the injection. Serial sections of striatal tissue from controls and METH-treated animals were stained with antibodies against choline acetyltransferase, somatostatin, parvalbumin, and DARPP-32. The number of cells positive for any of these markers was counted in both groups. The amount of cell death is expressed as percent of the total number of neurons in a given population.

NOTE: DARPP-32, dopamine- and cAMP-regulated phosphoprotein, of apparent Mr 32000; ChAT, choline acetyltransferase; [a]Wilson and Kawaguchi[38]; [b]Bolam *et al.* [39]; [c]Kita *et al.* [40]; [d]Kawaguchi *et al.*[34]

with immunofluorescence for DARPP-32 (dopamine- and cAMP-regulated phosphoprotein, of apparent Mr 32000) (projection neurons), choline acetyltransferase (cholinergic interneurons), somatostatin (somatostatin/ neuropeptide Y (NPY)/nitric oxide synthase (NOS) interneurons), and parvalbumin (γ-aminobutyric acid [GABA]-parvalbumin interneurons). We found that approximately 20% of the projection neurons are ablated by METH. Of the interneurons, 30% of the cholinergic and 50% of the GABA-parvalbumin is lost. Interestingly, the somatostatin/NPY/NOS interneurons are refractory to METH (TABLE 1).

Ablation of Striatal NK-1R-Expressing Interneurons with SSP-SAP

We asked if removal of the cells that express the NK-1Rs would have any effect on METH-induced striatal neuron apoptosis. For this study, a neurotoxin, SSP-SAP, which selectively eliminates NK-1R-bearing neurons was used. We first ensured that this neurotoxin was effective and selective by immunohistochemical methods. FIGURE 4 shows that there is a loss of NK-1R immunoreactivity in the side of the striatum that received the toxin, but no loss of NK-1R staining in the contralateral side, injected with SAP alone. To emphasize that all NK-1R-expressing interneurons are ablated in the core of the lesion, we showed that immunostaining for selective markers of these neurons, choline acetyltransferase and somatostatin, is absent on the side receiving the injection of SSP-SAP. In sharp contrast, after a similar SSP-SAP injection, the majority of the projection neurons (stained with DARPP-32 and representing approximately 90% of all striatal neurons) and GABA interneurons (GABA-parvalbumin) are spared (*Neuroscience*, submitted).

Next we administered a high dose of METH (30 mg/kg) to mice 3 weeks after they had received SSP-SAP. After 24 h they were euthanized and alternate serial sections were processed for TUNEL and for NK-1R immunostaining (on

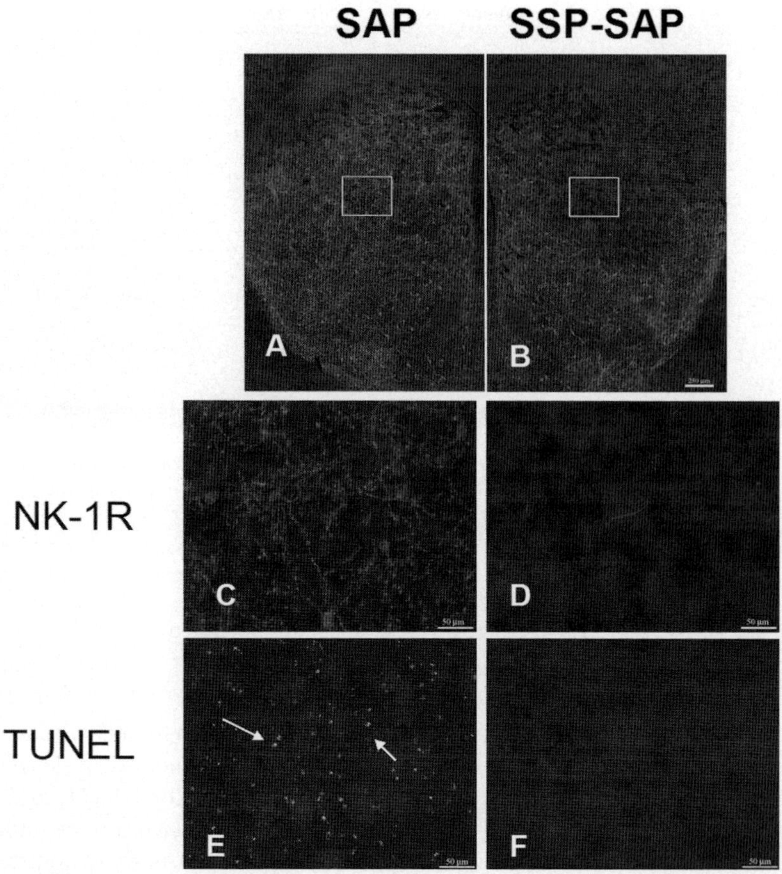

FIGURE 4. Intrastriatal injection of SSP-SAP (**B**) depletes immunostaining for the NK-1Rs (**D**) rendering the striatal tissue resistant to METH-induced apoptosis (TUNEL, **F**). The contralateral side that received SAP (**A**), retains NK-1R immunoreactivity (**C**) and remains vulnerable to METH (**E**). The mice ($n = 6$) received one intrastriatal injection of SSP-SAP or just SAP in the contralateral striatum. The animals received METH (30 mg/kg, i.p.) 3 weeks after the intrastriatal injection of SSP-SAP and were sacrificed 24 h after METH. NK-1Rs were visualized by immunofluorescence with an antibody conjugated to Cy3.

the same section). FIGURE 4 indicates that SSP-SAP had effectively eliminated NK-1R immunoreactivity. Importantly, in the absence of NK-1R-positive immunostaining, there was no detectable METH-induced apoptosis. In contrast, on the contralateral control side injected with SAP, there was little loss of NK-1R immunostaining but there was considerable apoptosis (FIG. 4).

In the light of these results, we hypothesized that ablation of the NK-1R-expressing interneurons would protect the dopamine terminals from METH. To

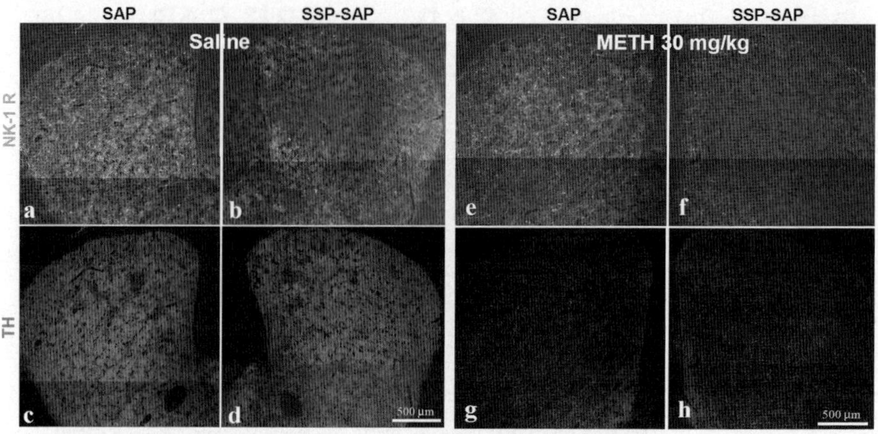

FIGURE 5. Ablation of striatal NK-1R-expressing interneurons does not prevent METH-induced depletion of TH. The mice ($n = 6$) received an intrastriatal injection of SSP-SAP into one side and SAP into the contralateral side. Then, 3 weeks later, the mice received a single injection of METH (30 mg/kg, i.p.) and were sacrificed 3 days after METH. Striatal sections were processed for NK-1R and TH immunofluorescence in the same section. Note that SSP-SAP abolishes NK-1R staining without affecting staining for TH (b and d). NK-1Rs were visualized with an antibody conjugated to FITC (a, b, e & f) and TH with Cy3 (c, d, g & h).

test this hypothesis, we administered METH (30 mg/kg) to mice 3 weeks after the intrastriatal injection of SSP-SAP. After 3 days, the mice were sacrificed and serial sections through the striatum were processed for NK-1R and TH immunostaining. The SSP-SAP injection eliminated NK-1R immunostaining without affecting immunostaining for TH (FIG. 5). However, in sharp contrast to the apoptosis, removal of the NK-1R-expressing interneurons failed to preserve immunostaining for TH in the group receiving METH (FIG. 5).

DISCUSSION

The data demonstrate that substance P signaling through the striatal NK-1R triggers the activation of a neurodegenerative cascade in the presence of METH. The apoptosis of some striatal neurons induced by METH requires the NK-1R-expressing interneurons because ablation of these neurons with SSP-SAP prevents the apoptosis. However, the toxicity of the dopamine terminals induced by METH can be attenuated by pretreatment with NK-1R antagonists,[23] but interestingly, does not require the presence of the NK-1R-bearing interneurons. This observation suggests that substance P may affect the METH-induced glutamate overflow in the striatum.

In the striatum, various lines of evidence point toward a connection between substance P and glutamate transmission. First, our results show that substance

P signals METH-induced damage of both the striatal dopamine terminals and some striatal neurons. Second, pharmacological studies demonstrate that blockade of the NMDA subtype of glutamate receptor protects the striatum from METH.[13,27] Third, the activity of the striatal-nigral-cortical loop regulates METH-induced glutamate release in the striatum and dopamine toxicity.[28] Finally, preprotachykinin-A knockout mice (lacking substance P) show resistance to kainic-acid-induced cell death in the hippocampus.[29] We hypothesize that pharmacological blockade of the NK-1R will attenuate NMDA-induced cell death and dopamine terminal toxicity in the striatum because an NK-1R antagonist protects both pre- and postsynaptic sites from METH-induced damage. Substance P may have a dual role in signaling degeneration in the striatum in the presence of METH. For example, on the one hand, substance P may activate nitric oxide formation via an intrastriatal mechanism while, on the other hand, substance P may activate striatal glutamate release via an extrastriatal mechanism through the substantia nigra.

Identifying the phenotype of the striatal neurons killed by METH is very important because subpopulations of striatal neurons affect differently the output of the basal ganglia. Our data suggest that approximately half of the GABA-parvalbumin interneurons of the dorsal striatum are killed by METH. These interneurons have a high content of GABA[30] and receive glutamatergic excitation from the cortex.[31] Thus, in the aftermath of cortical transmission these interneurons exert inhibition on striatal neurons via GABA, and it is noteworthy that METH ablates nearly half of this population of interneuron in the dorsal striatum. We demonstrate here that another population of striatal interneuron impacted by METH is the cholinergic interneuron. These interneurons affect the output of the projection neurons. For example, cholinergic transmission augments striatal dopamine release[32] and increases the responses of the medium spiny projection neurons to glutamate.[33] Because the GABA-parvalbumin interneurons mediate inhibition and the cholinergic interneurons facilitate excitation, and because both populations show deficits in the aftermath of METH, it would appear that the two effects cancel each other out. However, the post-METH striatum has the interneuron balance skewed in favor of transmission by the somatostatin/NPY/NOS interneurons because the latter population is refractory to METH. The nitric oxide made by these interneurons is known to increase the release of glutamate and dopamine in the striatum.[34]

In addition to the loss of some interneurons, METH also induces the loss of some projection neurons. The substantia nigra and the globus pallidum are targets of striatal projection neurons that exert inhibition via $GABA_A$ receptors.[35] Moreover, the recurrent collaterals within the striatum of the GABAergic medium spiny neurons provide the substrate for the mutual inhibition between these neurons.[36,37] Thus, the ablation of some projection neurons in the aftermath of METH could be interpreted to result in attenuation of inhibition within the striatum and in the targets of the projection neurons. More work is needed to describe the functional state of striatal neurons in the aftermath of METH.

In conclusion, our results demonstrate a role for the striatal neuropeptide substance P and its receptor in the neurodegenerative cascade induced by METH affecting the striatal dopamine terminals and some striatal neurons. More work in needed to describe the mechanism by which substance P signals METH-induced striatal injury, the functional state of the striatum in the aftermath of METH, and recovery from METH.

ACKNOWLEDGMENTS

This work was supported by a "Specialized Neuroscience Research Program" grant NS41073 from the *National Institute for Neurological Disorders and Stroke*. Support for the research infrastructure at Hunter College has come from a "Research Centers in Minority Institutions" award to Hunter College.

REFERENCES

1. KOGAN, F.J., W.K. NICHOLS & J.W. GIBB. 1976. Influence of methamphetamine on nigral and striatal tyrosine hydroxylase activity and on striatal dopamine levels. Eur. J. Pharmacol. **36**: 363–371.
2. SEIDEN, L.S., M.W. FISCHMAN & C.R. SCHUSTER. 1976. Long-term methamphetamine induced changes in brain catecholamines in tolerant rhesus monkeys. Drug Alcohol Depend. **1**: 215–219.
3. HOTCHKISS, A.J. & J.W. GIBB. 1980. Long-term effects of multiple doses of methamphetamine on tryptophan hydroxylase and tyrosine hydroxylase activity in rat brain. J. Pharmacol. Exp. Ther. **214**: 257–262.
4. RICAURTE, G.A., C.R. SCHUSTER & L.S. SEIDEN. 1980. Long-term effects of repeated methylamphetamine administration on dopamine and serotonin neurons in the rat brain: a regional study. Brain Res. **193**: 153–163.
5. AXT, K.J. & M.E. MOLLIVER. 1991. Immunocytochemical evidence for methamphetamine-induced serotonergic axon loss in the rat brain. Synapse **9**: 302–313.
6. ELLISON, G., M.S. EISON, H.S. HUBERMAN, *et al.* 1978. Long-term changes in dopaminergic innervation of caudate nucleus after continuous amphetamine administration. Science **201**: 276–278.
7. RICAURTE, G.A., R.W. GUILLERY, L.S. SEIDEN, *et al.* 1982. Dopamine nerve terminal degeneration produced by high doses of methylamphetamine in the rat brain. Brain Res. **235**: 93–103.
8. FLECKENSTEIN, A.E., R.R. METZGER, D.G. WILKINS, *et al.* 1997. Rapid and reversible effects of methamphetamine on dopamine transporters. J. Pharmacol. Exp. Ther. **282**: 834–838.
9. BAUCUM, A.J. II, K.S. RAU, E.L. RIDDLE, *et al.* 2004. Methamphetamine increases dopamine transporter higher molecular weight complex formation via

a dopamine- and hyperthermia-associated mechanism. J. Neurosci. **24**: 3436–3443.
10. Pu, C., H.W. Broening & C.V. Vorhees. 1996. Effect of methamphetamine on glutamate-positive neurons in the adult and developing rat somatosensory cortex. Synapse **23**: 328–334.
11. Eisch, A.J. & J.F. Marshall. 1998. Methamphetamine neurotoxicity: dissociation of striatal dopamine terminal damage from parietal cortical cell body injury. Synapse **30**: 433–445.
12. Deng, X., Y. Wang, J. Chou, *et al.* 2001. Methamphetamine causes widespread apoptosis in the mouse brain: evidence from using an improved TUNEL histochemical method. Brain Res. Mol. Brain Res. **93**: 64–69.
13. Sonsalla, P.K., D.E. Riordan & R.E. Heikkila. 1991. Competitive and noncompetitive antagonists at N-methyl-D-aspartate receptors protect against methamphetamine-induced dopaminergic damage in mice. J. Pharmacol. Exp. Ther. **256**: 506–512.
14. O'Dell, S.J., F.B. Weihmuller & J.F. Marshall. 1993. Methamphetamine-induced dopamine overflow and injury to striatal dopamine terminals: attenuation by dopamine D1 or D2 antagonists. J. Neurochem. **60**: 1792–1799.
15. Nash, J.F. & B.K. Yamamoto. 1992. Methamphetamine neurotoxicity and striatal glutamate release: comparison to 3,4-methylenedioxymethamphetamine. Brain Res. **581**: 237–243.
16. Stephans, S.E. & B.K. Yamamoto. 1994. Methamphetamine-induced neurotoxicity: roles for glutamate and dopamine efflux. Synapse **17**: 203–209.
17. Fridovich, I. 1983. Superoxide radical: an endogenous toxicant. Annu. Rev. Pharmacol. Toxicol. **23**: 239–257.
18. Fridovich, I. 1986. Biological effects of the superoxide radical. Arch. Biochem. Biophys. **247**: 1–11.
19. Cadet, J.L. & C. Brannock. 1998. Free radicals and the pathobiology of brain dopamine systems. Neurochem. Int. **32**: 117–131.
20. Itzhak, Y. & S.F. Ali. 1996. The neuronal nitric oxide synthase inhibitor, 7-nitroindazole, protects against methamphetamine-induced neurotoxicity in vivo. J. Neurochem. **67**: 1770–1773.
21. Imam, S.Z., G.D. Newport, Y. Itzhak, *et al.* 2001. Peroxynitrite plays a role in methamphetamine-induced dopaminergic neurotoxicity: evidence from mice lacking neuronal nitric oxide synthase gene or overexpressing copper-zinc superoxide dismutase. J. Neurochem. **76**: 745–749.
22. Li, J.L., T. Kaneko & N. Mizuno. 2001. Colocalization of neuronal nitric oxide synthase and neurokinin-1 receptor in striatal interneurons in the rat. Neurosci. Lett. **310**: 109–112.
23. Yu, J., J.L. Cadet & J.A. Angulo. 2002. Neurokinin-1 (NK-1) receptor antagonists abrogate methamphetamine-induced striatal dopaminergic neurotoxicity in the murine brain. J. Neurochem. **83**: 613–622.
24. Yu, J., J. Wang, J.L. Cadet, *et al.* 2004. Histological evidence supporting a role for the striatal neurokinin-1 receptor in methamphetamine-induced neurotoxicity in the mouse brain. Brain Res. **1007**: 124–131.
25. Franklin, K.B.J. & G. Paxinos. 1997. The Mouse Brain in Stereotaxic Coordinates. Academic Press. San Diego.
26. Zhu, J.P.Q., W. Xu & J.A. Angulo. 2005. Disparity in the temporal appearance of methamphetamine-induced apoptosis and depletion of dopamine terminal markers in the striatum of mice. Brain Res. **1049**: 171–181.

27. PU, C. & C.V. VORHEES. 1995. Protective effects of MK-801 on methamphetamine-induced depletion of dopaminergic and serotonergic terminals and striatal astrocytic response: an immunohistochemical study. Synapse **19**: 97–104.
28. MARK, K.A., J.J. SOGHOMONIAN & B.K. YAMAMOTO. 2004. High-dose methamphetamine acutely activates the striatonigral pathway to increase striatal glutamate and mediate long-term dopamine toxicity. J. Neurosci. **24**: 11449–11456.
29. LIU, H., Y. CAO, A.I. BASBAUM, *et al.* 1999. Resistance to excitotoxin-induced seizures and neuronal death in mice lacking the preprotachykinin A gene. Proc. Natl. Acad. Sci. USA **96**: 12096–12101.
30. BOLAM, J.P., D.J. CLARKE, A.D. SMITH, *et al.* 1983. A type of aspiny neuron in the rat neostriatum accumulates [3H]gamma-aminobutyric acid: combination of Golgi-staining, autoradiography, and electron microscopy. J. Comp. Neurol. **213**: 121–134.
31. KOOS, T. & J.M. TEPPER. 1999. Inhibitory control of neostriatal projection neurons by GABAergic interneurons. Nat. Neurosci. **2**: 467–472.
32. ZHOU, F.M., Y. LIANG & J.A. DANI. 2001. Endogenous nicotinic cholinergic activity regulates dopamine release in the striatum. Nat. Neurosci. **4**: 1224–1229.
33. CALABRESI, P., D. CENTONZE, P. GUBELLINI, *et al.* 1998. Endogenous ACh enhances striatal NMDA-responses via M1-like muscarinic receptors and PKC activation. Eur. J. Neurosci. **10**: 2887–2895.
34. KAWAGUCHI, Y., C.J. WILSON, S.J. AUGOOD, *et al.* 1995. Striatal interneurones: chemical, physiological and morphological characterization. Trends Neurosci. **18**: 527–535.
35. PRECHT, W. & M. YOSHIDA. 1971. Blockage of caudate-evoked inhibition of neurons in the substantia nigra by picrotoxin. Brain Res. **32**: 229–233.
36. WILSON, C.J. & P.M. GROVES. 1980. Fine structure and synaptic connections of the common spiny neuron of the rat neostriatum: a study employing intracellular inject of horseradish peroxidase. J. Comp. Neurol. **194**: 599–615.
37. YUNG, K.K., A.D. SMITH, A.I. LEVEY, *et al.* 1996. Synaptic connections between spiny neurons of the direct and indirect pathways in the neostriatum of the rat: evidence from dopamine receptor and neuropeptide immunostaining. Eur. J. Neurosci. **8**: 861–869.
38. WILSON, C.J. & Y. KAWAGUCHI. 1996. The origins of two-state spontaneous membrane potential fluctuations of neostriatal spiny neurons. J. Neurosci. **16**: 2397–2410.
39. BOLAM, J.P., B.H. WAINER & A.D. SMITH. 1984. Characterization of cholinergic neurons in the rat neostriatum. A combination of choline acetyltransferase immunocytochemistry, Golgi-impregnation and electron microscopy. Neuroscience **12**: 711–718.
40. KITA, H., T. KOSAKA & C.W. HEIZMANN. 1990. Parvalbumin-immunoreactive neurons in the rat neostriatum: a light and electron microscopic study. Brain Res. **536**: 1–15.

Effects of Methamphetamine on the Cerebellar Cortex

A Preliminary Study

MICHELA FERRUCCI,[a] CARLA L. BUSCETI,[b] ALESSANDRA FALLENI,[a] FILIPPO S. GIORGI,[a,c] STEFANO RUGGIERI,[b,d] AND FRANCESCO FORNAI[a,b]

[a]*Department of Human Morphology and Applied Biology, University of Pisa, Pisa, 56126 Italy*

[b]*Laboratory of Neurobiology of Movement Disorders, IRCCS INM Neuromed, 86077 Pozzilli, Isernia, Italy*

[c]*Department of Neuroscience, University of Pisa, 56126 Pisa, Italy*

[d]*University of Rome "La Sapienza," 00185 Rome, Italy*

ABSTRACT: Methamphetamine (METH) targets monoamine nerve terminals and produces motor effects, which are related to changes in catecholamine activity within the basal ganglia. Cerebellum plays an important role in motor control, nonetheless only a few studies investigated the effects of METH in this area. In this article, we report preliminary results on protein expression in the cerebellum following METH administration. In particular, we focused on the rate-limiting catecholamine-synthesizing enzyme tyrosine hydroxylase (TH). By using immunoblotting, we found that METH administration produces a dose-dependent increase of TH within the cerebellar cortex of mice, which is opposite to the decrease of TH within the striatum. Further investigations are needed in order to determine the time course, the cerebellar regions, the cellular (and subcellular) compartments, and the functional role related to these effects.

KEYWORDS: tyrosine hydroxylase; Western blot; cerebellum

INTRODUCTION

Methamphetamine (METH) is known to target monoamine systems where it produces a damage to dopaminergic (DA) and serotonergic (5-HT) nerve

Address for correspondence: Francesco Fornai, M.D., Department of Human Morphology and Applied Biology, University of Pisa, Via Roma, 55, I-56126 Pisa, Italy. Voice: +39-50-2218611; fax: +39-50-2218606.
e-mail: f.fornai@med.unipi.it

Ann. N.Y. Acad. Sci. 1074: 149–153 (2006). © 2006 New York Academy of Sciences.
doi: 10.1196/annals.1369.014

terminals depending on the animal species.[1–3] In particular, changes in catecholamine activity within the striatum are believed to be responsible for motor alterations produced by METH in rodents and primates,[3] and consist of a behavioral alteration and a Parkinsonian-like syndrome, which can occur as a consequence of the neurotoxic effect of METH on striatal DA terminals.[1,4,5] Nigrostriatal lesion produced by METH is typically featured by biochemical, morphological, and immunohistochemical changes within the striatal tissue, consisting of decreased DA levels and reduced immunostaining for typical DA markers, such as tyrosine hydroxylase (TH) and DA transporter (DAT).[3,6]

Despite the relevant role of the striatum in extrapyramidal motor control, there is another brain area, the cerebellum, which is known to play a significant effect on repetitive and stereotyped motor activity. The cerebellar cortex is reached by noradrenergic (NA) fibers, fully provided by locus coeruleus, and 5-HT nerve terminals deriving from raphe nuclei of the brain stem.[7,8] Furthermore, a few DA terminals arising directly from the ventral tegmental area were described in the cerebellar cortex of both rodents and primates.[9,10] However, despite the occurrence of a large variety of monoamine innervation, and the seminal role in motor control which make the cerebellum a potential target for METH, there are only a few studies investigating the effects of METH within the cerebellum.

Therefore, in the present article we decided to analyze the effect produced by METH in the cerebellar cortex in mice. This preliminary study reports semiquantitative immunoblotting of TH within cerebellar cortex and striatum following METH treatment.

METH INCREASES CEREBELLAR EXPRESSION OF TH

C57 Black mice ($n = 30$), 9–10 weeks old, were administered with various doses of METH, corresponding to either 5 mg/kg $\times$ 2 i.p., 2 h apart, or 5 mg/kg $\times$ 3 i.p., 2 h apart, in order to produce a mild or a frank striatal neurotoxicity, respectively.[4] Control mice received saline at the same time intervals as METH-treated mice. All mice were killed by cervical dislocation 5 days after METH administration and their brains assigned to immunoblotting assay for TH after dissection of striatum and cerebellar cortex. Blotting of TH protein carried out in striatal homogenates showed that METH produces a dose-dependent decrease in TH content, as shown by comparing lines corresponding to increasing doses of METH with control (FIG. 1 A). In contrast, immunoblotting for TH protein performed within cerebellar cortex of METH-treated mice showed a dose-dependent increase in TH expression, which becomes more evident after the higher dose of METH used (FIG. 1 B).

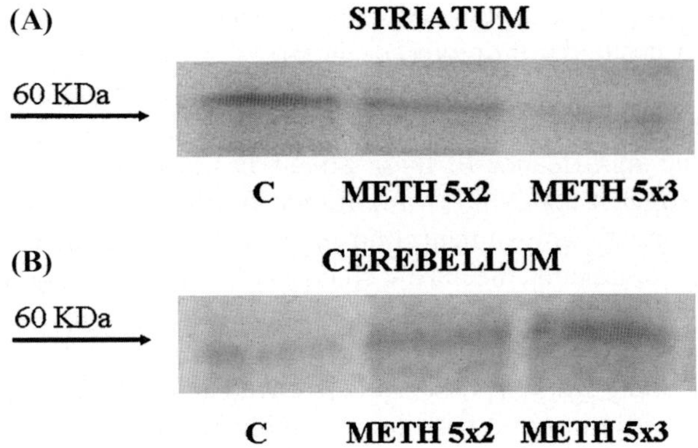

FIGURE 1. Immunoblotting of TH within striatal and cerebellar tissue. (**A**) Blotting of TH in striatal homogenates shows a progressive decrease in the signal intensity corresponding to treatment with increasing doses of METH. (**B**) The same regimen of METH administration produces an increase in TH expression within the cerebellar cortex, as revealed by the dose-dependent increased staining of the blotted TH following METH compared to control. C = control; METH 5×2 = METH 5 mg/kg ×2 i.p., 2 h apart; METH 5×3 = METH 5 mg/kg ×3 i.p., 2 h apart.

SUMMARY AND CONCLUSION

Our results demonstrate that METH does produce biochemical effects in the cerebellar cortex of mice since it increases the optical density of the blotted catecholamine-synthesizing enzyme TH. This effect is opposite to what induced in the dorsal striatum where the TH protein was found to be reduced. These effects of METH were both dose dependent.

A decrease in TH content observed in the striatal tissue is consistent with the loss of DA terminals, as shown by various studies using different markers (DA levels, TH and DAT immunohistochemistry, silver staining).[3,11] In contrast, the increase of TH immunoblotting within the cerebellum is not consistent with a loss of catecholamine nerve ending and it remains unexplained.

Only a very few studies analyzed the occurrence of morphological and/or functional alterations of the cerebellar cortex after METH administration. These studies analyzed the effects of METH on gene expression or electrophysiology of cerebellar neurons. In particular, within the Purkinje cells METH induces the early gene *c-fos*,[12] the corticosterone receptor,[13] and the aldolase C.[12]

Moreover, recent electrophysiological studies demonstrated that METH produces acute and long-term alteration in the efficacy of electrophysiological depression induced by GABA in the Purkinje cells.[14] These effects were attributed to short- and long-lasting changes in the NA transmission within the rat cerebellar cortex. Moreover, chronic METH administration produced a refractoriness to the electrophysiological effects induced by a selective NA uptake blocker desmethylimipramine (DMI).[15]

Our preliminary data joined with these previous findings indicate that METH can induce changes within the cerebellar cortex.

Although the significance of these effects has to be disclosed, in general these studies suggest that METH might modify cerebellar activity. Since the cerebellum is critical in movement control, repetitive motor patterns, and learning of motor automatisms, the plastic changes of cerebellum following METH might underlie long-term behavioral alterations. Interestingly, inherited cerebellar alterations are described in a variety of strains of mice (*weaver* mice, Rolling Mouse Nagoya, and *dilute-lethal* mice), in which the occurrence of motor disorders is associated with a comparable increase in TH immunoreactivity in cerebellar cortex,[16] suggesting that the expression pattern of cerebellar TH might be related to altered motor functions.

The increase in TH expression we found in the cerebellar cortex after METH leaves open many questions. For instance:

1. Does immunohistochemistry replicate the increase in TH immunostaining within the cerebellar cortex?
2. Is there a regional specificity (vermis, hemispheres) of the expression of TH within the cerebellum?
3. Which cellular and subcellular compartment are involved (fibers, cells)?
4. Is METH-induced TH expression a persistent cerebellar change?
5. Is the increase in TH expression accompanied by an increase in other catecholamine-synthesizing enzymes?
6. Is the increase in TH producing a change in the level of cerebellar catecholamines?

To ask these questions, various experiments, using histology and immunoelettronmicroscopy joined with biochemistry of the cerebellar cortex at various time intervals following METH, are needed.

REFERENCES

1. Ricaurte, G.A. *et al.* 1982. Dopamine nerve terminal degeneration produced by high doses of methylamphetamine in the rat brain. Brain Res. **235:** 93–103.
2. Woolverton, W.L. *et al.* 1989. Long-term effects of chronic methamphetamine administration in rhesus monkeys. Brain Res.**486:** 73–78.
3. O'Callaghan, J.P. & D.B. Miller. 1994. Neurotoxicity profiles of substituted amphetamines in the C57BL/6J mouse. J. Pharmacol. Exp. Ther. **270:** 741–751.
4. Fornai, F. *et al.* 1995. Norepinephrine loss exacerbates methamphetamine-induced striatal dopamine depletion in mice. Eur. J. Pharmacol. **283:** 99–102.
5. Hanson, G.R. *et al.* 2004. The methamphetamine experience: a NIDA partnership. Neuropharmacology **47:** 92–100.

6. KOGAN, F.J. *et al.* 1976. Influence of methamphetamine on nigral and striatal tyrosine hydroxylase activity and on striatal dopamine levels. Eur. J. Pharmacol. **36:** 363–371.
7. PAXINOS, G. 1995. The Rat Nervous System, 2nd ed. Academic Press, Inc. San Diego, CA.
8. PAXINOS, G. & J.K. MAI. 2004. The Human Nervous System, 2nd ed. Elsevier Academic Press. New York.
9. PANAGOPOULOS, N.T. *et al.* 1991. Dopaminergic innervation and binding in the rat cerebellum. Neurosci. Lett. **130:** 208–212.
10. MELCHITZKY, D.S. & D.A. LEWIS. 2000. Tyrosine hydroxylase- and dopamine transporter-immunoreactive axons in the primate cerebellum. Neuropsychopharmacology **22:** 466–472.
11. FORNAI, F. *et al.* 2004. Methamphetamine produces neuronal inclusions in the nigrostriatal system and in PC12 cells. J. Neurochem. **88:** 114–123.
12. HAMAMURA, M. *et al.* 1999. Differential decreases in c-fos and aldolase C mRNA expression in the rat cerebellum after repeated administration of methamphetamine. Mol. Brain Res. **64:** 119–131.
13. NUMACHI, Y. *et al.* 2000. Two inbred strains of rats, Fischer 344 and Lewis, showed differential behavior and brain expression of corticosterone receptor mRNA induced by methamphetamine. Ann. N. Y. Acad. Sci. **914:** 33–45.
14. JENG, C.H. & Y. WANG. 1998. Methamphetamine modulates GABA-induced electrophysiological depression by alternating noradrenergic actions in cerebellar Purkinje neurons. Psychopharmacology (Berl.) **136:** 132–138.
15. WANG, Y. *et al.* 2000. Chronic methamphetamine exposure decreases high affinity uptake function in norepinephrine afferents in the cerebellar cortex: an electrophysiological and electrochemical study. Psychopharmacology (Berl.) **39:** 2112–2123.
16. SAWADA, K. *et al.* 1999. Abnormal expression of tyrosine hydroxylase immunoreactivity in cerebellar cortex of ataxic mutant mice. Brain Res. **829:** 107–112.

Age-Dependent Effects of Methamphetamine on VMAT-2

KRISTI S. RAU, JANNINE G. TRUONG, DIANA G. WILKINS, ANNETTE E. FLECKENSTEIN, AND GLEN R. HANSON

Department of Pharmacology and Toxicology, University of Utah, Salt Lake City, Utah 84112, USA

ABSTRACT: Abuse of methamphetamine (METH) among adolescents and young adults is concerning since studies have demonstrated that multiple administrations of high-dose METH induce persistent dopaminergic deficits. METH has also been shown to reduce dopamine (DA) uptake by the vesicular monoamine transporter-2 (VMAT-2) and to reduce the amount of VMAT-2 protein in a purified vesicular fraction. VMAT-2 plays a critical role in the sequestration of DA in dopaminergic nerve terminals. This function is important since DA can oxidize rapidly to form highly reactive species. It is likely that disruption of this normal intracellular processing of DA contributes to oxidative sequences ultimately leading to persistent deficits. Interestingly, METH appears to be less toxic in adolescent rats compared to young adult rats. VMAT-2 is proposed to play an important role in the age-dependent difference. Since the effect of METH on the function and quantity of VMAT-2 has primarily been studied in young adult rats and since developmental changes in the dopaminergic system are reported to occur between adolescence and adulthood, it is important to determine if there is an age-dependent difference in response of VMAT-2 to METH.

KEYWORDS: methamphetamine; aging; dopamine; vesicular monoamine transporter-2; reactive oxygen species

INTRODUCTION

Abuse of psychoactive phenylethylamines, including methamphetamine (METH), is a major health problem worldwide. In the United States, it is estimated that nearly 1.3% of adolescents aged 12–17 and 5.3% of young adults aged 18–25 have illicitly used METH at least once in their lifetime.[1] This is of great concern since high-dose METH administration can cause persistent dopaminergic deficits associated with nerve terminal degeneration.

Address for correspondence: Glen R. Hanson, Ph.D., D.D.S., Department of Pharmacology and Toxicology, University of Utah, 30 South 2000 East, Skaggs Hall, Room 201, Salt Lake City, UT 84112. Voice: 801-581-3174; fax: 801-585-5111.
e-mail: glen.hanson@hsc.utah.edu

Ann. N.Y. Acad. Sci. 1074: 154–159 (2006).
doi: 10.1196/annals.1369.015

Mechanisms whereby METH-induced dopaminergic toxicity occurs are unclear, although dopamine (DA) is considered a critical mediator.[2–4] Previous reports have suggested that METH causes an excess of cytoplasmic DA accumulation which, in turn, gives rise to the formation of neurotoxic reactive oxygen species (ROS).[5–7] The vesicular monoamine transporter-2 (VMAT-2) is principally involved in regulating concentrations of cytoplasmic DA by sequestering free DA into synaptic vesicles thereby impacting levels of cytoplasmic and vesicular DA (i.e., amount of DA available for exocytotic release). Our laboratory previously demonstrated that METH reduces VMAT-2 function in a purified vesicular preparation,[8] an effect associated with a redistribution of VMAT-2 protein within dopaminergic nerve terminals from the subcellular vesicular fraction to a fraction that is not retained in the synaptosomal preparation.[9] These data suggest that by altering redistribution of VMAT-2 protein and its associated vesicles METH alters DA disposition within DA terminals resulting in neurotoxic effects.

The majority of studies investigating the potentially neurotoxic effects of METH have been performed primarily in adult animal models, consequently little is known about the influence of age on the response of VMAT-2 to METH. Because METH-induced toxicity may affect thousands of individuals, and because an understanding of its DA-involved toxicity may also be relevant to the study of other DA-involved disease processes, mechanism(s) whereby METH affects toxicity warrants investigation. In this article, the age-dependent differential effect of METH on VMAT-2 described previously[10] and the consequent implications will be reviewed.

MATERIALS AND METHODS

Animals and Treatment

Postnatal day (PND) 40 and PND 90 male Sprague-Dawley rats were maintained under conditions of controlled lighting and temperature as previously described.[10] These animals have been previously determined to be developmentally consistent with adolescent and young adult rats, respectively.[11] Food and water were available *ad libitum*. Either 1 h or 7 days following METH or saline treatments, animals were euthanized by decapitation. All procedures were conducted in accordance with the National Institutes of Health Guidelines and approved by the Institutional Animal Care and Use Committee at the University of Utah.

Tissue Preparation and Analysis

The striata dissected from treated animals were processed and separated into subcellular fractions that included whole synaptosomes and principal synaptosomal components, the plasmalemmal membrane-containing and the vesicular subcellular (presumably containing cytosolic elements) fractions. Western blot analysis was performed using these fractions and probed for VMAT-2 protein using a highly selective VMAT-2 antibody purchased from Chemicon International (Temecula, CA). Immunoreactive bands on the blots were measured by densitometry, and the intensity determined from each animal was averaged with other related values and compared with other treatment groups. The vesicular subcellular fraction was also evaluated for VMAT-2 activity. In addition, DA content or METH concentrations were measured in the whole striata taken from some of the animals. Details for tissue preparation and assays are described elsewhere.[10]

RESULTS

Data presented in TABLE 1 demonstrate greater VMAT-2 protein levels in the purified vesicular subcellular fraction of untreated PND 90 rats compared to untreated PND 40 animals. Levels of VMAT-2 protein did not significantly differ between the two age groups in either the plasmalemmal membrane-associated fraction or the whole synaptosomal fraction (TABLE 1).

Repeated injections of high-dose METH (4 injections; 5, 10, or 15 mg/kg, subcutaneous; 2-h intervals; with the 5 and 10 mg/kg doses determined such that striatal METH concentrations were relatively equivalent between the two age groups, see TABLE 2) were administered to PND 40 and PND 90 rats. Results presented in TABLE 2 demonstrate that 1 h following the last METH or saline injection, vesicular DA uptake, as assessed in a purified vesicular fraction, was significantly reduced in both PND 40 and PND 90 animals. Vesicular DA uptake remained significantly reduced 7 days post-injection in PND 90 rats but returned to control levels in PND 40 rats (TABLE 3). Likewise, striatal DA content was reduced in PND 90, but not in PND 40 rats, 7 day following METH treatment (TABLE 3).

TABLE 1. Densitometric analysis of striatal VMAT-2 immunoreactivity in the vesicular subcellular, plasmalemmal membrane, and whole synaptosomal fractions in untreated PND 40 and PND 90 rats

Group	Vesicular Subcellular Fraction	Plasmalemmal Membrane Fraction	Whole Synaptosomal Fraction
PND 40	570.9 ± 67.9	2,824.1 ± 229.9	7,811.7 ± 1,282.3
PND 90	1,824.6 ± 103.3*	2,921.4 ± 179.8	9,419.5 ± 1,091.5

Samples were prepared as described in Materials and Methods. Values are expressed as the means and 1 SEM calculated from the arbitrary units of densitometric determinations in six rats. *Indicates values significantly different from PND 40 rats.

TABLE 2. Effect of multiple injections of METH on striatal VMAT-2 activity in the purified vesicular subcellular fraction and on striatal METH concentrations in PND 40 and PND 90 rats 1 h after treatment

Group	Saline	METH 4 × 5 mg/kg	METH 4 × 10 mg/kg	METH 4 × 15 mg/kg
PND 40				
Vesicular DA uptake	163.7 ± 11.8	ND	90.32 ± 3.3*	81 ± 8.4*
Brain METH concentration	ND	ND	5.03 ± 0.38	10.70 ± 1.15
PND 90				
Vesicular DA uptake	257.2 ± 12.2#	91.5 ± 7.5*	ND	ND
Brain METH concentration	ND	4.31 ± 0.49	ND	ND

Animals were treated with 4 injections of saline (1 mL/kg/injection) or METH (see table for doses) at 2-h intervals and sacrificed 1 h following the last injection. Samples were prepared as described in Materials and Methods. Values are expressed as the means and ± 1 SEM of determinations in six rats. *Indicates values significantly different from age-matched saline-treated controls ($P \leq 0.05$). #Indicates values significantly different from saline-treated PND 40 rats ($P \leq 0.05$). Values that were not determined are indicated by ND.

DISCUSSION

Multiple injections of high-dose METH induce dopaminergic deficits via a mechanism that is not completely understood. DA, however, is thought to play a pivotal role.[2–4] It has been suggested that METH induces persistent DA deficits by causing an excess accumulation of unsequestered cytoplasmic DA which, in turn, gives rise to the formation of ROS.[5–7] It is possible that the increased formation of ROS overwhelms antioxidant systems of the neuron resulting in cytotoxic consequences. VMAT-2 is important for the se-

TABLE 3. Effect of multiple injections of METH on striatal VMAT-2 activity in the purified vesicular subcellular fraction and on striatal DA content 7 days after treatment in PND 40 and PND 90 rats

Group	Saline	METH 4 × 5 mg/kg	METH 4 × 10 mg/kg
PND 40			
Vesicular DA uptake	159.1 ± 14.3	ND	146.0 ± 15.9
Striatal DA concentration	83.6 ± 2.0	ND	71.4 ± 3.0
PND 90			
Vesicular DA uptake	347.2 ± 34.7#	241.6 ± 30.3*	99.3 ± 24.3*
Striatal DA concentration	110.7 ± 7.1#	63.1 ± 5.7*	17.3 ± 3.2*

Animals were treated with 4 injections of saline (1 mL/kg/injection) or METH (see table for doses) at 2-h intervals and sacrificed 7 days following the last injection. Samples were prepared as described in Materials and Methods. Values are expressed as the means and ± 1 SEM of determinations in six rats. *Indicates values significantly different from age-matched saline-treated controls ($P \leq 0.05$). #Indicates values significantly different from saline-treated PND 40 rats ($P \leq 0.05$). Values that were not determined are indicated by ND.

questration of cytosolic DA protecting this catecholamine from oxidation, and likely preventing excessive production of DA-related free radicals. Reduced function and/or quantity of VMAT-2 would presumably compromise normal functioning of the nerve terminal. Consistent with this hypothesis, this laboratory previously demonstrated that in a purified vesicular preparation, VMAT-2 function[8] and VMAT-2 protein levels[9] are rapidly reduced following multiple administrations of high-dose METH in rats. While these effects of METH on the dopaminergic system have primarily been studied in young adult rats (typically PND 60–90), it is important to study the impact of METH on adolescent rats (PND 40) in order to appreciate the possible consequences, both short- and long-term.

Interestingly, the amount of VMAT-2 protein measured by densitometric analysis of VMAT-2 Western blots demonstrated that adolescent animals (i.e., PND 40) had less VMAT-2 protein in the subcellular vesicular fraction compared to PND 90 (i.e., young adult) rats (TABLE 1). Basal DA content in this subcellular fraction was also lower in the adolescent rats compared to the young adult rats as illustrated in TABLE 3 and as previously reported.[10,12,13] These data suggest that older rats may have more VMAT-2 in the subcellular vesicular fraction in order to sequester the greater concentrations of striatal DA. As would be predicted based on the greater level of VMAT-2 protein in the vesicular fraction of PND 90 rats, basal vesicular DA uptake in saline-treated animals was also greater in the young adult rats compared to the adolescent rats (TABLE 2). It cannot be elucidated from these studies, however, whether older animals have more VMAT-2 per DA terminal and/or whether there is an age-dependent development of new terminals that contain VMAT-2.

In both PND 40 and PND 90 rats, multiple injections of METH reduced VMAT-2 uptake 1 h following the last METH injection (TABLE 2). Of significance is the finding that the magnitude of the METH-induced reduction was much greater in the older rats possibly suggesting the presence of a larger susceptible pool of VMAT-2 that develops with age. The METH-induced decrease in VMAT-2 uptake persisted 7 days following the last injection of METH in PND 90 rats. In contrast, in PND 40 rats the acute (1 h) reduction in vesicular uptake completely reversed to control levels 7 days post-injection. These data suggest the existence of at least three pools of VMAT-2: (a) VMAT-2 resistant to the acute and persistent effects of METH present in both age groups; (b) VMAT-2 in PND 40 rats resistant to the long-term but not the short-term effects of METH; and (c) VMAT-2 that develops with age and is susceptible to both the acute and persistent effects of METH.

Taken together, these data demonstrate age-related differential short- and long-term responses in vesicular DA uptake to METH. These findings may aid in understanding the mechanistic factors responsible for the age-related differences in the dopaminergic responses by adolescent and young adult rats elucidating the nature of METH-induced short- and long-term consequences. In addition, these findings may provide insight into possible mechanisms associated with DA-linked functions and neurological disorders, such as Parkinson's disease.

ACKNOWLEDGMENTS

This study was supported by Public Health Service Grants DA00869, DA11389, DA00378, and DA04222.

REFERENCES

1. SUBSTANCE ABUSE AND MENTAL HEALTH SERVICES ADMINISTRATION. 2004. Results from the 2003 National Survey on Drug Use and Health (NSDUH): National Findings. Series H-25, Department of Health and Human Services publication number SMA 04-3964, Office of Applied Studies, National Institutes of Health, Rockville, MD.
2. GIBB, J.W. & F.J. KOGAN. 1979. Influence of dopamine synthesis on methamphetamine-induced changes in striatal and adrenal tyrosine hydroxylase activity. Nauny-Schmiedebergs Arch. Pharmacol. **310:** 185–187.
3. SCHMIDT, C.J. & J.W. GIBB. 1985. Role of dopamine uptake carrier in the neurochemical response to methamphetamine: effects of amfonelic acid. Eur. J. Pharmacol. **109:** 73–80.
4. SONSALLA, P.K., J.W. GIBB & G.R. HANSON. 1986. Roles of D1 and D2 dopamine receptor subtypes in mediating the methamphetamine-induced changes in monoamine systems. J. Pharmacol. Exp. Ther. **283:** 932–937.
5. DE VITO, M.J. & G.C. WAGNER. 1989. Methamphetamine-induced neuronal damage: a possible role for free radicals. Neuropharmacology **28:** 1145–1150.
6. CUBELLS, J.F., S. RAYPORT, G. RAJENDRAN & D. SULZER. 1994. Methamphetamine neurotoxicity involves vacuolation of endocytic organelles and dopamine-dependent intracellular oxidative stress. J. Neurosci. **14:** 2260–2271.
7. CADET, J.L. & C. BRANNOCK. 1998. Free radicals and the pathobiology of brain dopamine systems. Neurochem. Int. **32:** 117–132.
8. BROWN, J.M., G.R. HANSON & A.E. FLECKENSTEIN. 2000. Methamphetamine rapidly decreases vesicular dopamine uptake. J. Neurochem. **74:** 2221–2223.
9. RIDDLE, E.L., M.K. TOPHAM, J.W. HAYCOCK, *et al.* 2002. Differential trafficking of the vesicular monoamine transporter-2 by methamphetamine and cocaine. Eur. J. Pharmacol. **449:** 71–74.
10. TRUONG, J.G., D.G. WILKINS, J. BAUDYS, *et al.* 2005. Age-dependent methamphetamine-induced alterations in vesicular monoamine transporter-2 function: implications for neurotoxicity. J. Pharmacol. Exp. Ther. **314:** 1087–1092.
11. OJEDA, S.R., W.W. ANDREWS, J.P. ADVIS & S.S. WHITE. 1980. Recent advances in the endocrinology of puberty. Endocr. Rev. **3:** 228–257.
12. NOMURA, Y., F. NAITOH & T. SEGAWA. 1976. Regional changes in monoamine content and uptake of the rat brain during postnatal development. Brain Res. **101:** 305–315.
13. GIORGI, O., G. DE MONTIS, M.L. PORCEDDU, *et al.* 1987. Developmental and age-related changes in D1-dopamine receptors and dopamine content in the rat striatum. Brain Res. **432:** 283–290.

Methamphetamine, Morphine, and Their Combination

Acute Changes in Striatal Dopaminergic Transmission Evaluated by Microdialysis in Awake Rats

FREDERICO C. PEREIRA,[a] ELITA LOURENÇO,[a] NUNO MILHAZES,[b] TERESA MORGADINHO,[a] CARLOS F. RIBEIRO,[a] SYED F. ALI,[c] AND TICE R. MACEDO[a]

[a]*Instituto de Farmacologia e Terapêutica, Medical School, University of Coimbra 3004-504, Portugal*

[b]*CEQOFFUP, Organic Chemistry Department, Faculty of Pharmacy, University of Porto 4050-047, Portugal*

[c]*Neurochemistry Laboratory, Division of Neurotoxicology, NCTR, Jefferson, Arkansas 72079-9502, USA*

ABSTRACT: The co-administration of methamphetamine (METH) and MOR (MOR)-like compounds is becoming increasingly popular among drug abusers. Recently, it was demonstrated that rats would self-inject METH–heroin combination and that this combination produced a greater rewarding effect than the identical doses of METH alone and it was further suggested that enhanced reward might underlie the popularity of this combination. However, there is null information on the effects of the MOR–METH combination on striatal dopaminergic transmission. In the present article, *in vivo* brain microdialysis was used to examine the effects of two METH doses (1 and 5 mg/kg, i.p.; [METH1: hyperlocomotion-inducing] and [METH5: stereotypy-inducing], respectively) and MOR (10 mg/kg, i.p. [MOR10]) either alone or in combination on dopamine (DA) and 3,4-dihydroxyphenylacetic acid (DOPAC) release in caudate putamen (CPu) in freely moving rats. METH1 evoked a transient threefold increase in DA overflow in only one-third of dosed rats. On the contrary, METH5 elicited a 11-fold increase in the extracellular DA levels 30 min after dosing and stayed significantly ($P < 0.05$) above control levels up to 1.5 h. On the other hand, MOR10 did not significantly change DA extracellular levels. MOR10–METH1 combination prolonged DA outflow for 1 h in all rats dosed without changing peak effect

Address for correspondence: Frederico C. Pereira, Instituto de Farmacologia e Terapêutica, Medical School, University of Coimbra, Rua Larga, Coimbra 3004-504, Portugal. Voice: 351-239857700; fax: 351-239823236.
e-mail: fredcp@ci.uc.pt

Ann. N.Y. Acad. Sci. 1074: 160–173 (2006). © 2006 New York Academy of Sciences.
doi: 10.1196/annals.1369.016

compared to METH1. On the other hand, MOR10–METH5 combination did not change the peak effect nor the DA outflow profile compared to METH5 alone. Consistently, there is a concentration-dependent decrease in DOPAC efflux evoked by METH: METH1 evoked a smaller decrease in DOPAC outflow showing a tendency for returning to basal values whereas METH5 kept DOPAC extracellular levels reduced throughout the experiment. Again, MOR10 did not significantly change DOPAC extracellular levels. MOR delayed the onset without changing METH effect on the DOPAC output. These findings provide suggestive evidence that MOR potentiated the increase in extracellular DA levels induced by a low dose of METH. Thus, this combination yields a profile of action that might underlie the reinforcing properties sought by drug addicts.

KEYWORDS: morphine–methamphetamine combination; caudate putamen; dopamine neurotransmission; microdialysis

INTRODUCTION

METH (METH) abuse has been associated with psychosis and damage to dopamine (DA) terminals resulting in potentially long-lasting effects.[1,2] Opioid μ-receptor agonists, such as MOR (MOR) and heroin are considered to have high dependence potential.[3] Although these two drugs have opposite pharmacological effects (amphetamines produce hypertension, tachycardia, arrhythmia, hyperpyrexia, mydriasis, whereas opiates induce hypotension, bradycardia, hypothermia, and pinpoint pupils), METH and MOR share the common feature of increasing extracellular concentration of DA in the striatal complex and precipitating addiction.[4–6] Polydrug abuse is a major problem around the world. Of particular interest is the incidence in concurrent use of amphetamines and opiates.[7,8] Amphetamine and MOR mixture produced greater euphoria than that produced by either drug alone in male non-dependent substance abusers. In contrast, this mixture lessened each side effects.[9] Recently, it was demonstrated that rats would self-inject METH–heroin combination and that this combination produced a greater rewarding effect than the identical doses of METH alone and it was further suggested that enhanced reward might underlie the popularity of this combination.[10] Also, behavioral studies have demonstrated that conditioned place preference for METH was enhanced in combination with MOR.[11] However, there is null information on the effects of the MOR–METH combination on brain dopaminergic chemistry. Therefore, the purpose of the present article was to investigate the effect of MOR–METH combination effect on nigrostriatal dopaminergic transmission. To this end, *in vivo* microdialysis was used to monitor changes in extracellular concentrations of DA and 3,4-dihydroxyphenylacetic acid (DOPAC) in the caudate putamen (CPu) in response to the combination of the opiate and the stimulant.

MATERIALS AND METHODS

Subjects

Adult male Sprague-Dawley rats (Charles River Laboratories Inc., Barcelona, Spain), weighing 250–380 g, were housed two per cage under controlled environmental conditions (12-h light/dark schedule, at room temperature of 21 ± 1°C) with food and water supplied *ad libitum* and subsequently housed individually after surgery. All experiments were performed under the rules of the European Convention on Animal Care.

Drugs and Dosage Regimen

Drugs were dissolved in physiological saline. All injections were given intraperitoneally (i.p.) in a volume of 1.0 mL/kg. METH was administered at two different doses (1 and 5 mg/kg; hyperlocomotion and stereotypy-inducing doses, respectively) while MOR was administered at a dose of 10 mg/kg. This dose was selected based on a recent study showing that a single exposure to 10 mg/kg MOR induced long-lasting hyporeactivity of caudate nucleus dopaminergic nerve terminals through μ receptors.[12] When MOR and METH were administered in combination, the two drugs were administered in two separate injections within approximately 30 s. Both drugs were administered at the identical doses used in the single drug studies. Control animals were injected with saline. METH–HCl was synthesized in the Organic Chemistry Department, University of Porto, Portugal. MOR–HCl (1%) was kindly gifted by University Hospital of Coimbra. DA and DOPAC were purchased from Sigma-Aldrich Fine Chemicals (St. Louis, MO) All other reagents were purchased from both Sigma-Aldrich and Merck (Darmstadt, Germany).

In Vivo *Microdialysis*

DA and DOPAC release in freely moving rats were measured by microdialysis. Rats were anesthetized with sodium pentobarbital and placed into a stereotaxic frame. The dorsal skull was exposed and a small hole was drilled to allow implantation of intracerebral guide cannula (CMA/12, Carnegie Medicine, Stockholm, Sweden) into the caudate (AP, +0.5; Lat, –3; DV, –3). The cannula was fixed to the skull with dental acrylic and two anchor screws. To avoid effects of surgery and anesthesia, the dialysis experiments were started 1 week after surgery. On the day of tests, animals were hand held and a 4.0 × 0.5 mm dialysis probe (CMA/12) was slowly inserted through the guide cannula into the CPu. The probes were perfused at 1.3 μL/min with a microperfusion pump

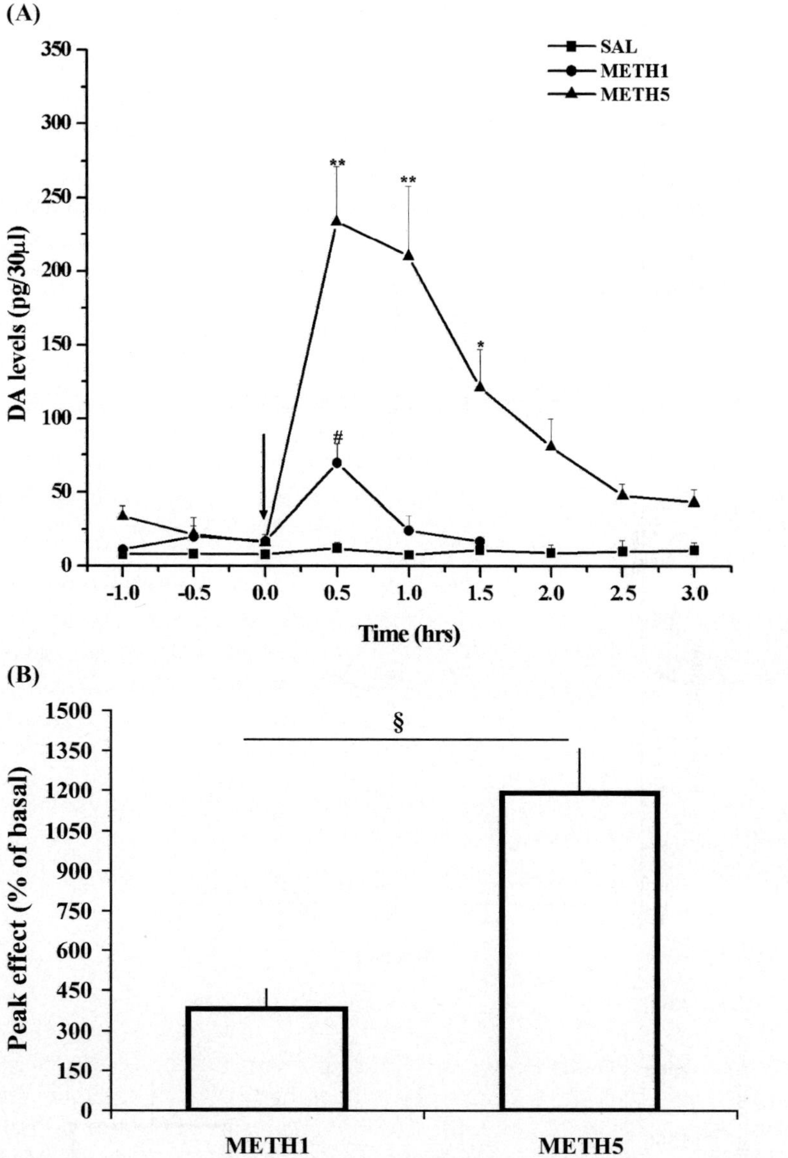

FIGURE 1. (**A**) The effect of METH on extracellular levels of DA in CPu. Extracellular levels of DA were measured in CPu by *in vivo* microdialysis following i.p. injections of 1, 5 mg/kg METH and saline [METH1 ($n = 2/6$), METH5 ($n = 7$), and SAL ($n = 4$), respectively] at the time point (0 h) indicated by the arrow. Each value is mean ± SEM (**B**) The effect of METH1 and METH5 on DA peak effect in CPu. Data are mean ± SEM and are expressed as percentage of the basal values. $^{\#,*}P < 0.05$ versus basal values from METH1 and METH5 groups, respectively; $^{**}P < 0.001$ versus basal values from METH5 group; $^{\S}P < 0.05$ METH1 compared to METH5.

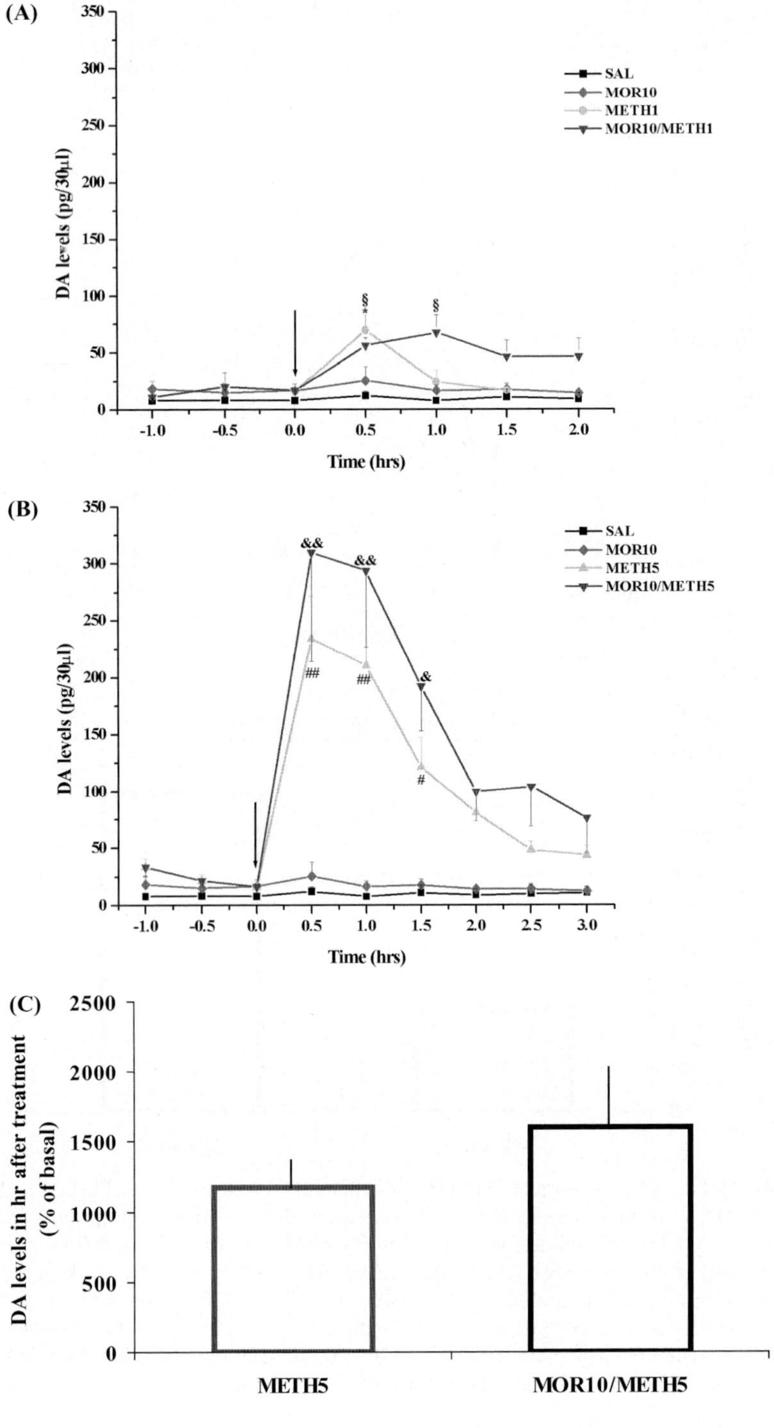
(A)
SAL
MOR10
METH1
MOR10/METH1
DA levels (pg/30μl)
Time (hrs)
(B)
SAL
MOR10
METH5
MOR10/METH5
DA levels (pg/30μl)
Time (hrs)
(C)
DA levels in hr after treatment (% of basal)
METH5
MOR10/METH5

(CMA/100) with artificial cerebrospinal fluid (ACSF) containing in (mM): 140 NaCl, 2.4 KCl, 2.4 $CaCl_2$, 1.0 $MgCl_2$, 1.2 Na_2HPO_4, 0.27 NaH_2PO_4 adjusted to pH 7.2. Dialysate samples were collected in 30-min intervals on ice and their content in DA and DOPAC was analyzed by HPLC-ED. Three samples were taken to establish baseline levels of extracellular DA and DOPAC before drug administration which ocurred ~5 h following probe insertion. Extracellular DA basal values for METH1 and MOR10/METH1 on one hand and METH5 and MOR10/METH5 on the other hand were pooled.

Measurement of Extracellular DA and DOPAC by HPLC-EC

Extracellular concentrations of DA and DOPAC were separated on a reverse-phase Supelcosil LC-18 (SUPELCO, Bellefonte, PA) (4.6 mm; 7.5 cm; 3 μM particle size) with a mobile phase (pH = 3.0) consisting of 0.07 M KH_2PO_4, 2.85 mM L-heptanesulfonic acid, 0.12 mM Na-EDTA, and 7% Methanol (v/v). A flow rate of 1.2 mL/min was mantained and detection of the chromatographed compounds achieved by using a glassy carbon working electrode set at 0.75 V. The settings of sensitivity used were 0.05 and 0.5 nA/V for DA and DOPAC, respectively. Thirty microliters were injected to chromatograph.

Statistical Analysis

Statistical analysis were performed applying one-way repeated measures ANOVAs to each drug condition with time as the repeated measures factor followed by post hoc comparison (Dunnett's multiple comparison test between groups). Student's two-tailed *t*-test was used for statistical comparisons between two drug conditions and one-way ANOVA followed by post hoc Bonferroni's test for comparisons between more than two drug conditions. Significant differences were defined at $P < 0.05$.

FIGURE 2. (**A**) The effect of METH1, MOR10, and their combination on extracellular levels of DA in CPu. Extracellular levels of DA were measured in CPu by *in vivo* microdialysis following i.p. injections of METH1, 10 mg/kg MOR (MOR10; $n = 5$), their combination (MOR10/METH1; $n = 4$), and SAL. (**B**) The effect of METH5, MOR10, and their combination on extracellular levels of DA in CPu. Extracellular levels of DA were measured in CPu by *in vivo* microdialysis following i.p. injections of METH5, MOR10, their combination (MOR10/METH5; $n = 7$), and SAL. Each value is mean ± SEM Time point (0 h) of injection is indicated by the arrow. (**C**) The effect of METH5 and MOR10/METH5 on mean levels of extracellular DA across the 1st hour in CPu. Data are mean ± SEM and are expressed as percentage of the basal values. $^{*,\S,\#,\&}P < 0.05$, $^{\#\#,\&\&}P < 0.001$ versus basal values from METH1, MOR10/METH1, METH5, and MOR10/METH5 groups, respectively. METH1 and METH5 groups are plotted as shown in FIGURE 1 A.

RESULTS

Extracellular DA Levels

METH-induced changes in extracellular DA levels were monitored by microdialysis after doses of 1 and 5 mg/kg i.p. (METH1 and METH5, respectively; FIG. 1 A). Administration of METH1 evoked a transient and modest release of DA in CPu in only two out of six dosed animals. Extracellular DA levels peaked 30 min after injection ($P < 0.05$) and returned to basal levels 1 h following treatment. On the contrary, METH5 induced a robust increase in extracellular CPu DA levels that peaked 30 min after dosing and stayed significantly ($P < 0.05$) above control levels up to 1.5 h. Although extracellular DA levels from 2 to 3 h following METH5 treatment were higher than basal levels, they did not reach significance. Extracellular levels of DA stayed constant throughout the experiment in the saline-treated animals. METH1 and METH5 peak effects are presented in FIGURE 1 B to facilitate comparison of dose–response relationships. METH5 produced an 11-fold increase in DA release, which was significantly higher than the threefold increase produced by METH1 ($P < 0.05$). MOR (10 mg/kg i.p.; MOR10) did not produce a detectable change from baseline in extracellular DA levels in rat CPu (FIG. 2 A). The combination of MOR10 and METH1 (MOR10/MERH1) evoked DA release in all treated rats ($n = 4$) that lasted longer than the one produced by METH1 alone (60 versus 30 min). Although extracellular DA levels from 90 to 120 min following MOR10/METH1 treatment were higher than basal levels, they did not reach significance. The combination of MOR10 and METH5 (MOR10/METH5) produced extracellular DA levels that were not significantly different than METH5 alone did (FIG. 2 B). Average extracellular DA levels over 1 h post-treatment are presented in FIGURE 2 C to facilitate comparison between METH5 and MOR10/METH5. This MOR/METH combination produced a 15-fold increase in DA release over 1 h following treatment which was not significantly different than the increase evoked by METH5 over the same period.

Extracellular DOPAC Levels

METH-induced changes in extracellular DOPAC levels were monitored by microdialysis after METH1 and METH5 treatments (FIG. 3 A). Administration of METH1 produced a significant decrease in dialysate DOPAC levels ($P < 0.05$) that started at 30 min, peaked at 1 h and showed a clear tendency to return to basal levels onwards. On the other hand, DOPAC levels showed a significant decrease peaking within 2 h following METH5 treatment and staying significantly decreased up to 3 h. The extracellular levels of DOPAC

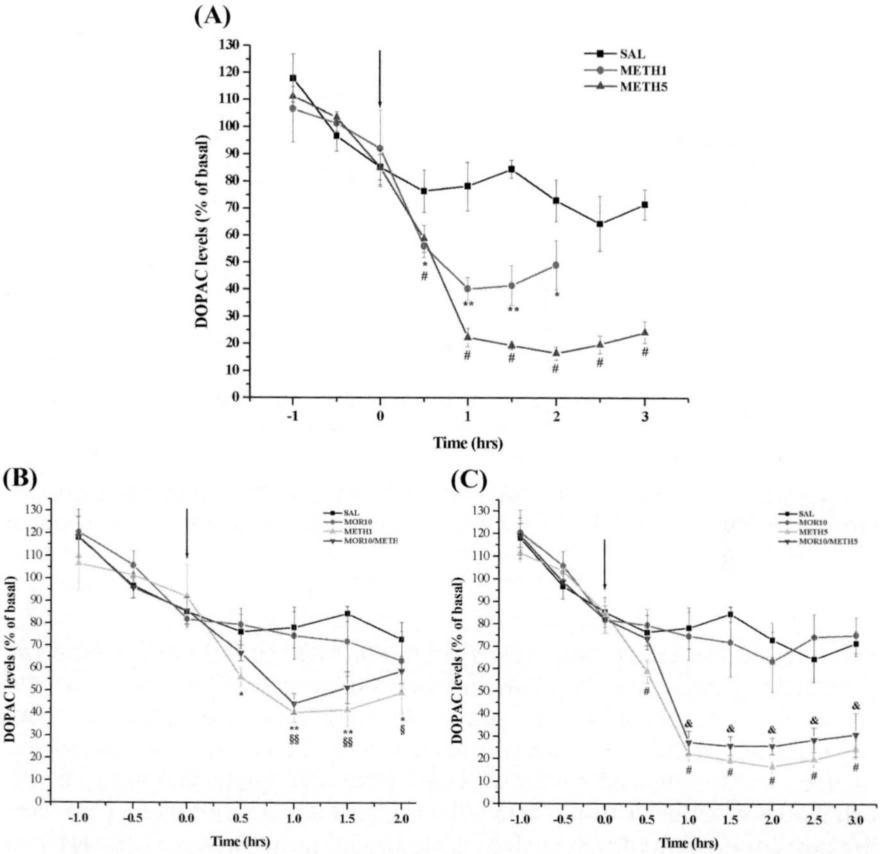

FIGURE 3. (**A**) The effect of METH on extracellular levels of DOPAC in CPu. Extracellular levels of DOPAC were measured in CPu by *in vivo* microdialysis following i.p. injections of METH1, METH5, and SAL. (**B**) The effect of METH1, MOR10, and their combination on extracellular levels of DOPAC in CPu. Extracellular levels of DOPAC were measured in CPu by *in vivo* microdialysis following i.p. injections of METH1, MOR10, MOR10/METH1, and SAL. (**C**)j The effect of METH5, MOR10, and their combination on extracellular levels of DOPAC in CPu. Extracellular levels of DOPAC were measured in CPu by *in vivo* microdialysis following i.p. injections of METH5, MOR10, MOR10/METH5, and SAL. Each value is mean ± SEM Time point (0 h) of injection is indicated by the arrow. $^{*,\S}P < 0.05$; $^{**,\S\S,\#,\&}P < 0.001$ versus time-zero value from METH1, MOR10/METH1, METH5, and MOR10/METH5 groups, respectively.

in the saline-treated animals stayed constant throughout the experiment. To facilitate comparison of dose–response relationship, mean DOPAC levels from 1 h to 1.5 h evoked by both METH1 and METH5 are presented in FIGURE 4. The decrease in DOPAC extracellular levels induced by METH5 was bigger

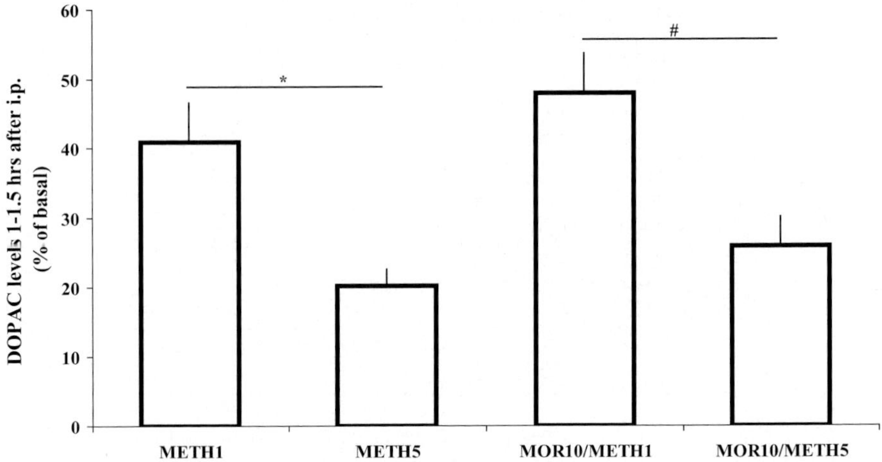

FIGURE 4. The effect of METH1, METH5, MOR10/METH1, and MOR10/METH5 on mean DOPAC levels 1–1.5 h following treatment in CPu. Data are mean ± SEM and are expressed as percentage of the basal values. $^{*}P < 0.05$ METH1 compared to METH5; $^{\#}P < 0.05$ MOR10/METH1 compared to MOR10/METH5.

than the one evoked by METH1 ($P < 0.05$). MOR10 did not produce any detectable changes from baseline in extracellular DOPAC levels in rat CPu (FIG. 3 B, C). Although MOR10 delayed the onset of the effect evoked by both METH doses, it did not change the amplitude of the decrease in extracelular DOPAC levels produced by the stimulant (FIG. 3 B, C). In fact, mean extracellular DOPAC levels from 1 h to 1.5 h evoked by both METH1 and METH5 are not significantly different than those produced by MOR10/METH1 and MOR10/METH5 (FIG. 4).

DISCUSSION

Our study clearly demonstrates for the first time that whereas 10 mg/kg MOR prolongs DA efflux evoked by a low dose of METH (1 mg/kg), it does not change DA efflux profile evoked by a higher METH dose (5 mg/kg) in rat CPu. Firsty, it is shown that the acute administration of increasing doses of METH over the range of 1–5 mg/kg resulted in progressively enhanced extracellular concentrations of DA, proportional both in magnitude and duration to the dose of the drug. This is consistent with results obtained also using the microdialysis technique showing that METH promotes a dose-dependent increase in the extracellular concentration of DA.[13] There appears to be a wide range of individual differences in responsiveness to both amphetamine and METH.[13,14] This may, in part, account for METH1 having induced DA release in only two out of six dosed rats. Human narcotic addicts typically admin-

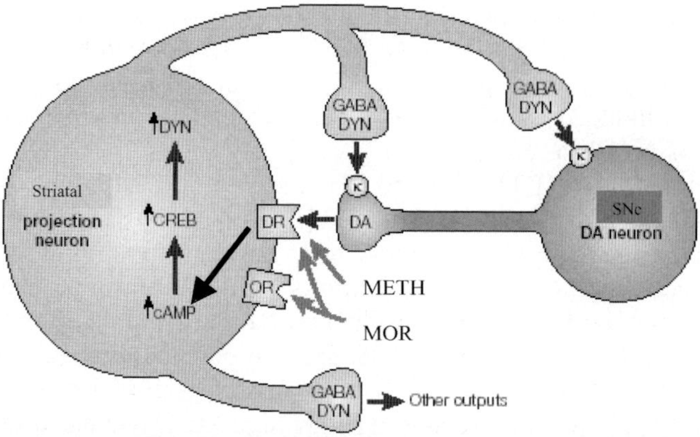

FIGURE 5. The figure shows an SNc dopamine (DA) neuron innervating a striatal GABAergic projection neuron, specifically, a subtype of such neurons that expresses DYN. DYN serves a negative feedback mechanism in this circuit: High METH concentration would release DYN from terminals of the striatal neurons via upregulation of the cAMP pathway. This peptide would act on k-opioid receptors located on nerve terminals and cell bodies of the DA neurons to inhibit their functioning. (Adapted from Nestler[36]).

ister bolus doses of opioids rather than intermittent small doses. Hence, the present results concerning 10 mg/kg MOR may be relevant to mechanisms of addiction. In this study, we show that in contrast with METH, MOR10, a dose inducing the typical opiate catalepsy,[15] did not produce any significant change in extracellular DA levels. Some previous studies also showed that acute systemic administration of opioids did not increase the release of nigrostriatal DA.[16,17] However, the results presented here are contradictory with 10 mg/kg MOR increasing HVA/DA in rat caudate nucleus.[12] First, we should be cautious when comparing different rat strains: Sprague-Dawley (present study) versus Wistar (former study). Second, it is noteworthy that differences between *in vivo* extracellular measurements and post-mortem tissue levels are not unusual and have been noted by other authors.[18,19] Finally, it could be speculated that a putative relatively small increase in DA release induced by MOR would not be sufficient to overcome the highly efficient intrasynaptic DA uptake system,[20] hence not measurable using microdialysis in our conditions. Polydrug abuse is a major problem around the world. Of particular interest is the incidence in concurrent use of amphetamines and opiates (see Introduction). Opioids, besides playing a role in modulating dopaminergic pathways in the central nervous system (CNS),[21] can also modulate the effects of drugs that act via brain DA systems, such as amphetamines. In fact, opioid receptor agonists attenuate METH negative impact in nigrostriatal pathway.[22,23] In addition, some studies suggest that naloxone attenuates the amphetamine-induced increases in extracellular DA levels in the rat striatum.[24] Extracellular DA levels are an adequate marker for demonstrating an interaction between MOR and drugs that affect DA transporters (DATs) (e.g., METH). Therefore, in the present study we aimed to characterize the effect of MOR on dopaminergic nigrastriatal transmission induced by METH to further understand the increasing popularity of this polydrug combination. It is clearly shown that MOR increased the duration of low METH-induced DA release in the striatum. In addition, all rats responded to the low MOR/METH combination. These observations may reflect an increase in the activity of DA neurons, resulting mostly from opioid-induced inhibition of local inhibitory GABAergic interneurons upon μ-receptor stimulation.[25,26] Our results point in the same direction suggested by Kimmel *et al.*[27]: namely, that MOR induced potentiation of DA release by amphetamine in the contralateral striatum from nigrally lesioned rats. Interestingly, MOR did not significantly change high METH-induced DA release. Taking into consideration the magnitude and the duration of the dopaminergic signal evoked by METH5 *versus* METH1 (4 times as high and 3 times as long when compared to the one induced by METH1), one should admit that this dopaminergic signal could contribute to dynorphin (DYN) release and consequently to decreased activity of dopaminergic neurons (see FIG. 5 for details). This suggestion is consistent with METH dose dependently increasing preprodynorphin (PPD) mRNA expression in striatum[28] and with a single systemic high dose of METH increasing DYN levels in both striatum and substantia nigra (SN).[29] Therefore, DYN action through k-opioid receptors would counteract the increase in the activity of DA neurons produced by MOR10. The net effect being the lack of modulatory action of MOR10 on dopaminergic transmission induced by METH5. In fact, Xi *et al.*[30] suggested that kappa agonists reduce the dopaminergic effects of opioid agents. To fully confirm our hypothesis, one could use k-opioid antagonist, such as nor-binaltorphimine (nor-BNI) to antagonize DYN action on our experimental model.

In addition to its effects at the DAT, thus inhibiting DA uptake, it has also been demonstrated that METH decreases intraneuronal oxidative metabolism of DA through monoamine oxidase (MAO) inhibition.[31,32] Accordingly, in our study, METH decreased dose dependently extracellular DOPAC levels. We further showed that systemically administered 10 mg/kg MOR did not significantly change the output of DOPAC. Since extracellular DOPAC is closely related to the amount of newly synthesized DA, no alterations in DOPAC levels may be explained by an unaltered DA synthesis. Alternatively, it could be suggested that a putative relatively small increase in DOPAC release induced by MOR would not be sufficient to overcome the highly efficient DOPAC clearance rate. Although MOR shortly delayed the onset of the effect of both METH treatments on extracellular DOPAC levels, it did not change the magnitude of DOPAC decrease produced by the stimulant. These results suggest that MOR did not modulate the action of METH on intracellular DA metabolism. In summary, this is the first recording demonstrating that MOR-induced potentiation of DA release evoked by METH. Nigrostriatal DA neurons innervating the dorsal striatum have been implicated in habit-based learning that may drive compulsive behavior in addiction.[33,34] Moreover, alterations in cell signaling in the striatum may be particularly important in the response to both acute and chronic administration of drugs of abuse, resulting in maladaptative changes in the reward-based associative learning involved in addiction.[35] Therefore, MOR prolonging striatal DA efflux evoked by a low dose of METH might justify the abuse potential attributed to MOR–METH combination.

ACKNOWLEDGMENTS

This work has been partially supported by IPDT (Portugal).

REFERENCES

1. WILSON, J.M., K.S. KALASINSKY, A.I. LEVEY, *et al.* 1996. Striatal dopamine nerve terminal markers in human, chronic METH users. Nat. Med. **2:** 699–703.
2. VILLEMAGNE, V., J. YUAN, D.F. WONG, *et al.* 1988. Brain dopamine neurotoxicity in baboons treated with doses of METH comparable to those recreationally abused by humans: evidence from [11C]WIN-35,428 positron emission tomography studies and direct in vitro determinations. J. Neurosci. **18:** 419–427.
3. HEISHMAN, S.J., K.J. SCHUH, C.R. SCHUSTER, *et al.* 2000. Reinforcing and subjective effects of MOR in human opioid abusers: effect of dose and alternative reinforcer. Psychopharmacology **148:** 272–280.
4. BERKE, J.D. & S.E. HYMAN. 2000. Addiction, dopamine, and the molecular mechanisms of memory. Neuron **25:** 515–532.
5. PEREIRA, F.C., S.Z. IMAM, B. GOUGH, *et al.* 2002. Acute changes in dopamine release and turnover in rat caudate nucleus following a single dose of METH. J. Neural Transm. **109:** 1151–1158.
6. PEREIRA, F.C., T.R. MACEDO, S.Z. IMAM, *et al.* 2004. Lack of hydroxyl radical generation upon central administration of METH in rat caudate nucleus: a microdialysis study. Neurotox. Res. **6:** 149–152.
7. RICHARDS, J.R., S.W. BRETZ, E.B. JOHNSON, *et al.* 1999. METH abuse and emergency department utilization. West. J. Med. **170:** 198–202.
8. LERI, F., J. BRUNEAU & J. STEWART. 2003. Understanding polydrug use: review of heroin and cocaine co-use. Addiction **98:** 7–22.
9. JASISNKI, D.R. & K.L. PRESTON. 1986. Evaluation of mixtures of MOR and d-amphetamine for subjective and physiological effects. Drug Alcohol Depend. **17:** 1–13.
10. RANALDI, R. & R.A. WISE. 2000. Intravenous self-administration of methamphetamine-heroin (speedball) combinations under a progressive-ratio schedule of reinforcement in rats. Neuroreport **11:** 2621–2623.
11. MASUKAWA, Y., T. SUZUKI & M. MISAWA. 1993. Differential modification of the rewarding effects of METH and cocaine by opioids and antihistamines. Psychopharmacology **111:** 139–143.
12. PEREIRA, F.C., S.D. SANTOS, C.F. RIBEIRO, *et al.* 2004. A single exposure to MOR induces long-lasting hyporeactivity of rat caudate putamen dopaminergic nerve terminals. Ann. N. Y. Acad. Sci. **1025:** 414–423.

13. MELEGA, W.P., A.E. WILLIAMS, D.A. SCHMITZ, *et al.* 1995. Pharmacokinetic and pharmacodynamic analysis of the actions of D-amphetamine and D-METH on the dopamine terminal. J. Pharmacol. Exp. Ther. **274:** 90–96.
14. SEGAL, D.S. & R. KUCZENSKI. 1987. Individual differences in responsiveness to single and repeated amphetamine administration: behavioral characteristics and neurochemical correlates. J. Pharmacol. Exp. Ther. **242:** 917–926.
15. Di CHIARA, G. & A. IMPERATO. 1988. Opposite effects of mu and kappa opiate agonists on dopamine release in the nucleus accumbens and in the dorsal caudate of freely moving rats. J. Pharmacol. Exp. Ther. **244:** 1067–1080.
16. WOOD, P.L. & T.S. RAO. 1991. MOR stimulation of mesolimbic and mesocortical but not nigrostriatal dopamine release in the rat as reflected by changes in 3-methoxytyramine levels. Neuropharmacology **30:** 399–401.
17. YONEHARA, N. & D.H. CLOUET. 1984. Effects of delta and mu opiopeptides on the turnover and release of dopamine in rat striatum. J. Pharmacol. Exp. Ther. **231:** 38–42.
18. MAISONNEUVE, I.M., R.W. KELLER JR. & S.D. GLICK. 1991. Interactions between ibogaine, a potential anti-addictive agent, and MOR: an *in vivo* microdialysis study. Eur. J. Pharmacol. **199:** 35–42.
19. MAISONNEUVE, I.M., K.L. ROSSMAN, R.W. KELLER JR. & S.D. GLICK. 1992. Acute and prolonged effects of ibogaine on brain dopamine metabolism and MOR-induced locomotor activity in rats. Brain Res. **575:** 69–73.
20. WESTERINK, B.H. 1995. Brain microdialysis and its application for the study of animal behaviour. Behav. Brain Res. **70:** 103–124.
21. WOOD, P.L. 1983. Opioid regulation of CNS dopaminergic pathways: a review of methodology, receptor types, regional variations and species differences. Peptides **4:** 595–601.
22. TSAO, L-I., B. LANDENHEIM, A.M. ANDREWS, *et al.* 1998. Delta opiod peptide [D-Ala2, D-Leu5] enkephalin blocks the long-term loss of dopamine transporters induced by multiple administrations of METH: involvement of opioid receptors and reactive oxygen species. J. Pharmacol. Exp. Ther. **287:** 322–331.
23. EL DAILY, E. *et al.* 2000. Modulation of the neurotoxic effects of METH by the selective kappa-opiod receptor agonist U69593. J. Neurochem. **74:** 1553–1562.
24. HOOKS, M.S., D.N. JONES, J.B. JUSTICE JR. & S.G. HOLTZMAN. 1992. Naloxone reduces amphetamine-induced stimulation of locomotor activity and in vivo dopamine release in the striatum and nucleus accumbens. Pharmacol. Biochem. Behav. **42:** 765–770.
25. DI CHIARA, G. & R.A. NORTH. 1992. Neurobiology of opiate abuse. Trends Pharmacol. Sci. **13:** 185–193.
26. JOHNSON, S.W. & R.A. NORTH. 1992. Opioids excite dopamine neurons by hyperpolarization of local interneurons. J. Neurosci. **12:** 483–488.
27. KIMMEL, H.L., J.B. JUSTICE JR. & S.G. HOLTZMAN. 1998. Dissociation of MOR-induced potentiation of turning and striatal dopamine release by amphetamine in the nigrally-lesioned rat. Eur. J. Pharmacol. **346:** 203–208.
28. ADAMS, D.H., G.R. HANSON & K.A. KEEFE. 2003. Distinct effects of METH and cocaine on preprodynorphin messenger RNA in rat striatal patch and matrix. J. Neurochem. **84:** 87–93.
29. BUSTAMANTE, D., Z.B. YOU, M.N. CASTEL, *et al.* 2002. Effect of single and repeated METH treatment on neurotransmitter release in substantia nigra and neostriatum of the rat. J. Neurochem. **83:** 645–654.

30. XI, Z.X., S.A. FULLER & E.A. STEIN. 1988. Dopamine release in the nucleus accumbens during heroin self-administration is modulated by kappa opiod receptors: an *in vivo* fast-cyclic voltametry study. J. Pharmacol. Exp. Ther. **284:** 151–161.
31. JONES, S.R., R.R. GAINETDINOV, R.M. WIGHTMAN & M.G. CARON. 1998. Mechanisms of amphetamine action revealed in mice lacking the dopamine transporter. J. Neurosci. **18:** 1979–1986.
32. METZGER, R.R., H.M. HAUGHEY, D.G. WILKINS, *et al.* 2000. METH-induced rapid decrease in dopamine transporter function: role of dopamine and hyperthermia. J. Pharmacol. Exp. Ther. **295:** 1077–1085.
33. EVERITT, B.J. & M.E. WOLF. 2002. Psychomotor stimulant addiction: a neural systems perspective. J. Neurosci. **22:** 3312–3320.
34. GERDEMAN, G.L., J.G. PARTRIDGE, C.R. LUPICA & D.M. LOVINGER. 2003. It could be habit forming: drugs of abuse and striatal synaptic plasticity. Trends Neurosci. **26:** 184–192.
35. FASANO, S. & R. BRAMBILLA. 2002. Cellular mechanisms of striatum-dependent behavioral plasticity and drug addiction. Curr. Mol. Med. **2:** 649–665.
36. NESTLER, E.J. 2001. molecular basis of long-term plasticty underlying addiction. Nat. Rev. Neurosci. **2:** 119–128.

In PC12 Cells Neurotoxicity Induced by Methamphetamine Is Related to Proteasome Inhibition

GLORIA LAZZERI,[a] PAOLA LENZI,[a] MARCO GESI,[a]
MICHELA FERRUCCI,[a] FEDERICA FULCERI,[a] STEFANO RUGGIERI,[b,c]
VALERIA BRUNO,[b] AND FRANCESCO FORNAI[a,b]

[a]*Department of Human Morphology and Applied Biology, University of Pisa, 56126 Pisa, Italy*

[b]*Laboratory of Neurobiology of Movement Disorders, IRCCS INM Neuromed, 86077 Pozzilli, Isernia, Italy*

[c]*University of Rome "La Sapienza," 00185 Rome, Italy*

ABSTRACT: Neurodegenerative disorders are featured by a variety of pathological hallmarks, and very often they are characterized by neuronal inclusions in specific brain nuclei. Occurrence of neuronal inclusions has been often related to the onset of cell death. Recent studies demonstrated that amphetamine derivatives produce intracellular inclusions, which are reminiscent of those occurring in degenerative disorders. In the present article, we analyzed the correlation between neuronal inclusions and cell death using methamphetamine (METH) in PC12 cell cultures. We found that the dose necessary to induce cell death is higher compared with that required to induce inclusions formation. Our results demonstrate a dissociation between formation of inclusion bodies and cell death suggesting that neuronal inclusions do not necessarily lead to cell death. The conclusions of the present article suggest that the onset of inclusion bodies represents a slight consequence of toxicity, which requires a prolonged cell viability to take place.

KEYWORDS: methamphetamine; neuronal inclusions; cell death; proteasome inhibition

INTRODUCTION

Amphetamine derivatives, such as methamphetamine (METH) and 3,4-methylenedioxymethamphetamine (MDMA), act as monaminergic neuro-

Address for correspondence: Francesco Fornai, M.D., Department of Human Morphology and Applied Biology, University of Pisa, Via Roma, 55, 56126 Pisa, Italy. Voice: +39-050-2218611; fax: +39-050-2218606.
e-mail: f.fornai@med.unipi.it

Ann. N.Y. Acad. Sci. 1074: 174–177 (2006).
doi: 10.1196/annals.1369.017

toxins in the central nervous system (CNS). Recent studies in mice have demonstrated that METH and MDMA produce *in vivo* within the cytoplasm of neurons of the substantia nigra pars compacta inclusions which are reminiscent of those occurring in degenerative disorders.[1–3] These consist of neuronal bodies staining for ubiquitin, the ubiquitin-activating enzyme (E1), parkin (an ubiquitin protein ligase E3-like), and other antigens belonging to the ubiquitin-proteasome (UP) pathway. In keeping with this, intracellular inclusions known as Lewy bodies, a pathological hallmark of Parkinson's disease (PD), stain specifically for proteins associated with UP-system,[4,5] including α-synuclein.[6,7] This suggests that neurotoxicity induced by amphetamine derivatives involves the UP-system and indicates that a failure of this multi-enzymatic system might represent a final common pathway in the pathogenesis of nigrostriatal alterations occurring during PD and following treatment with amphetamine derivatives. In fact, intrastriatal injections of UP inhibitors, such as lactacystin/epoxomycyn, lead to retrograde degenerative processes in the substantia nigra accompanied by neuronal inclusions.[8] Inclusion bodies can be reproduced by METH in cultured PC12 cells.[1] Similar to those observed *in vivo*, inclusion bodies are exclusively localized in the cytoplasm and are stained for ubiquitin and α-synuclein.[1]

In the present article, by using PC12 cell cultures we took the advantage of a simple cellular model to study the correlation between cell death and inclusion formation induced by METH. In addition, we correlated the occurrence of UP inhibition with the occurrence of inclusion bodies and cell death. We treated PC12 cells, obtained from the American Type Culture Collection and grown in RPMI 1640 medium supplemented with 10% heat-inactivated horse serum and 5% fetal bovine serum, with various doses of METH and measured cell survival and the fine morphology by using light and electron microscopy. In addition, we measured proteasome activity by a fluorimetric assay. Cellular pellets were collected after various time intervals and different doses and were processed for morphological and biochemical investigation.

The treatment with METH led to morphological changes within the cytoplasm of PC12 cells, consisting of inclusion bodies shaped as whorls of concentric membranes, which stained for various components of the UP-system. The effect of METH was concentration dependent with almost the entire cell population developing the inclusions to 1 μM. Higher doses of METH of up to 10 μM did not allow recovery of viable cells in the pellet and the cell remnants did not seem to contain inclusions (FIG. 1). However, the dose necessary to induce cell death was constantly higher compared with that required to induce inclusions formation. Moreover, when we measured the proteasome activity, we found that both the effects induced by METH correlated with inhibition of the UP-system (FIG. 2).

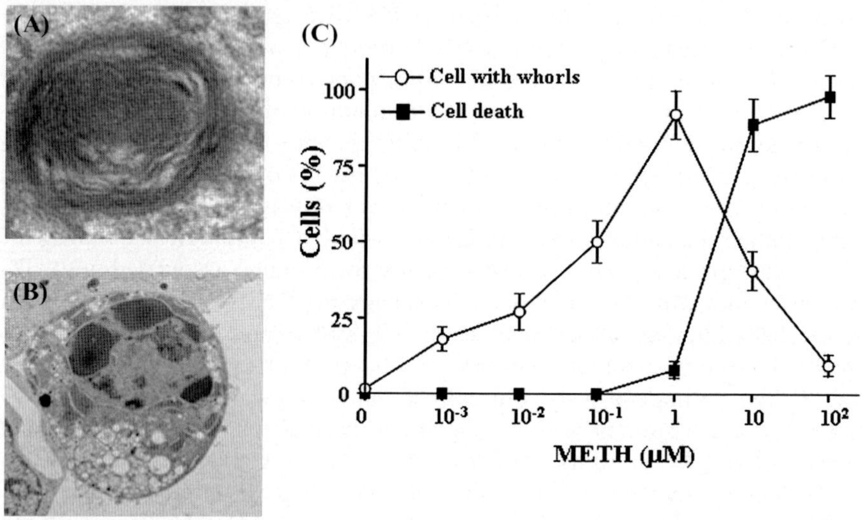

FIGURE 1. METH produces neuronal inclusions and cell death. Electron microscopic analysis of an inclusion (**A**) and apoptotic cell (**B**) in PC12 cells exposed to METH. (**C**) Correlation between neuronal inclusions and cell death induced by METH. High doses of METH produces a decrease of inclusion-containing cells and concomitantly produce a progressive onset of cell death.

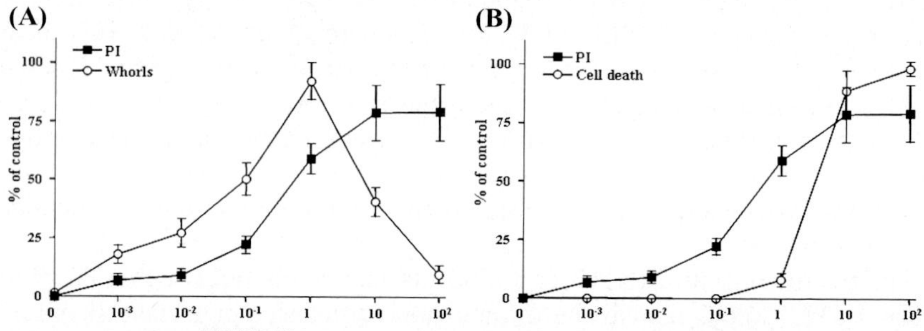

FIGURE 2. Correlation between inclusion formation, cell death, and proteasome inhibition after METH. Inclusion bodies formation (**A**) or cell death (**B**) couple with proteasome inhibition. Low doses of METH induce formation of cytoplasmic inclusions and low inhibition of the UP-system, while raising doses of METH up to 10 μM, induce massive cell loss accompanied by a severe inhibition of proteasome activity with no evidence of inclusions.

CONCLUSIONS

Our findings demonstrate that neuronal inclusions and cell death induced by METH in PC12 cells are related with inhibition of the UP-system. However, we have observed that high doses of METH produce a decrease of inclusions-containing cells and concomitantly produce a severe cell death. This suggests that impairment of the UP-system by METH is involved both in the pathogenesis of neuronal inclusions and cell death, but these effects occur with a different dose–response curve. Thus, a negative correlation between formation of inclusion bodies and cell death support the hypothesis that neuronal inclusions are beneficial for the cell. Nonetheless, both phenomena are related to various degree of UP inhibition which leads to postulate that neuronal inclusions and cell death represent different stages of the cellular response to a neurotoxic insult.

In keeping with recent data,[9] formation of inclusion bodies might represent a defense mechanism which is recruited when a slight insult, allowing cell viability, is generated. This effect may eventually recover once the neurotoxic agent is removed or lead to cell death once the neurotoxic activity overcomes the defense mechanisms.

REFERENCES

1. FORNAI, F. *et al.* 2004. Methamphetamine produces neuronal inclusions in the nigrostriatal system and in PC12 cells. J. Neurochem. **88**: 114–123.
2. FORNAI, F. *et al.* 2004a. DNA damage and ubiquitinated neuronal inclusions in the substantia nigra and striatum of mice following MDMA (ecstasy). Psychopharmacology (Berl.) **173**: 353–363.
3. FORNAI, F. *et al.* 2002. Striatal postsynaptic ultrastructural alterations following methylenedioxymethamphetamine administration. Ann. N. Y. Acad. Sci. **965**: 381–398.
4. GAI, W.P. *et al.* 2000. In situ and in vitro study of colocalization and segregation of α-synuclein, ubiquitin, and lipids in Lewy bodies. Exp. Neurol. **166**: 324–333.
5. MCNAUGHT, K.S. *et al.* 2002. Aggresome-related biogenesis of Lewy bodies. Eur. J. Neurosci. **16**: 2136–2148.
6. SPILLANTINI, M.G. *et al.* 1997. Alpha-synuclein in Lewy bodies. Nature **388**: 839–840.
7. FORNAI, F. *et al.* 2005. Occurrence of neuronal inclusions combined with increased nigral expression of alpha-synuclein within dopaminergic neurons following treatment with amphetamine derivatives in mice. Brain Res. Bull. **65**: 405–413.
8. FORNAI, F. *et al.* 2003. Fine structure and biochemical mechanisms underlying nigrostriatal inclusions and cell death after proteasome inhibition. J Neurosci. **23**: 8955–8966.
9. FORNAI, F. *et al.* 2005. Parkinson-like syndrome induced by continuous MPTP infusion: convergent roles of the ubiquitin-proteasome system and alpha-synuclein. Proc. Natl. Acad. Sci. USA **102**: 3413–3418.

Human Immunodeficiency Virus-1 Protein Tat and Methamphetamine Interactions

SHAJI THEODORE,[a] STEPHANIE STOLBERG,[a] WAYNE A. CASS,[b] AND WILLIAM F. MARAGOS[a,b,c,d]

[a]*Graduate Center for Toxicology, University of Kentucky, Lexington, Kentucky 40536, USA*

[b]*Department of Anatomy and Neurobiology, University of Kentucky, Lexington, Kentucky 40536, USA*

[c]*Department of Neurology, University of Kentucky, Lexington, Kentucky 40536, USA*

[d]*Sanders Brown Center on Aging, University of Kentucky, Lexington, Kentucky 40536, USA*

ABSTRACT: The human immunodeficiency virus-1 (HIV-1) affects the central nervous system (CNS) in ∼30% of infected individuals and basal ganglia structures seem to be most affected. The HIV-1-transactivating protein, Tat, has been suggested to be pathogenically relevant in HIV-1-induced neuronal injury. The abuse of methamphetamine (METH), which is great among this patient population, also affects the basal ganglia, causing degeneration of dopaminergic terminals. In previous studies, we demonstrated that coexposure to these two toxins caused a synergistic loss of striatal dopamine and binding to the dopamine transporter (DAT), suggesting a loss of dopamine terminals. Because the loss of dopamine and DAT, however, do not necessarily reflect dopamine terminal degeneration, we have used silver staining and TH immunohistochemistry to further examine this issue. We have also examined the glial reaction using GFAP as a marker of astrocyte activation and OX-42 as a marker of activated microglia. Lastly, we have begun to explore the mechanism of synergy by investigating the role that the cytokine TNF-α might play in Tat + METH synergy. Our data indicate that the synergistic loss of dopamine is likely the result of dopamine terminal degeneration. This injury is not a direct result of the number of activated glia but does involve TNF-α.

KEYWORDS: AIDS; cytokines; dopamine; drug abuse; glia; neurodegeneration

Address for correspondence: William F. Maragos, Department of Neurology, University of Kentucky, 260 Health Science Research Building, 1095 V.A. Drive, Lexington, KY 40536-0305. Voice: 859-323-2522; fax: 859-257-9700.
e-mail: maragos@uky.edu

**Ann. N.Y. Acad. Sci. 1074: 178–190 (2006). © 2006 New York Academy of Sciences.
doi: 10.1196/annals.1369.018**

INTRODUCTION

Methamphetamine (METH) is currently being abused worldwide in epidemic proportions. Through needle-sharing and increased sexual practices, it has become the single greatest risk factor for contracting human immunodeficiency virus-1 (HIV-1) infection.[1,2] Approximately, one-third of HIV-1-infected individuals develop a constellation of symptoms referred to as HIV-1-associated dementia.[3,4] In addition to cognitive impairment, these individuals may develop motor abnormalities reminiscent of Parkinson's disease. Consistent with this latter observation, postmortem studies of brain tissue from patients who died with HIV-1 infection have revealed severe neuropathology in basal ganglia structures and reductions in both striatal and nigral dopamine (and metabolite) levels.[4,5] In at least one study, a reduction of dopaminergic neurons in the substantia nigra was reported.[5] Like HIV-1, METH also has a propensity to injure basal ganglia structures. Loss of dopamine and its synthetic enzyme tyrosine hydroxylase have been consistently observed in animal models of METH toxicity and are thought to result from the degeneration of dopamine terminals in the striatum.[6–8] Mechanisms of action of both HIV-1-induced neuronal injury and that of METH include oxidative stress, cytokine production, and excitotoxicity.[9–11]

Based on the vulnerability of the basal ganglia to injury caused by both HIV-1 and METH, we hypothesized that exposure to both of these insults would have a synergistic effect on dopaminergic function in the striatum. In support of this notion, HIV-1-positive drug-abusing patients acquire a more severe form of central nervous system (CNS) inflammation (i.e., encephalitis) than nondrug-abusing HIV-1-positive patients[12] and in some instances, have developed movement disorders characteristic of severe basal ganglia dysfunction.[13] In a previous study, we examined the potential interactions between METH and HIV-1 "virotoxin" Tat.[14] Tat is a transactivating protein essential for HIV-1 replication.[15] It is actively secreted by infected cells[16] and after either gaining entrance to a cell or interacting at the membrane surface, can cause neuronal damage and even cell death.[17] Importantly, Tat has been demonstrated in the striatum of HIV-1 postmortem brain tissue.[18,19] In our earlier study, we reported that rats administered intraparenchymal Tat followed by systemic administration of METH showed a synergistic loss of striatal dopamine and its metabolites.[14] Specifically, we showed that in rats exposed to both Tat and METH, dopamine levels were decreased 60% compared to the 7–8% reduction in dopamine following administration of METH or Tat alone, respectively. In this study, we have investigated whether the reduction in striatal dopamine following exposure to both METH and Tat is the result of dopamine terminal degeneration. We have also begun to study the involvement of activated glial elements and the cytokine tumor necrosis factor-α (TNF-α) in the enhanced neurotoxicity induced by Tat + METH.

METHODS

Surgery

Adult male Sprague-Dawley rats (3–4 months old) were used for all experiments except that in which Tat + METH toxicity was examined in C57BL/6 mice lacking TNF-receptors (double knockouts [DKOs]). These C57BL/6, mice which are genetically deficient in both p55 and p75 TNF receptors, were generated and characterized as previously described.[20] All experimental procedures were carried out according to the NIH *Guide for the Care and Use of Laboratory Animals* and were approved by the University of Kentucky Institutional Animal Care and Use Committee. Four treatment groups were used in the rat studies. Group I was administered normal saline intraperitoneal (i.p.) (1 mL/kg every 2 h × 4 injections). Group 2 received 20 μg recombinant $Tat_{1\text{–}72}$ (in 1 μL sterile water) into the right striatum and 24 h later was administered saline in an identical fashion as group I. Group 3 received systemic injections of METH (Sigma-Aldrich, St. Louis, MO, USA; 4 mg/kg every 2 h × 4 injections). Finally, group 4 was administered 20 μg Tat into the right striatum and 24 h later received METH i.p. (4 mg/kg) every 2 h × 4 injections. In studies using DKO mice, only groups 1 and 4 were generated and animals received 3 mg/kg METH. The doses of Tat and METH chosen were previously determined to be "threshold" and not cause significant decreases in dopamine levels nor cause hyperthermia when administered alone.[14]

Animals were anesthetized with isoflurane and placed in a small animal stereotactic apparatus. Following exposure of the cortical surface, Tat was injected into the right striatum over a 1-min period, using a Hamilton syringe. For rats the coordinates were AP = +0.5 mm, ML = −2.5 mm, and DV = −4.5 mm relative to bregma and the incisor bar was 3.4 mm below the interaural line. For TNF-receptor knockout mice the coordinates were AP = +0.7 mm, ML = −2.0 mm, and DV = −4.0 mm relative to bregma and the incisor bar was 1.7 mm below the interaural line. To prevent the adsorption of Tat to the glass barrel, the syringe was pretreated with a 5% solution of dimethyldichlorosilane before administration of Tat using a procedure previously described.[21]

Silver Staining

One week following treatment, animals were deeply anesthetized with 50 mg/kg pentobarbital sodium and perfused transcardially with 100 mL of phosphate-buffered saline, pH 7.4 followed by 250 mL of 4% paraformaldehyde in phosphate-buffered saline, pH 7.4. Following postfixation in 4% paraformaldehyde at 4°C for at least 1 week, the brains were immersed in 30% sucrose for 48 h. The brains were rapidly frozen in isopentane on dry ice and 40 μm thick sections of striatum were collected in a cryoprotectant solution and stored at −20°C until use. Silver staining of sections was carried out using FD Neurosilver kit (FD Neurotechnologies, Gaithersburg, MD, USA) with modifications. The silver-stained sections were mounted on glass slides, dehydrated in 100% ethanol, cleared in xylene, and coverslipped.

TH, GFAP, and OX-42 Immunohistochemistry

Forty micrometer paraformaldehyde fixed tissue sections were rinsed in Tris-buffered saline (TBS, pH 7.6), blocked with 10% normal goat serum in TBS containing 0.1% Triton X-100 for 30 min. Sections were incubated with either a 1:1000 dilution of rabbit polyclonal antibody for TH (Pelfreez Biologicals, Rogers, AK, USA), a 1:1000 dilution of mouse monoclonal OX-42 antibody for microglia (Serotec, Oxford, UK), or 1:500 dilution of rabbit polyclonal antibody for GFAP (Chemicon, Temecula, CA, USA). Sections were then processed with either Vectastain ABC reagent (Vector Labs, Burlingame, CA, USA) or the appropriate peroxidase-conjugated antibodies and immunoreactivity visualized with diaminobenzidine.

HPLC

Animals were sacrificed by decapitation and a 2 mm slab of striatum, which contained the center of the injection site, was dissected on ice, weighed and stored at −80°C until analysis. Frozen tissue samples were processed and analyzed by HPLC using previously described methods.[22] Tissue levels of dopamine and DOPAC are expressed as pg/mg wet weight tissue.

TNF-α ELISA

Tissue (2 mm thick slabs of striatum) was homogenized in a buffer (0.32 M sucrose, 20 mM HEPES, 2 mM EDTA, 2 mM EGTA) at a concentration of 10 mg tissue/150 μL buffer. After centrifugation at 13,200 rpm for 30 min the supernatant was collected and 50 μL was incubated for 2 h in 96-well plates that were coated with 1 μg/mL of monoclonal rat anti-TNF capture antibody (R&D systems, Minneapolis, MN, USA). The samples were then exposed to 200 ng/mL biotinylated goat anti-rat detection antibody for 2 h at 22°C followed by incubation with 2 μg/mL streptavidin-conjugated horseradish peroxidase for 30 min at 37°C and finally reacted with tetramethylbenzidine for 30 min at 22°C. The reaction was terminated with 1N sulfuric acid and samples scanned at 450 nm. A standard curve was generated using known concentrations of recombinant TNF-α.

RESULTS

Silver Staining

In an earlier study, we demonstrated a profound synergistic loss of dopamine in animals treated with Tat + METH compared to animals treated with either toxin alone and this was confirmed (not shown). One week following treatment, saline-treated animals (group 1) revealed very slight silver stain in the striatum (FIG. 1). Similarly, there was little reaction product in animals exposed to METH (group 2) and in those animals receiving Tat (group 3), there was modest staining in the region immediately surrounding the injection site. In contrast, the striata from animals exposed to both Tat and METH (group 4) were replete with silver grains, indicative of widespread terminal degeneration.

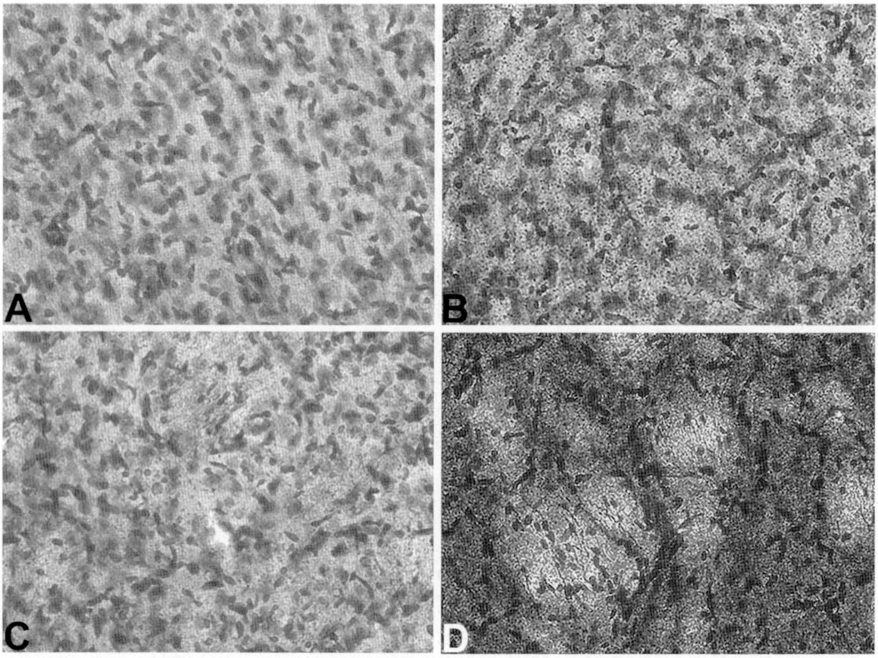

FIGURE 1. Effect of Tat + METH treatment on striatal silver staining. Striatum from saline control group (**A**) showed little silver staining. Sections from the METH-treated group (**B**) showed very mild silver staining, which was detectable only under high magnification while Tat-treated animals showed silver staining, which was confined to the region immediately adjacent to the needle tract (**C**). In the Tat + METH-treated group (**D**), extensive silver staining typified by the presence of minute, black, punctate silver granules was observed throughout the entire striatal parenchyma (40x magnification, $n = 4$/group).

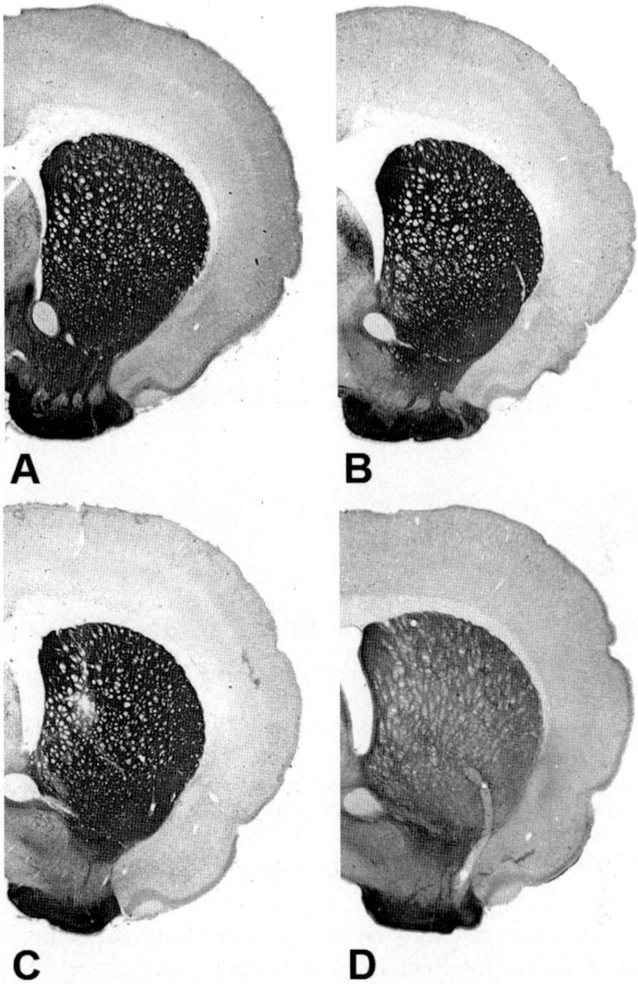

FIGURE 2. Effect of Tat + METH treatment on striatal TH immunoreactivity. Treatment with saline (**A**), METH (**B**), or Tat (**C**) did not cause any change in the striatal TH immunoreactivity. In contrast, treatment with Tat + METH (**D**) produced a severe loss of TH immunoreactivity in the ipsilateral striatum ($n = 4$/group).

TH Immunoreactivity

Consistent with our finding using the silver stain method, little to no changes in the intensity of TH immunoreactivity was observed in the striatum taken from animals in groups 1, 2, or 3 one week after treatment (FIG. 2). On the other hand, there was an obvious depletion of TH immunoreactivity in animals exposed to both Tat and METH.

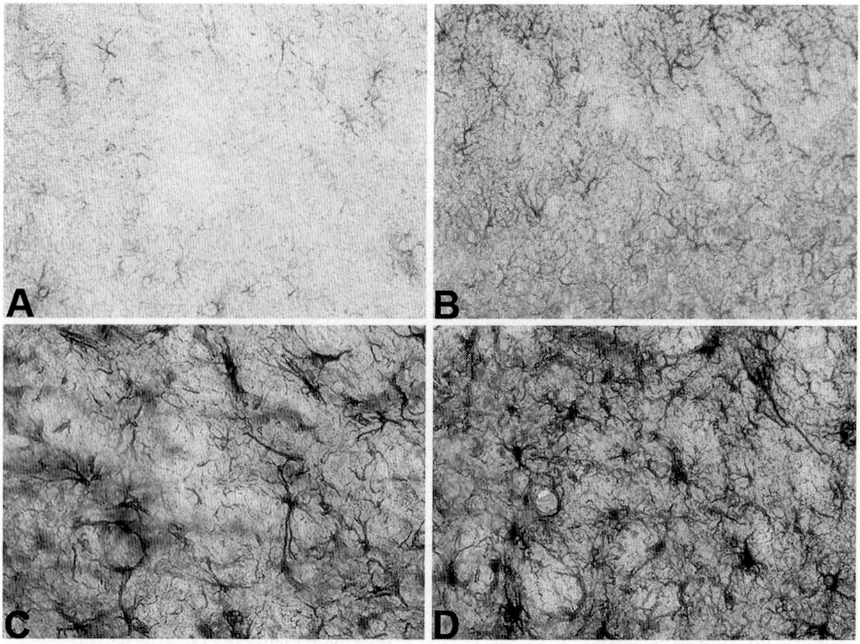

FIGURE 3. Effect of Tat + METH treatment on striatal GFAP immunoreactivity. The striatum of saline-treated group (**A**) was essentially void of any GFAP-positive cells. The METH-treated group (**B**) showed a few GFAP-positive astrocytes scattered throughout the striatum. On the other hand, Tat (**C**) and Tat + METH (**D**) treatment-induced extensive astrocyte activation indicated by an increase in the intensity and number of GFAP immunoreactive cells throughout the striatum (n = 4/group).

Glial Reaction

Previous studies have revealed the release of cytokines following administration of either METH or Tat. Because glia are the likely sources of these factors, we examined the activation of astrocytes using the marker GFAP and microglia using OX-42 at 48 h. As expected, the striatum from group 1 animals was essentially void of activated astrocytes while a few scattered GFAP-positive cells were observed in METH-treated animals (FIG. 3). In animals injected with Tat, there was an extensive syncitium of GFAP immunoreactivity comprised cell bodies and processes. The pattern of GFAP immunoreactivity was essentially the same in Tat + METH-treated animals. When the number of GFAP-positive astrocytes was quantified, there was no difference from the number seen in Tat-treated animals (not shown). Similarly, there were essentially no OX-42-labeled microglia in control striatum and a few scattered microglia with the typical "cigar-shaped" morphology in the striatum from METH-treated animals (FIG. 4). In Tat-treated animals, these was widespread OX-42 immunoreactivity, however, these cells were round, suggestive of infiltrating monocytes.

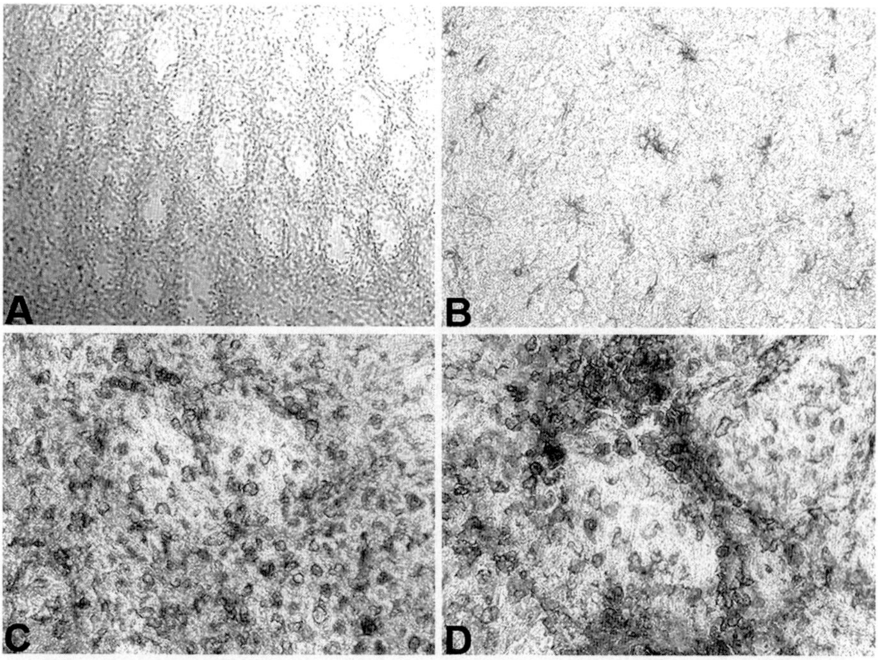

FIGURE 4. Effect of Tat + METH treatment on striatal OX-42 immunoreactivity. Saline treatment (**A**) did not reveal any OX-42 immunoreactivity in the striatum. Following METH treatment (**B**), there appeared a few scattered microglia with the typical "cigar-shaped" morphology in the striatum. Treatment with Tat (**C**) and Tat + METH (**D**) caused a more intense OX-42 immunoreactivity in the striatum, but the OX-42 immunoreactive cells had a round morphology suggesting increased infiltration of monocytes and macrophages from the circulation into the striatum. The Tat + METH-treated group did not reveal any overt increase in OX-42 immunoreactivity over that of Tat-treated group ($n = 4$/group).

Exposure to both Tat and METH had no overt effect on the intensity of staining or cell morphology compared to Tat-treated animals alone.

TNF Studies

As both Tat and METH cause an early rise in TNF-α levels, we sought to determine whether this cytokine mediated the Tat + METH synergy. As a first approach, we examined whether Tat + METH caused a synergistic increase in striatal TNF-α levels. While Tat and Tat + METH treatment induced a small but significant increase in TNF-α compared to saline- and METH-treated animals, there was no significant difference in TNF-α levels between Tat and Tat + METH-treated groups (FIG. 5). We next examined Tat + METH toxicity in TNF-α DKO mice. In wild-type mice exposed to Tat + METH, there was an

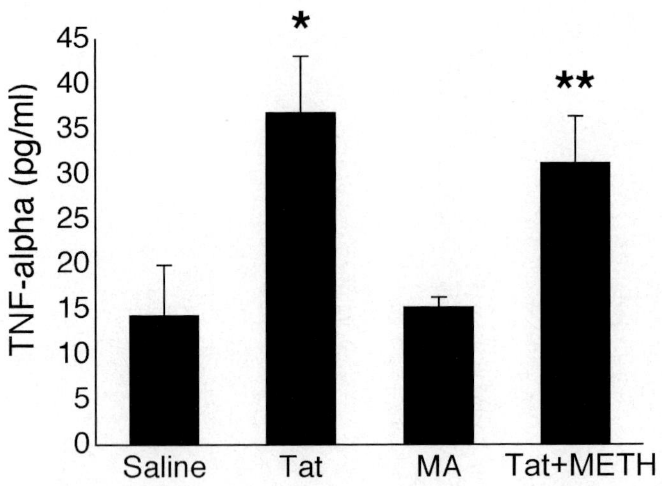

FIGURE 5. Effect of Tat + METH treatment on striatal TNF-α levels. Compared to saline-treated animals, there was a greater than two fold increase in striatal TNF-α. Systemic administration of METH had no effect on striatal TNF-α levels. Administration of both Tat and METH to animals resulted in the same increase in TNF-α observed in animals treated with Tat alone. $^{*}P < 0.01$, Tat versus saline control; $^{**}P < 0.01$, Tat + METH versus saline control (one-way ANOVA with Fisher's PLSD *post hoc* testing, $n = 3$/group).

approximately 50% reduction in striatal dopamine compared to basal dopamine levels in untreated wild-type controls (FIG. 6). In DKO, however, Tat + METH caused only an ~20% loss of striatal dopamine indicating the possibility that the enhanced neurotoxicity seen with Tat + METH might be mediated by a Tat-induced increase in TNF-α.

DISCUSSION

In a previous study, we demonstrated that exposure to the street drug METH and HIV-1 protein Tat results in a synergistic loss of striatal dopamine and DOPAC levels. We measured an ~50% reduction in radioligand binding to the dopamine transporter, which suggested the possibility that the loss of dopamine was the result of dopamine terminal degeneration.[14] In this study, we have extended our findings and now reveal that 1 week following exposure to both Tat and METH, there is prominent silver staining in the striatum compared to exposure to either Tat or METH alone. As silver staining does not reveal the transmitter phenotype of the degenerating processes, we also performed tyrosine hydroxylase immunohistochemistry, which revealed a widespread loss in TH immunoreactivity in Tat + METH-treated animals compared to that seen in either Tat- or METH-treated rats. These findings, in addition to the observed loss of DAT, provide compelling evidence that Tat + METH interact in such a way as to destroy dopamine terminals.

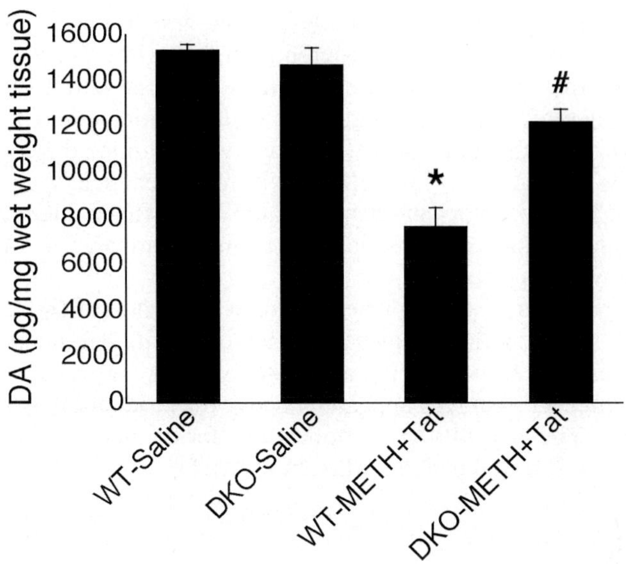

FIGURE 6. Effect of Tat + METH treatment in TNF receptor knockout mice. Seven days after treatment, wild-type mice exposed to both Tat and METH showed a significant reduction (50%) in striatal dopamine levels compared to untreated wild-type controls. In DKO, however, METH + Tat caused only an ~20% loss of striatal dopamine indicating a significant attenuation of TNF-α -mediated neurotoxicity induced by METH + Tat. $^{*}P < 0.01$, WT-METH + Tat versus WT-saline control; $^{\#}P < 0.01$ DKO-METH + Tat versus WT-METH + Tat (one-way ANOVA with Fisher's PLSD *post hoc* testing, $n = 3$/group).

Glial cell activation is a common feature associated with both METH-induced neurodegeneration and HIV-1 infection.[23–26] In light of these observations, we speculated that the synergistic loss of dopamine caused by Tat + METH might be associated with an increase in the glial response. Using GFAP as a marker of activated astrocytes and OX-42 to label activated microglia, we were unable to identify any overt change in the number of either of these cell types. While these findings indicate that the number of activated glia does not increase following Tat + METH exposure, our findings demonstrate a "disconnect" between dopamine terminal degeneration and microglial activation, the latter of which has been shown to be a pharmacological marker of METH toxicity.[27]

Despite the lack of change in the number of activated glia, it is conceivable that factors elaborated by these cell types are enhanced following Tat and METH treatment. TNF-α is a cytokine that is increased following exposure to either Tat or METH and has been correlated to the severity of CNS damage following HIV-1 infection.[28] To begin to understand the role of TNF-α, we first examined whether Tat + METH administration caused a synergistic increase in striatal TNF-α levels. Interestingly, although there was a significant increase in TNF-α produced in animals injected with Tat alone, this was not enhanced when METH was administered 24 h following Tat. We considered the possibility that an early increase in TNF-α after Tat administration could exert a priming effect on the dopaminergic system, which could make the terminals more vulnerable to METH. Therefore, we examined the dopaminergic neurotoxicity conferred by Tat + METH in mice genetically engineered to lack both the TNF receptors and demonstrated a significant attenuation of Tat + METH-induced dopamine loss in these animals compared to the reduction measured in wild-type controls.

In summary, we have shown that exposure to the virotoxin Tat and the street drug METH, results in the enhanced degeneration of dopaminergic terminals in the striatum. This damage is not associated with an increase in the number of activated glial cells but may appear to involve the production of the cytokine TNF-α by Tat. These results have implications for the neuropathogenesis observed in HIV-1-infected patients who abuse METH.

ACKNOWLEDGMENTS

This work was supported by grants DA13144 to WFM and AG17963 to WAC. The authors thank Dr. Avindra Nath for generously providing Tat and Laura Peters for technical support.

REFERENCES

1. Halkitis, P.N., J.T. Parsons & M.J. Stirratt. 2001. A double epidemic: crystal methamphetamine drug use in relation to HIV transmission among gay men. J. Homosex. **41:** 17–35.
2. Molitor, F. *et al.* 1998. Association of methamphetamine use during sex with risky sexual behaviors and HIV infection among non-injection drug users. West J. Med. **168:** 93–97.
3. McArthur, J.C., *et al.* 1993. Dementia in AIDS patients: incidence and risk factors. Multicenter AIDS Cohort Study. Neurology **43:** 2245–2252.
4. Navia, B.A., B.D. Jordan & R.W. Price. 1986. The AIDS dementia complex: I. Clinical features. Ann. Neurol. **19:** 517–524.
5. Sardar, A.M., C. Czudek & G.P. Reynolds. 1996. Dopamine deficits in the brain: the neurochemical basis of Parkinsonian symptoms in AIDS. Neuroreport **7:** 910–912.
6. Cass, W.A., M.W. Manning & M.T. Dugan. 1998. Effects of neurotoxic doses of methamphetamine on potassium and amphetamine evoked overflow of dopamine in the striatum of awake rats. Neurosci. Lett. **248:** 175–178.
7. Hotchkiss, A.J. & J.W. Gibb. 1980. Long-term effects of multiple doses of methamphetamine on tryptophan hydroxylase and tyrosine hydroxylase activity in rat brain. J. Pharmacol. Exp. Ther. **214:** 257–262.

8. Kogan, F.J., W.K. Nichols & J.W. Gibb. 1976. Influence of methamphetamine on nigral and striatal tyrosine hydroxylase activity and on striatal dopamine levels. Eur. J. Pharmacol. **36:** 363–371.
9. Cubells, J.F. *et al.* 1994. Methamphetamine neurotoxicity involves vacuolation of endocytic organelles and dopamine-dependent intracellular oxidative stress. J. Neurosci. **14:** 2260–2271.
10. Imam, S.Z. *et al.* 2001. Methamphetamine-induced dopaminergic neurotoxicity: role of peroxynitrite and neuroprotective role of antioxidants and peroxynitrite decomposition catalysts. Ann. N. Y. Acad. Sci. **939:** 366–380.
11. Nath, A. & J. Geiger. 1998. Neurobiological aspects of human immunodeficiency virus infection: neurotoxic mechanisms. Prog. Neurobiol. **54:** 19–33.
12. Bell, J.E. *et al.* 1998. HIV encephalitis, proviral load and dementia in drug users and homosexuals with AIDS. Effect of neocortical involvement. Brain **121:** 2043–2052.
13. Nath, A. *et al.* 2001. Acceleration of HIV dementia with methamphetamine and cocaine. J. Neurovirol. **7:** 66–71.
14. Maragos, W.F. *et al.* 2002. Human immunodeficiency virus-1 Tat protein and methamphetamine interact synergistically to impair striatal dopaminergic function. J. Neurochem. **83:** 955–963.
15. Marciniak, R.A. *et al.* 1990. HIV-1 Tat protein trans-activates transcription in vitro. Cell **63:** 791–802.
16. Ensoli, B. *et al.* 1993. Release, uptake, and effects of extracellular human immunodeficiency virus type 1 Tat protein on cell growth and viral transactivation. J. Virol. **67:** 277–287.
17. Jones, M. *et al.* 1998. Intraventricular injection of human immunodeficiency virus type 1 (HIV-1) tat protein causes inflammation, gliosis, apoptosis, and ventricular enlargement. J. Neuropathol. Exp. Neurol. **57:** 563–570.
18. Hudson, L. *et al.* 2000. Detection of the human immunodeficiency virus regulatory protein tat in CNS tissues. J. Neurovirol. **6:** 145–155.
19. Parmentier, H.K. *et al.* 1992. Epitopes of human immunodeficiency virus regulatory proteins tat, nef, and rev are expressed in normal human tissue. Am. J. Pathol. **141:** 1209–1216.
20. Bruce, A.J. *et al.* 1996. Altered neuronal and microglial responses to excitotoxic and ischemic brain injury in mice lacking TNF receptors. Nat. Med. **2:** 788–794.
21. Maragos, W.F. *et al.* 2003. Neuronal injury in hippocampus with human immunodeficiency virus transactivating protein. Tat. Neuroscience **117:** 43–53.
22. Cass, W.A. & M.W. Manning. 1999. Recovery of presynaptic dopaminergic functioning in rats treated with neurotoxic doses of methamphetamine. J. Neurosci. **19:** 7653–7660.
23. Brana, C. *et al.* 1999. A soluble factor produced by macrophages mediates the neurotoxic effects of HIV-1 Tat in vitro. Aids **13:** 1443–1452.
24. Bruce-Keller, A.J. *et al.* 2003. Synaptic transport of human immunodeficiency virus-Tat protein causes neurotoxicity and gliosis in rat brain. J. Neurosci. **23:** 8417–8422.
25. LaVoie, M.J., J.P. Card & T.G. Hastings. 2004. Microglial activation precedes dopamine terminal pathology in methamphetamine-induced neurotoxicity. Exp. Neurol. **187:** 47–57.
26. Thomas, D.M. *et al.* 2004. Methamphetamine neurotoxicity in dopamine nerve endings of the striatum is associated with microglial activation. J. Pharmacol. Exp. Ther. **311:** 1–7.

27. THOMAS, D.M. *et al.* 2004. Microglial activation is a pharmacologically specific marker for the neurotoxic amphetamines. Neurosci. Lett. **367:** 349–354.
28. GLASS, J.D. *et al.* 1993. Clinical-neuropathologic correlation in HIV-associated dementia. Neurology **43:** 2230–2237.

Overexpression of α-Synuclein following Methamphetamine

Is It Good or Bad?

GIUSEPPE MAUCELI,[a] CARLA I. BUSCETI,[b] ANTONIO PELLEGRINI,[a] PAOLA SOLDANI,[a] PAOLA LENZI,[a] ANTONIO PAPARELLI,[a] AND FRANCESCO FORNAI[a,b]

[a]*Department of Human Morphology and Applied Biology, University of Pisa, I-56126 Pisa, Italy*

[b]*Laboratory of Neurobiology of Movement Disorders I.R.C.C.S., I.N.M. Neuromed 86077 Pozzilli, Isernia, Italy*

ABSTRACT: α-Synuclein is a presynaptic protein involved in various degenerative disorders now defined as synucleinopathies. These include neurological diseases that share a few pathological features consisting of aggregates of both normal and altered α-synuclein within specific neuronal populations and/or glial cells. The prototype of synucleinopathies is represented by Parkinson's disease (PD) in which α-synuclein is identified as a constant component of neuronal pale eosinophilic inclusions: "the Lewy Bodies." In the present article, we discuss the potential significance of amphetamine-induced overexpression of α-synuclein in light of clinical findings showing neurodegeneration following overexpression of α-synuclein and recent experimental studies that measured increased expression of α-synuclein following amphetamine derivatives.

KEYWORDS: α-synuclein; amphetamine derivatives; dopaminergic neuron; neurotoxicity

INTRODUCTION

In a recent paper,[1] we demonstrated that treatment of mice with amphetamine derivatives (methamphetamine [METH], or methylenedioxymethamphetamine [MDMA] ecstasy) produces increased expression of α-synuclein in the substantia nigra. Interestingly, this occurs mainly within tyrosine hydroxylase (TH) immunopositive dopamine (DA)-containing neurons without any significant increase in the GABAergic population of the substantia nigra pars

Address for correspondence: Francesco Fornai, M.D., Department of Human Morphology and Applied Biology, University of Pisa, Via Roma, 55, I-56126 Pisa, Italy. Voice: +39-50-2218611; fax: +39-50-2218606.
e-mail: f.fornai@med.unipi.it

Ann. N.Y. Acad. Sci. 1074: 191–197 (2006). © 2006 New York Academy of Sciences.
doi: 10.1196/annals.1369.019

reticulata. Increased levels of α-synuclein also occur in humans chronically abusing cocaine.[2] The role of α-synuclein has been recently investigated in relation with Parkinson's disease (PD). In fact, both point mutation (producing normal amount of structurally altered α-synuclein) and gene overexpression (producing increased amount of structurally normal α-synuclein) cause inherited nigrostriatal damage, which, from a clinical point of view, represents a form of inherited parkinsonism. Despite such a clinical relevance, the bulk of the available data did not allow to attribute a specific function to this widespread presynaptic protein.

DETRIMENTAL ROLE OF MUTATION OF GENE CODING FOR α-SYNUCLEIN

Data reported above, suggest that α-synuclein is detrimental for DA neurons, in fact an increased amount of α-synuclein with a normal structure is sufficient *per se* to cause DA neuronal cell death. Again, the occurrence of autosomal dominant parkinsonism following point mutation of the α-synuclein gene indicates that the mechanism of α-synuclein-induced neurotoxicity is a result of a detrimental gain of function. Confirming this point, when α-synuclein is overexpressed with a normal structure the clinical parkinsonism is worse and involves additional area in the degenerative process.

OVEREXPRESSION OF α-SYNUCLEIN FOLLOWING AMPHETAMINES

In a recent paper, we found that treatment with amphetamine derivatives (METH and MDMA) produces an increased expression of α-synuclein within the DA neurons of the substantia nigra pars compacta. These finding were related to the occurrence of toxic effects in the terminals of these neurons projecting to the striatum. In light of the findings reported in the previous paragraph and the correlation between neurotoxicity and increased expression of α-synuclein following amphetamines, we considered the possibility that the occurrence of increased amount of α-synuclein following exposure to drugs of abuse affecting the DA system (e.g., amphetamine, cocaine) might be part of the neurotoxic process generated by these compounds within this class of neurons.

FOCUS ON THE DETRIMENTAL EFFECTS

Looking at the potential mechanisms of action, we recently demonstrated that α-synuclein might participate in the impairment of the proteasome activity, and as shown in a paper of the present issue, we found that METH produces an impairment of the catalytic activity of the proteasome. In fact, α-synuclein is

TABLE 1. Clinical and experimental studies showing correlation between neuronal inclusions and α-synuclein

Correlation between neuronal inclusion and α-synuclein (clinical studies)	Correlation between neuronal inclusion and α-synuclein (experimental studies)
Punctiform mutation of α-synuclein (altered protein and normal level of expression):	Punctiform mutation of α-synuclein (altered protein and normal level of expression):
Contursi/Greek kindred (Polymeropoulos, 1997)[14]	PC12 cell line (Stefanis *et al.*, 2001)[19]
German kindred (Kruger *et al.*, 1998)[15]	Drosophila (Takahashi *et al.*, 2003)[20]
Spanish kindred (Zarranz *et al.*, 2004)[16]	Mouse (Richfield *et al.*, 2002)[21]
	Drosophila (Feany & Bender, 2000)[25]
Gene triplication of α-synuclein (normal structure and increased expression):	Gene triplication of α-synuclein (normal structure and increased expression):
Iowa kindred (Singleton *et al.*, 2003)[17]	Mouse (Song *et al.*, 2004)[22]
Swedish-American kindred (Farrer *et al.*, 2004)[18]	Drosophila (Takahashi *et al.*, 2003)[20]
	Rat (Yamada *et al.*, 2004)[23]
	Mouse (Yazawa *et al.*, 2005)[24]

known to interact with the ubiquitin-proteasome system and to alter its catalytic function. In line with this, mice knockout for the α-synuclein gene, or carrying a spontaneous deletion of the same gene, are protected against experimental parkinsonism induced by MPTP.[3] Again, when MPTP is administered continuously, this produces neuronal inclusions that can be attenuated in α-synuclein knockout mice. Despite the lack of knowledge of its physiological function, α-synuclein is a constant component of the neuronal inclusions occurring during the sporadic degeneration of nigrostriatal DA neurons.[4] An exhaustive list of clinical and experimental studies about α-synuclein and neuronal inclusions is reported in TABLE 1. Altogether these data suggest that α-synuclein is a protein in search for a function, which, on the other hand, seems to be related only to neurotoxicity.

FOCUS ON NOVEL POTENTIAL NEUROPROTECTIVE EFFECTS

Despite the amount of data substantiating a detrimental effect of α-synuclein overexpression, a recent paper by the group of Hattori was able to show that the lack of α-synuclein worsens the detrimental effect produced by knocking out the parkin gene; on the other hand, reinstating normal α-synuclein level, was able to rescue neurotoxicity related to the loss of parkin.[5] Thus the α-synuclein, when expressed at normal levels, might play a protective effect for the cell. This new hypothesis is difficult to reconcile with data on MPTP toxicity reported above. Nonetheless, there are a variety of proteins that play a fundamental role in the cell physiology, which, at the same time, promote MPTP toxicity. For instance, the dopamine transporter (DAT) is a fundamental protein for the physiology of the DA neuron and knocking out DAT gene protects from MPTP toxicity.[6] Similarly, monoamine oxidase (MAO) type B is crucial for the physiological DA metabolism but the blockade[7] or knocking out of this protein[8] prevents MPTP toxicity. α-Synuclein overexpression resembles what is found in the overexpression of the protein Cu-Zn superoxide dismutase (SOD 1), which is commonly believed to possess a protective activity against oxidative stress. In fact, SOD 1 overexpression produces neuronal damage. This is the case of inherited amyotrophic lateral sclerosis (ALS), which features the loss of motor neurons, neurons of the motor cortex and, in addition, loss of nigral DA cells. This insight coming from other research fields showed new light on the potential role of α-synuclein as a neuroprotective protein.

POTENTIAL SIGNIFICANCE OF α-SYNUCLEIN IN METH TOXICITY

In keeping with the neurotoxic effect induced by amphetamines, while it is true that this occurs in the DA neurons, this concerns only the axon terminals while the cell body is generally spared. Again, cocaine despite affecting the physiology of DA neuron was never shown to induce DA neuronal cell death. Therefore, as an alternative hypothesis one might consider that the increase in α-synuclein observed concomitantly with amphetamine administration might represent a compensatory mechanism aimed at preserving the DA cell body. Interestingly, when METH is administered repetitively following long-time intervals (allowing the subsequent expression of α-synuclein), the neurotoxicity for the DA terminals is much less pronounced compared with multiple dosing at short (2 h) time intervals, which does not allow the expression of newly synthesized α-synuclein. In this article we wish to pose the hypothesis that the protective or detrimental role of α-synuclein is insult-dependent. In particular, in the case of METH we found the occurrence of α-synuclein aggregates *in vivo* within DA neurons, without concomitant cell death. Thus the integrity of the DA neurons is affected, since the striatal DA terminals are lost but the cell body survives, again, similar inclusions are produced by METH within striatal GABAergic cells that do not undergo any neurotoxic phenomena. The opposite roles of a given protein depending on the specific neurotoxin affecting the DA neurons is not a novelty; for instance MAO promotes MPTP toxicity while it prevents METH toxicity.

THE ISSUE OF TOXIN DEPENDENCY

Therefore, we think it is critical to interpret the potential neuroprotective/detrimental activity within the context of the specific mechanism of action of the neurotoxin. When examining the most robust effects of METH for the

DA neuron, this is represented by a massive increase of free cytosolic DA, which never occurs following MPTP toxicity (which targets the mitochondrial complex I). As a consequence, all those molecules that contribute to increase free cytosolic DA are believed to worsen METH toxicity. This explains why MAO by metabolizing DA is able to reduce METH toxicity and, conversely, when blocking MAO activity[9] or knocking out the MAO gene,[10] amphetamine toxicity can be exacerbated. In an interesting paper, the Lansbury group demonstrated a critical interaction between DA and α-synuclein.[11] They showed that α-synuclein was able to interact with DA derivatives produced by auto-oxidation (DA-quinones). In light of these findings, it was commented that DA might interact with α-synuclein, thus stabilizing a bad situation.[12] In fact, the interaction between α-synuclein and DA-quinones was shown to occlude the polymerization of α-synuclein protofibrils, thus promoting the formation of α-synuclein aggregates. A point that remains to be solved is whether the binding of α-synuclein with DA-quinones and the subsequent formation of precipitates is really toxic for the cell. Alternatively, one might hypothesize that this interaction might prevent DA-quinones to produce a greater oxidative damage for the DA neurons. In light of this latter hypothesis, α-synuclein may act as a buffer that prevents DA-derived oxidative species to cause further oxidative damage. Thus, by trapping DA-quinones within non-soluble aggregates, α-synuclein protofibrils might segregate a substantial part of the offensive mechanism derived from high levels of free cytosolic DA. This applies to the case of METH, since this compound is known to disrupt the storage of DA within the presynaptic vesicles and to competitively inhibit MAO activity. This results in an unbearable amount of cytosolic DA, which is directly responsible for the neuronal damage. In fact, inhibiting the DA synthesis as well as promoting a DA depletion before administering METH is known to prevent neurotoxicity.[13] In this way, α-synuclein might be viewed as a chaperone protein that alleviates the effects of an excess of DA, such as what was promoted by METH. This is not the case of other DA neurotoxins (i.e., MPTP) whose neurotoxic mechanism is not grounded on increasing cytosolic DA. In this case, α-synuclein might represent accidentally a detrimental factor adding further substrates for the ubiquitin proteasome system, which is impaired by the adenosine triphosphate (ATP) depletion caused by the blockade of the mitochondrial complex I. To verify this hypothesis, an experiment that is necessary to be carried out is the administration of METH to α-synuclein knockout mice and *vice versa* to give the same treatment to transgenic mice overexpressing this presynaptic protein. If the "buffering hypothesis" is correct, one should expect that METH toxicity is prevented in the latter group of mice while it is worsened in the knockout animals. This experiment is critical in order to interpret the significance of METH-induced overexpression of α-synuclein as well as to unravel the physiological role of this protein as a potential chaperone. This would reconcile the recent literature on the detrimental effect of α-synuclein with the very recent finding that discloses a neuroprotective activity.

REFERENCES

1. FORNAI, F. *et al.* 2005. Occurrence of neuronal inclusions combined with increased nigral expression of alpha-synuclein within dopaminergic neurons following treatment with amphetamine derivatives in mice. Brain Res. Bull. **65:** 405–413.
2. MASH, D.C. *et al.* 2003. Cocaine abusers have an overexpression of alpha-synuclein in dopamine neurons. J. Neurosci. **23:** 2564–2571.
3. FORNAI, F. *et al.* 2005. Parkinson-like syndrome induced by continuous MPTP infusion: convergent roles of the ubiquitin proteasome system and alpha synuclein. Proc. Natl. Acad. Sci. USA **102:** 3413–3418.
4. SPILLANTINI, M.L. *et al.* 1997. Synuclein in Lewy bodies. Nature **388:** 839–840.
5. MACHIDA, Y. *et al.* 2005. Common anti-apoptotic roles of parkin and alpha-synuclein in human dopaminergic cells. Biochem. Biophys. Res. Commun. **332:** 233–240.
6. GAINETDINOV, R.R. *et al.* 1997. Dopamine transporter is required for in vivo MPTP neurotoxicity: evidence from mice lacking the transporter. J. Neurochem. **69:** 1322–1325.
7. HEIKKILA, R.E. *et al.* 1985. Studies on the oxidation of the dopaminergic neurotoxin 1-methyl-4-phenyl-1,2,5,6-tetrahydropyridine by monoamine oxidase B. J. Neurochem. **45:** 1049–1054.
8. GRIMSBY, J. *et al.* 1997. Increased stress response and beta-phenylethylamine in MAOB-deficient mice. Nat. Genet. **17:** 206–210.
9. KITA, T. *et al.* 1995. Effects of pargyline and pyrogallol on the methamphetamine-induced dopamine depletion. Mol. Chem. Neuropathol. **24:** 31–41.
10. FORNAI, F. *et al.* 2001. Biochemical effects of monoamine neurotoxins DSP-4 and MDMA in specific brain regions of MAO-B deficient mice. Synapse **39:** 213–221.
11. CONWAY, K.A. *et al.* 2001. Kinetic stabilization of the alpha-synuclein protofibril by a dopaminealpha-synuclein adduct. Science **294:** 1346–1349.
12. SULZER, D. 2001. Alpha-synuclein and cytosolic dopamine: stabilizing a bad situation. Nat. Med. **7:** 1280–1282.
13. GIBB, J.W. *et al.* 1990. Neurochemical basis of neurotoxicity. Neurotoxicology **11:** 317–321.
14. POLYMEROPOULOS, M.H. *et al.* 1997. Mutation in the alpha-synuclein gene identified in families with Parkinson's disease. Science **276:** 2045–2047.
15. KRUGER, R. *et al.* 1998. Ala30Pro mutation in the gene encoding alpha-synuclein in Parkinson's disease. Nat. Genet. **18:** 106–108.
16. ZARRANZ, J.J. *et al.* 2004. The new mutation, E46K, of alpha-synuclein causes Parkinson and Lewy body dementia. Ann. Neurol. **55:** 164–173.
17. SINGLETON, A.B. *et al.* 2003. alpha-Synuclein locus triplication causes Parkinson's disease. Science **302:** 841.
18. FARRER, M. *et al.* 2004. Comparison of kindreds with parkinsonism and alpha-synuclein genomic multiplications. Ann. Neurol. **55:** 174–179.
19. STEFANIS, L. *et al.* 2001. Expression of A53T mutant but not wild-type alpha-synuclein in PC12 cells induces alterations of the ubiquitin-dependent degradation system, loss of dopamine release, and autophagic cell death. J. Neurosci. **21:** 9549–9560.
20. TAKAHASHI, M. *et al.* 2003. Phosphorylation of alpha-synuclein characteristic of synucleinopathy lesions is recapitulated in alpha-synuclein transgenic Drosophila. Neurosci. Lett. **336:** 155–158.

21. RICHFIELD, E.K. *et al.* 2002. Behavioral and neurochemical effects of wild-type and mutated human alpha-synuclein in transgenic mice. Exp. Neurol. **175:** 35–48.
22. SONG, D.D. *et al.* 2004. Enhanced substantia nigra mitochondrial pathology in human alpha-synuclein transgenic mice after treatment with MPTP. Exp. Neurol. **186:** 158–172.
23. YAMADA, M. *et al.* 2004. Overexpression of alpha-synuclein in rat substantia nigra results in loss of dopaminergic neurons, phosphorylation of alpha-synuclein and activation of caspase-9: resemblance to pathogenetic changes in Parkinson's disease. J. Neurochem. **91:** 451–461.
24. YAZAWA, I. *et al.* 2005. Mouse model of multiple system atrophy alpha-synuclein expression in oligodendrocytes causes glial and neuronal degeneration. Neuron **45:** 847–859.
25. FEANY, M.B. & W.W. BENDER. 2000. A Drosophila model of Parkinson's disease. Nature **404:** 394–398.

Alterations in Blood–Brain Barrier Function by Morphine and Methamphetamine

HARI SHANKER SHARMA[a,b] AND SYED F. ALI[b]

[a]*Laboratory of Cerebrovascular Research, Department of Surgical Sciences, Anesthesiology & Intensive Care Medicine, University Hospital, Uppsala University, SE-75185 Uppsala, Sweden*

[b]*Neurochemistry Laboratory, Division of Neurotoxicology, National Center for Toxicological Research/FDA, Jefferson, Arkansas 72079, USA*

Abstract: The possibility that stress associated with morphine and amphetamine administration or withdrawal will influence the blood–brain barrier (BBB) and brain dysfunction was examined in a rodent model. Repeated daily administration of morphine (10 mg/kg, i.p.) resulted in drug dependence in rats on the sixth day and onwards. Measurement of the BBB permeability to large molecule tracers normally bound to proteins, e.g., Evans blue albumin and radioiodine ([$^{131]}$Iodine) did not show any leakage on the 12th day of drug dependence. On the other hand, spontaneous withdrawal of morphine on day 1 resulted in profound stress symptoms. These symptoms were much more intense on the second day of morphine withdrawal. Alterations in the BBB to protein tracers were seen in several regions of the brain. This increase in BBB to protein tracers was most pronounced on the second day of morphine withdrawal. These rats also exhibited abnormal neuronal, glial and stress protein, the heat-shock protein 72 kD (HSP-72 kD) response. On the other hand, acute administration of methamphetamine (40 mg/kg, i.p.) in mice resulted in marked extravasation of endogenous serum protein as seen with increased expression of albumin immunohistochemistry. These observations suggest that psychostimulants and associated stress are capable to influence the brain function, probably through modifying the BBB function, not reported earlier.

Keywords: morphine; methamphetamine; rats; mice; stress; blood–brain barrier; brain dysfunction; heat shock protein; glial cells; nerve cells; Evans blue; radioiodine

Address for correspondence: Hari Shanker Sharma, Dr. Med. Sci., Frödingsgatan 12:28, SE-75421 Uppsala, Sweden. Voice & fax: +46-18-243899.
e-mail: Sharma@surgsci.uu.se

Ann. N.Y. Acad. Sci. 1074: 198–224 (2006). © 2006 New York Academy of Sciences.
doi: 10.1196/annals.1369.020

INTRODUCTION

There are reasons to believe that psychostimulant drugs, such as morphine and methamphetamine administration, and/or their withdrawal induces severe stress situations in humans as well as in animals.[1–3] Morphine and methamphetamine are well-known drugs of abuse that cause a huge burden on our society. Thus, efforts should be made to expand our knowledge to understand the cellular and molecular mechanisms of action of these psychostimulants in the central nervous system (CNS) in order to develop suitable therapeutic strategies to treat this menace of the society.

Our knowledge and awareness on the dependence caused by opioids or opioid-like drugs dates back to the advent of pharmacological sciences in early 19th century. The "withdrawal symptoms" caused by an abrupt cessation of these drugs leading to intense biological reactions was described by Himmelsbach about 62 years ago.[4] However, the consequences of withdrawal symptoms-induced alterations in the brain fluid microenvironment are still not well known (see TABLE 1). Recent investigations suggest that both spontaneous and drug-precipitated withdrawals induce alterations in the cellular and receptor levels in the CNS[3,5] and induce severe stressful situations. Thus, it is likely

TABLE 1. Shows studies on morphine withdrawal and blood–brain barrier (BBB) breakdown are still lacking

Subject headings	Number of hits	% of Morphine withdrawal
Morphine withdrawal symptoms	2,737	
Morphine dependence	2,615	
Morphine withdrawal	3,882	
+serotonin	150	4%
+serotonin2 receptor	8	0.2%
+serotonin3 receptor	12	2%
+nitric oxide	69	2%
+naloxone	1,959	50%
+gene expression	94	2%
+cAMP	120	3%
+Ca2+	98	1%
+BBB breakdown	0	
+BBB disruption	0	
+BBB damage	0	0
+BBB dysfunction#	12	
+cerebral blood flow	7	0.2%
+brain edema	0	0
+heat shock proteins	1	0
+glial fibrillary acidic protein	2	
+brain damage	2	0.05%

= limited to BBB permeability of ligands used in the abstract.
SOURCE: PubMed, November 2005.

that these psychostimulants may have some influence on the microvascular permeability function.

Experiments carried out in our laboratory in the last 25 years suggest that various kinds of emotional or environmental stressors depending on their magnitude and duration are able to alter the BBB permeability and induce brain dysfunction.[6–20] The BBB is a physiological dynamic barrier that regulates the composition of the fluid microenvironment within a narrow limit.[18] A slight alteration in the composition of the brain fluid microenvironment, in which neurons and glial cells bath, leads to abnormal brain function.[19] However, the BBB function and cellular reactions in the brain during administration or withdrawal of potential drugs of abuses have not been investigated so far.

Keeping these views in consideration, the present investigation is focused to examine the potential efficacy of morphine and methamphetamine on their ability to influence the BBB function in rodents. Furthermore, whether the alteration in the BBB function is associated with abnormal reactions in neuronal and glial cell was also examined using a morphological approach.

MATERIALS AND METHODS

Animals

Experiments were carried out on male Sprague-Dawley rats (250–300 g) and B57 mice (35–50 g) housed at controlled ambient temperature of $21 \pm 1°C$ with 12-h light and 12-h dark schedule. The food and tap water were supplied *ad libitum*.

The Model

We used rat model to study morphine dependence and spontaneous withdrawal[20–22] induced changes in the microvascular permeability disturbances in the brain.[20] The influence of acute methamphetamine administration (40 mg/kg, intraperitoneally once) on the BBB function was evaluated in mice model.[21] All experiments were carried out according to the NIH Guidelines for Care and Maintenance of Laboratory Animals.

Administration of Morphine and Development of Tolerance

In rat model, morphine tolerance was developed by injecting morphine hydrochloride (10 mg/kg, i.p) under aseptic conditions once daily at 8:00 AM for 12 days. The development of tolerance appeared from the 4th day and full tolerance was developed on the 12th day of morphine administration. The tail flick latency to thermal stimulus was examined 30 min after the administration of morphine daily.[22]

Administration of Methamphetamine

Methamphetamine (40 mg/kg) was administered into inbred B57 mice (35–50 g body weight). This dose of the compound induces marked hyperthermia and behavioral consequences (see Refs. 21 and 23). The BBB permeability was examined in these mice 4 h after drug administration using albumin immunohistochemistry (see below).

Measurement of Morphine Analgesia

The analgesic response to thermal stimulus was carried out by placing the middle part of the tail (keratinized scales were already removed 24 h before) on an electrically heated tungsten wire (50°C). The cutoff latency for tail-flick response was kept to 15 s (see FIG. 1). The control tail-flick response was determined in each animal before the morphine administration. The analgesic tests after morphine administration were carried out at every 10–15 min for about 120 min.[22,24]

Changes in Body Temperature

Changes in the deep core body temperature following morphine administration was recorded using a thermistor probe (Yellow Spring Co., St. Louis, MO) inserted into the rectum (about 6 cm) and connected to a 6-channel telethermometer (Electromed, London UK).[7]

Morphine Withdrawal Symptoms

To induce spontaneous morphine withdrawal symptoms, the morphine administration was withdrawn on the day 12 and the symptoms were noted daily for 72 h. Each rat was observed for 30 min and the gross abnormal behavior as described by Gianutsos *et al.*[25,26]

Wet-Shakes

These are vigorous shaking movements of the head and/or body of the rat similar to those produced by an animal when wetted with water.

Piloerection

This is the condition in which the fur on the body surface stood erect.

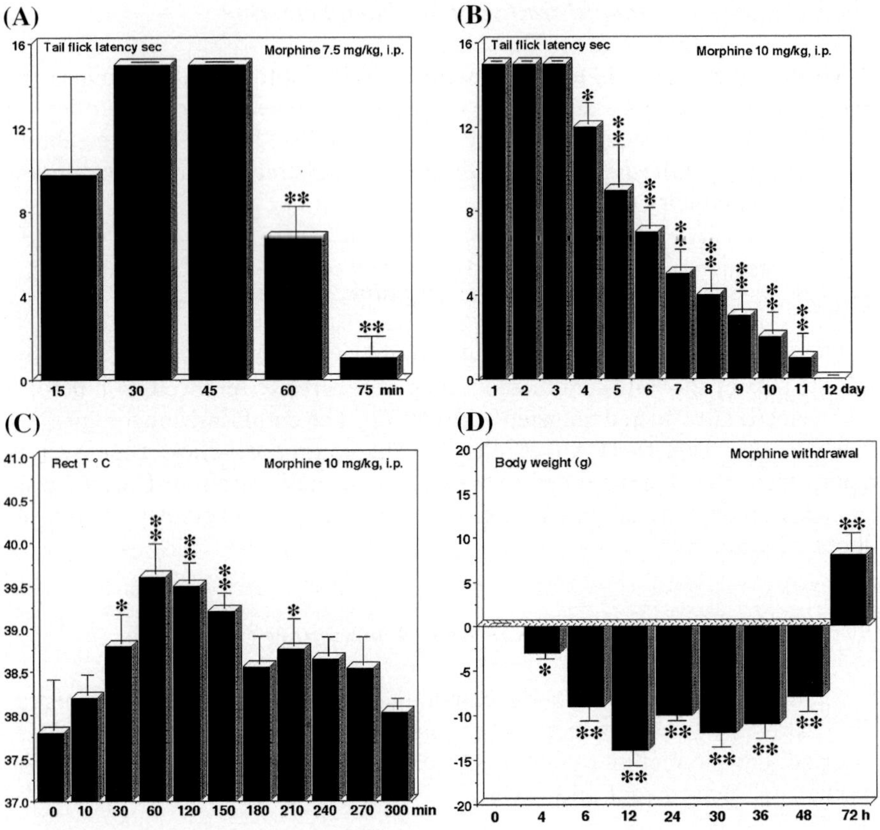

FIGURE 1. Morphine analgesia (**A**), dependence (**B**), hyperthermia (**C**), and body weight changes (**D**) in rats. Intraperitoneal administration of morphine (7.5 mg/kg) results in analgesia in naïve animals within 30 min and lasted up to 75 min (**A**). During chronic treatment with morphine (10 mg/kg, i.p.), tolerance to morphine appeared from the day 4 and onwards and on the day 12, all animals showed complete tolerance to morphine analgesia (**B**). Morphine administration (10 mg/kg, i.p.) resulted in hyperthermia in naive animals that reached its peak (+2.5°C) at 60 min and lasted up to 240 min (**C**). Loss of body weight following spontaneous withdrawal can be seen as early as 4 h after cessation of morphine that reached its peak at 12 h (−14 g) and lasted up to 48 h (−8 g). The body weight showed a significant gain at 72 h (+8 g) after discontinuation of morphine administration * = $P < 0.05$; ** = $P < 0.01$, ANOVA followed by Dunnet's test (data modified after Sharma *et al.*[24]).

Writhing

This syndrome consists of dragging of the abdomen along the floor of the cage with "sucking in" the abdominal wall or stretching and arching of the back, neither of which was accompanied with yawning.

Teeth Chattering

This is an audible distinct sound and was identical to the gnawing sound produced by a rat while eating food pellets.

Diarrhea

The presence or absence of formless stool generally adhered to the base of the tail was noted during 30-min observation period.

Aggressive Behavior

The aggressive behavior of the animal was explored by placing an untreated rat in the cage of the morphine-*withdrawn* rats for 5 min. Immediately after placement, the animals started fighting with squeaking and biting attempts. Animals often show erect posture and facing each other like a boxing stance. The morphine-withdrawn rats exhibiting such symptoms were termed as aggressive.

Loss of Body Weight

The weight of the morphine withdrawal rats was compared with the weight of animals immediately before morphine withdrawal.[20]

Physiological Variables

The mean arterial blood pressure (MABP), heart rate, arterial pH, and blood gases were examined in controls, morphine-treated, and-dependent rats as well as in rats subjected to morphine withdrawal according to standard procedures.[9,10]

Measurement of BBB Permeability to Intravascular Tracers

The BBB permeability was measured *in vivo* using two protein tracers, i.e., Evans blue (Mol. diam 0.60 nm) and $^{[131]}$Iodine (Mol diam 0.40 nm).[27] These tracers when administered into the circulation bind to the serum albumin.[27] Leakage of these tracers across the microvessels, thus represents extravasation of tracer-protein complexes.[28–30] Both tracers were administered into the right femoral vein at the end of experiments under anesthesia as described earlier[29,30] and allowed to circulate for 10 min. The intravascular tracer was washed out with sterile 0.9% saline perfused through heart (at 90 torr). After perfusion, the brains were removed, examined for Evans blue leakage, and the radioactivity determined in selected brain regions.[30]

Morphological Investigations

The morphological investigation of morphine-depended and-withdrawal rats were done using light and electron microscopy according to the standard protocol.[24] In addition, detection of specific markers or BBB dysfunction or nerve cell reaction or glial cell changes was examined using immunohistochemistry.

Light Microscopy

Selected brain regions from control and morphine-treated or-withdrawal rats were embedded in paraffin and examined for nerve cell changes reaction using routine haemotoxylin and eosin or Nissl staining at light microscopy.[16]

Immunohistochemistry

In separate group of animals, immunohistochemistry was employed to study leakage to the BBB, activation of astrocytes as well as upregulation of heat shock protein (HSP-72 kD), a marker of stress reaction using standard procedures. The integrity of the BBB was examined using a sheep polyclonal anti-rat albumin antibody (Sigma, St. Louis, MO) with immunostaining of albumin.[31,32] The state of glial activation was examined using antibodies to glial fibrillary acidic protein (GFAP), a specific marker of astrocytes.[33,34] The HSP expression was examined in the using antibodies directed against HSP-72 kD (Amersham, England, UK).[35–37]

Immunostaining was detected using the streptavidin-HRP-biotin technique as described previously.[36,37] Reagent controls (omitting the primary antibody or substituting nonimmune serum for the primary antibody in the staining protocol) on tissue sections revealed no staining, thus confirming the specificity of the primary antibodies used.

Microphotography and Processing of Digital Images

Microphotographs were taken on Kodak Supra 100 ASA Color negative film under a Leica bright field microscope. The digital images (size 52 cm × 32 cm, 80 pixels/inch) were processed on a CD by Kodak Color Laboratories

(Stockholm, Sweden). These digital images were modified using Adobe Photoshop 3.5 program on a G-4 Macintosh computer. The images obtained from the control or experimental groups were processed (final image size 8 × 13 cm, 300 pixels/inch) using identical color filter and color balance.[16]

Semiquantitative Analysis of Immunohistochemical Data

The semiquantitative analysis of immunostaining in the controls and experimental groups were done manually in a blinded fashion. The number of immunostained cells per section was counted in the desired anatomical region in each slide obtained from each group of minimum five rats as described earlier.[16]

Electron Microscopy

For ultrastructural investigation, selected tissue pieces were postfixed in osmium and embedded in Epon as described earlier.[37] The ultrathin sections from the desired area were cut using a diamond knife (LKB, Ultramicrotome, Stockholm, Sweden) and collected on one hole grid. The sections were examined under transmission electron microscope (Phillips Amsterdam 400) after counterstaining with uranyl acetate and lead citrate. Some of the sections were examined unstained.[36,37]

Lanthanum Extravasation Across the BBB

The passage of tracer transfer across the BBB was examined at the ultrastructural level using a small molecule ionic tracer, lanthanum ($La3+$ ionic form, hydrated; Mol. diameter <10 Å).[13,27,28] This tracer under normal conditions does not penetrate CNS microvessels.[30]

The lanthanum was added to the fixative (2.5%) during perfusion followed by saline rinse in some group of animals.[28–30] After perfusion, the brain tissue pieces were processed according to standard transmission electron microscopy.[13,28,37,38]

Statistical Analysis of Data

The quantitative data obtained were analyzed using ANOVA followed by Dunnet's test for multiple group comparison using one control group. The semiquamtitiave data were analyzed using non-parametric chi-square test. A P value <0.05 was considered significant.

RESULTS

Morphine Analgesia and Dependence

In naïve rats, administration of morphine (7.5 mg/kg, i.p.) induced analgesia to thermal stimulus within 30 min that lasted for 75 min (FIG. 1). Thus, for the development of tolerance and dependence, a 10 mg/kg, i.p. dose of morphine was used (FIG. 1). The development of tolerance to analgesic response of morphine in rats occurred with a single daily injection of morphine (10 mg/kg, i.p.). The onset of development of tolerance was found to commence from the fourth day onwards. The full tolerance was developed by the 12th day of morphine treatment (FIG. 1).

Morphine-Induced Hyperthermia

Administration of morphine (10 mg/kg, i.p.) induced profound hyperthermia (+1.8°C; from 37.6 ± 0.43 to 39.4 ± 0.23°C) at 60 min and continued until 90 min. The body temperature remained elevated (>1°C) even 5 h after the morphine administration (FIG. 1). Morphine hyperthermia was diminished in chronic morphine-treated rats. Thus, from the day 6 to 8 and onwards, hyperthermia is largely absent in the morphine dependent animals (results not shown).

Morphine Withdrawal Symptoms

The withdrawal symptoms were examined after the development of complete morphine tolerance to analgesia was developed on the day 12 as evident with their analgesic response. In these morphine-dependent rats, cessation of morphine injection resulted in the appearance of spontaneous withdrawal symptoms within 12 h (TABLE 2). The withdrawal symptoms were mainly observed to be the loss of body weight (FIG. 1), "wet-shake" phenomena, piloerection, writhing, teeth chattering, diarrhea, and aggressive behavior and jumping (TABLE 2). These withdrawal symptoms continue to worsen with advancement of time. Thus, the withdrawal symptoms were aggravated at 24 and 48 h after the cessation of morphine. No apparent reduction in the withdrawal symptoms was observed until 72 h later the cessation of morphine administration (TABLE 2, FIG. 1).

Physiological Variables

Morphine-dependent rats on the 10th and the 12th day exhibited profound hyperthermia and an increase in the MABP compared to the control group

TABLE 2. Effect of morphine dependence and withdrawal on stress symptoms and physiological variables

		Morphine dependence		Morphine withdrawal		
Parameters	Control	1st day	12th day	12 h	24 h	48 h
Physiological variables	$n = 6$	$n = 8$	$n = 6$	$n = 8$	$n = 8$	$n = 6$
MABP torr	110 ± 8	122 ± 8**	140 ± 6**	90 ± 4**	128 ± 6**	146 ± 14**
Arterial pH	7.38 ± 0.02	7.36 ± 0.08	7.36 ± 0.05	7.35 ± 0.06	7.36 ± 0.08	7.34 ± 0.05
PaO^2 torr	81.56 ± 0.23	80.34 ± 0.32	78.34 ± 1.34	81.87 ± 0.23	82.45 ± 0.34**a	82.67 ± 0.31**a
$PaCO^2$ torr	34.62 ± 0.34	33.32 ± 0.22	33.10 ± 0.43	33.21 ± 0.43	31.54 ± 1.24	32.06 ± 1.34
Body temp °C	37.61 ± 0.42	39.42 ± 0.41**	38.42 ± 0.31	39.54 ± 0.23**	40.23 ± 0.18**a	39.28 ± 0.11**a
Heart rate beats/min	280 ± 12	320 ± 18* 330 ± 12**	338 ± 10**	304 ± 8*	310 ± 8*a	308 ± 7*
Respiration cycles/min	76 ± 6	80 ± 8	86 ± 7**	89 ± 5*	94 ± 4**a	92 ± 5**
Stress symptoms	$n = 6$	$n = 6$	$n = 8$	$n = 8$	$n = 14$	$n = 16$
Wet-shakes	Nil	Nil	Nil	4 ± 2	8 ± 3a	6 ± 2
Piloerection	Nil	Nil	Nil	+++	+++++	++++
Writhing	Nil	Nil	Nil	+++	+++++	++++
Teeth chattering	Nil	Nil	Nil	+++	+++++	+++++
Diarrhea	Nil	Nil	Nil	+++	+++++	+++
Aggressive behavior	Nil	Nil	?	+++	+++++	+++++
Microhemorrhages in stomach	Nil	6 ± 5	12 ± 8	48 ± 12	68 ± 18#	85 ± 14#

Values are mean ± SD.

= many microhemorrhages; a = significantly different ($P < 0.05$) from morphine withdrawal 12 h; +++ = mild; ++++ = moderate; +++++ = severe; ? = unclear; Nil = absent; * = $P < 0.05$; ** = $P < 0.01$

Data modified after Sharma.[18]

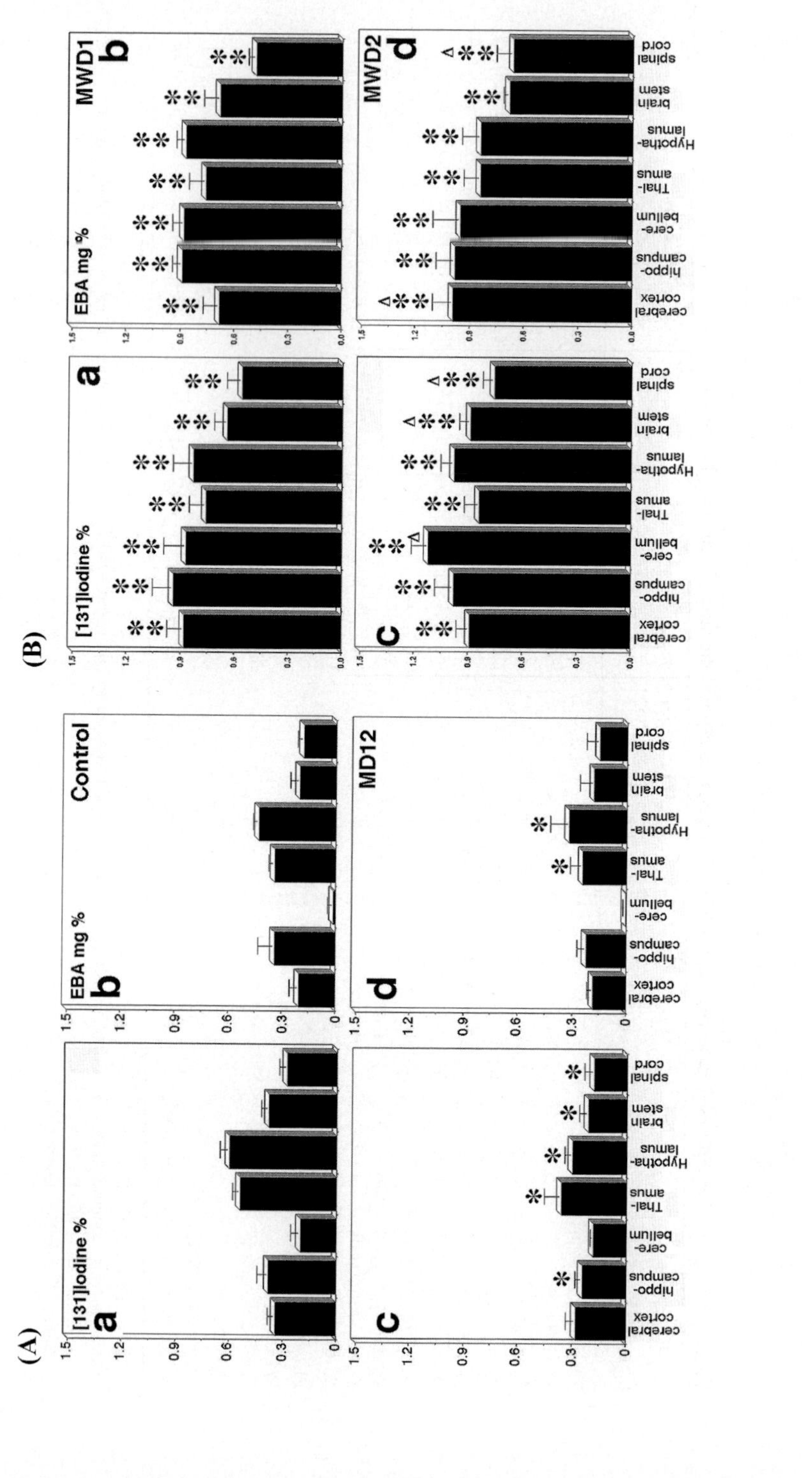
(A)
(B)
[131]Iodine %
EBA mg %
Control
MD12
MWD1
MWD2
a
b
c
d
cerebral cortex
hippo-campus
cere-bellum
Thal-amus
Hypotha-lamus
brain stem
spinal cord
1.5
1.2
0.9
0.6
0.3
0

(TABLE 2). In these animals, the heart rate and respiration cycles were increased significantly compared to the control rats (TABLE 2). The arterial pH did not differ from the controls, however, there was a significant increase in the arterial $PaCO^2$ in morphine-withdrawal rats compared to the control group. On the other hand, the PaO^2 values were slightly but significantly decreased (TABLE 2).

Spontaneous withdrawal of morphine treatment showed a significant increase in the MABP at 24 h that remained stable until 48 h of cessation of the morphine treatment. The heart rate did not altered; however the respiration rate was slightly increased from the chronic morphine treatment. The blood gases showed marked increase in $PaCO^2$ and a slight decrease in PaO^2 without any changes in the arterial pH. Chronic treatment with morphine alone did not alter these variables, however, significantly.

Stress Symptoms

In morphine-withdrawal rats, the stress symptoms were most severe following 24 and 48 h after the cessation of morphine administration. These animals showed profound hyperthermia. In these animals, the body weight decreased significantly and the food and water intake was also considerably reduced. These symptoms are most prominent in animals subjected to 48 h of morphine withdrawal.

FIGURE 2. BBB permeability to $^{[131]}$Iodine (a,c) and Evans blue (b,d) tracers in the control, morphine dependent (**A**) and following morphine withdrawal (**B**) in various brain regions in the rat. The BBB permeability to Evans blue and radioiodine varies in different brain regions and was significantly lower in the cerebellum, brain stem, and spinal cord (A.a,b) compared to the cerebral cortex. However, a slight increase in the BBB permeability to these tracers was seen in the thalamus and hypothalamus (A.a,b) compared to the cerebral cortex. Chronic treatment with morphine in rats resulted in a slight but significant decline in the BBB permeability to the tracers that was most significant in the hippocampus, thalamus, hypothalamus, brain stem, and the spinal cord to radioiodine tracer (A.c). Whereas, only thalamus and hypothalamus showed significant decline in morphine dependent (MD) rats on the day 12 to Evans blue (A.d). Morphine withdrawal for 1 day (MWD1) resulted in profound increase in the BBB permeability to these protein tracers (B.a,b) in all the regions examined (B.a–d). This increase in the regional BBB permeability was further enhanced on the second day of morphine withdrawal (MWD2, B.c,d). This increase in the rBBB to iodine was significant in the cerebellum in MWD2 group compared to MWD1 rats, whereas the increase in Evans blue extravasation was found to be higher in the cerebral cortex and the spinal cord in MWD2 rats compared to the corresponding MWD1 group. Values are mean ± SD of 5 to 8 rats. ANOVA followed by Dunnet's test for multiple group comparison from one control. ** $= P < 0.01$; * $= P < 0.05$, compared from control group. $\Delta = P < 0.05$ compared to corresponding MED1 group. EBA = Evans blue albumin; MD12 = morphine-dependent day 12; MWD1 = morphine withdrawal day 1; MWD2 = morphine withdrawal day 2. Data modified after Sharma *et al.*[24]

The symptoms of jumping, teeth chattering, writhing, circular motion, and restlessness in the cages as evident with hyper-locomotor activity were most pronounced during 24-h withdrawal period. The occurrence of diarrhea was most prominent on the second day of morphine withdrawal. At post-mortem, many microhemorrhages were noted in the mucosal wall of the stomach indicating formation of stress ulcers (TABLE 2).

BBB Permeability

Using intravascular tracers, such as Evans blue albumin and radioactive iodine, changes in the BBB permeability during morphine dependence or morphine withdrawal in rats are shown in FIGURE 2.

Normal Animals

The BBB permeability to Evans blue and $^{[131]}$Iodine in normal animals remained very low in several brain regions (FIG. 2), although the magnitude and tracer extravasation varied in different CNS regions. The cerebellum, brain stem, and spinal exhibited least extravasation of the Evans blue and radioactive iodine tracers, whereas thalamus and hypothalamus showed moderately high concentration compared to the cerebral cortex (FIG. 2).

Morphine-Dependent Animals

Chronic morphine treatment did not result in any increase in the tracer extravasation in the CNS. However, in some brain regions, a significant decrease in the tracer extravasation was observed. This decrease was significant in the thalamus, hypothalamus, and in the cerebral cortex (FIG. 2).

Morphine-Withdrawal Animals

Morphine-withdrawal animals exhibited significant increase in the permeability of the BBB to Evans blue and radioactive iodine in the cerebral cortex, hippocampus, and the cerebellum. The hypothalamus and thalamus showed only moderate increase in the permeability (FIG. 2).

On the second day, a significantly higher increase in the permeability to these tracers was noted in all the brain regions (FIG. 2). The most significant increase in the BBB permeability was noted in the cerebellum followed by cerebral cortex, thalamus, and hypothalamus at this time compared to the other regions (FIG. 2).

Extravasation of Lanthanum at the Ultrastructural Level

Lanthanum extravasation was examined in animals following second day of morphine withdrawal in the cerebral cortex, cerebellum, and the spinal cord (see TABLE 3). The lanthanum was mainly infiltrated into the endothelial cell cytoplasm, whereas in some cases, the tracer was found in the basal lamina as well. However, the tight junctions remained intact to lanthanum (FIG. 3). Occasionally, the tracer was also seen in vesicular profiles located within the endothelial cell cytoplasm in some large superficial vessels.

The endothelial cell membrane permeability to lanthanum appears to be very selective and specific following morphine withdrawal. The most marked endothelial cell infiltration was seen in the cerebellar capillaries. Several microvessels, often comprising only one endothelial cell, show only a part of the membrane permeable to lanthanum leaving other areas of the endothelial cell completely normal.

Leakage of Albumin across the BBB During Morphine Withdrawal

Rats subjected to morphine withdrawal showed profound leakage of albumin as seen using immunohistochemistry in several brain areas (FIG. 3). The albumin immunoreactivity was mainly seen in the neuropil. However, in several brain regions, few nerve cells exhibited albumin immunoreactivity, whereas some glial cells, possibly astrocytes, exhibited albumin immunostaining. The intensity of albumin immunoreactivity was much more pronounced on the second and third day of morphine withdrawal. The nerve cells showing albumin immunoreactivity were largely distorted and edematous in appearance. Most pronounced extravasation of albumin was seen in edematous areas of the brain or spinal cord (results not shown).

Leakage of Albumin across the BBB in Methamphetamine-Treated Mice

Mice subjected to methamphetamine treatment showed profound leakage of albumin as seen in the cerebral cortex of animals (FIG. 3). The leakage of albumin was mainly seen within the neuropil. Few nerve cells took albumin staining as well. However, the magnitude and intensity of albumin immunostaining was much less severe compared to the rats subjected to morphine withdrawal (FIG. 3). Interestingly, the area showing BBB disruption also exhibited pronounced nerve cell damage, sponginess, and edema (FIG. 3).

Morphological Changes in Morphine Dependent or Withdrawal

Rats subjected to spontaneous morphine treatment or withdrawal showed mild to moderate degree of nerve cell and glial cell reaction at both light and electron microscopy.

TABLE 3. Semiquantitative data on lanthanum extravasation in 120 vascular profiles from the cerebellum and the cerebral cortex

		Lanthanum distribution in 80 microvascular profiles (no.)							
		Endothelial cell cytoplasm		Basal lamina		Vesivular profile		Between the tight junctions#	
Type of Experiment	*n*	Cerebellum	Cortex	Cerebellum	Cortex	Cerebellum	Cortex	Cerebellum	Cortex
Control	5	0	0	0	0	6 ± 4	8 ± 5	0	0
Morphine 12th day	6	16 ± 8*	10 ± 4*	10 ± 6*	8 ± 4*	22 ± 6*	18 ± 6	1 ± 1	1 ± 2
Morphine withdrawal 24 h	6	38 ± 10*	306 ± 12*	24 ± 6*	22 ± 8*	40 ± 12*	38 ± 10*	2 ± 2	3 ± 2
Morphine withdrawal 48 h	6	51 ± 6*	46 ± 9*	48 ± 9*	38 ± 8*	48 ± 9*	418 ± 12*	2 ± 2	2 ± 3

Data from 5 to 6 animals in each group; values are mean ± SD.
* = $P < 0.01$; chi-square test, significantly different from control group; # = lanthanum is seen between the two tight junctions and stopped at the second one.
Data modified after Sharma.[18]

Nerve Cell Reaction

Few nerve cells showed degenerative changes in animals subjected to either acute methamphetamine administration or chronic morphine treatment in the regions showing BBB leakage as seen using albumin extravasation (FIG. 3). During morphine withdrawal, most pronounced nerve cell damage was seen in the brain stem reticular formation (FIG. 3). However, scattered damaged nerve cells were also present in the cerebral cortex, hippocampus, thalamus, and hypothalamus (Sharma, unpublished observations).

These changes in nerve cell further enhanced during morphine withdrawal and were most prominent on the second day compared to morphine dependent rats (FIG. 3). The damaged nerve cells were largely present in the regions showing leakage of albumin, sponginess, and edema. Perivascular regions around large vessels often show profound degeneration of the neuropil (FIG. 3). The epithelial cell layers of the choroid plexus also exhibited profound degenerative changes following morphine withdrawal (FIG. 3).

Glial Cell Reaction

Light microscopy revealed pronounced cell damage around the perivascular regions containing astrocytes. Thus, in selected brain regions GFAP immunoreactivity, a specific marker of astrocytes, was used in animals during morphine dependence and withdrawal experiments. Chronic morphine treatment resulted in mild to moderate activation of astrocytes in different brain or spinal cord regions compared to controls (FIG. 3). This activation of astrocytes is much more pronounced during 2nd day of spontaneous morphine withdrawal (FIG. 3).

HSP Expression

We examined HSP-72 expression to determine the magnitude and severity of cellular stress during second day of morphine withdrawal. Chronic treatment with morphine resulted in a mild upregulation of HSP in selected CNS regions. This effect was most pronounced following morphine withdrawal on the second day (FIG. 3) that continued until 72 h after cessation of morphine treatment (results not shown). The magnitude and intensity of HSP expression was most pronounced in the damaged nerve cells and probably glial cells located in the edematous areas showing extravasation of albumin (Sharma and Ali, unpublished observations).

Ultrastructural Changes in the Neuropil

In morphine-dependent animals, vacuolation, membrane disruption, and damage to cellular structures are seen in some regions of the brain. These

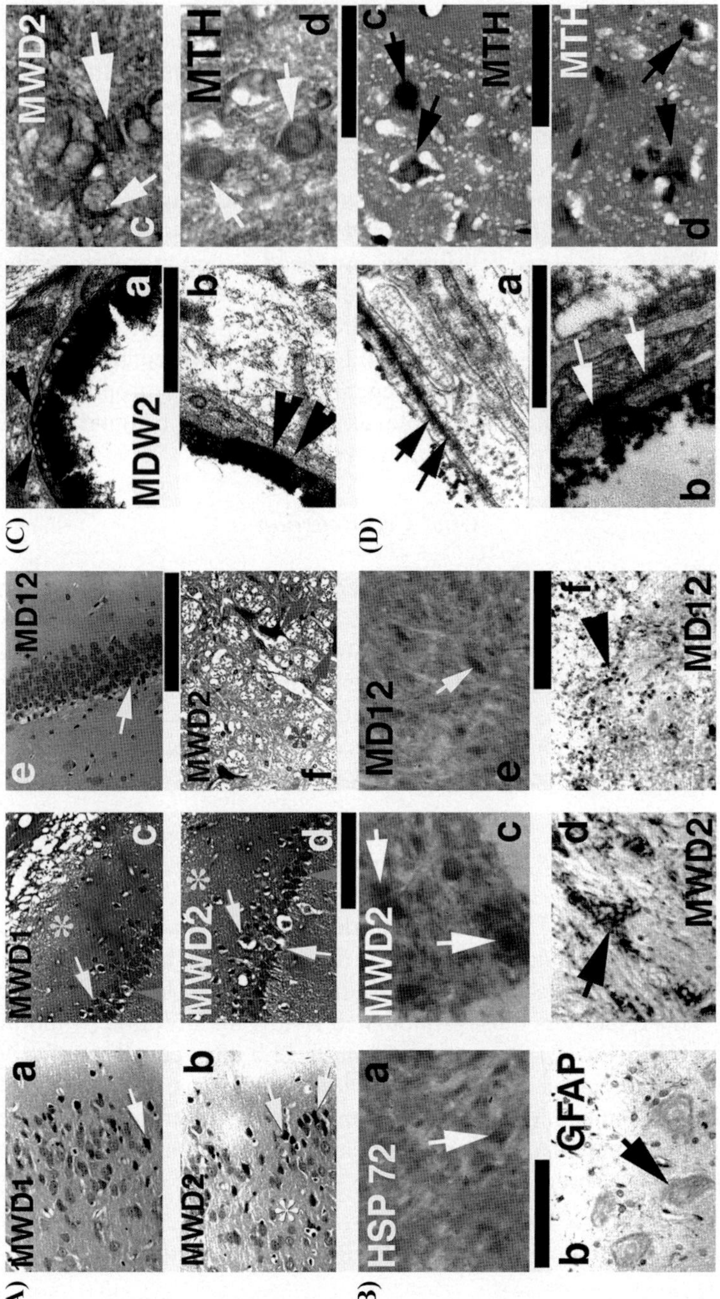
(A)
MWD1
MWD2
MD12
(B)
HSP 72
GFAP
MWD2
MD12
(C)
MDW2
MWD2
MTH
(D)
MTH

FIGURE 3. Changes in nerve cell (**A**), HSP-72 and GFAP expression (**B**), lanthanum and albumin extravasation (**C, D**) in rodents following morphine and methamphetamine administration. (**A**) Nerve cell changes in the rat brain following morphine dependence (day 12; MD12) or after its spontaneous withdrawal following day 1 (MWD1) or day 2 (MWD2). A. Nissl stained paraffin sections (3 μM thick) from rat brain passing through piriform area (−3.70 mm from bregma) shows marked selective nerve cell damage following 1 day after morphine withdrawal (MWD1; arrows, A.a). The magnitude and intensity of nerve cell damage appear to be increased following second day of morphine withdrawal (MWD2; arrows, A.b). Haematoxylin and eosin (H & E) stained 3 μM thick paraffin sections passing through hippocampus (−3.25 mm from bregma) showing selective cell damage in the CA-1 subfield from rats following morphine withdrawal (day 1, MWD1, A.c and day 2, MWD2, A.d). Sponginess and edema (*) are clearly visible. In morphine-dependent rats on the day 12 (MD 12, A.e), damage to hippocampal dentate granule cells (−4.20 mm from bregma) are clearly seen (Nissl stain, arrows). Paraffin section passing through the mesencephalic reticular nucleus (−7.10 mm from bregma) show many damaged nerve cells (H& E stain, arrows), sponginess, and edema (*) on the second day of spontaneous morphine withdrawal in dependent rats (MWD2, A.f). Bars: A.a,b,c,d = 25 μM; A.e,f = 30 μM. Data modified after Sharma *et al.*[24] (**B**) Immunoreactivity of heat shock protein (HSP, arrows) 72 kD, a marker of cellular stress in the spinal cord (C-5) of morphine dependent rats in the ventral (B.a) and in lateral (B.e) horns in the morphine dependent rat on the day 12 (MD12,) and in the ventral horn (B.c) and following second day of spontaneous morphine withdrawal (MWD2). Increased intensity of HSP expression is evident in rat subjected to morphine withdrawal (MWD2, c,d, arrows). The HSP immunostaining is largely present in the cell cytoplasm, however in some cases nerve cell nucleus also exhibited HSP expression. Bars = B.a,e = 40 μM; B.c = 30 μM. Data modified after Sharma *et al.*[24] Increased expression of GFAP (a marker of astrocytes activation) immunoreactivity in the spinal cord of in one 12-day morphine-dependent (MD 12, B.f) rat and following second day of morphine withdrawal (MWD2, B.d) rat compared to control (B.b). Activation of astrocytes as seen using expression of GFAP is much more intense in rats following second day of morphine withdrawal (MWD2). Bar: B.b = 25 μM, d = 30 μM, f = 40 μM. Data modified after Sharma *et al.*[24] (**C–D**) Lanthanum infiltration is seen (arrowheads) across the endothelial cell of one microvessel from the cerebral cortex (C.b) and from the cervical spinal cord (C.a) following 48 h after spontaneous morphine withdrawal in dependent rat. Several microvesicular profiles within the endothelium are clearly seen (C.a). The tight junctions are still closed for lanthanum (arrows) in the cerebral (D.b) and spinal cord (D.a) microvessel. Edematous swelling of perivascular astrocytes is also evident (C.b; D.b). Bars = 500 nm (C.a); 600 nm (C.b); 300 nm (D.a); 400 nm (D.b). Data modified after Sharma *et al.*[24] Extravasation of albumin as seen using immunohistochemistry is evident in the cerebral cortex of the rat subjected to 48 h of spontaneous morphine withdrawal. Leakage of albumin is seen around the nerve cell and within the nerve cell cytoplasm (arrows) located within the edematous region (C.c). Leakage of albumin is also evident in the nerve cell cytoplasm and in the neuropil (arrows) of mouse cerebral cortex following single injection of methamphetamine (C.b). The magnitude and intensity of albumin leakage however is much less compared to the rats subjected top spontaneous morphine withdrawal (for details, see text). Methamphetamine showed pronounced neurotoxicity in brain regions showing breakdown of the BBB function as seen by leakage of albumin (D.c,d). Thus, perineuronal edema, distorted and damaged nerve cells (arrows) are quite frequent in the edematous regions showing sponginess and edema (D.c,d). Bars: C.c,d = 50 μM; D.c,d = 40 μM.

cellular changes are most prominent in the brain stem reticular information (results not shown). Morphine withdrawal further aggravated these changes and thus vacuolation, edema, cell membrane damage, and appearance of swollen cells are much more frequent in the neuropil in several brain regions (results not shown).

DISCUSSION

The present investigation for the first time shows the spontaneous morphine withdrawal in rats, and acute amphetamine administration in mice is associated with a selective and specific breakdown of the BBB to proteins. Our observations further show that this breakdown of the BBB to large molecules, such as albumin is largely seen in the regions showing distortion of neuronal, endothelial, and glial cells structure and function. This indicates that leakage of proteins across the BBB is mainly responsible for the altered brain function and neurotoxicity commonly seen during usage of these drugs of abuse. An increased expression of HSP-72 in nerve cells and probably glial cells in the areas showing extravasation of serum proteins is in line with this hypothesis.

Another important finding of this investigation is marked activation of astrocytes, as seen using GFAP immunostaining during morphine dependence caused by single low dose of the morphine administration. This observation suggests that morphine somehow activates glial cells when administered repeatedly and is in line with one previous study showing similar activation of GFAP following 8–10 days after high dose of twice daily morphine (15 mg/kg, s.c. for 8–10 days) administration in rats.[39] Our observations further revealed a massive upregulation of GFAP following morphine withdrawal indicating that astrocytes actively participate in the process of withdrawal symptoms as well, not reported earlier.

Taken together, these novel observations indicate that drugs of abuse are capable to alter almost all neural and non-neural components within the CNS by influencing its fluid microenvironment leading to brain pathology and/or neurodegeneration.

Morphine Dependence and CNS Function

Our results clearly show that morphine dependence can be developed in rats by daily single injection of the compound for 12 days. This observation is in line with previous studies showing that both chronic administration of the exogenous or endogenous opioids for pain relief results in the development of tolerance to both their analgesic and pharmacological actions that is probably mediated through the μ-receptors (for details, see Refs. 3, 40–42).

It appears that disturbances in the CNS homeostasis by opioids are somehow responsible for the development of dependence as suggested by Himmelsbach about 62 years ago[4] (for review, see Refs. 3 and 24). Our observations further support this idea and demonstrate that chronic administration of morphine is associated with alterations in the neuronal microenvironment as well as profound neuronal, glial, and endothelial cell reactions. Whether these changes are reversible or permanent in nature is still unclear and require additional investigation.

Spontaneous Withdrawal Precipitates Symptoms

Another important observation from our study shows that an abrupt cessation of morphine injection on the day 12 resulted in profound withdrawal symptoms within 24 h. The symptoms of morphine withdrawal can be induced either by abrupt cessation of morphine or by administration of opioid receptor antagonists, e.g., naloxone, naltrexone, nalorphine, and other related compounds.[40] The withdrawal symptoms following abrupt or antagonist-induced withdrawal differ particularly in their onset, intensity, and duration. In general, the spontaneous withdrawal symptoms take long time to appear, e.g., 24 h after or later. While the drug-induced withdrawal can be precipitated within few hours depending on the nature of induced withdrawals, the symptoms and apparently the stress associated with withdrawal may also differ.

Our observations suggest that the magnitude and intensity of spontaneous withdrawal symptoms are progressive in nature, i.e., from 24 h up to 48 h and then declined slightly at 72 h. The breakdown of the BBB function closely corresponds to the intensity of withdrawal symptoms. Thus, it would be interesting to find out whether drug-induced withdrawal is also associated with BBB disturbances and cellular alterations in the CNS. This aspect is particularly important to investigate as most of the opioid antagonists, e.g., naloxone and naltrexone that are used to precipitate drug-induced withdrawal symptoms, are also known to attenuate stress response and BBB disturbances in other animal models.[18,43,44]

Psychostimulants Versus Cellular Stress

Repeated morphine administration appears to activate the hypothalamic-pituitary-adrenal (HPA) axis and thus are able to induce considerable stress response in both experimental and in clinical situations.[41,42,45–47] Activation of HPA axis in stressful situation[18] is quite comparable to that seen in humans using drug abuse and is in line with this idea.[18,24] There are evidences that acute morphine treatment increases corticotrophin-releasing hormone (CRH) release which, in turn, induces the secretions of adrenocorticotrophic hormone (ACTH) and corticosterone.[18,24,48] Similar activation of HPA as observed during other chronic stress conditions are also seen following repeated exposure to morphine.[18,24] Thus, like other chronic stressors, long-term morphine treatment results in a decrease in body weight, thymus involution, hypertrophy of the adrenal glands, and an elevated level of the basal corticosteroids concentration.[41,42,48] Our studies provide new lines of evidences that support the idea that chronic morphine treatment induced profound cellular stress as evident with the overexpression of HSP as well as massive alterations in the neuronal and glial cell function.

Withdrawal Symptoms Versus Stress

There are indications that withdrawal of morphine in chronically morphine-intoxicated rats also induces profound and severe stress reactions.[24,41,42,48,49] This is apparent from the findings that rats undergoing 12-h spontaneous morphine withdrawal exhibited a potentiated and prolonged corticosterone response following restraint despite of a high basal corticosterone levels in their plasma during chronic morphine treatment.[41] Normally, elevated hormone level will act as negative feedback for further release of corticosterone under stressful situations.[18,24,41,42]

It appears that the enhanced response of stress in rats undergoing morphine withdrawal is quite comparable to the HPA response during an acute novel stressor applied to any chronically stressed rats.[48,49] An enhanced activity of paraventricular thalamic and hypothalamic nuclei, activation of CRH neurons in the hypothalamus, increased sensitivity of adrenal to ACTH, and reduced glucocorticoid receptor (GR) expression in the hippocampus[50–52] following morphine withdrawal is in line with this idea. However, the anatomical neural network behind morphine withdrawal-induced stress response is still unclear and requires further investigation.

Mechanisms of Increased Vascular Permeability

The detailed mechanisms of increased BBB permeability following morphine withdrawal or methamphetamine administration are not fully understood. However, there are reasons to believe that drug-induced hyperthermia, release of several neurochemical mediators, cytokines, immunomodulators, and/or signal transduction molecules are playing important roles (see Refs. 18 and 24).

Alterations in serotonin, neuropeptides, nitric oxide, histamine, and other vasoactive agents that are known mediators of BBB breakdown occur during morphine withdrawal or methamphetamine administration. It is quite likely that these neurochemicals or vasoactive agents act on cerebral microvessels through a receptor-mediated events and through several secondary mechanisms of signal transduction agents leading to the opening of the BBB.[53–57] An increase in cAMP following morphine withdrawal can lead to increase in the BBB permeability.[13–15,29,35,37,55] Likewise NO-mediated stimulation of cGMP can also increase the BBB function (see Refs. 58 and 59). Many neurochemicals act through opening of Ca^{2+} channels.[18,57,60] An opening of Ca^{2+} channel during trauma or disease condition will cause alteration in the BBB permeability.[56,57] Blockade of Ca^{2+} channel in several conditions is known to attenuate BBB dysfunction.[18,57] Thus, it appears that several molecular mechanisms of cellular transduction play important role in BBB dysfunction during morphine withdrawal.

It seems likely that the mechanism of BBB opening in morphine withdrawal is very similar to that seen during stress and trauma. Thus, NOS inhibitors or Ca^{2+} channel blockers that attenuated heat stress or spinal cord injury-induced microvascular permeability disturbances[13–15,19,28,38,44,58,59] are able to reduce morphine withdrawal-induced BBB dysfunction (Sharma and Ali, unpublished observations). These observations indicate that the cellular and molecular mechanisms of BBB breakdown in many diverse situations are quite similar in nature. Obviously, opening of the BBB in several diseases or in experimental conditions is instrumental in cell injury.

Possible Significance of BBB Dysfunction and Unanswered Questions

This is not yet clear whether the increased BBB permeability during morphine withdrawal is necessary for the altered physiological demand or may represent adverse pathological condition leading to brain damage. Structural alterations in the CNS during morphine withdrawal suggest that opening of the BBB appears to contribute to the adverse cell reaction in the CNS. Whether these cell changes and the BBB dysfunction are reversible in nature still remains to be investigated.

Interestingly, we found that chronic morphine treatment decreases the BBB function and induces neuronal damage. The mechanism behind a decrease in the BBB and its possible significance is unclear. It seems quite likely that if the barrier is tightened enough to influence normal transport mechanisms, the CNS functions appear to be disturbed. Likewise, if the barrier function is increased to unwanted substances, it can also lead to the adverse cell reaction. Thus, a normal function of the BBB is needed for optimal function of the CNS, a feature that requires further investigation.

Thus, the opioid dependence is associated with tightening of the barrier and withdrawal is associated with the opposite effects, i.e., breakdown of the barrier. Under both conditions, adverse neuronal changes and cell damage are evident. At that time, no increase in the BBB permeability is seen. However, blood flow studies showed profound ischemia during morphine dependence. Thus, the cell changes seen during morphine dependence may represent selective neuronal injury due to morphine toxicity and/or ischemia associated with opioid administration. Morphine withdrawal aggravates neuronal damage in these animals probably due to breakdown of the BBB function. It may be that during morphine dependence, the cell changes seen could be due to local alterations in neuronal energy metabolism, toxicity, or alteration in cellular membrane function.[60] Similar cellular damage during early phase of ischemic injuries without clear disruption of the BBB to large molecular tracers[57,60] supports this idea.

There are reasons to believe that drugs that reduced the morphine withdrawal symptoms and brain damage are able to attenuate BBB disruption (see Refs. 18, 54, and 59). This indicates that the withdrawal symptoms, opening of the BBB, and brain damage are interrelated. However, it is still unclear whether opening of the BBB results in withdrawal symptoms or the stress associated with withdrawal symptoms is capable to induce BBB dysfunction. To clarify these points, additional studies using pharmacological blockade of withdrawal symptoms and/or BBB at various time intervals after morphine withdrawal is needed, a feature that is currently being investigated in our laboratory.

Future Directions

Our laboratory is now engaged to study selective expression of immediate early gene expression and apoptotic pathways in relation to alterations in various neurotransmitters and their receptors in our model of morphine dependence and withdrawal. These investigations will definitely expand our knowledge on the cellular and molecular mechanism of opioid-induced tolerance and dependence with regard to the breakdown of the BBB function and brain pathology.

ACKNOWLEDGMENTS

This study is supported by grants from Swedish Medical Research Council No. 2710, Göran Gustafsson Foundation, Sweden, Astra-Zeneca Mölndal, Sweden, The University Grants Commission, New Delhi, India, and The Alexander von Humboldt Foundation, Bonn, Germany. The skillful technical assistance of Kärstin Flink, Ingmarie Olsson, Inga Hörte, Madeleine Järild, and Gunilla Tibling; the computer assistance of Leif Ljung and Suraj Sharma; and the secretarial assistance of Angela Ludwig and Aruna Sharma is highly appreciated.

REFERENCES

1. BUCKINGHAM, J.C. & T.A. COOPER. 1984. Differences in hypothalamo-pituitary-adrenocortical activity in the rat after acute and prolonged treatment with morphine. Neuroendocrinology **38:** 411–417.

2. BHATNAGAR, S. & M. DALLMAN. 1998. Neuroanatomical basis for facilitation of hypothalamic-pituitary-adrenal responses to a novel stressor after chronic stress. Neuroscience **84:** 1025–1039.
3. WILLIAMS, J.T., M.J. CHRISTIE & O. MANZONI. 2001. Cellular and synaptic adaptations mediating opioid dependence. Physiol. Rev. **81:** 299–343.
4. HIMMELSBACH, C.K. 1943. With reference to physical dependence. Fed. Proc. **2:** 201–203.
5. MITCHELL, J.M., A.I. BASBAUM & H.L. FIELDS. 2000. A locus and mechanism of action for associative morphine tolerance. Nat. Neurosci. **3:** 47–53.
6. SHARMA, H.S. & P.K. DEY. 1981. Impairment of blood-brain barrier by immobilization stress: role of serotonin. Indian J. Physiol. Pharmacol. **25:** 111–122.
7. SHARMA, H.S. 1982. Blood-brain barrier in stress. Ph. D. thesis, Banaras Hindu University, Varanasi, India. pp. 1–85.
8. SHARMA, H.S. & P.K. DEY. 1984. Role of 5-HT on increased permeability of blood-brain barrier under heat stress. Indian J. Physiol. Pharmacol. **28:** 259–267.
9. SHARMA, H.S. & P.K. DEY. 1986a. Probable involvement of 5-hydroxytryptamine in increased permeability of blood-brain barrier under heat stress. Neuropharmacology **25:** 161–167.
10. SHARMA, H.S. & P.K. DEY. 1986b. Influence of long-term immobilization stress on regional blood-brain barrier permeability, cerebral blood flow and 5-HT level in conscious normotensive young rats. J. Neurol. Sci. **72:** 61–76.
11. SHARMA, H.S. & P.K. DEY. 1987a. Increased blood-brain and blood-CSF barrier permeability following long-term immobilization stress in conscious rats. Wissenschaftliche Zeitschrift Karl-Marx Universität Leipzig. Mathematisch-Naturwissenschaftliche Reihe **36:** 104–106.
12. SHARMA, H.S. & P.K. DEY. 1987b. Influence of long-term acute heat exposure on regional blood-brain barrier permeability, cerebral blood flow and 5-HT level in conscious normotensive young rats. Brain Res. **424:** 153–162.
13. SHARMA, H.S., J. WESTMAN & F. NYBERG. 1998a. Pathophysiology of brain edema and cell changes following hyperthermic brain injury. *In* Brain Functions in Hot Environment. H.S. Sharma & J. Westman, Eds.: Prog. Brain Res. **115:** 351–412.
14. SHARMA, H.S., P. ALM & J. WESTMAN. 1998b. Nitric oxide and carbon monoxide in the pathophysiology of brain functions in heat stress. *In* Brain Functions in Hot Environment. H.S. Sharma & J. Westman, Eds.: Prog. Brain Res. **115:** 297–333.
15. SHARMA, H.S., J. WESTMAN, J. CERVÓS-NAVARRO, *et al.* 1998c. Blood-brain barrier in stress: a gateway to various brain diseases. *In* New Frontiers of Stress Research: modulation of Brain Function. A. Levy, E. Grauer, D. Ben-Nathan & E.R. de Kloet, Eds.: 259–276. Harwood Academic Publishers Inc. Amsterdam.
16. SHARMA, H.S. 1999. Pathophysiology of blood-brain barrier, brain edema and cell injury following hyperthermia: new role of heat shock protein, nitric oxide and carbon monoxide. An experimental study in the rat using light and electron microscopy. Acta Universitatis Upsaliensis **830:** 1–94.
17. SHARMA, H.S. & P.J. HOOPES. 2003. Hyperthermia induced pathophysiology of the central nervous system. Int. J. Hypertherm. **19:** 325–354.
18. SHARMA, H.S. 2004. Blood-brain and spinal cord barriers in stress. *In* The Blood-Spinal Cord and Brain Barriers in Health and Disease. H.S. Sharma & J. Westman, Eds.: 231–298. Elsevier Academic Press. San Diego.
19. SHARMA, H.S. & J. WESTMAN. 2004. The Blood-Spinal Cord and Brain Barriers in Health and Disease. Academic Press. San Diego.

20. SHARMA, H.S. 2000/2002. Role of nitric oxide in morphine withdrawal stress induced increased permeability of the blood-brain and the blood-CSF barriers in the rat. Endothelium **8:** 302.
21. ALI, S.F., R.R. NEWPORT, W. HOLSON, *et al.* 1995. Low environmental temperatures or pharmacologic agents that produce hyperthermia decrease methamphetamine neurotoxicity in mice. Ann. N. Y. Acad. Sci. **765:** 338–341.
22. RAY, A.K. & P.K. DEY. 1980. Morphine analgesia following its infusion into different liquor spaces in rat brain. Arch. Int. Pharmacodyn. Ther. **246:** 108–117.
23. ITZHAK, Y. & S.F. ALI. 2002. Behavioral consequences of methamphetamine-induced neurotoxicity in mice: relevance to the psychopathology of methamphetamine addiction. Ann. N. Y. Acad. Sci. **965:** 127–135.
24. SHARMA, H.S., R. PATNAIK, A.K. RAY & P.K. DEY. 2004. Blood-central nervous system barriers in morphine dependence and withdrawal. *In* The Blood-Spinal Cord and Brain Barriers in Health and Disease. H.S. Sharma & J. Westman, Eds.: 299–328. Elsevier Academic Press. San Diego.
25. GIANUTSOS, G., M.D. HYNES, R.B. DRAWBAUGH & H. LAL. 1975a. Paradoxical absence of aggression during naloxone-precipitated morphine withdrawal. Psychopharmacologia **43:** 43–46.
26. GIANUTSOS, G., M.D. HYNES, R.B. DRAWBAUGH & H. LAL. 1975b. The narcotic withdrawal syndrome in rats. *In* Methods in Narcotic Research. S. Ehrenpreis & A. Neidle, Eds.: 293–309. Marcel Dekker Inc. New York.
27. RAPOPORT, S.I. 1976. Blood-Brain Barrier in Physiology and Medicine. Raven Press. New York.
28. OLSSON, Y., H.S. SHARMA & C.A. PETTERSSON. 1990. Effects of p-chlorophenylalanine on microvascular permeability changes in spinal cord trauma. An experimental study in the rat using 131I-sodium and lanthanum tracers. Acta Neuropathol. (Berl.) **79:** 595–603.
29. SHARMA, H.S., Y. OLSSON & P.K. DEY. 1990. Early accumulation of serotonin in rat spinal cord subjected to traumatic injury. Relation to edema and blood flow changes. Neuroscience **36:** 725–730.
30. SHARMA, H.S. & J. CERVÓS-NAVARRO. 1990. Brain oedema and cellular changes induced by acute heat stress in young rats. Acta Neurochir. Suppl. (Wien) **51:** 383–386.
31. NAG, S. 2003. Blood-brain barrier permeability using tracers and immunohistochemistry. Methods Mol. Med. **89:** 133–144.
32. ZEA-ARAGON, Z., N. TERADA, N. OHNO, *et al.* 2004. Effects of anoxia on serum immunoglobulin and albumin leakage through blood-brain barrier in mouse cerebellum as revealed by cryotechniques. J. Neurosci. Methods **138:** 89–95.
33. SHARMA, H.S., C. ZIMMER, J. WESTMAN & J. CERVÓS-NAVARRO. 1992. Acute systemic heat stress increases glial fibrillary acidic protein immunoreactivity in brain. An experimental study in the conscious normotensive young rats. Neuroscience **48:** 889–901.
34. SHARMA, H.S., Y. OLSSON & J. CERVOS-NAVARRO. 1993. p-Chlorophenylalanine, a serotonin synthesis inhibitor, reduces the response of glial fibrillary acidic protein induced by trauma to the spinal cord. An immunohistochemical investigation in the rat. Acta Neuropathol. (Berl.) **86:** 422–427.
35. SHARMA, H.S., J. WESTMAN, J.C. NAVARRO, *et al.* 1995. Probable involvement of serotonin in the increased permeability of the blood-brain barrier by forced

swimming. An experimental study using Evans blue and 131I-sodium tracers in the rat. Behav. Brain Res. **72:** 189–196.
36. WESTMAN, J. & H.S. SHARMA. 1998. Heat shock protein response in the central nervous system following hyperthermia. Prog. Brain Res. **115:** 207–239.
37. SHARMA, H.S., Y. OLSSON & J. WESTMAN. 1995. A serotonin synthesis inhibitor, p-chlorophenylalanine reduces the heat shock protein response following trauma to the spinal cord: an immunohistochemical and ultrastructural study in the rat. Neurosci. Res. **21:** 241–249.
38. OLSSON, Y., H.S. SHARMA, A. PETTERSSON & J. CERVOS-NAVARRO. 1992. Release of endogenous neurochemicals may increase vascular permeability, induce edema and influence cell changes in trauma to the spinal cord. Prog. Brain Res. **91:** 197–203.
39. SONG, P. & Z.-Q. ZHAP. 2001. The involvement of glial cells in the development of morphine tolerance. Neurosci. Res. **39:** 281–286.
40. BHARGAVA, H.N. 1994. Diversity of agents that modify opioid tolerance, physical dependence, abstinence syndrome, and self-administrative behavior. Pharmacol. Rev. **46:** 293–324.
41. HOUSHYAR, H., M.D. GALIGNIANA, W.B. PRATT & J.H. WOODS. 2001a. Differential responsivity of the hypothalamic-pituitary-adrenal axis to glucocorticoid negative-feedback and corticotropin releasing hormone in rats undergoing morphine withdrawal: possible mechanisms involved in facilitated and attenuated stress responses. J. Neuroendocrinol. **13:** 875–886.
42. HOUSHYAR, H., Z.D. COOPER & J.H. WOODS. 2001b. Paradoxical effects of chronic morphine treatment on the temperature and pituitary-adrenal responses to acute restraint stress: a chronic stress paradigm. J. Neuroendocrinol. **13:** 862–874.
43. SHARMA, H.S., J. WESTMAN, J. CERVÓS-NAVARRO & F. NYBERG. 1997. Role of neurochemicals in brain edema and cell changes following hyperthermic brain injury in the rat. Acta Neurochir. **70:** 269–274.
44. OLSSON, Y., H.S. SHARMA, F. NYBERG & J. WESTMAN. 1995. The opioid receptor antagonist naloxone influences the pathophysiology of spinal cord injury. Prog. Brain Res. **104:** 381–399.
45. KOSTEN, T.R., M.J. KREEK, J. RAGUNATH & H.D. KLEBER. 1986. Cortisol levels during chronic naltrexone maintenance treatment in ex-opiate addicts. Biol. Psychiatry **21:** 217–220.
46. O'DOHERTY, F. 1991. Is drug use a response to stress? Drug Alcohol Depend. **29:** 97–106.
47. CHILDRESS, A.R., R. EHRMAN, A.T. MCLELLAN, *et al.* 1994. Can induced moods trigger drug-related responses in opiate abuse patients? J. Subst. Abuse Treat. **11:** 17–23.
48. DALLMAN, M.J., O. SHIHO, T.H. PAGE, *et al.* 1991. Peripheral tolerance to alloantigen results from altered regulation of the interleukin 2 pathway. J. Exp. Med. **173:** 79–87.
49. BHATNAGAR, S., J.B. MITCHELL, K. BETITO, *et al.* 1995. Effects of chronic intermittent cold stress on pituitary adrenocortical and sympathetic adrenomedullary functioning. Physiol. Behav. **57:** 633–639.
50. YOUNG, E. & H. AKIL. 1985. Changes in releasability of ACTH and beta-endorphin with chronic stress. Neuropeptides **5:** 545–548.
51. ANDERSSON, K., A. JANSSON, F. KUYLENSTIERNA & P. ENEROTH. 1993. Nicotine and its major metabolite cotinine have different effects on aldosterone and prolactin serum levels in the normal male rat. Eur. J. Pharmacol. **228:** 305–312.

52. MARTI, O., A. GAVALDA, F. GOMEZ & A. ARMARIO. 1994. Direct evidence for chronic stress-induced facilitation of the adrenocorticotropin response to a novel acute stressor. Neuroendocrinology **60:** 1–7.
53. SHARMA, H.S., J. WESTMAN, F. NYBERG, *et al.* 1994. Role of serotonin and prostaglandins in brain edema induced by heat stress. An experimental study in the young rat. Acta Neurochir. Suppl. (Wien) **60:** 65–70.
54. SHARMA, H.S., T. LUNDSTEDT, A. BOMAN, *et al.* 2005. A potent serotonin modulating compound AP-267 attenuates morphine withdrawal induced blood-brain barrier dysfunction in rats. Ann. N. Y. Acad. Sci. (in this volume).
55. SHARMA, H.S., J. CERVOS-NAVARRO & P.K. DEY. 1991. Increased blood-brain barrier permeability following acute short-term swimming exercise in conscious normotensive young rats. Neurosci. Res. **10:** 211–221.
56. SHARMA, H.S. 2005. Pathophysiology of blood-spinal cord barrier in traumatic injury and repair. Curr. Pharm. Des. **11:** 1353–1389.
57. SHARMA, H.S. 2004. Pathophysiology of the blood-spinal cord barrier in traumatic injury. *In* The Blood-Spinal Cord and Brain Barriers in Health and Disease. H.S. Sharma & J Westman, Eds.: 437–518. Elsevier Academic Press. San Diego.
58. SHARMA, H.S., J. WESTMAN, Y. OLSSON & P. ALM. 1996. Involvement of nitric oxide in acute spinal cord injury: an immunocytochemical study using light and electron microscopy in the rat. Neurosci. Res. **24:** 373–384.
59. SHARMA, H.S., R.D. BADGAIYAN, P. ALM, *et al.* 2005a. Neuroprotective effects of nitric oxide synthase inhibitors in spinal cord injury-induced pathophysiology and motor functions: an experimental study in the rat. Ann. N. Y. Acad. Sci. **1053:** 422–434.
60. KRISTIAN, T. & B.K. SIESJO. 1998. Calcium in ischemic cell death. Stroke **29:** 705–718.

Methamphetamine-Induced Selective Dopaminergic Neurotoxicity Is Accompanied by an Increase in Striatal Nitrate in the Mouse

KAREN L. ANDERSON AND YOSSEF ITZHAK

Department of Psychiatry and Behavioral Sciences, University of Miami School of Medicine Miami, Florida 33136, USA

ABSTRACT: Exposure to high doses of methamphetamine (METH), a major drug of abuse, may cause neuronal damage. Previous studies have implicated the role of peroxynitrite, produced by nitric oxide (NO) and reactive oxygen species, in dopaminergic neurotoxicity produced by METH in mice. The present article was undertaken to investigate if a neurotoxic regimen of METH is associated with changes in tissue levels of nitrate and nitrite, which are the stable products of NO. Administration of METH (5 mg/kg $\times$ 3) to Swiss Webster mice resulted in marked depletion of dopamine (DA) and DA transporter (DAT) binding sites but no change in 5-hydroxytryptamine (5-HT) and 5-HT transporter (5-HTT) binding sites in the striatum, amygdala, frontal cortex, and hippocampus, suggesting that METH causes selective neurotoxicity to DA nerve terminals. The concentration of nitrate in the striatum was increased by about two-fold after METH administration; however, no changes in nitrate concentration were detected in other brain regions that endured dopaminergic neurotoxicity. These findings suggest that (*a*) a neurotoxic regimen of METH produces selective increase in NO in the striatum, which may generate toxic species such as peroxynitrite, and (*b*) toxins other than NO-related derivatives may mediate dopaminergic neurotoxicity in the amygdala and frontal cortex.

KEYWORDS: methamphetamine; dopamine; serotonin; neurotoxicity; nitric oxide (NO); nitrate; nitrite; peroxynitrite

Address for correspondence: Y. Itzhak, Ph.D., Department of Psychiatry and Behavioral Sciences, University of Miami School of Medicine, Gautier Building 503, 1011 NW 15th Street, Miami, FL 33136. Voice: 305-243-4635; fax: 305-243-2989.
e-mail: yitzhak@med.miami.edu

Ann. N.Y. Acad. Sci. 1074: 225–233 (2006).
doi: 10.1196/annals.1369.021

INTRODUCTION

Methamphetamine (METH) is a major drug of abuse that may cause long-lasting neuronal damage in animal models and humans. Early reports on the neurotoxic potential of METH came from studies in rats[1] and monkeys.[2] In rats, a high dose of METH caused degeneration of dopamine (DA) nerve terminals, loss of tyrosine hydroxylase (TH), DA transporter (DAT), tryptophan hydroxylase (TPH), and 5-hydroxytryptamine (5-HT)-immunoreactive axon terminals.[3–6] Further support for the neurotoxic potential of METH stems from evidence that (*a*) high doses of METH cause gliosis in rats and mice [7–9] and (*b*) apoptotic pathways are involved in METH-induced neuronal injury.[10] Species differences in response to the neurotoxic effects of amphetamine derivatives have been reported. For instance, METH causes concurrent DA and 5-HT neurotoxicity in rats but rather selective dopaminergic neurotoxicity in mice.[11]

In human METH abusers, selective deficits in dopaminergic markers have been observed. Positron emission tomography (PET) studies in METH users showed a significant reduction in DAT density in the caudate and putamen; this reduction was associated with motor slowing and memory impairment. [12,13] Similar findings were observed in abstinent METH users.[14] Postmortem studies showed that caudate and putamen DA were decreased by 61 and 50%, respectively, in chronic METH users.[15] The finding that METH selectively reduces dopaminergic markers in mice and humans, suggests the relevance of the mouse model for further investigation the mechanisms underlying METH neurotoxicity.

The roles of various neurotransmitters (DA, 5-HT, and glutamate), free radicals (reactive oxygen species), apoptotic proteins, and inflammatory cytokines in amphetamines neurotoxicity have been described in several reviews.[10,11,16] Nitric oxide (NO) has a role in interneuronal communication and excitotoxic neuronal injury. Specifically, peroxynitrite ($ONOO^-$) formed by the interaction of NO with superoxide radicals is a major neurotoxin.[17] Several lines of evidence support the role of NO in METH-induced neurotoxicity.[18] Inhibition of neuronal NO synthase (nNOS) by various selective nNOS inhibitors[19–21] and deletion of the nNOS gene (e.g., nNOS knockout mice)[22] protected against METH-induced dopaminergic neurotoxicity. METH-induced neurotoxicity in mice has been associated with a marked increase in striatal peroxynitrite[23] and 3-nitrotyrosine,[24] the latter a marker for peroxynitrite formation. Administration of high doses of METH to nNOS KO mice did not cause production of 3-nitrotyrosine as it did in wild-type mice.[25] To further investigate the role of NO in METH neurotoxicity, the effect of high doses of METH on the accumulation of NO by-products, e.g., nitrate/nitrite in various brain regions of the mouse brain was investigated.

MATERIALS AND METHODS

Animals and Drug Administration

Male Swiss Webster mice (9–10 weeks old; Charles River, Wilmington, MA) were maintained on a 12-h light/dark cycle at a room temperature of 22±0.5°C, with free access to food and water. Animal care was in accordance with the Guide for the Care and Use of Laboratory Animals (National Research Council, National Academy Press, 1996) and approved by the University of Miami Animal Care and Use Committee. (+)Methamphetamine-HCl (Sigma, St. Louis, MO) was dissolved in saline. Mice received three intraperitoneal (i.p.) injections of either saline ($n = 30$) or METH (5 mg/kg; $n = 30$) in 3-h intervals at a room temperature of 22±0.5°C. Mice were sacrificed after 72 h for the determination of monoamine concentrations, monoamine transporter densities, and nitrate/nitrite concentrations.

Determination of Monoaminergic Markers in Brain

The striatum, frontal cortex, hippocampus, and amygdala were freshly dissected and frozen at −80°C. Routinely, tissue from one hemisphere was used for monoamine and nitrate/nitrite assays, and tissue from the other hemisphere was used for determination of the density of DAT and 5-HT transporter (5-HTT) binding sites. High-performance liquid chromatography (HPLC) combined with electrochemical detection[22] was used to determine the concentrations of DA and 5-HT. The densities of DAT and 5-HTT binding sites were determined by saturation binding assays using [^{3}H]mazindol (1.0–20.0 nm) and [^{3}H]citalopram (0.5–5.0 nm), respectively, as we described previously.[22,26]

Determination of Nitrate/Nitrite in Brain

Brain nitrate (NO_3^-) was determined after its reduction to nitrite (NO_2^-), followed by the Griess reaction. Frontal cortex, hippocampus, amygdala, and striatum were removed and immediately frozen at −80°C. Tissue from groups of 3–4 mice was homogenized in 10 volumes ice-cold potassium phosphate buffer (50 mM) containing sucrose (0.25 M) and EDTA (0.1 mM). The homogenate was centrifuged at 8000*g* (30 min at 4°C) and the supernatant was re-centrifuged (12,000*g*; 30 min; 4°C). Supernatant aliquots were incubated in the dark (30 min; 24°C) with NADPH (4 mM) and nitrate reductase (0.04 U) in a final volume of 100 μL potassium phosphate buffer. Thereafter, a Griess reagent containing 50 μL sulfanilamide (1.5% in 1 N HCl) and 50 μL *N*-(1-naphthyl) ethylenediamine–HCl (0.15%) was added to the samples. Following 20-min incubation, samples were centrifuged (12,000*g*; 5 min; 4°C) and absorbance was measured at 540 nm with a reference wavelength of 620 nm. A sodium-nitrite standard curve was generated for calculation of nitrite concentrations. Protein concentration was assayed using a standard Bio-Rad kit.

Statistics

Results were analyzed by one-way ANOVA followed by post-hoc Newman-Keuls' test. A P-value <0.05 was considered statistically significant.

RESULTS

FIGURE 1 depicts the effect of METH (5 mg/kg $\times$ 3) on DA, DAT, 5-HT, and 5-HTT levels in the striatum, amygdala, frontal cortex, and hippocampus. A significant reduction in DA and DAT was observed in striatum (43–56%), amygdala (40–45%), and frontal cortex (44–61%) of METH treated mice compared to saline treated mice ($P < 0.001$). Notably, METH had no effect on 5-HT or 5-HTT levels in all four brain regions investigated. While DA and DAT in the hippocampus of Swiss Webster mice were below detection levels; the concentration of 5-HT and 5-HTT in both control and METH treated mice were measurable (5-HT: $\sim$28$\pm$2 ng/100 mg tissue and 5-HTT: $\sim$442$\pm$32 fmole/mg protein); METH had no significant effect on 5-HT and 5-HTT levels.

In the second set of experiments, the concentration of nitrate/nitrite in various brain regions was determined. Preliminary studies have shown no detectable tissue levels of nitrite (NO_2^-) when assays were carried out in the absence of nitrate reductase. Therefore, all experiments were carried out in the presence of reductase, which converts NO_3^- to NO_2^-; the latter forms a stable complex with the Griess reagent. Results in FIGURE 2 show that the level of nitrate in the striatum was increased by about twofold in METH pretreated mice compared to saline pretreated mice. Despite the finding that dopaminergic neurotoxicity was detected in the amygdala and frontal cortex (FIG. 1), the levels of nitrate in the amygdala, frontal cortex, and hippocampus of METH pretreated mice were not significantly different from control (FIG. 2).

DISCUSSION

The major finding of the present study is that METH-induced dopaminergic neurotoxicity was accompanied by a large increase in striatal nitrate concentration, suggesting that overproduction of NO is associated with dopaminergic neurotoxicity. Administration of high doses of METH to Swiss Webster mice resulted in selective depletion of DA and DAT in the striatum, amygdala, and frontal cortex; no change in 5-HT or 5-HTT levels was detected. The selective injury to DA nerve terminals in mouse brain is akin to the selective dopaminergic deficits observed in human METH abuser.[12–15] This finding and the observation that in rats METH produces concurrent dopaminergic and serotonergic

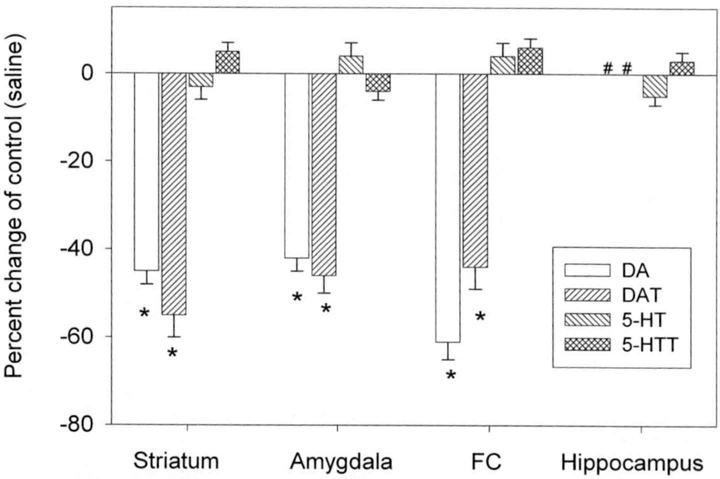

FIGURE 1. Effect of METH (5 mg/kg × 3) on dopaminergic and serotonergic markers in mouse brain. Levels of DA, DAT, 5-HT, and 5-HTT were determined 72 h after the last treatment of METH ($n = 15$) and saline ($n = 15$) was given. Results represent the mean ± SEM of percentage change in monoamine markers compared to control (*$P < 0.05$ METH, $n = 15$ versus control). METH produced significant reduction of DA and DAT in striatum, amygdala, and frontal cortex (FC) and had no significant effect on 5-HT and 5-HTT levels. The following are the control values of DA (ng/100 mg tissue) and DAT binding sites (fmole/mg protein) in striatum: 629±21 and 1734±101; in amygdala: 42±2 and 232±17; in frontal cortex: 53±5 and 189±21. The following are the control values of 5-HT (ng/100 mg tissue) and 5-HTT binding sites (fmole/mg protein) in striatum: 55±3 and 449±31; in amygdala: 32±4 and 895±71; in frontal cortex: 27±2 and 432±22; in hippocampus: 39±5 and 467±39.

neurotoxicity,[3–6] suggests that the mouse model is more relevant than the rat model for investigation of the mechanisms underlying METH neurotoxicity and the physiological significance of such insult.

Interestingly, although depletion of DA and DAT was observed in several brain regions, a significant change in nitrate concentration was detected only in the striatum (FIG. 2). Although a time course study for nitrate production was not conducted, it is noticeable that nitrate conjugates in the striatum were stable and detectable at least for 3 days after METH administration. The mechanism by which NO/peroxynitrite mediates dopaminergic neurotoxicity is unclear. However, inactivation of TH[27] and DAT[28] by peroxynitrite-induced nitration and increased vulnerability of dopaminergic neurons to cell loss after exposure to peroxynitrite[29] have been implicated in METH neurotoxicity.

If overproduction of NO, as determined by nitrate levels, leads to dopaminergic neurotoxicity, it is expected that a similar increase in NO would occur in all brain regions that sustained dopaminergic neurotoxicity. The reason why nitrate levels in the amygdala and frontal cortex were similar in control and METH treated mice is not clear. This result cannot be attributed to

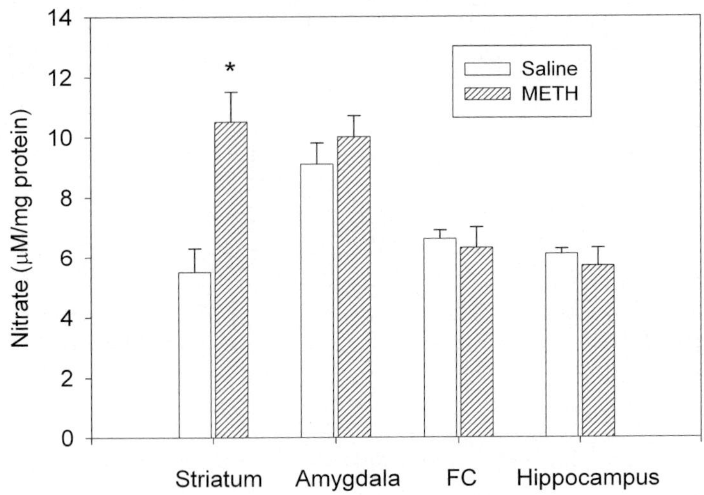

FIGURE 2. Effect of METH (5 mg/kg × 3) on nitrate level in mouse brain. The level of nitrate was determined by Griess reaction 72 h after the last treatment of METH ($n = 15$) and saline ($n = 15$) was given. Results represent the mean ± SEM of nitrate in the various brain regions. A significant increase in nitrate was observed only in the striatum ($^*P < 0.005$).

differences in the extent of dopaminergic depletion in the various substrates because no such differences were observed (FIG. 1). One explanation could be that different mechanisms underlie dopaminergic neurotoxicity in various brain regions. In the striatum, overproduction of NO and a favorable oxidative stress milieu could generate peroxynitrite which leads to neurotoxicity in DA nerve terminals. While the striatum receives dense dopaminergic innervation from the midbrain, the frontal cortex, amygdala, and hippocampus receive relatively sparse dopaminergic projections from the midbrain. As summarized in the legend to FIGURE 1, the density of striatal DAT is about eightfold higher than that in the amygdala and frontal cortex, while DAT in hippocampus was undetectable by [^{3}H]mazindol binding assays. Interestingly, immunohistochemical studies have recently shown high density of nNOS immunoreactive (ir) neurons in the striatum, but sparse staining of these neurons in the hippocampus and amygdala.[30] It has been suggested that NO release is regulated by direct synaptic input from dopaminergic neurons; likewise, TH-ir terminals that are associated with the dendrites of NO-containing neurons provide the locus where NO affects DA release from neighboring terminals.[31] These findings suggest interaction between nNOS containing neurons and DA nerve terminals in the striatum. Thus, it is likely that overproduction of NO and peroxynitrite mediates dopaminergic neurotoxicity in the striatum, but oxygen species other than peroxynitrite mediate dopaminergic neurotoxicity in other brain regions (frontal cortex and amygdala).

Several lines of evidence suggest dopaminergic modulation of the nitrergic system. Activation of striatal D1 receptors increased NO release[32] by stimulating NOS-positive interneurons.[33] A high dose of amphetamine increased striatal nNOS mRNA expression[34] as well as striatal nNOS enzymatic activity.[35] On the other hand, 6-hydroxydopamine (6-OHDA) lesions markedly reduced nNOS activity in the striatum and frontal cortex,[36] and decreased the numbers of NADPH-d/NOS-ir neurons in the nucleus accumbens.[37] *In vivo* administration of the D1/D2 dopamine receptor antagonist haloperidol attenuated expression of nNOS-ir neurons in the pituitary gland, while *in vitro* application of DA increased the expression.[38] Although nNOS is considered a constitutively expressed protein, these findings suggest that nNOS is subject to expressional regulation in response to activity-dependent plasticity.

In summary, results show that METH produces selective dopaminergic neurotoxicity in mice. Striatal dopaminergic neurotoxicity is associated with enhanced levels of nitrate, suggesting a mechanism by which increased production of striatal NO and peroxynitrite may cause damage to DA nerve terminals. In other brain regions, however, toxic species other than NO/peroxynitrite may be involved in METH-induced dopaminergic neurotoxicity.

ACKNOWLEDGMENTS

This work was supported by RO1DA 012867 and RO1DA 019107 from the National Institute on Drug Abuse, National Institutes of Health.

REFERENCES

1. Kogan, F.J., W.K. Nichols & J.W. Gibb. 1976. Influence of methamphetamine on nigral and striatal tyrosine hydroxylase activity and on striatal dopamine levels. Eur. J. Pharmacol. **36**: 363–371.
2. Seiden, L.S., M.W. Fischman & C.R. Schuster. 1976. Long-term methamphetamine induced changes in brain catecholamines in tolerant rhesus monkeys. Drug Alcohol Depend. **1**: 215–219.
3. Axt, K.J. & M.E. Molliver. 1991. Immunocytochemical evidence for methamphetamine-induced serotonergic axon loss in the rat brain. Synapse **9**: 302–313.
4. Gibb, J.W., M. Johnson & G.R. Hanson. 1990. Neurochemical basis of neurotoxicity. NeuroToxicol. **11**: 317–322.
5. Ricaurte, G.A., R.W. Guillery, L.S. Seiden, *et al.* 1982. Dopamine nerve terminal degeneration produced by high doses of methylamphetamine in the rat brain. Brain Res. **235**: 93–103.
6. Seiden, L.S. & K.E. Sabol. 1996. Methamphetamine and methylenedioxymethamphetamine neurotoxicity: possible mechanisms of cell destruction. NIDA Res. Monogr. **163**: 251–276.
7. Johnson, E.A., J.P. O'Callaghan & D.B. Miller. 2002. Chronic treatment with supraphysiological levels of corticosterone enhances D-MDMA-induced

dopaminergic neurotoxicity in the C57BL/6J female mouse. Brain Res. **933**: 130–138.

8. O'CALLAGHAN, J.P. & D.B. MILLER. 1994. Neurotoxicity profiles of substituted amphetamines in the C57BL/6J mouse. J. Pharmacol. Exp. Ther. **270**: 741–751.
9. SHENG, P., C. CERRUTI & J.L. CADET. 1994. Methamphetamine (METH) causes reactive gliosis in vitro: attenuation by the ADP-ribosylation (ADPR) inhibitor, benzamide. Life Sci. **55**: PL51-54.
10. CADET, J.L., S. JAYANTHI & X. DENG. 2003. Speed kills: cellular and molecular bases of methamphetamine-induced nerve terminal degeneration and neuronal apoptosis. FASEB J. **17**: 1775–1788.
11. ITZHAK, Y. & C. ACHAT-MENDES. 2004. Methamphetamine and MDMA (ecstasy) neurotoxicity: 'of mice and men.' IUBMB Life **56**: 249–255.
12. VOLKOW, N.D., L. CHANG, G.J. WANG, *et al.* 2001. Loss of dopamine transporters in methamphetamine abusers recovers with protracted abstinence. J. Neurosci. **21**: 9414–9418.
13. VOLKOW, N.D., L. CHANG, G.J. WANG, *et al.* 2001. Association of dopamine transporter reduction with psychomotor impairment in methamphetamine abusers. Am. J. Psychiatry **158**: 377–382.
14. MCCANN, U.D., D.F. WONG, F. YOKOI, *et al.* 1998. Reduced striatal dopamine transporter density in abstinent methamphetamine and methcathinone users: evidence from positron emission tomography studies with [11C]WIN-35,428. J. Neurosci. **18**: 8417–8422.
15. MOSZCZYNSKA, A., P. FITZMAURICE, L. ANG, *et al.* 2004. Why is parkinsonism not a feature of human methamphetamine users? Brain **127**: 363–370.
16. MCCANN, U.D. & G.A. RICAURTE. 2004. Amphetamine neurotoxicity: accomplishments and remaining challenges. Neurosci. Biobehav. Rev. **27**: 821–826.
17. BECKMAN, J.S., T.W. BECKMAN, J. CHEN, *et al.* 1990. Apparent hydroxyl radical production by peroxynitrite: implications for endothelial injury from nitric oxide and superoxide. Proc. Natl. Acad. Sci. USA **87**: 1620–1624.
18. ITZHAK, Y. & S.F. ALI. 2006. Role of nitrergic system in the behavioral and neurotoxic effects of amphetamine analogs. Pharmacol. Ther. **109**: 246–262.
19. DI MONTE, D.A., J.E. ROYLAND, M.W. JAKOWEC & J.W. LANGSTON. 1996. Role of nitric oxide in methamphetamine neurotoxicity: protection by 7-nitroindazole, an inhibitor of neuronal nitric oxide synthase. J. Neurochem. **67**: 2443–2450.
20. ITZHAK, Y. & S.F. ALI. 1996. The neuronal nitric oxide synthase inhibitor, 7-nitroindazole, protects against methamphetamine-induced neurotoxicity in vivo. J. Neurochem. **67**: 1770–1773.
21. ITZHAK, Y., J.L. MARTIN & S.F. ALI. 2000. nNOS inhibitors attenuate methamphetamine-induced dopaminergic neurotoxicity but not hyperthermia in mice. Neuroreport **11**: 2943–2946.
22. ITZHAK, Y., C. GANDIA, P.L. HUANG & S.F. ALI. 1998. Resistance of neuronal nitric oxide synthase-deficient mice to methamphetamine-induced dopaminergic neurotoxicity. J. Pharmacol. Exp. Ther. **284**: 1040–1047.
23. IMAM, S.Z., J.P. CROW, G.D. NEWPORT, *et al.*. 1999. Methamphetamine generates peroxynitrite and produces dopaminergic neurotoxicity in mice: protective effects of peroxynitrite decomposition catalyst. Brain Res. **837**: 15–21.
24. IMAM, S.Z. & S.F. ALI. 2000. Selenium, an antioxidant, attenuates methamphetamine-induced dopaminergic toxicity and peroxynitrite generation. Brain Res. **855**: 186–191.

25. IMAM, S.Z., G.D. NEWPORT, Y. ITZHAK, *et al.* 2001. Peroxynitrite plays a role in methamphetamine-induced dopaminergic neurotoxicity: evidence from mice lacking neuronal nitric oxide synthase gene or overexpressing copper-zinc superoxide dismutase. J. Neurochem. **76**: 745–749.
26. ITZHAK, Y., S.F. ALI, C.N. ACHAT & K.L. ANDERSON. 2003. Relevance of MDMA ("ecstasy")-induced neurotoxicity to long-lasting psychomotor stimulation in mice. Psychopharmacol. **166**: 241–248.
27. KUHN, D.M., C.W. ARETHA & T.J. GEDDES. 1999. Peroxynitrite inactivation of tyrosine hydroxylase: mediation by sulfhydryl oxidation, not tyrosine nitration. J. Neurosci. **19**: 10289–10294.
28. PARK, S.U., J.V. FERRER, J.A. JAVITCH & D.M. KUHN. 2002. Peroxynitrite inactivates the human dopamine transporter by modification of cysteine 342: potential mechanism of neurotoxicity in dopamine neurons. J. Neurosci. **22**: 4399–4405.
29. LA VOIE, M.J. & T.G. HASTINGS. 1999. Peroxynitrite- and nitrite-induced oxidation of dopamine: implications for nitric oxide in dopaminergic cell loss. J. Neurochem. **73**: 2546–2554.
30. GOTTI, S., M. SICA, C. VIGLIETTI-PANZICA & G. PANZICA. 2005. Distribution of nitric oxide synthase immunoreactivity in the mouse brain. Microsc. Res. Tech. **68**: 13–35.
31. FUJIYAMA, F. & S. MASUKO. 1996. Association of dopaminergic terminals and neurons releasing nitric oxide in the rat striatum: an electron microscopic study using NADPH-diaphorase histochemistry and tyrosine hydroxylase immunohistochemistry. Brain Res. Bull. **40**: 121–127.
32. MORRIS, B.J., C.S. SIMPSON, S. MUNDELL, *et al.* 1997. Dynamic changes in NADPH-diaphorase staining reflect activity in nitric oxide synthase: evidence for a dopaminergic regulation of striatal nitric oxide release. Neuropharmacology **36**: 1589–1599.
33. CENTONZE, D., E. BRACCI, A. PISANI, *et al.* 2002. Activation of dopamine D1-like receptors excites LTS interneurons of the striatum. Eur. J. Neurosci. **15**: 2049–2052.
34. WANG, J.Q. & Y-S LAU. 2001. Dose-related alteration in nitric oxide synthase mRNA expression induced by amphetamine and the full D1 dopamine receptor agonist SKF-82958 in mouse striatum. Neurosci. Lett. **311**: 5–8.
35. LIN, H.-C., B.-H. KANG, C.-S. WONG, *et al.* 1999. Systemic administration of D-amphetamine induced a delayed production of nitric oxide in the striatum of rats. Neurosci Lett **276**: 141–144.
36. DE VENTE, J., M. MARKERINK-VAN ITTERSUM, J. VAN ABEELEN, *et al.* 2000. NO-mediated cGMP synthesis in cholinergic neurons in the rat forebrain: effects of lesioning dopaminergic or serotonergic pathways on nNOS and cGMP synthesis. Eur. J. Neurosci **12**: 507–519.
37. GOMEZ, M.Z. & E.A. DEL BEL. 2003. Effects of electrolytic and 6-hydroxydopamine lesions of rat nigrostriatal pathway on nitric oxide synthase and nicotinamide adenine dinucleotide phosphate diaphorase. Brain Res. Bull. **62**: 107–115.
38. CARRETERO, J., E. WERUAGA, E. HERNANDEZ, *et al.* 2003. Dopaminergic modulation of nNOS expression in the pituitary gland of the rat. Anat. Embryol. **207**: 381–388.

Methamphetamine Induces Autophagy and Apoptosis in a Mesencephalic Dopaminergic Neuronal Culture Model

Role of Cathepsin-D in Methamphetamine-Induced Apoptotic Cell Death

ARTHI KANTHASAMY,[a] V. ANANTHARAM,[a] SYED F. ALI,[b] AND A.G. KANTHASAMY[a]

[a]*Parkinson Disorders Research Laboratory, Department of Biomedical Sciences, Iowa State University, Ames, Iowa 50011-1250, USA*

[b]*Neurochemistry Laboratory, Division of Neurotoxicology, National Center for Toxicological Research/US FDA, Jefferson, Arkansas 72079, USA*

ABSTRACT: Autophagy is a phylogenetically conserved process that plays a critical role in the degradation of oxidatively damaged proteins and organelle turnover. The role of oxidative stress and apoptosis in methamphetamine (METH)-induced neurotoxicity is well known; however, the potential contribution of autophagy to METH-induced oxidative damage in dopaminergic neuronal systems remains unclear. The goals of the present article were twofold: (*a*) to develop an *in vitro* dopaminergic cell culture model to study cellular and molecular mechanisms underlying METH-ind-uced autophagy and apoptosis, and (*b*) to determine whether lysosomal protease cathepsin-D activation, resulting from the loss of lysosomal membrane integrity, contributes to METH-induced apoptosis. To accomplish these goals, we characterized morphological and biochemical changes in an immortalized mesencephalic dopaminergic neuronal cell line (N27 cells) following treatment with METH. Exposure of METH (2 mM) to N27 cells resulted in the appearance of cytoplasmic vacuolar structures reminiscent of autophagic vacuoles within 3 h. In order to ascertain the identity of the vacuolar structures that are formed following METH exposure, immunohistochemical staining for markers of autophagy were performed. LAMP 2, a classical marker of autophagolysosomes, revealed an extensive punctuate pattern of distribution on the vacuolar membrane surface, with exclusive localization in the cytoplasm. Additionally, using DNA fragmentation analysis we showed

Address for correspondence: Dr. A. Kanthasamy, Parkinson Disorders Research Laboratory, Department of Biomedical Sciences, 2062 Veterinary Medicine Building, Iowa State University, Ames, IA 50011. Voice: 515-294-7238; fax: 515-294-2315.
e-mail: arthik@iastate.edu

**Ann. N.Y. Acad. Sci. 1074: 234–244 (2006). © 2006 New York Academy of Sciences.
doi: 10.1196/annals.1369.022**

a dose-dependent increase in fragmented DNA in METH treated N27 cells. Since METH-induced autophagy preceded DNA fragmentation, we tested whether dysfunction of the autophagolysosomal system contributes to nuclear damage. Immunofluorescence studies with cathepsin-D demonstrated a granular pattern of staining in untreated cells, whereas an increased cathepsin- D immunoreactivity with a globular pattern of staining was observed in METH-treated cells. Nevertheless, blockade of cathepsin-D activation by pepstatin-A, cathepsin-D inhibitor, failed to alter METH-induced DNA fragmentation. Collectively, these results demonstrate that N27 dopaminergic neuronal cell model may serve as an excellent *in vitro* model to study the mechanisms of METH-induced autophagy and apoptosis. Furthermore, it is less likely that cathepsin-D may serve as a trigger for the induction of apoptosis subsequent to exposure of N27 dopaminergic neuronal cells to METH.

KEYWORDS: methamphetamine; neurotoxicity; autophagy; cathepsin-D; DNA fragmentation

INTRODUCTION

Methamphetamine (METH) is a widely used potent psychostimulant drug of abuse,[1–3] in recent years increased incidence of abuse in rural communities has raised great concerns regarding its potential neurotoxicity. It is well known that METH is a potent monoaminergic neurotoxin in animal models of METH-induced neuronal degeneration.[4,5] The biochemical manifestations of repeated exposure to METH in rodents include decrease in tyrosine hydroxylase activity, loss of dopamine transporter, and persistent depletion of dopamine and 5 serotonin.[5] The nigrostriatal damage that is evidenced after METH exposure resembles some of the cardinal features of Parkinson's disease, making it a putative experimental model for drug-induced Parkinsonism.[6] Although the cellular mechanisms underlying METH-induced dopaminergic degenerative processes are not entirely clear, oxidative stress[7–11] and apoptosis have been implicated in METH-induced neurodegenerative changes. In our recent studies, we showed that activation of nitric oxide, caspases, and various transcription factors may play roles in the METH-induced neurotoxicity.[8–12] Additionally, Deng *et al.*,[13] using rat striatal cells, demonstrated that METH-induced activation of mitochondria-mediated intrinsic cell death signaling events was associated with the loss of mitochondrial membrane potential, release of apoptogenic factors including cytochrome *c* into the cytosol, and subsequent activation of the caspase-dependent apoptotic cascade. In an analogous finding, Jayanthi *et al.*[14] demonstrated a functional interaction between endoplasmic (ER) and mitochondrial-mediated cell death pathways in METH-induced striatal damage in a mouse model. Thus, the possibility remains that the oxidative stress-mediated apoptotic cell death pathway may play a critical role in METH-induced nigrostriatal dopaminergic neuronal damage.

Autophagic cell death or type-II cell death is a cellular process characterized by engulfment of bulk cytoplasm and organelles within double or multilamellar autophagic vesicles and delivery to the cell's lysosomal system for subsequent degradation.[15,16] It is believed that autophagic activity in dying cells is far more active than which occur under normal homeostatic conditions. The consequence of such an event leads to self cannibalization, allowing the cells to degrade the damaged proteins or organelles and thereby limiting the accumulation of oxidatively damaged proteins and subsequent progression of cellular damage and loss of cell viability. In addition, depletion of energy resources subsequent to exposure to oxidizing stimulus has been proposed to signal the activation of autophagic mechanism possibly to restore the depleted energy levels that are observed in dying cells.[17] Despite these evidences, the exact role of autophagy in normal and diseased states remain poorly understood. Interestingly, METH-induced loss of dopaminergic neurons in ventral midbrain cultures derived from VMAT-2 knockout mice was accompanied by a time-dependent increase in the accumulation of autophagic vacuoles in the cell body.[18] In an analogous finding,[19] MA was found to induce accumulation of multilamellar bodies resembling autophagic granules exclusively in the cytoplasm of METH-treated PC-12 cells and in the nigrostrial system but not in the frontal cortex. Thus, impact of autophagy on apoptotic cell death dependent process subsequent to METH exposure remains to be clarified.

It is well known that caspases play a central role in apoptotic cell death,[19,20] however; an emerging body of evidence supports noncaspase protease, including cathepsin proteases, in the cell death process. The cathepsins are primarily localized to lysosomes and endosomes [21] and are classified based on their catalytic amino acid sequences: (*a*) the aspartate proteases (cathepsins D and E), (*b*) the cysteine proteases (CAT-B,C,H,K,L,O,S,T,V,W, and X), and (*c*) serine proteases (cathepsins A and G). Although, it was originally thought to play a central role in protein degradation within the lysosomal compartment, recent reports indicate that apoptotic stimuli-mediated disruption of the lysosomal membrane leads to the relocalization of cathepsins from the lysosomal compartment to the cytosol, which in turn may serve as a trigger for the execution of the cell death process.[22,23] Furthermore, cathepsin-D release into the cytosol was observed in cells undergoing oxidative stress mediated cell death and in cells treated with anti-cancer agents.[26] Furthermore, pharmacological inhibitors of cathepsin-D and siRNA-mediated suppression of cathepsin-D was found to ameliorate cell death.[29] Taken together, these studies establish an important role for cathepsin-D in apoptotic cell death.

The search for a useful dopaminergic neuronal cell model continues, as neurodegenerative mechanisms underlying dopaminergic degenerative conditions remain uncharacterized. The non-neuronal origin of PC12 cells and lack of sufficient homogenous population of nigral dopaminergic neurons from primary cultures warrant an alternative *in vitro* model system to investigate the cell mechanisms underlying METH-neurotoxicity. Herein, we used an immortalized mesencephalic dopaminergic neuronal cell line (N27 cells) to further understand the functional interactions between METH-induced autophagy and apoptotic cell death. In particular, using the present cell model, we sought to investigate whether METH-induced DNA damage and impairment of the lysosomal system are inexorably linked and whether DNA damage is secondary to increased lysosomal membrane permeability.

MATERIALS AND METHODS

Drugs and Chemicals

METH–hydrochloric acid (HCl) was kindly provided by NIDA drug distribution program. METH–HCl was prepared in PBS.

Cell Cultures

Immortalized rat mesencephalic cells (N27) were grown in RPMI medium supplemented with 10% fetal bovine serum, 1% L-glutamine, penicillin, and streptomycin (100 units/mL), and maintained at 37°C in a humidified atmosphere of 5% CO_2 as described previously.[24,26]

Assessment of DNA Fragmentation

DNA fragmentation was measured using a Cell Death Detection ELISA Plus Assay Kit, as described previously. Briefly, N27 cells (30,000 cells) were subcultured in 24-well culture plates the previous day. The following day cells were exposed to METH (1–2 mM) with or without 200 μM pepstatin-A (Calbiochem, San Diego, CA). N27 cells were pretreated with pepstatin-A prior to the addition of METH. At the end of 24 h, cells were processed to determine the extent of DNA fragmentation. Quantitative determination of the amount of fragmented DNA retained by anti-DNA-HRP in the immunocomplex was determined spectrophotometrically with ABTS as an HRP substrate (supplied with the kit). Colorimetric measurements were made at 405 and 490 nm using a SpectroMax 190 spectrophotomer (molecular Devices; molecular Probes; Sunnyvale, CA). The magnitude of DNA fragmentation in the cell lysate was quantified by measuring the difference in absorbance between OD_{405} and OD_{490} nm.

Immunofluorescence for the Assessment of Autophagy and Modulation of Lysosomal Membrane Permeability

For immunohistochemical studies N27 cells were treated with 2 mM METH for 12–24 h and subsequently fixed with 4% paraformaldehyde for 30 min at room temperature and rinsed three times in PBS. In order to block nonspecific binding, the cells were incubated for 1 h with 5% goat serum in 0.3% triton X-100/PBS followed by incubation with the primary antibody overnight at 4°C. Specific antibodies used were rabbit with goat anti-lamp-2a antibody (1:500) (Santacruz, SC 8100; Santacruz, Santacruz, CA) or rabbit anti-cathepsin-D antibody (1:200) (Santzcruz, SC 10725) and were suspended in PBS. Following incubation with the primary antibody, the cells were labeled with the fluorescent secondary antibody Cy-3 coupled goat anti-rabbit IgG (1:600) (Jackson immunoresearch; Jackson, West Grove, PA). At the end of incubation, the cells were rinsed three times in PBS and mounted with antifade agent (Molecular Probes, Eugene, OR). For nuclear counter staining cells were incubated with 10 μg/mL Hoechst 33342 for 5 min before the final rinse in PBS. Images were examined in a Nikon fluorescence microscope, and pictures were taken using a SPOT-RT digital camera (Diagnostic Instruments, Sterling Heights, MI) as described previously.[28] Images were quantified using MetaMorph image analysis software version 5.0 (Universal Imaging Corporation, Downingtown, PA).

RESULTS AND DISCUSSION

We used an immortalized N27 dopaminergic cell model to systematically characterize METH-induced neurodegenerative changes. N27 cells are a homogenous population of TH positive neuronal cells that synthesize and release dopamine.[26] First, we examined the feasibility of using N27 cells as a model system to study METH-induced autophagy and apoptosis. Immunohistochemical staining was performed using antibody directed against LAMP-2 to identify METH-induced autophagy. LAMP-2 is a lysosomal associated membrane glycoprotein that has been successfully used as a marker to identify cells undergoing lysosomal dependent autophagic degradation.[29,30]

Treatment of N27 cells with 2 mM METH resulted in the induction of autophagy within 3 h post-treatment as evidenced by an exclusive punctuate pattern of distribution of LAMP-2 positive structures on vacuolar membranes (FIG. 1 B). Additionally, the volume and surface density of autophagic vacuoles continued to increase in a time-dependent manner. Conversely, accumulation of autophagic vacuoles was absent in cells that received the vehicle alone, instead a uniform diffuse pattern of LAMP-2 staining was observed.

In order to correlate autophagy with the extent of apoptosis, we also performed DNA fragmentation analysis in METH-treated N27 cells. As shown in FIGURE 2, dose-dependent increase in DNA fragmentation was observed at 12 and 24 h post-METH treatment indicating a delayed onset of apoptotic cell death. Although the concentration of METH used in the present study is high, the present data are consistent with other studies[10,13] that have demonstrated the need for higher doses of the drug to reproduce METH-induced neurodegenerative changes in an *in vitro* environment.

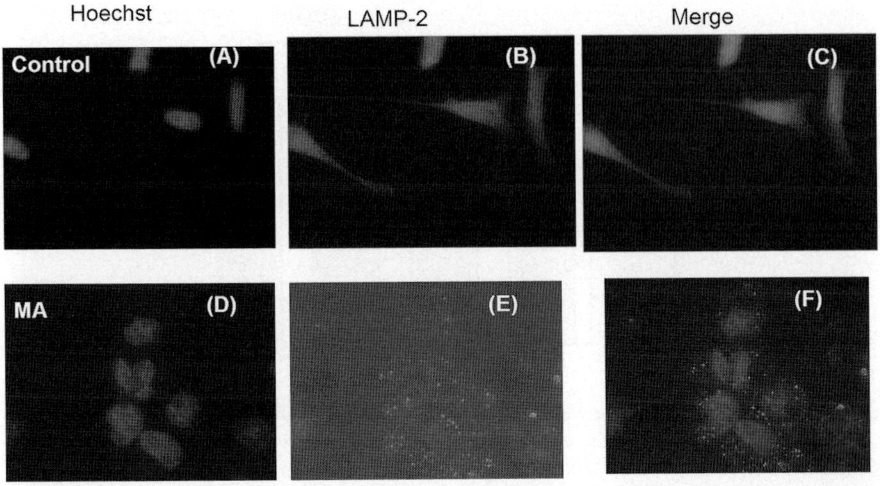

FIGURE 1. METH-induced autophagy in N27 mesencephalic do-paminergic cells. N27 cells were incubated with METH-2 mM or vehicle for 24 h and then cells were fixed and dual stained with LAMP-2 antibody and Hoechst. A diffused pattern of LAMP-2 staining was observed in untreated N27 cells (panel B), whereas massive accumulation of punctate structures were noted in the cytoplasm of METH-2 treated cells (panels E and F), indicating the induction of autophagy.

After the characterization of autophagic granules in METH-treated dopaminergic cells, we examined the integrity of the lysosomal system by assessing the relative distribution of cathepsin-D in METH-treated cells using immunohistochemical studies. Cat-D-expression levels were more intense in METH-treated cells and were found to cohlocalize with inclusions distinctly in the nucleus and perinuclear regions whereas in control cells that received the vehicle alone, a more grainy pattern of distribution was observed (FIG. 3). In order to determine the significance of nuclear accumulation of cat-D and to examine the inter-relationship between METH-induced autophagy and apoptosis, we tested the neuroprotective effects of a cathepsin-D inhibition on METH-induced DNA fragmentation in N27 cells. Following pretreatment with a known cathepsin-D inhibitor, pepstatin-A (200 μM) for 2 h, the cells were exposed to METH and assayed for DNA fragmentation. As shown in FIGURE 4, pepstatin pretreatment was ineffective in attenuating METH-induced DNA fragmentation, suggesting that cat-D may not play a role in METH-induced DNA fragmentation. However, the role of other cathepsin isoforms in mediating increased dopaminergic neuronal vulnerability to METH-neurotoxicity cannot be entirely ruled out.

Recent evidence indicates that cellular oxidative stress,[11] mitochondrial and ER dysfunction, and accumulation of neuronal inclusions in the substantia nigra compacta neuronal population but not in the frontal cortex,[19] indicating

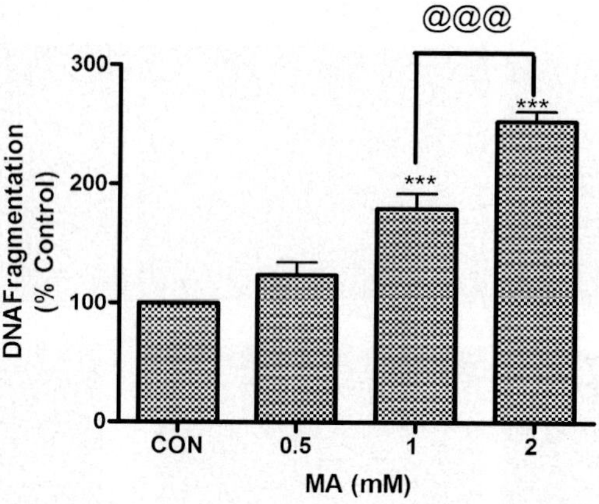

FIGURE 2. METH-induced apoptosis in N27 dopaminergic cells. Apoptotic cell death was determined by measuring the degree of DNA fragmentation. Cells were treated with increasing concentrations of METH for 24 h and then the levels of fragmented DNA was measured using a DNA ELISA kit. Each bar represents mean ± SEM ($n = 6$–9). $^{***}P < 0.001$ in comparison with vehicle treated cells;$^{@@@}$ $P< 0.001$ indicate a significant difference between two different concentrations of METH treatments.

distinct region-specific cell death signaling events, might mediate METH-induced neurodegenerative changes. The appearance of massive vacuolization in cells undergoing apoptotic cell death further prompted us to investigate the functional interaction between autophagy and apoptosis. In fact, induction of autophagolysosomes may represent, at least in part, a protective mechanism to eliminate oxidatively damaged proteins and organelles that may be deleterious to dopaminergic neuronal survival.[19] Additionally, owing to methamphetamines's weak base properties that results in the collapse of intracellular pH gradients in acidic organelles such as endosomes, lysosomes, and synaptic vesicles, it is possible that acidotropic uptake of METH[31] might have resulted in osmotic swelling and release of the lysosomal enzymatic contents into the cytoplasm, hence resulting in the induction of apoptotic cell death signaling events.[21,22] Consistent with this hypothesis it is well known that cat-D relocalization to cytosol provides an oxidative environment that is conducive to the shift toward cell death via activation of mitochondria dependent caspase dependent cell signaling events. In order to address that possibility, we determined METH-induced loss of lysosomal membrane integrity by investigating the effects of cat-D on METH-induced DNA fragmentation. Interestingly, pepstatin-mediated cat-D inhibition failed to influence the outcome of METH-induced DNA fragmentation, indicating that cathepsin-D is an unlikely candidate in the acceleration of mitochondria-mediated cell death signaling events in METH-induced neurodegeneration.

Another important finding in the present study is that N27 cells served as an excellent dopaminergic neuronal cell line for studying mechanisms

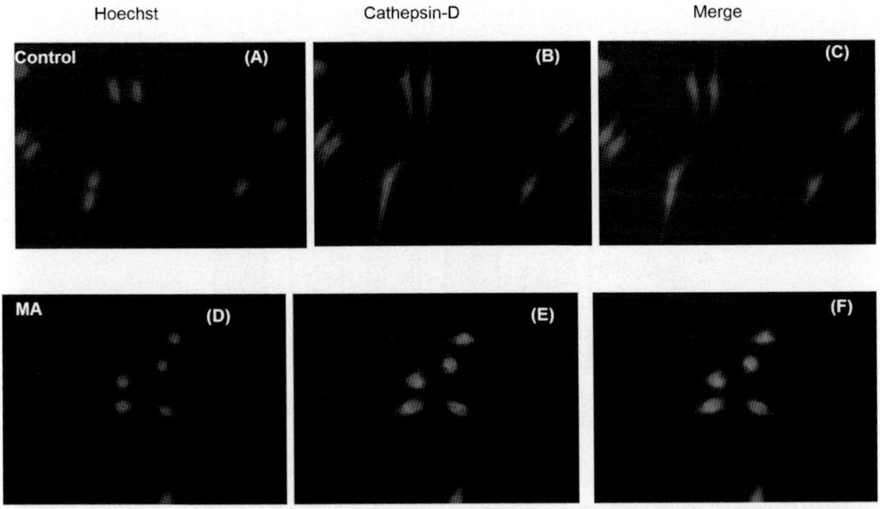

FIGURE 3. METH-induced co-localization of cathepsin-D in inclusion like structures in the nucleus. N_{27} cells were exposed to METH or vehicle for 12 h. Immunofluorescence studies were performed using cathepsin-D antibody followed by nuclear counter staining with Hoechst. In the untreated cells, a uniform pattern of cathepsin-D staining was observed (B and C). However, in the METH-treated cells, cathepsin-D staining displayed an intense staining pattern that co-localized with inclusion like structures in and around the nucleus (E and F).

underlying autophagy and apoptotic cell death. We and others have shown that this dopaminergic neuronal cell line is highly sensitive to MPP^+ induced apoptotic cell death and serves as a useful model *in vitro* model of Parkinson's disease.[25–27] MPP^+ at concentrations between 100 and 300 μM consistently activated the apoptotic cascade in N27.[25,26] Furthermore, we found that the experimental results obtained from N27 cells were readily reproducible in primary mesencephalic dopaminergic neuronal cultures and mid-brain slices.[25,26] Also, the N27 dopaminergic cell line is easily transfectable and is convenient for establishing stable cell lines compared to hard-to-transfect PC12 cells. Together, this neuronal cell line has been recognized by many investigators, including us, as a highly useful cell culture model for studying dopaminergic degenerative mechanisms in Parkinson's disease and METH neurotoxicity.

In conclusion, our study indicates that immortalized N27 dopaminergic neuronal cells may serve as an experimental tool to study cellular events underlying METH-induced dopaminergic neurodegenerative changes in a simplified yet a biologically relevant model. In addition, this model will allow us to gain further knowledge into the functional interaction between the two different modes of cell death in mediating dopaminergic neurodegenerative process.

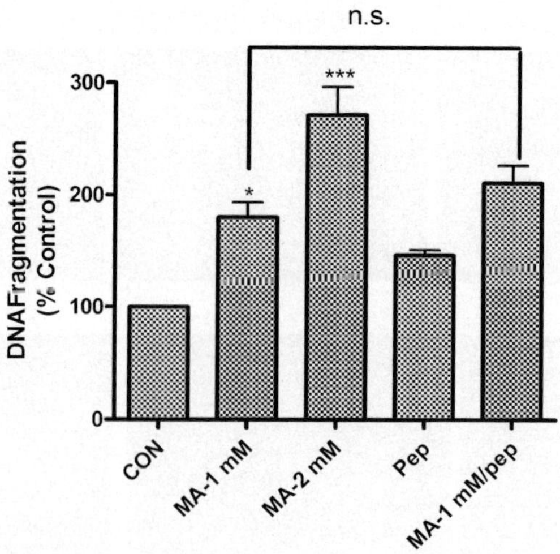

FIGURE 4. Blockade of cathepsin-D does not prevent METH-induced DNA fragmentation in N_{27} dopaminergic cells. N27 cells were treated for 12 h with vehicle, METH alone or in combination with pepstatin-A (200 μM). Following drug treatment, DNA fragmentation was measured using DNA ELISA kit. Results are reported as mean ± SEM ($n = 5$–6);$^{*}P < 0.05$; $^{***}P < 0.001$; n.s.= not significant from METH-1 mM.

Furthermore, the present studies indicate that cathepsin-D is less likely to play a central role in METH-induced neurotoxicity, at least in immortalized N27 dopaminergic neuronal cells.

ACKNOWLEDGMENTS

This study was supported by the National Institute of Health (NIH) grant ES 10586, Iowa State University Biotech Start-up fund.

REFERENCES

1. Wilson, J.M., K.S. Kalasinsky, A.I. Levey, *et al.* 1996a. Striatal dopamine nerve terminal markers in human, chronic methamphetamine users. Nat. Med. **2:** 699–703.
2. Volkow, N.D., L. Chang, G.J. Wang, *et al.* 2001. Loss of dopamine transporters in methamphetamine abusers recovers with protracted abstinence. J. Neurosci. **21:** 9414–9418.
3. Wilson, J.M., A.I. Levey, A. Rajput, *et al.* 1996c. Differential changes in neurochemical markers of striatal dopamine nerve terminals in idiopathic Parkinson's disease. Neurology **47:** 718–726.

4. CADET, J.L., S.V. ORDONEZ, J.V. ORDONEZ. 1997. Methamphetamine induces apoptosis in immortalized neural cells: protection by the proto-oncogene, bcl-2. Synapse **25:** 176–184.
5. SEIDEN, L.S. & K.E. SABOL. 1996. Methamphetamine and methylenedioxymethamphetamine neurotoxicity: possible mechanisms of cell destruction. NIDA Res. Monogr. **163:** 251–276.
6. GERLACH, M. & P. RIEDERER. 1996. Animal models of Parkinson's disease: an empirical comparison with the phenomenology of the disease in man. J. Neural Transm. **103:** 987–1041.
7. CADET, J.L., S. JAYANTHI & X. DENG. 2003. Speed kills: cellular and molecular bases of methamphetamine-induced nerve terminal degeneration and neuronal apoptosis. FASEB J. **17:** 1775–1788.
8. DE VITO, M.J. & G.C. WAGNER. 1989. Methamphetamine-induced neuronal damage: a possible role for free radicals. Neuropharmacology **28:** 1145–1150.
9. IMAM, S.Z., F. ISLAM, Y. ITZHAK, *et al.* 2000. Prevention of dopaminergic neurotoxicity by targeting nitric oxide and peroxynitrite: implications for the prevention of methamphetamine-induced neurotoxic damage. Ann. N. Y. Acad. Sci. **914:** 157–171.
10. IMAM, S.Z., J. JANKOVIC, S.F. ALI, *et al.* 2005. Nitric oxide mediates increased susceptibility to dopaminergic damage in Nurr1 heterozygous mice. FASEB J. **19:** 1441–1450.
11. IMAM, S.Z., G.D. NEWPORT, H.M. DUHART, *et al.* 2002. Methamphetamine-induced dopaminergic neurotoxicity and production of peroxynitrite are potentiated in nerve growth factor differentiated pheochromocytoma 12 cells. Ann. N. Y. Acad. Sci. **965:** 204–213.
12. IMAM, S.Z., M. OETINGER, J. SKINNER, *et al.* 2003. The role of caspase III inhibition in methamphetamine-induced alterations in p53 and bcl-2 expression: correlation with dopaminergic neurotoxicity. Ann. N. Y. Acad. Sci. **993:** 350–393.
13. DENG, X., N.S. CAI, M.T. MCCOY, *et al.* 2002. Methamphetamine induces apoptosis in an immortalized rat striatal cell line by activating the mitochondrial cell death pathway. Neuropharmacology **42:** 837–845.
14. JAYANTHI, S., X. DENG, P.A. NOAILLES, *et al.* 2004. Methamphetamine induces neuronal apoptosis via cross-talks between endoplasmic reticulum and mitochondria-dependent death cascades. FASEB J. **18:** 238–251.
15. ABRAHAM, M.C. & S. SHAHAM. 2004. Death without caspases, caspases without death. Trends Cell. Biol. **14:** 184–193.
16. YOSHIMORI, T. 2004. Autophagy: a regulated bulk degradation process inside cells. Biochem. Biophys. Res. Commun. **313:** 453–458.
17. LEMASTERS, J.J., T. QIAN, L. HE, *et al.* 2002. Role of mitochondrial inner membrane permeabilization in necrotic cell death, apoptosis, and autophagy. Antioxid. Redox. Signal **4:** 769–781.
18. LARSEN, K.E., E.A. FON, T.G. HASTINGS, *et al.* 2002. Methamphetamine-induced degeneration of dopaminergic neurons involves autophagy and upregulation of dopamine synthesis. J. Neurosci. **22:** 8951–8960.
19. FORNAI, F., P. LENZI, M. GESI, *et al.* 2004b. Methamphetamine produces neuronal inclusions in the nigrostriatal system and in PC12 cells. J. Neurochem. **88:** 114–123.
20. KORSMEYER, S.J. 2004. Cell death: critical control points. Cell **116:** 205–219.
21. CHAPMAN, H.A., R.J. RIESE & G.P. SHI. 1997. Emerging roles for cysteine proteases in human biology. Annu. Rev. Physiol. **59:** 63–88.

22. GUICCIARDI, M.E., M. LEIST & G.J. GORES. 2004. Lysosomes in cell death. Oncogene **23:** 2881–2890.
23. JOHNSON, D.E. 2000. Noncaspase proteases in apoptosis. Leukemia **14:** 1695–1703.
24. EMERT-SEDLAK, L., S. SHANGARY, A. RABINOVITZ, *et al.* 2005b. Involvement of cathepsin D in chemotherapy-induced cytochrome *c* release, caspase activation, and cell death. Mol. Cancer Ther. **4:** 733–742.
25. KAUL, S., V. ANANTHARAM, Y. YANG, *et al.* 2005b. Tyrosine phosphorylation regulates the proteolytic activation of protcin kinase Cdelta in dopaminergic neuronal cells. J. Biol. Chem. **280:** 28721–28730.
26. KITAZAWA, M., V. ANANTHARAM, Y. YANG, *et al.* 2005. Activation of protein kinase C delta by proteolytic cleavage contributes to manganese-induced apoptosis in dopaminergic cells: protective role of Bcl-2. Biochem. Pharmacol. **69:** 133–146.
27. PRASAD, K.N., E.D. CLARKSON, F.G. La ROSA, *et al.* 1998. Efficacy of grafted immortalized dopamine neurons in an animal model of parkinsonism: a review. Mol. Genet. Metab. **65:** 1–9.
28. YANG, Y., S. KAUL, D. ZHANG, *et al.* 2004. Suppression of caspase-3-dependent proteolytic activation of protein kinase C delta by small interfering RNA prevents MPP+-induced dopaminergic degeneration. Mol. Cell. Neurosci. **25:** 406–421.
29. LAJOIE, P., G. GUAY, J.W. DENNIS & I.R. NABI. 2005. The lipid composition of autophagic vacuoles regulates expression of multilamellar bodies. J. Cell Sci. **118:** 1991–2003.
30. MIZUSHIMA, N., A. YAMAMOTO, M. MATSUI, *et al.* 2004. *In vivo* analysis of autophagy in response to nutrient starvation using transgenic mice expressing a fluorescent autophagosome marker. Mol. Biol. Cell **15:** 1101–1111.
31. CUBELLS, J.F., S. RAYPORT, G. RAJENDRAN & D. SULZER. 1994. Methamphetamine neurotoxicity involves vacuolation of endocytic organelles and dopamine-dependent intracellular oxidative stress. J. Neurosci. **14:** 2260–2271.

Balance between Dopamine and Serotonin Release Modulates Behavioral Effects of Amphetamine-Type Drugs

RICHARD B. ROTHMAN AND MICHAEL H. BAUMANN

Clinical Psychopharmacology Section, IRP, NIDA, NIH, DHHS, Baltimore, Maryland 21224, USA

ABSTRACT: The abuse of illicit stimulants is a worldwide crisis, yet few medicines are available for treating stimulant addiction. We have advocated the idea of "agonist therapy" for cocaine dependence. This strategy involves administration of stimulant-like medications (e.g., monoamine releasers) to alleviate cocaine withdrawal symptoms and prevent relapse. A chief limitation of this strategy is that many candidate medicines possess high abuse liability due to activation of mesolimbic dopamine (DA) neurons in reward pathways. Evidence suggests that serotonin (5-HT) neurons can provide an inhibitory influence over mesolimbic DA neurons. Thus, it might be predicted that the balance between DA and 5-HT transmission is a critical variable when developing medications with reduced stimulant side effects. In this article, we review recent studies from our laboratory that examined neurochemical and behavioral effects of a series of monoamine releasers which displayed different potencies at DA and 5-HT transporters. The data show that increasing 5-HT release can attenuate stimulant effects mediated by DA release, such as motor stimulation and drug self-administration. Our findings support the work of others and indicate that elevated synaptic 5-HT can dampen certain behavioral effects of DA-releasing agents. Moreover, the relationship between DA and 5-HT releasing potency is an important determinant in developing new agonist medications with reduced stimulant properties.

KEYWORDS: agonist therapy; dopamine (DA); serotonin (5-HT); releasing agent; stimulant dependence

INTRODUCTION

The abuse of illicit stimulants, such as cocaine and methamphetamine, remains a major public health concern in the United States and elsewhere.[1] In particular, the intravenous (i.v.) use of stimulant drugs negatively impacts public health through the spread of HIV-1, hepatitis B and C, and drug resistant

Address for correspondence: Richard B. Rothman, M.D., Ph.D., CPS, IRP, NIDA, NIH, 5500 Nathan Shock Drive, Baltimore, MD 21224. Voice: 410-550-1487; fax: 410-550-2997.
e-mail: rrothman@mail.nih.gov

Ann. N.Y. Acad. Sci. 1074: 245–260 (2006). © 2006 New York Academy of Sciences.
doi: 10.1196/annals.1369.064

tuberculosis.[2] Despite the extent of the stimulant abuse crisis, development of medications to treat stimulant dependence has been largely unsuccessful.[3]

The use of stimulant-like medications to treat stimulant addictions is an approach described as "agonist therapy." This strategy involves administration of medications that share neurobiological mechanisms of action with cocaine and methamphetamine, but are less potent and less addictive.[4,5] From one perspective, agonist therapy might be viewed as "neurochemical normalization"—i.e., the treatment drug normalizes dysregulated neurochemistry by replacing the abused drug. Neurochemical normalization therapy has provided effective treatment options for nicotine dependence[6] and opioid dependence.[7,8] With regard to stimulant addiction, considerable evidence suggests that chronic cocaine exposure produces neurochemical deficits in dopamine (DA) and serotonin (5-HT) systems in the central nervous system (CNS).[9] Accordingly, the ideal agonist therapy in this case would be expected to normalize DA and 5-HT dysfunction.

Along with other researchers, we have advocated the use of amphetamine-type monoamine releasers as agonist therapies for cocaine dependence.[10,11] Similar to cocaine, these compounds target monoamine transporters to elevate synaptic levels of norepinephrine (NE), DA, and 5-HT.[9,12] Preclinical studies support the utility of amphetamines as agonist treatments.[13,14] For example, Negus and Mello[15] demonstrated that slow infusion of the DA releaser (+)-amphetamine decreases cocaine self-administration behavior in monkeys, with minimal effects on food-maintained behavior. Perhaps more importantly, Grabowski *et al.*[16] and Shearer *et al.*[17] showed that (+)-amphetamine is an effective treatment adjunct for reducing illicit cocaine use in cocaine-dependent human patients. Unfortunately, the use of amphetamine as a medication is limited by at least two problems. First, pure DA releasers possess significant abuse potential due to activation of mesolimbic DA neurons in reward pathways.[18] Second, DA releasers will not correct 5-HT deficits that accompany long-term cocaine abuse.

We have suggested the possibility of designing dual DA/5-HT releasers that can overcome both of the aforementioned limitations.[19] The purpose of the present article is to review our published findings, and new unpublished data, addressing the hypothesis that 5-HT release can antagonize the stimulant and reinforcing effects mediated by DA release. To this end, we examined the neurochemical and behavioral effects produced by a series of monoamine-releasing agents that display varying degrees of potency for DA and 5-HT transporters.

MATERIALS AND METHODS

Animals

Male Sprague-Dawley rats weighing 280–320 g were housed at the animal facility of the National Institute on Drug Abuse (NIDA), Intramural Research

Program (IRP). Food and water were freely available. For *in vitro* release experiments, rats were housed three per cage. For *in vivo* microdialysis and behavioral experiments, rats were single-housed post-surgery. Facilities are accredited by the American Association of the Accreditation of Laboratory Animal Care, and procedures were carried out in accordance with the Animal Care and Use Committee of the NIDA IRP. Male rhesus monkeys (*Macaca mulatta*) weighing 9–11 kg were individually housed in 1 m^3 cubicles at the animal facility of the University of Mississippi Medical Center and were maintained in accordance with guidelines provided by the National Institutes of Health (NIH) Committee on Laboratory Animal Resources. Monkeys were provided with sufficient food to maintain stable body weight and water was freely available.

Drugs

FIGURE 1 depicts the various compounds discussed in this paper. (+)-Amphetamine is a phenylethylamine analog, whereas PAL-287 is a naphthylethylamine analog. PAL-313, -314, -303, and -353 are ring-substituted amphetamines.

In Vitro *Release Assays*

In vitro assays measuring the release of [^{3}H]DA and [^{3}H]5-HT were carried out according to published methods.[20] Synaptosomes were prepared from rat caudate (DA release) or whole brain minus caudate (5-HT release). Assays were performed in a Krebs-phosphate buffer (pH 7.4) containing 154.4 mM NaCl, 2.9 mM KCl, 1.1 mM $CaCl_2$, 0.83 mM $MgCl_2$, 5 mM glucose, 1 mg/ml ascorbic acid, 50 μM pargyline, and 1 μM reserpine. [^{3}H]5-HT release assays were performed in the presence of 100 nM nomifensine and 100 nM GBR12909 to prevent reuptake of tritium into NE and DA nerves. Synaptosomes were incubated to steady state with 5 nM [^{3}H]DA (30 min) or [^{3}H]5-HT (60 min). Preloaded synaptosomes were added to tubes containing test drugs and were incubated for 5 min. Assays were stopped by filtration and residual tritium in the tissue was counted. Non-displaceable tritium was measured in the presence of 10 μM tyramine for [^{3}H]DA release and 100 μM tyramine for [^{3}H]5-HT release. Data from three experiments were pooled and fit to the two-parameter logistic equation of best-fit estimates for EC_{50} and E_{max} using MLAB-PC.

In Vivo *Microdialysis in Rats*

In vivo microdialysis sampling was carried out as previously described.[20] Indwelling jugular catheters and intracerebral guide cannulae were surgically

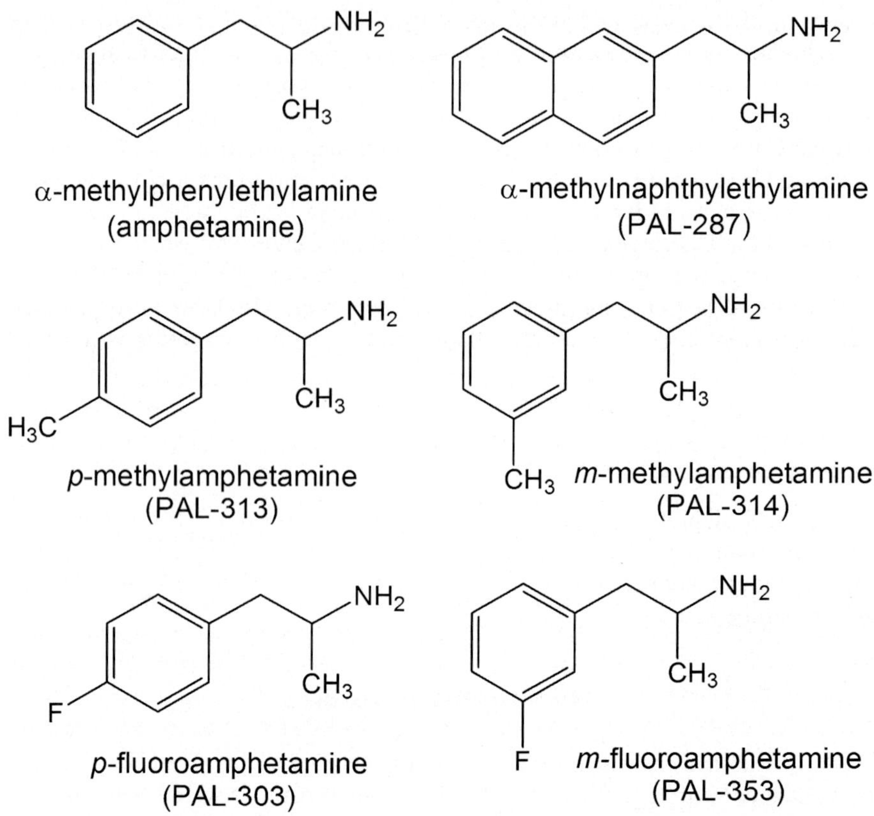

FIGURE 1. Chemical structures of (+)-amphetamine, PAL-287, and PAL amphetamines.

implanted into rats anesthetized with 60 mg/kg i.p. pentobarbital. Guide cannulae were aimed at the prefrontal cortex according to coordinates ML-2.5 mm and AP+3.0 mm relative to bregma, DV-0.8 mm relative to dura. After a week of recovery, extension tubes attached to 1-mL syringes were connected to catheters, and microdialysis probes (3 mm × 0.5 mm exchange surface, CMA/12, CMA/Microdialysis; Solna, Sweden) were inserted into guide cannulae. Each rat was attached to a tether and placed into a 40 cm^3 Plexiglas arena equipped with photobeams for automated assessment of motor activity (TruScan, Coulborn Instruments, Allentown, PA). Probes were perfused with Ringers' solution overnight at 1 μL/min.

On the next morning, samples were collected at 20-min intervals and assayed for DA and 5-HT by microbore HPLC with electrochemical detection (HPLC-ECD). Three baseline samples were collected, averaged, and subsequent DA and 5-HT measures were expressed as a percent of mean baseline. Motor activity was monitored by beam-break analysis during dialysis sampling.

Specifically, distance traveled in the horizontal plane (i.e., ambulation) and episodes of repetitive movements (i.e., stereotypic events) were quantified in 20-min bins and recorded using a computer. The neurochemical and locomotor data were evaluated using one-factor (drug treatment) repeated measures analysis of variance (rANOVA) followed by Duncan's post hoc tests.

Behavioral Observations in Rats

Rats were anesthetized with 60 mg/kg i.p. pentobarbital and indwelling jugular catheters were implanted. After a week of recovery, rats were brought into the testing room in their home cages. Extension tubes attached to 1-mL syringes were connected to catheters, and 0.5 mL of saline was flushed into the catheters. After 1 h of acclimation, rats received i.v. infusions of either PAL amphetamines or saline (1 mL/kg over 5 s). Drugs were dissolved in saline and administered at 1.0 and 3.0 mg/kg. DA-mediated behaviors including forward ambulation (all 4 feet move), rearing (forepaws off the floor), and stereotypy (vertical head-bobbing) were assessed every 10 min by an observer blind to the treatment. Behaviors were scored during 60-s intervals using a graded scale where 0: absent, 1: equivocal, 2: present, and 3: continuous or intense. Each rat was given a single behavioral score consisting of the summed scores for all behaviors over the first 30 min post-injection (i.e., three observation intervals). Behavioral data were analyzed by one-factor (drug treatment) ANOVA followed by Duncan's tests.

Drug Self-Administration in Monkeys

Details of the self-administration procedure have been previously published.[21] Each monkey was fitted with a stainless-steel harness attached by a tether to the rear wall of the chamber. The front door of the chamber was transparent plastic while remaining walls were opaque. Two response levers were mounted on the inside of the door and four stimulus lights, two red and two white, were mounted above each lever. A peristaltic infusion pump delivered drug injections. A Macintosh computer with custom interface and software controlled all events in an experimental session.

Monkeys were implanted with i.v. catheters and allowed to self-administer drugs by pressing the right lever on the chamber door (25 lever presses/injection; FR25) for 2 h/day, beginning at noon, 7 days/week. At the start of a session, the white lights were illuminated above both levers and responding on the right lever resulted in the delivery of a drug injection for 10 s. During the injection, the white lights were extinguished and the red lights were illuminated. Pressing the left lever was counted but had no other programmed consequence. In baseline sessions, cocaine (0.01–0.03 mg/kg/injection) or saline was made available. Once stable cocaine- and saline-maintained responding was established, sessions with test drugs were introduced randomly among baseline sessions. A test session was identical to a baseline session, except that saline or one of various doses of cocaine (0.001–1.0 mg/kg/injection) or PAL compounds (0.001–1.0 mg/kg/injection) were made available for self-administration. After a test session, monkeys were returned to baseline conditions until cocaine- and saline-maintained responding were again stable.

Mean injection rates per session for each monkey were calculated from two test sessions as a function of dose. A dose of drug was considered reinforcing when the mean number of injections exceeded the levels seen with saline and the ranges did not overlap. For the PAL amphetamine drugs, group mean dose-effect functions for each drug were collapsed across monkeys with respect to the dose maintaining maximum injections; this was done to account for individual variations in the dose producing maximal responding. A statistical analysis was performed on group means normalized to dose using rANOVA followed by Newman–Keul's tests.

RESULTS

In Vitro *Release Data*

TABLE 1 summarizes *in vitro* potencies of test drugs as releasers of [^{3}H]DA and [^{3}H]5-HT. The DA/5-HT ratio for each drug was calculated by dividing the EC_{50} value for DA release by the corresponding value for 5-HT release. With this method, ratios greater than 1 indicate increasing 5-HT selectivity while ratios less than 1 indicate DA selectivity. All of the drugs are substrate-type releasers that cause efflux of preloaded tritiated transmitter via transporter-mediated mechanisms. The selectivity of drugs for DA and 5-HT transporters differs substantially. (+)-Amphetamine is often considered the prototypical monoamine releaser, and this compound has much higher potency for DA

TABLE 1. Effects of test compounds on the release of [^{3}H]DA and [^{3}H]5-HT from rat brain synaptosomes. Data are mean ± SD for $n = 3$ experiments

Test drug	[^{3}H]DA release EC_{50} (nM)	[^{3}H]5-HT release EC_{50} (nM)	DA/5-HT ratio
(+)-Amphetamine[a]	8.0 ± 0.4	1756 ± 94	0.005
PAL-287 [a]	12.6 ± 0.4	3.4 ± 0.2	3.706
PAL-313 [b]	44.1 ± 2.6	53.4 ± 4.1	0.824
PAL-314 [b]	33.3 ± 1.3	218 ± 22	0.154
PAL-303 [b]	51.5 ± 1.7	939 ± 76	0.055
PAL-353 [b]	24.2 ± 1.1	1937 ± 202	0.012

[a]Data taken from Ref. 20.
[b]Data taken from Ref. 21.

release when compared to 5-HT release (DA/5-HT ratio = 0.005). The naphthalene derivative PAL-287 has 500-fold greater potency for 5-HT release when compared to amphetamine, while effects on DA are comparable (DA/5-HT ratio = 3.706). The substituted amphetamines, PAL-313, -314, -303, and -353, display roughly equivalent potency as DA releasers, but these compounds have varying potencies as 5-HT releasers, with PAL-313 exhibiting highest potency and PAL-353 exhibiting lowest potency.

In Vivo *Effects of PAL-287*

In our initial investigations, we sought to identify and characterize non-amphetamine monoamine releasing agents.[20] The first lead compound discovered from this search was PAL-287, and we compared the *in vivo* effects of PAL-287 to those of (+)-amphetamine. FIGURE 2 shows the effects of (+)-amphetamine on extracellular DA and 5-HT in rat prefrontal cortex as determined by *in vivo* microdialysis. Consistent with *in vitro* data, (+)-amphetamine stimulates the release of endogenous DA, with little effect on endogenous 5-HT. In rats undergoing dialysis, (+)-amphetamine causes dose-related increases in ambulation and stereotypy as depicted in FIGURE 3. Amphetamine-induced hyperactivity increases in parallel with elevations in extracellular DA. After a 1 mg/kg i.v. dose of amphetamine, dialysate DA levels rise eightfold above baseline in conjunction with an ambulation distance of nearly 6000 cm.

FIGURE 4 shows the effects of PAL-287 on extracellular DA and 5-HT in rat prefrontal cortex.[20] In agreement with *in vitro* data, PAL-287 increases

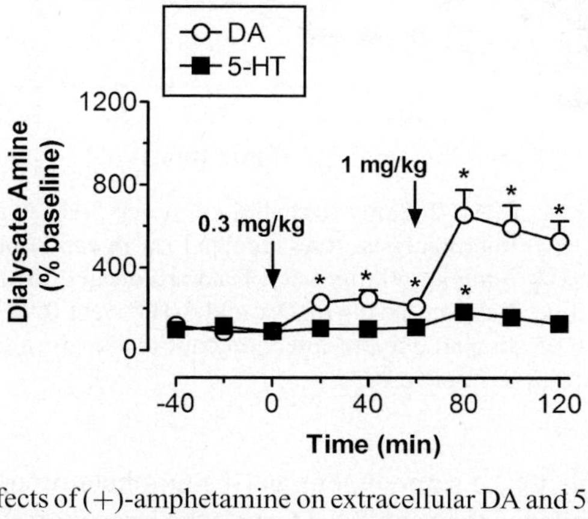

FIGURE 2. Effects of (+)-amphetamine on extracellular DA and 5-HT in rat prefrontal cortex as determined by *in vivo* microdialysis. Rats received i.v. injection of 0.3 mg/kg (+)-amphetamine at time zero, followed by 1 mg/kg 60 min later. Data are mean ± SEM for 7 rats/ group, expressed as % baseline. Baseline levels of DA and 5-HT were 0.38 ± 0.07 and 0.24 ± 0.06 pg/5 μl. $^*P < 0.05$ compared to pre-injection control at a given time point, Duncan's post hoc test. Taken from Reference 20.

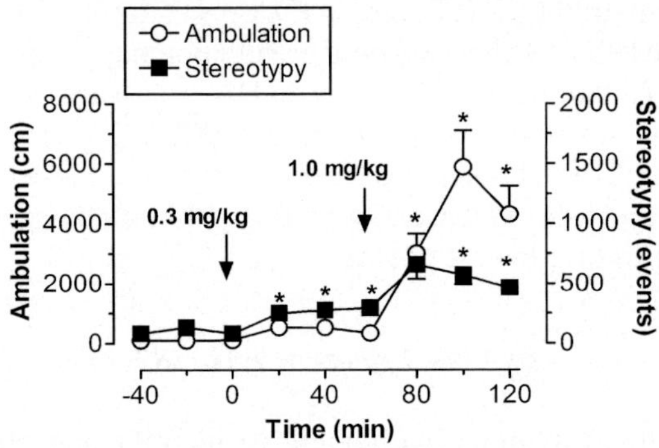

FIGURE 3. Effects of (+)-amphetamine on ambulation and stereotypy in rats undergoing microdialysis sampling. Rats received i.v. injections of 0.3 mg/kg (+)-amphetamine at time zero, followed by 1 mg/kg 60 min later. Data are mean ± SEM for 7 rats/ group, expressed as distance traveled in cm (ambulation) and number of repetitive movements (stereotypy). $^*P < 0.05$ compared to pre-injection control, Duncan's post hoc test. Taken from Reference 20.

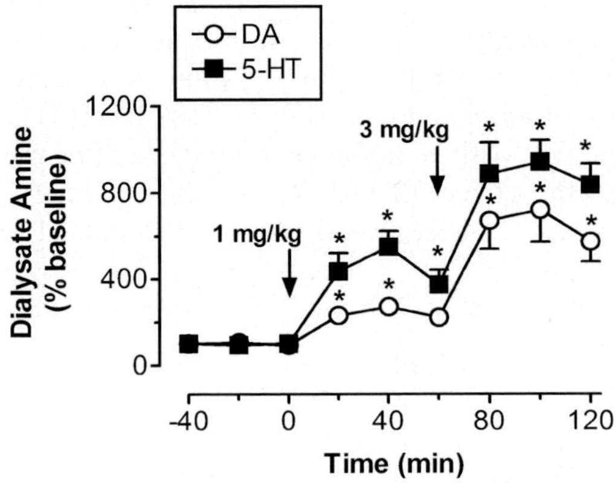

FIGURE 4. Effects of PAL-287 on extracellular DA and 5-HT in rat prefrontal cortex as determined by *in vivo* microdialysis. Rats received i.v. injection of 1 mg/kg PAL-287 at time zero, followed by 3 mg/kg 60 min later. Data are mean ± SEM for 7 rats/ group, expressed as % baseline. Baseline levels of DA and 5-HT were 0.43 ± 0.07 and 0.27 ± 0.06 pg/5 μL. $^*P < 0.05$ compared to pre-injection control at a given time point, Duncan's post hoc test. Taken from Reference 20.

dialysate DA levels to the same extent as (+)-amphetamine, while elevations in dialysate 5-HT exceed those of DA. Despite the large increase in extracellular DA produced by PAL-287, this drug produces very little ambulation as illustrated in FIGURE 5. Specifically, after a 3 mg/kg i.v. dose of PAL-287, dialysate DA levels are increased eight-fold above baseline but ambulation distance is only 1000 cm. One simple interpretation of these data is that marked release of

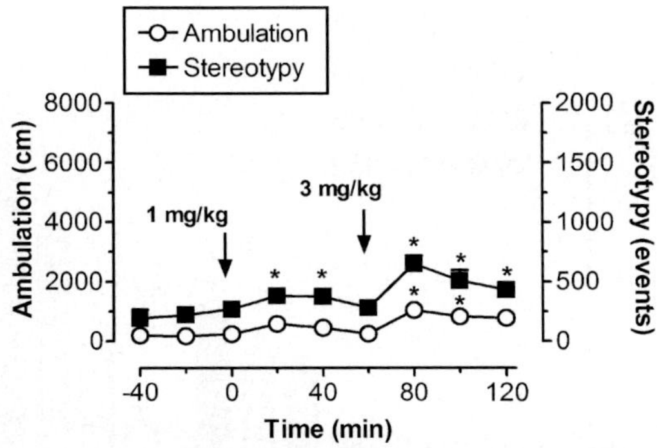

FIGURE 5. Effects of PAL-287 on ambulation and stereotypy in rats undergoing microdialysis sampling. Rats received i.v. injections of 1 mg/kg PAL-287 at time zero, followed by 3 mg/kg 60 min later. Data are mean ± SEM for 7 rats/group, expressed as distance traveled in cm (ambulation) and number of repetitive movements (stereotypy). $^*P < 0.05$ compared to pre-injection control, Duncan's post hoc test. Taken from Reference 20.

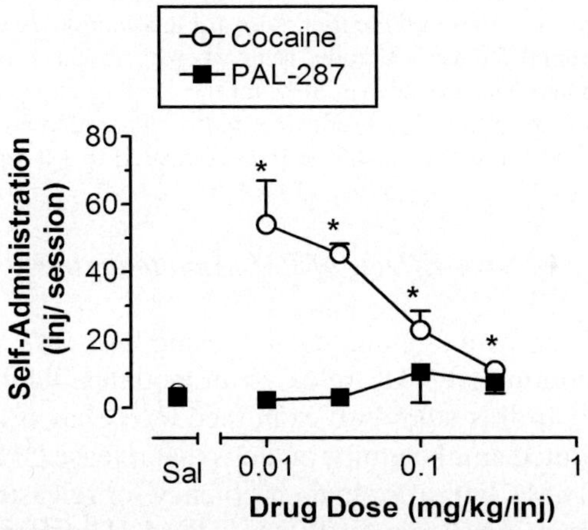

FIGURE 6. Self-administration of cocaine and PAL 287 by rhesus monkeys. Drugs were available under an FR25 schedule of reinforcement for 2 hours/day. Each point is the mean of two sessions of access to each dose of the drugs. Data are mean ± SEM for $n = 4$ monkeys. Symbols without bars have variability smaller than the points. $^*P < 0.05$ compared to saline-injected control, Newman–Keul's post hoc test. Taken from Reference 20.

5-HT produced by PAL-287 attenuates stimulant effects normally produced by release of DA. Importantly, the findings in FIGURE 6 demonstrate that PAL-287 is not readily self-administered by rhesus monkeys, suggesting that serotonergic effects of PAL-287 blunt the reinforcing effects normally associated with release of DA.

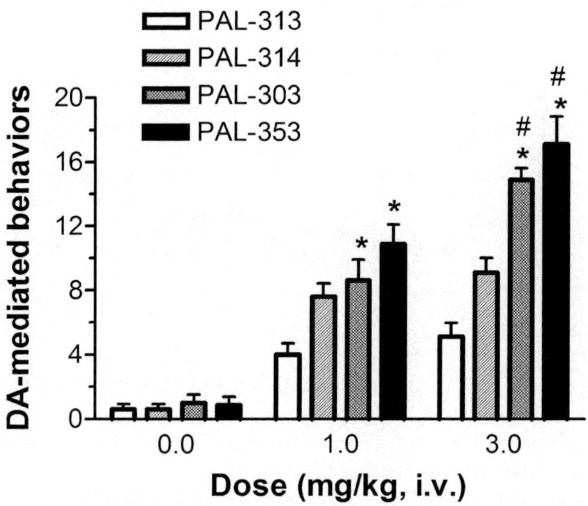

FIGURE 7. Effects of PAL amphetamines on DA-mediated behaviors in rats. Saline or drug injections were administered i.v. via indwelling catheters, and specific behaviors were assessed every 10 min for 30 min thereafter. Forward locomotion, rearing and stereotypic head bobbing were quantified using a graded scale where 0: absent, 1: equivocal, 2: present, 3: intense or continuous. Data are mean ± SEM for $n = 7$ rats/group expressed as the single summed scores for all behaviors measured. $^{*}P < 0.05$ compared to PAL-313 and PAL-314 at a given dose, Duncan's post hoc test. $p < 0.05$ compared to 1.0 mg/kg dose, Duncan's post hoc test.

In Vivo *Effects of PAL Amphetamines*

Given our findings with (+)-amphetamine and PAL-287, we wished to further explore the notion that 5-HT release can modulate the behavioral effects of DA releasers.[21] In this study, we examined the behavioral effects of a series of ring-substituted amphetamine analogs that release [^{3}H]DA with similar potency (~25–50 nM), but differ in their potency for releasing [^{3}H]5-HT (see FIG. 1 for structures). As shown on TABLE 1, the 5-HT-releasing potencies for these drugs range from 53 nM for PAL-313 to 1937 nM for PAL-353. Upon i.v. administration, all PAL amphetamines cause increases in DA-mediated hyperactivity as illustrated in FIGURE 7. Specifically, the drugs elicit dose-related increases in ambulation, rearing, and stereotypy. Interestingly, the rank-order of potency for stimulating DA-mediated behaviors is inversely related to the potency for [^{3}H]5-HT release. PAL-313 and PAL-314, the most potent 5-HT releasers, produced significantly less motor activation when compared to the other two drugs.

The data in FIGURE 8 show that all PAL amphetamines are readily self-administered by rhesus monkeys, confirming that these agents function as positive reinforcers. However, the rank-order of efficacy, as measured by maximal number of injections, was inversely related to potency for [^{3}H]5-HT release.

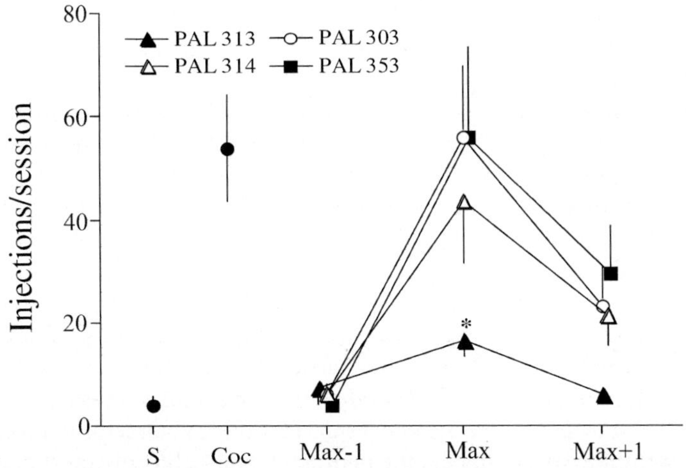

FIGURE 8. Self-administration of PAL amphetamines under an FR25 schedule of reinforcement. Drugs were available for self-administration for 2 h/day. Each data point represents the mean injections/session of each dose for four rhesus monkeys, and vertical error bars represent the SEM. values. The point above *Sal* or Coc represents self-administration of saline or the baseline dose of cocaine in test sessions, respectively. Data were normalized as to dose to adjust for individual differences in sensitivity. Max, dose that maintained maximum injections in each animal; Max−1, half-log dose lower than Max; Max+1, half-log dose higher than Max. $^{*}P < 0.05$ compared with PAL-314, PAL-303, or PAL-353, Duncan's post hoc test. Taken from Reference 21.

The most potent 5-HT releaser, PAL-313, maintained significantly less injections than the other drugs. Thus, the monkey self-administration data indicate that 5-HT release can reduce the reinforcing efficacy attributable to concurrent DA release.

DISCUSSION

The findings presented in this paper support the hypothesis that 5-HT release antagonizes the stimulant properties of DA-releasing drugs. The ability of 5-HT to diminish DA-mediated effects was demonstrated in several behavioral paradigms carried out in phylogenetically distinct mammalian species (i.e., rat and monkey), indicating a generalized phenomenon. Our data contribute to the growing body of knowledge that shows elevations in synaptic 5-HT can counteract stimulant and reinforcing effects mediated by elevations in synaptic DA.[22–25] Self-administration studies provide ample evidence for the "antistimulant" actions of 5-HT. 5-HT precursor loading with dietary tryptophan attenuates amphetamine self-administration in rats.[26] Similarly, pretreatment with 5-HT reuptake inhibitors reduces intravenous cocaine self-administration in rats[27] and squirrel monkeys.[28] Cocaine analogs with high 5-HT transporter affinity support less self-administration behavior than analogs with low 5-HT transporter affinity.[29]

The *in vivo* microdialysis data comparing PAL-287 with (+)-amphetamine offer direct evidence that 5-HT release dampens the effects mediated by DA release. PAL-287 (3 mg/kg, i.v.) and (+)-amphetamine (1 mg/kg, i.v.) increase extracellular DA to the same extent, yet the locomotor stimulant effects of PAL-287 are much less than those of (+)-amphetamine. We believe that weak locomotor and reinforcing effects afforded by PAL-287 are related to the marked increase in extracellular 5-HT produced by this drug, an effect which is not shared by (+)-amphetamine. The findings with PAL-287 are similar to those observed with PAL-313, the substituted amphetamine with greatest 5-HT-releasing potency. PAL-313 produced the least amount of motor activity in rats and supported the weakest self-administration behavior in monkeys. A pertinent correlate of our data is the anorectic agent chlorphentermine, which releases 5-HT to a greater extent than DA but does not increase locomotor activity and is weakly self-administered.[30,31] It seems likely that 5-HT release counteracts the stimulant effects of amphetamine in humans, since fenfluramine administration decreases amphetamine-induced subjective effects in humans,[32] and chlorphentermine is devoid of amphetamine-like subjective effects.[33]

Part of our initial rationale for the development of dual DA/5-HT releasers was based on the knowledge that selective 5-HT releasing agents, such as fenfluramine, lack stimulant properties and are not self-administered.[34] Additionally, fenfluramine antagonizes locomotor and rewarding actions of DA releasers.[19,30,35] Studies using co-administered phentermine and fenfluramine show that drug treatments producing simultaneous elevations in extracellular DA and 5-HT produce minimal motor activity,[30] are not rewarding,[36] and are not reinforcing.[37] Unfortunately, interpreting the effects of fenfluramine is hampered by the complex pharmacology of the drug, and *N*-dealkylation produces a bioactive metabolite with potent agonist activity at 5-HT_{2C} receptors (for review, see Ref. 38). PAL-287 also displays activity at various 5-HT_2 receptor subtypes including 5-HT_{2C} sites.[20] It is not clear to what extent direct agonist activities contribute to the ability of PAL-287 to attenuate DA-mediated behavioral effects, especially since transporter-mediated increases in synaptic 5-HT would be expected to "globally" activate all 5-HT receptors throughout the CNS. Nonetheless, 5-HT_{2C} receptors could be involved in the suppression of DA-mediated effects observed in our studies, as this receptor site has been shown to inhibit DA transmission under a variety of conditions.[39–41] Obviously, it will be interesting to determine which 5-HT receptor subtypes are responsible for the anti-stimulant effects of PAL-287 and related agents.[23] On the other hand, "selectively" non-selective drugs have proven to be superior treatments for mood disorders and schizophrenia,[42] and the same may hold true for developing treatment agents for stimulant dependence.

The ideal monoamine releaser for treating stimulant dependence should reduce drug-seeking behavior and correct neurochemical deficits produced by the abused drug. In this regard, cocaine abstinence in humans is accompanied by major depressive-like symptoms[43,44] and increased suicide attempts,[45,46] consistent with 5-HT dysfunction in the CNS. Neuroendocrine and behavioral studies in rats demonstrate that cocaine withdrawal produces serotonergic deficits.[47–50] Importantly, the spectrum of endocrine and behavioral abnormalities in rats withdrawn from cocaine resembles that of humans diagnosed with major depression.[51–54] Direct evidence for cocaine-induced 5-HT deficits in rats comes from electrophysiological[55] and *in vivo* microdialysis experiments.[56,57]

Based on the findings mentioned above, we proposed a dual deficit model of stimulant withdrawal in which drug-induced DA and 5-HT dysfunction contributes to withdrawal symptoms, drug craving, and relapse.[30,51,58,59] According to the model, decreased synaptic DA during stimulant withdrawal underlies anhedonia and psychomotor retardation, whereas decreased synaptic 5-HT gives rise to depressed mood, obsessive thoughts, and lack of impulse control. The dual deficit model predicts that pharmacotherapies capable of reversing abnormalities in DA and 5-HT function should be effective in treating stimulant dependence. The findings reviewed here support the feasibility of developing non-amphetamine releasers with low abuse potential, by designing dual DA and 5-HT releasing activity into a single molecule. We believe that drugs with a similar mode of action will provide neurochemical normalization therapy for the treatment of cocaine addiction, and such medications might also be useful for treating depression, obsessive compulsive disorder, attention deficit disorder, and obesity. .

ACKNOWLEDGMENT

This research was generously supported in part by the Intramural Research Program of the NIH, NIDA.

REFERENCES

1. Banken, J.A. 2004. Drug abuse trends among youth in the United States. Ann. N. Y. Acad. Sci. **1025:** 465–471.
2. Kresina, T.F. *et al.* 2004. Addressing the need for treatment paradigms for drug-abusing patients with multiple morbidities. Clin. Infect. Dis. **38:** S398–S401.
3. Shearer, J. & L.R. Gowing. 2004. Pharmacotherapies for problematic psychostimulant use: a review of current research. Drug Alcohol Rev. **23:** 203–211.
4. Grabowski, J. *et al.* 2004. Agonist-like, replacement pharmacotherapy for stimulant abuse and dependence. Addict Behav. **29:** 1439–1464.
5. Gorelick, D.A. 1998. The rate hypothesis and agonist substitution approaches to cocaine abuse treatment. Adv. Pharmacol. **42:** 995–997.

6. HENNINGFIELD, J.E. 1995. Nicotine medications for smoking cessation. N. Engl. J. Med. **333:** 1196–1203.
7. KREEK, M.J. 1996. Opiates, opioids and addiction. Mol. Psychiatry. **1:** 232–254.
8. LING, W., R.A. RAWSON & M.A. COMPTON. 1994. Substitution pharmacotherapies for opioid addiction: from methadone to LAAM and buprenorphine. J. Psychoactive Drugs. **26:** 119–128.
9. ROTHMAN, R.B. & M.H. BAUMANN. 2003. Monoamine transporters and psychostimulant drugs. Eur. J. Pharmacol. **479:** 23–40.
10. ROTHMAN, R.B., B.E. BLOUGH & M.H. BAUMANN. 2002. Appetite suppressants as agonist substitution therapies for stimulant dependence. Ann. N. Y. Acad. Sci. **965:** 109–126.
11. GRABOWSKI, J. *et al.* 2004. Agonist-like or antagonist-like treatment for cocaine dependence with methadone for heroin dependence: two double-blind randomized clinical trials. Neuropsychopharmacology. **29:** 969–981.
12. AMARA, S.G. & M.S. SONDERS. 1998. Neurotransmitter transporters as molecular targets for addictive drugs. Drug Alcohol Depend. **51:** 87–96.
13. NEGUS, S.S. & N.K. MELLO. 2003. Effects of chronic d-amphetamine treatment on cocaine- and food-maintained responding under a second-order schedule in rhesus monkeys. Drug Alcohol Depend. **70:** 39–52.
14. WOJNICKI, F.H.E. *et al.* 1999. Effects of phentermine on responding maintained under multiple fixed-ratio schedules of food-presentation and cocaine-delivery in the rhesus monkey. J. Pharmacol. Exp. Ther. **288:** 550–560.
15. NEGUS, S.S. & N.K. MELLO. 2003. Effects of chronic d-amphetamine treatment on cocaine- and food-maintained responding under a progressive-ratio schedule in rhesus monkeys. Psychopharmacology (Berl.) **167:** 324–332.
16. GRABOWSKI, J. *et al.* 2001. Dextroamphetamine for cocaine-dependence treatment: a double-blind randomized clinical trial. J. Clin. Psychopharmacol. **21:** 522–526.
17. SHEARER, J. *et al.* 2003. Pilot randomized double blind placebo-controlled study of dexamphetamine for cocaine dependence. Addiction. **98:** 1137–1141.
18. WISE, R.A. 1981. Brain dopamine and reward. *In* Theory in Psychopharmacology. S.J. Cooper, Ed.: 103–122. Academic Press. London, NY.
19. ROTHMAN, R.B. & M.H. BAUMANN. 2000. Neurochemical mechanisms of phentermine and fenfluramine: therapeutic and adverse effects. Drug Dev. Res. **51:** 52–65.
20. ROTHMAN, R.B. *et al.* 2005. Development of a rationally designed, low abuse potential, biogenic amine releaser that suppresses cocaine self-administration. J. Pharmacol. Exp. Ther. **313:** 1361–1369.
21. WEE, S. *et al.* 2005. Relationship between the serotonergic activity and reinforcing effects of a series of amphetamine analogs. J. Pharmacol. Exp. Ther. **313:** 848–854.
22. DAW, N.D., S. KAKADE & P. DAYAN. 2002. Opponent interactions between serotonin and dopamine. Neural Netw. **15:** 603–616.
23. BURMEISTER, J.J. *et al.* 2004. Differential roles of 5-HT receptor subtypes in cue and cocaine reinstatement of cocaine-seeking behavior in rats. Neuropsychopharmacology. **29:** 660–668.
24. HOWELL, L.L., P.W. CZOTY & L.D. BYRD. 1997. Pharmacological interactions between serotonin and dopamine on behavior in the squirrel monkey. Psychopharmacology (Berl.) **131:** 40–48.

25. CZOTY, P.W., B.C. GINSBURG & L.L. HOWELL. 2002. Serotonergic attenuation of the reinforcing and neurochemical effects of cocaine in squirrel monkeys. J. Pharmacol. Exp. Ther. **300:** 831–837.
26. SMITH, F.L. *et al.* 1986. Dietary tryptophan supplements attenuate amphetamine self-administration in the rat. Pharmacol. Biochem. Behav. **25:** 849–855.
27. CARROLL, M.E. *et al.* 1990. Fluoxetine reduces intravenous cocaine self-administration in rats. Pharmacol. Biochem. Behav. **35:** 237–244.
28. HOWELL, L.L. & L.D. BYRD. 1995. Serotonergic modulation of the behavioral effects of cocaine in the squirrel monkey. J. Pharmacol. Exp. Ther. **275:** 1551–1559.
29. ROBERTS, D.C. *et al.* 1999. Self-administration of cocaine analogs by rats. Psychopharmacology (Berl.) **144:** 389–397.
30. BAUMANN, M.H. *et al.* 2000. Effects of phentermine and fenfluramine on extracellular dopamine and serotonin in rat nucleus accumbens: therapeutic implications. Synapse. **36:** 102–113.
31. GRIFFITHS, R.R. *et al.* 1976. Comparison of behavior maintained by infusions of eight phenylethylamines in baboons. Psychopharmacology **50:** 251–258.
32. BRAUER, L.H. *et al.* 1996. Evaluation of phentermine and fenfluramine, alone and in combination, in normal, healthy volunteers. Neuropsychopharmacology **14:** 233–241.
33. GRIFFITH, J.D., D.R. JASINSKI & J.S. PEVNICK. 1976. Chlorphentermine: absence of amphetamine-like profile in man [abstract]. Clin. Pharmacol. Ther. **19:** 107.
34. WOODS, J.H. & R.E. TESSEL. 1974. Fenfluramine: amphetamine congener that fails to maintain drug-taking behavior in the rhesus monkey. Science **185:** 1067–1069.
35. BENDOTTI, C. *et al.* 1980. Effect of fenfluramine and norfenfluramine stereoisomers on stimulant effects of d-amphetamine and apomorphine in the rat. Pharmacol. Res. Commun. **12:** 567–574.
36. REA, W.P., R.B. ROTHMAN & T.S. SHIPPENBERG. 1998. Evaluation of the conditioned reinforcing effects of phentermine and fenfluramine in the rat: concordance with clinical studies. Synapse **30:** 107–111.
37. GLATZ, A.C. *et al.* 2002. Inhibition of cocaine self-administration by fluoxetine or D-fenfluramine combined with phentermine. Pharmacol. Biochem. Behav. **71:** 197–204.
38. ROTHMAN, R.B. *et al.* 2003. (+)-fenfluramine and its major metabolite, (+)-norfenfluramine, are potent substrates for norepinephrine transporters. J. Pharmacol. Exp. Ther. **305:** 1191–1199.
39. DI MATTEO, V. *et al.* 2001. Role of 5-HT(2C) receptors in the control of central dopamine function. Trends Pharmacol. Sci. **22:** 229–232.
40. FLETCHER, P.J. *et al.* 2004. Injection of the 5-HT2C receptor agonist Ro60-0175 into the ventral tegmental area reduces cocaine-induced locomotor activity and cocaine self-administration. Neuropsychopharmacology **29:** 308–318.
41. DE DEURWAERDERE, P. *et al.* 2004. Constitutive activity of the serotonin2C receptor inhibits *in vivo* dopamine release in the rat striatum and nucleus accumbens. J. Neurosci. **24:** 3235–3241.
42. ROTH, B.L., D.J. SHEFFLER & W.K. KROEZE. 2004. Magic shotguns versus magic bullets: selectively non-selective drugs for mood disorders and schizophrenia. Nat. Rev. Drug Discov. **3:** 353–359.
43. DACKIS, C.A. & M.S. GOLD. 1985. New concepts in cocaine addiction: the dopamine depletion hypothesis. Neurosci. Biobehav. Rev. **9:** 469–477.

44. GAWIN, F.H. & H.D. KLEBER. 1986. Abstinence symptomatology and psychiatric diagnosis in cocaine abusers. Arch. Gen. Psychiatry **43:** 107–113.
45. GARLOW, S.J., D. PURSELLE & B. D'ORIO. 2003. Cocaine use disorders and suicidal ideation. Drug Alcohol Depend. **70:** 101–104.
46. PETRONIS, K.R. *et al.* 1990. An epidemiologic investigation of potential risk factors for suicide attempts. Soc. Psychiatry Psychiatr Epidemiol. **25:** 193–199.
47. LEVY, A.D., M.H. BAUMANN & L.D. VAN DE KAR. 1994. Monoaminergic regulation of neuroendocrine function and its modification by cocaine. Front Neuroendocrinol. **15:** 85–156.
48. BAUMANN, M.H., K.M. BECKETTS & R.B. ROTHMAN. 1995. Evidence for alterations in presynaptic serotonergic function during withdrawal from cocaine in rats. Eur. J. Pharmacol. **282:** 87–93.
49. BAUMANN, M.H. & R.B. ROTHMAN. 1995. Repeated cocaine administration reduces 5-HT1A-mediated prolactin secretion in rats. Neurosci. Lett. **193:** 9–12.
50. BAUMANN, M.H. & R.B. ROTHMAN. 1996. Chronic cocaine exposure potentiates prolactin and head shake responses to 5-HT2 receptor stimulation in rats. Neuropharmacology **35:** 295–301.
51. BAUMANN, M.H. & R.B. ROTHMAN. 1998. Alterations in serotonergic responsiveness during cocaine withdrawal in rats: similarities to major depression in humans. Biol. Psychiatry **44:** 578–591.
52. LIN, D., G.F. KOOB & A. MARKOU. 1999. Differential effects of withdrawal from chronic amphetamine or fluoxetine administration on brain stimulation reward in the rat—interactions between the two drugs. Psychopharmacology (Berl.) **145:** 283–294.
53. MARKOU, A. & G.F. KOOB. 1991. Postcocaine anhedonia. An animal model of cocaine withdrawal. Neuropsychopharmacology **4:** 17–26.
54. BARR, A.M., A. MARKOU & A.G. PHILLIPS. 2002. A 'crash' course on psychostimulant withdrawal as a model of depression. Trends Pharmacol. Sci. **23:** 475–482.
55. CUNNINGHAM, K.A., J.M. PARIS & N.E. GOEDERS. 1992. Chronic cocaine enhances serotonin autoregulation and serotonin uptake binding. Synapse. **11:** 112–123.
56. WEISS, F. *et al.* 1992. Neurochemical correlates of cocaine and ethanol self-administration. Ann. N. Y. Acad. Sci. **654:** 220–241.
57. PARSONS, L.H., G.F. KOOB & F. WEISS. 1995. Serotonin dysfunction in the nucleus accumbens of rats during withdrawal after unlimited access to intravenous cocaine. J. Pharmacol. Exp. Ther. **274:** 1182–1191.
58. ROTHMAN, R.B. *et al.* 1998. Phentermine and fenfluramine: preclinical studies in animal models of cocaine addiction. Ann. N. Y. Acad. Sci. **844:** 59–74.
59. BAUMANN, M.H. & R.B. ROTHMAN. 1998. Serotonergic dysfunction during cocaine withdrawal: Implications for cocaine-induced depression. *In* Drug Abuse Handbook. S.B. Karch, Ed.: 463–484. CRC Press. Boca Raton.

Calcitriol Protects against the Dopamine- and Serotonin-Depleting Effects of Neurotoxic Doses of Methamphetamine

WAYNE A. CASS, MICHAEL P. SMITH, AND LAURA E. PETERS

Department of Anatomy and Neurobiology, University of Kentucky College of Medicine, Lexington, Kentucky 40536-0298, USA

ABSTRACT: Repeated methamphetamine (METH) administration to animals can result in long-lasting decreases in brain dopamine (DA) and serotonin (5-HT) content. Calcitriol, the active metabolite of vitamin D, has potent effects on brain cells, both *in vitro* and *in vivo*, including the ability to upregulate trophic factors and protect against various lesions. The present experiments were designed to examine the ability of calcitriol to protect against METH-induced reductions in striatal and nucleus accumbens levels of DA and 5-HT. Male Fischer-344 rats were administered vehicle or calcitriol (1μg/kg, s.c.) once a day for eight consecutive days. After the seventh day of treatment the animals were given METH (5 mg/kg, s.c.) or saline four times in 1 day at 2-h intervals. Seven days later the striata and accumbens were harvested from the animals for high-performance liquid chromatography (HPLC) analysis of monoamines and metabolites. In animals treated with vehicle and METH, there were significant reductions in DA, 5-HT, and their metabolites in both the striatum and accumbens. In animals treated with calcitriol and METH, the magnitude of the METH-induced reductions in DA, 5-HT, and metabolites was substantially and significantly attenuated. The calcitriol treatments did not reduce the hyperthermia associated with multiple injections of METH, indicating that the neuroprotective effects of calcitriol are not due to the prevention of increases in body temperature. These results suggest that calcitriol can provide significant protection against the DA- and 5-HT-depleting effects of neurotoxic doses of METH.

KEYWORDS: calcitriol; vitamin D; methamphetamine; neurotoxicity; striatum; accumbens; dopamine; serotonin

Address for correspondence: Wayne A. Cass, Ph.D., Department of Anatomy and Neurobiology, MN-225 Chandler Medical Center, University of KY, Lexington, KY 40536-0298. Voice: 859-323-1142; fax: 859-323-5946.
e-mail: wacass1@uky.edu

**Ann. N.Y. Acad. Sci. 1074: 261–271 (2006). © 2006 New York Academy of Sciences.
doi: 10.1196/annals.1369.023**

INTRODUCTION

Calcitriol (1,25-dihydroxyvitamin D_3) is the active metabolite of vitamin D_3. It is presently used clinically in humans to treat several conditions, such as rickets, hypoparathyroidism, and hypocalcemia. While its role in calcium metabolism and bone development are well established, there is increasing evidence for a role for calcitriol in central nervous system (CNS) physiology. The receptor for calcitriol belongs to the same supergene family as the steroid and thyroid hormone receptors,[1] and specific binding of calcitriol occurs throughout the brain, including the striatum.[2] Vitamin D metabolites are present in human cerebrospinal fluid,[3] and several studies have indicated that calcitriol regulates the expression of trophic factors in glial and neuroblastoma cell lines.[4–6] In addition, vitamin D_3 metabolites can cross the blood–brain barrier,[7] and activated microglial cells can produce calcitriol.[8] Taken together, these results suggest that calcitriol has CNS functions and may act as a modulator in the brain for trophic factor expression.

One of the trophic factors that appears to be regulated by calcitriol is glial cell line-derived neurotrophic factor (GDNF). GDNF has been shown to have potent effects on brain dopamine (DA) neurons. Depending on several factors, such as dose and timing of administration, GDNF has neuroprotective and restorative effects against the neurochemical and behavioral deficits associated with administration of the dopaminergic toxins 6-hydroxydopamine (6-OHDA),[9–14] 1-methyl-4-phenyl-1,2,3,6-tetrahydropyridine,[15–17] and methamphetamine (METH).[18–20] Calcitriol has been shown to increase expression of GDNF *in vitro* in C6 glioma cells,[21] and increase release of GDNF in human glioblastoma cells.[22] *In vivo*, calcitriol administration increases GDNF protein levels in the cortex[23] and striatum,[24] and provides partial protection against cortical infarction induced by middle cerebral artery ligation[23] and against 6-OHDA-induced lesions.[25]

It is possible that the calcitriol-induced protection mentioned above is due in part to upregulation of GDNF levels in the brain. We have previously shown that GDNF, if injected into the striatum 1 day prior to treatment with neurotoxic doses METH, can completely protect against METH-induced reductions in striatal DA content and release.[18] Melega and colleagues have also shown a similar protective effect of GDNF against the toxic effects of METH in monkeys.[20] While this protective effect of GDNF is impressive, the administration of GDNF is problematic as it does not cross the blood–brain barrier and must be injected directly into the brain. However, since calcitriol can cross the blood–brain barrier,[7] it upregulates GDNF levels in the brain,[23,24] and the striatum appears to contain receptors for calcitriol,[2] it is possible that systemic administration of calcitriol could provide significant protection against the toxic effects of METH without the need for more invasive intracerebral injections. The purpose of the present study was to determine if treatment with calcitriol can protect against the DA- and serotonin (5-HT)-depleting effects of neurotoxic doses of METH.

MATERIALS AND METHODS

Animals

Male Fischer-344 rats (Harlan Sprague Dawley, Indianapolis, IN) weighing 240–280 g were used for all experiments. They were housed in groups of two under a 12-h light–dark cycle with food and water freely available. All animal use procedures were in strict accordance with the NIH *Guide for the Care and Use of Laboratory Animals* and were approved by the Animal Care and Use Committee at the University of Kentucky.

Calcitriol Administration

Animals were injected once daily for eight consecutive days with calcitriol at a dose of 1 μg/kg body weight. The calcitriol (Sigma Chemical Co., St. Louis, MO) was first dissolved in propylene glycol at a concentration of 100 μg/mL of propylene glycol. For injections the calcitriol in propylene glycol was then diluted into 0.9% saline so that the final volume given was 1 mL/kg of body weight. Vehicle-treated animals were injected with propylene glycol diluted in 0.9% saline. All injections were administered subcutaneously and were given in the morning at the same time each day.

METH Treatment

METH or saline treatments were given on the seventh day of calcitriol administration. The rats were injected subcutaneously with 5 mg/kg METH-hydrochloride (Sigma Chemical Co.) in saline (1 mL/kg), or saline alone (1 mL/kg), four times in 1 day at 2-h intervals. Animals were housed individually during the injections. Body temperature was taken with a rectal probe prior to the first injection of saline or METH, at 1 h after each injection, and at 2 h after the last injection.

Tissue Collection and High-Performance Liquid Chromatography (HPLC)

Seven days after the METH treatments the animals were anesthetized with carbon dioxide and killed by decapitation. The brains were rapidly removed, chilled, and a coronal slice of brain approximately 2 mm thick was made at the level of the striatum and nucleus accumbens. The striatum and accumbens were then dissected from both sides of the slice. The tissue pieces were frozen and stored at −80°C until assayed for DA, 5-HT, and metabolites using HPLC coupled with electrochemical detection.[26]

Data Analysis

DA, 5-HT, and metabolite levels from the right and left sides of the brain were averaged to obtain a single value for each biogenic amine from the striatum and accumbens of each animal. The results were analyzed statistically using analysis of variance (ANOVA) followed by Newman Keuls *post hoc* comparisons as indicated in the results.

RESULTS

Hyperthermia

Body temperatures during the METH or saline treatments are shown in FIGURE 1. The METH treatments led to a significant rise in body temperature in both the animal groups treated with calcitriol or vehicle, and there were no differences between the two METH-treated groups.

Tissue Levels of DA

In the animals treated with vehicle and then given METH there was a 69% decrease in striatal DA levels (FIG. 2). The calcitriol treatment by itself had no effect on striatal DA, but the calcitriol did significantly reduce METH-induced decreases in DA to only 28%. A similar effect was observed with nucleus accumbens DA levels. The METH by itself led to a 45% decrease in accumbens DA content. However, in the calcitriol-treated rats the METH produced only a 15% reduction in accumbens DA.

Tissue Levels of 5-HT

Changes in striatal and accumbens 5-HT content were similar to those for DA. The METH alone led to a 52% decrease in striatal 5-HT levels (FIG. 3). In the calcitriol-treated rats the METH led to a nonsignificant 6.4% reduction in striatal 5-HT. Similarly, in the nucleus accumbens the METH led to a 42% decrease in 5-HT levels in the control animals treated with vehicle. However, the calcitriol treatment completely prevented METH-induced reductions in accumbens 5-HT levels.

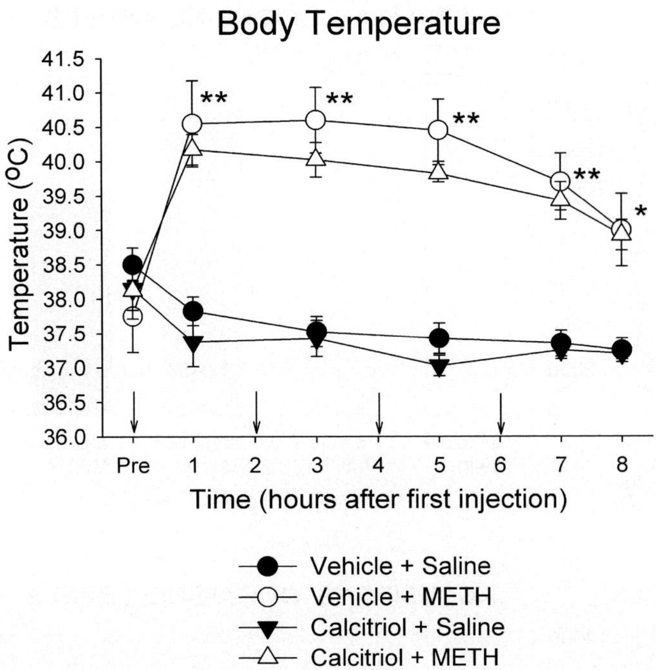

FIGURE 1. Body temperatures of animals during treatment with saline or METH. Animals were treated for eight consecutive days with vehicle or calcitriol. Saline or METH injections were administered on the seventh day of treatment. The timing for the saline and METH injections is indicated by arrows on the x axis. The data shown are mean values ± SD for eight animals per group. $^{*}P < 0.01$; $^{**}P < 0.001$ for both METH groups versus both saline groups at the same time point (two-factor ANOVA with time after injection as a within-factor and treatment group as a between factor followed by Newman Keuls *post hoc* comparisons).

Tissue Levels of Metabolites

In the vehicle-treated control animals the METH injections led to significant reductions in 3,4-dihydroxyphenylacetic acid (DOPAC) and homovanillic acid (HVA), the primary metabolites of DA; and in 5-hydroxyindoleacetic acid (5-HIAA), the primary metabolite of 5-HT (TABLE 1). The calcitriol by itself led to a significant increase in striatal and accumbens DOPAC levels of 25–31%; however, neither HVA nor 5-HIAA levels were elevated. The calcitriol treatments substantially attenuated the METH-induced reductions in DOPAC, HVA, and 5-HIAA in both the striatum and nucleus accumbens. The extent of protection against metabolite loss reflected the extent of protection against parent neurotransmitter loss. That is, there was partial protection against DOPAC and HVA loss, but nearly complete protection against 5-HIAA loss.

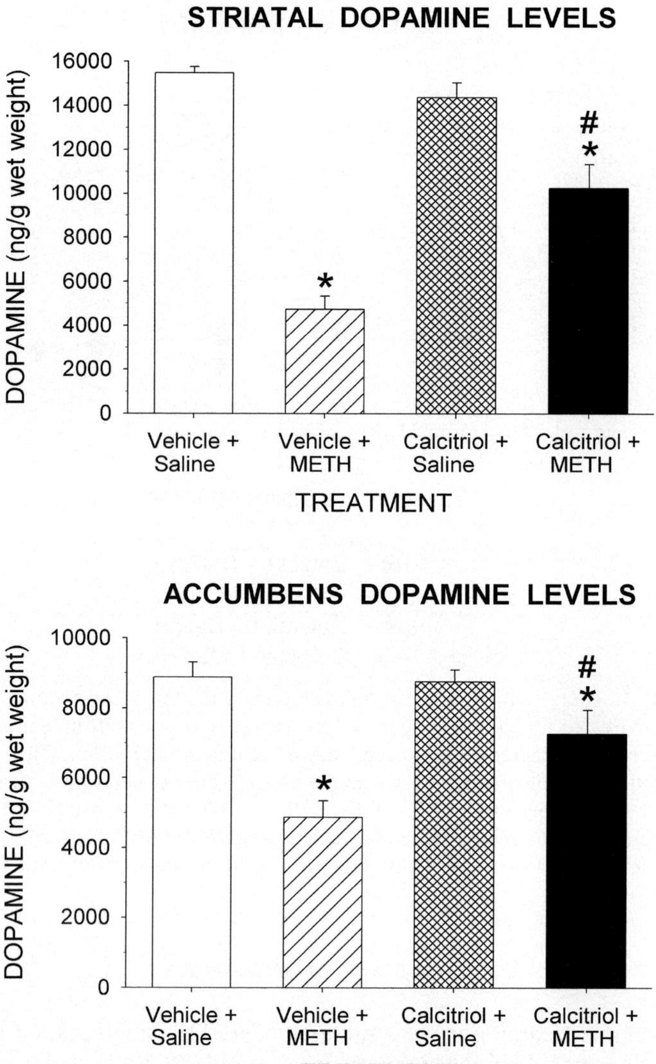

FIGURE 2. Postmortem tissue levels of DA from rats treated with vehicle or calcitriol followed by saline or METH. Animals were treated for eight consecutive days with vehicle or calcitriol. Saline or METH injections were administered on the seventh day of treatment. Striatal (upper graph) and nucleus accumbens (lower graph) levels of DA were determined 7 days after METH or saline administration. Values are mean ± SEM from eight animals per group. $^{*}P < 0.05$ versus respective saline group, $^{\#}P < 0.05$ versus vehicle + METH group (two-way ANOVA followed by Newman Keuls *post hoc* comparisons).

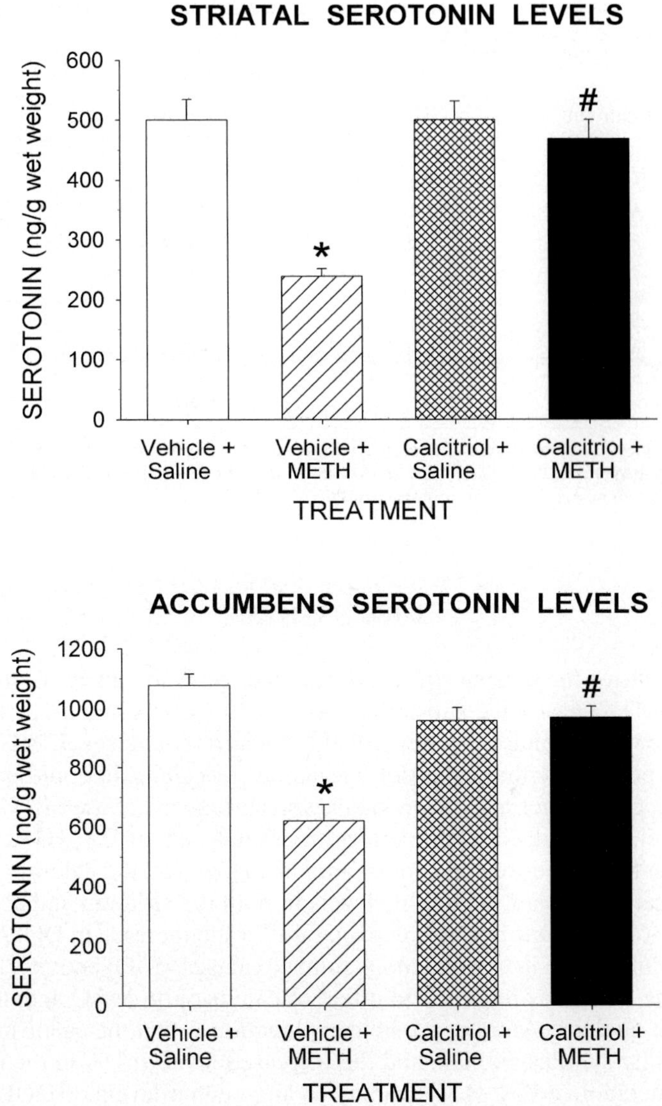

FIGURE 3. Postmortem tissue levels of 5-HT from rats treated with vehicle or calcitriol followed by saline or METH. Animals were treated for eight consecutive days with vehicle or calcitriol. Saline or METH injections were administered on the seventh day of treatment. Striatal (upper graph) and nucleus accumbens (lower graph) levels of 5-HT were determined 7 days after METH or saline administration. Values are mean ± SEM from eight animals per group. $^{*}P < 0.05$ versus respective saline group, $^{\#}P < 0.05$ versus vehicle + METH group (two-way ANOVA followed by Newman Keuls *post hoc* comparisons).

TABLE 1. Tissue levels of DOPAC, HVA, and 5-HIAA from rats treated with vehicle or calcitriol followed by saline or METH

	Metabolite (ng/g wet weight)		
Region and treatment	DOPAC	HVA	5-HIAA
Striatum			
Vehicle + Saline	2,324 ± 93	1,083 ± 28	589 ± 16
Vehicle + METH	804 ± 135*	385 ± 36*	366 ± 12*
Calcitriol + Saline	2,906 ± 151+	1,024 ± 32	571 ± 26
Calcitriol + METH	1,951 ± 272*#	655 ± 48*#	522 ± 34#
Nucleus accumbens			
Vehicle + Saline	2,055 ± 147	785 ± 38	836 ± 19
Vehicle + METH	1,022 ± 130*	342 ± 26*	516 ± 44*
Calcitriol + Saline	2,703 ± 138+	807 ± 34	834 ± 29
Calcitriol + METH	1,911 ± 161*#	546 ± 37*#	763 ± 60#

Values are mean ± SEM from eight animals per group. $^*P < 0.05$ versus respective saline group, $^{\#}P < 0.05$ versus vehicle + METH group, $^{+}P < 0.05$ versus vehicle + saline group (two-way ANOVA followed by Newman Keuls *post hoc* comparisons).

DISCUSSION

The results of the present study indicate that calcitriol, an active metabolite of vitamin D, can provide substantial protection for DA and 5-HT terminals against the monoamine-depleting effects of neurotoxic doses of METH. This raises the possibility that calcitriol, or analogs of calcitriol, could potentially have therapeutic benefits for individuals who chronically abuse METH.

The calcitriol by itself had no effect on tissue levels of DA, HVA, 5-HT, or 5-HIAA in the saline-treated control animals. However, the calcitriol did lead to significant increases in DOPAC levels in both the striatum and accumbens of the control rats. One possible explanation for the increase in DOPAC is that the calcitriol may be increasing monoamine oxidase (MAO) activity. However, at least one study has reported no effect of calcitriol on MAO activity in discrete brain nuclei.[27] Another possible explanation is that the calcitriol may be an increasing synthesis of DA and the increased level of DA in the terminals is being metabolized by MAO leading to augmented levels of DOPAC. Calcitriol has been reported to increase tyrosine hydroxylase mRNA expression in adrenal medulla cells.[28] If a similar phenomenon occurs in the brain then this could lead to increases in DA synthesis and to increases in levels of DOPAC. Further studies will be needed to investigate this and other effects of calcitriol on normal dopaminergic processes in the brain.

There are several possible mechanisms by which calcitriol could be acting to protect against METH-induced reductions in striatal and accumbens DA and 5-HT levels. Hyperthermia is important for METH-induced depletions of brain monoamines, and compounds that prevent hyperthermia are protective. In the present study the calcitriol treatments had no significant effect on METH-induced hyperthermia. This at least rules out a hypothermic effect of calcitriol as its mechanism of neuroprotection.

Another possible mechanism is upregulation of GDNF in the striatum. The dose and timing for calcitriol administration were chosen on the basis of published literature indicating that 1.0 μg/kg/day of calcitriol given for 7 or 8 days leads to an upregulation of cortical and striatal levels of GDNF protein.[23,24] Furthermore, this dosing schedule is partially protective against the lesions produced by middle cerebral artery ligation[23] or by injection of 6-OHDA into the medial forebrain bundle.[25] It has previously been reported that intrastriatal GDNF is protective for DA terminals against neurotoxic doses of METH.[18,20] Thus, if the calcitriol treatments were increasing GDNF levels in the striatum and accumbens, this could explain, in part, its protective effects. On the other hand, with our previous work with GDNF protection against METH we found that GDNF protected against loss of striatal DA content and release, but not 5-HT, in animals administered neurotoxic doses of METH (Ref. 18 and unpublished observations). However, in the present study we found that calcitriol provided protection against loss of 5-HT as well as against loss of DA. This suggests that others mechanisms, in addition to or instead of, an increase in GDNF are involved with calcitriol's protective effects. Calcitriol can also increase several other trophic factors, at least *in vitro*,[4–6] and this may play a role in its neuroprotective ability. Additionally, calcitriol has several other effects that could be involved with its protective actions. For instance, it can increase levels of glutathione[29] and inhibit iNOS production,[30] both of which could reduce METH-induced production of free radicals and thus reduce toxicity to DA and 5-HT terminals. Along these lines calcitriol has been reported to reduce oxidative damage to neurons both *in vitro*[31] and *in vivo*.[32] Further studies will need to be carried out to define the mechanisms by which calcitriol protects against METH-induced reductions in brain DA and 5-HT levels.

ACKNOWLEDGMENTS

This work was supported in part by USPHS Grants DA10115 and AG17963.

REFERENCES

1. Marcus, R. 1996. Agents affecting calcification and bone turnover. *In* The Pharmacological Basis of Therapeutics, 9th ed. J.G. Hardman & L.E. Limbird, Eds.: 1519–1546. McGraw-Hill. New York, NY.
2. Stumpf, W.E. & L.P. O'Brien. 1987. 1,25$(OH)_2$ vitamin D_3 sites of action in the brain. An autoradiographic study. Histochemistry **87:** 393–406.

3. BALABANOVA, S., H.P. RICHTER, G. ANTONIADIS, *et al.* 1984. 25-Hydroxyvitamin D, 24,25-dihydroxyvitamin D and 1,25-dihydroxyvitamin D in human cerebrospinal fluid. Klin. Wochenschr. **62:** 1086–1090.
4. NEVEU, I., P. NAVEILHAN, C. BAUDET, *et al.* 1994. 1,25-Dihydroxyvitamin D_3 regulates NT-3, NT-4 but not BDNF mRNA in astrocytes. Neuroreport **6:** 124–126.
5. VEENSTRA, T.D., J.M. LONDOWSKI, A.J. WINDEBANK, *et al.* 1997. Effects of 1,25-dihydroxyvitamin D3 on growth of mouse neuroblastoma cells. Dev. Brain Res. **99:** 53–60.
6. VEENSTRA, T.D., A.J. WINDEBANK & R. KUMAR. 1997. 1,25-Dihydroxyvitamin D3 regulates expression of N-myc, c-myc, protein kinase C, and transforming growth factor-beta2 in neuroblastoma cells. Biochem. Biophys. Res. Commun. **235:** 15–18.
7. GASCON-BARRE, M. & P.M. HUET. 1983. Apparent [^{3}H]1,25-dihydroxyvitamin D_3 uptake by canine and rodent brain. Am. J. Physiol. **244:** E266–E271.
8. NEVEU, I., P. NAVEILHAN, C. MENAA, *et al.* 1994. Synthesis of 1,25-dihydroxyvitamin D_3 by rat brain macrophages in vitro. J. Neurosci. Res. **38:** 214–220.
9. HOFFER, B.J., A. HOFFMAN, K. BOWENKAMP, *et al.* 1994. Glial cell line-derived neurotrophic factor reverses toxin-induced injury to midbrain dopaminergic neurons in vivo. Neurosci. Lett. **182:** 107–111.
10. WINKLER, C., H. SAUER, C.S. LEE, *et al.* 1996. Short-term GDNF treatment provides long-term rescue of lesioned nigral dopaminergic neurons in a rat model of Parkinson's disease. J. Neurosci. **16:** 7206–7215.
11. KEARNS, C.M., W.A. CASS, K. SMOOT, *et al.* 1997. GDNF protection against 6-OHDA: time dependence and requirement for protein synthesis. J. Neurosci. **17:** 7111–7118.
12. ROSENBLAD, C., A. MARTINEZ-SERRANO & A. BJÖRKLUND. 1998. Intrastriatal glial cell line-derived neurotrophic factor promotes sprouting of spared nigrostriatal dopaminergic afferents and induces recovery of function in a rat model of Parkinson's disease. Neuroscience **82:** 129–137.
13. SULLIVAN, A.M., J. OPACKA-JUFFRY & S.B. BLUNT. 1998. Long-term protection of the rat nigrostriatal dopaminergic system by glial cell line-derived neurotrophic factor against 6-hydroxydopamine in vivo. Eur. J. Neurosci. **10:** 57–63.
14. CASS, W.A. & M.W. MANNING. 1999. GDNF protection against 6-OHDA-induced reductions in potassium-evoked overflow of striatal dopamine. J. Neurosci. **19:** 1416–1423.
15. TOMAC, A., E. LINDQVIST, L.-F.H. LIN, *et al.* 1995. Protection and repair of the nigrostriatal dopaminergic system by GDNF in vivo. Nature **373:** 335–339.
16. GASH, D.M., Z. ZHANG, A. OVADIA, *et al.* 1996. Functional recovery in GDNF-treated parkinsonian monkeys. Nature **380:** 252–255.
17. KOJIMA, H., Y. ABIRU, K. SAKAJIRI, *et al.* 1997. Adenovirus-mediated transduction with human glial cell line-derived neurotrophic factor gene prevents 1-methyl-4-phenyl-1,2,3,6-tetrahydropyridine-induced dopamine depletion in striatum of mouse brain. Biochem. Biophys. Res. Commun. **238:** 569–573.
18. CASS, W.A. 1996. GDNF selectively protects dopamine neurons over serotonin neurons against the neurotoxic effects of methamphetamine. J. Neurosci. **16:** 8132–8139.
19. CASS, W.A., M.W. MANNING & S.L. BAILEY. 2000. Restorative effects of GDNF on striatal dopamine release in rats treated with neurotoxic doses of methamphetamine. Ann. N.Y. Acad. Sci. **914:** 127–136.

20. MELEGA, W.P., G. LACAN, A.A.F. DESALLES, *et al.* 2000. Long-term methamphetamine-induced decreases of [^{11}C]WIN 35,428 binding in striatum are reduced by GDNF: PET studies in the vervet monkey. Synapse **35:** 243–249.
21. NAVEILHAN, P., I. NEVEU, D. WION, *et al.* 1996. 1,25-Dihydroxyvitamin D_3, an inducer of glial cell line-derived neurotrophic factor. Neuroreport **7:** 2171–2175.
22. VERITY, A.N., T.L. WYATT, W. LEE, *et al.* 1999. Differential regulation of glial cell line-derived neurotrophic factor (GDNF) expression in human neuroblastoma and glioblastoma cell lines. J. Neurosci. Res. **55:** 187–197.
23. WANG, Y., Y.-H. CHIANG, T.-P. SU, *et al.* 2000. Vitamin D_3 attenuates cortical infarction induced by middle cerebral artery ligation in rats. Neuropharmacology **39:** 873–880.
24. SANCHEZ, B., E. LOPEZ-MARTIN, C. SEGURA, *et al.* 2002. 1,25-Dihydroxyvitamin D_3 increases striatal GDNF mRNA and protein expression in adult rats. Mol. Brain Res. **108:** 143–146.
25. WANG, J.-Y., J.-N. WU, T.-L. CHERNG, *et al.* 2001. Vitamin D3 attenuates 6-hydroxydopmaine-induced neurotoxicity in rats. Brain Res. **904:** 67–75.
26. CASS, W.A., M.E. HARNED, L.E. PETERS, *et al.* 2003. HIV-1 protein Tat potentiation of methamphetamine-induced decreases in evoked overflow of dopamine in the striatum of the rat. Brain Res. **984:** 133–142.
27. SONNENBERG, J., V.N. LUINE, L.C. KREY, *et al.* 1986. 1,25-Dihydroxyvitamin D_3 treatment results in increased choline acetyltransferase activity in specific brain nuclei. Endocrinology **118:** 1433–1439.
28. PUCHACZ, E., W.E. STUMPF, E.K. STACHOWIAK, *et al.* 1996. Vitamin D increases expression of the tyrosine hydroxylase gene in adrenal medullary cells. Mol. Brain Res. **36:** 193–196.
29. GARCION, E., L. SINDJI, G. LEBLONDEL, *et al.* 1999. 1,25-Dihydroxyvitamin D_3 regulates the synthesis of gamma-glutamyl transpeptidase and glutathione levels in rat primary astrocytes. J. Neurochem. **73:** 859–866.
30. GARCION, E., L. SINDJI, C. MONTERO-MENEI, *et al.* 1998. Expression of inducible nitric oxide synthase during rat brain inflammation: regulation by 1,25-dihydroxyvitamin D3. Glia **22:** 282–294.
31. IBI, M., H. SAWADA, M. NAKANISHI, *et al.* 2001. Protective effects of 1α,25-$(OH)_2D_3$ against the neurotoxicity of glutamate and reactive oxygen species in mesencephalic culture. Neuropharmacology **40:** 761–771.
32. CHEN, K.-B., A.M.-Y. LIN & T.-H. CHIU. 2003. Systemic vitamin D3 attenuated oxidative injuries in the locus coeruleus of rat brain. Ann. N. Y. Acad. Sci. **993:** 313–324.

Protection by GDNF and Other Trophic Factors Against the Dopamine-Depleting Effects of Neurotoxic Doses of Methamphetamine

WAYNE A. CASS,[a] LAURA E. PETERS,[a] MICHAEL E. HARNED,[a] AND KIM B. SEROOGY[b]

[a]*Department of Anatomy and Neurobiology, University of Kentucky College of Medicine, Lexington, Kentucky 40536–0298, USA*

[b]*Department of Neurology, University of Cincinnati College of Medicine, Cincinnati, Ohio 45267-0536, USA*

ABSTRACT: Repeated methamphetamine (METH) administration to animals can result in long-lasting decreases in striatal dopamine (DA) content. It has previously been shown that glial cell line-derived neurotrophic factor (GDNF) can reduce the DA-depleting effects of neurotoxic doses of METH. However, there are several other trophic factors that are protective against dopaminergic toxins. Thus, the present experiments further investigated the protective effect of GDNF as well as the protective effects of several other trophic factors. Male Fischer-344 rats were given an intracerebral injection of trophic factor (2–10 μg) 1 day before METH (5 mg/kg, s.c., 4 injections at 2-h intervals). Seven days later DA levels in the striatum were measured using high-performance liquid chromatography (HPLC). Initial experiments indicated that only intrastriatal GDNF, and not intranigral GDNF, was protective. Thereafter, all other trophic factors were administered into the striatum. Members of the GDNF family (GDNF, neurturin, and artemin) all provided significant protection against the DA-depleting effects of METH, with GDNF providing the greatest protection. Brain-derived neurotrophic factor, neurotrophin-3, acidic fibroblast growth factor, basic fibroblast growth factor, ciliary neurotrophic factor, transforming growth factor-α (TGF-α), heregulin β1 (HRG-β1), and amphiregulin (AR) provided no significant protection at the doses examined. These results suggest that the GDNF family of trophic factors can provide significant protection against the DA-depleting effects of neurotoxic doses of METH.

KEYWORDS: GDNF; trophic factors; neuroprotection; methamphetamine; neurotoxicity; striatum; dopamine

Address for correspondence: Wayne A. Cass, Ph.D., Department of Anatomy and Neurobiology, MN-225 Chandler Medical Center, University of Kentucky, Lexington, KY 40536-0298. Voice: 859-323-1142; fax: 859-323-5946.
e-mail: wacass1@uky.edu

**Ann. N.Y. Acad. Sci. 1074: 272–281 (2006). © 2006 New York Academy of Sciences.
doi: 10.1196/annals.1369.024**

INTRODUCTION

Methamphetamine (METH) is a potent psychomotor stimulant that has high potential for abuse in humans. METH can also act as a neurotoxin[1–4] and several regions of the brain, including the striatum, are affected in animals treated with neurotoxic doses of METH. METH-induced changes in the striatum include, but are not limited to, decreases in dopamine (DA) content, DA release, DA uptake, and tyrosine hydroxylase activity.[1,2,5,6] These changes in striatal DA terminals can last for months to years[1,7]; however, several studies have indicated that there may be partial recovery over extended periods of time.[8–10] It is likely that the extent and severity of METH treatment play a significant role in the degree of recovery possible after METH. Similar to the animal studies, postmortem and imaging studies in humans have indicated neurochemical deficits in the brains of METH abusers.[11–15] The abuse potential of METH, together with its neurotoxic effects, make METH an important drug from the standpoint that chronic use by humans may lead to long-term or permanent changes in brain neurochemistry and function.

Glial cell line-derived neurotrophic factor (GDNF) has been shown to have potent *in vitro* and *in vivo* effects on DA neurons.[16,17] These effects include both neuroprotective and neurorestorative properties for DA cell bodies and terminals lesioned with the toxins 6-hydroxydopamine (6-OHDA)[18–20] and 1-methyl-4-phenyl-1,2,3,6-tetrahydropyridine (MPTP).[21,22] We have previously demonstrated that GDNF, when injected into the striatum 24 h prior to treatment with neurotoxic doses of METH, can protect against METH-induced reductions in striatal DA content.[23] Similarly, intrastriatal GDNF is protective in monkeys against METH-induced reductions in ligand binding to the DA transporter.[24] While the neuroprotective effects of GDNF have been evaluated in many models, there are numerous other trophic factors that have been shown to provide protection to DA neurons against various lesions.[25–27] The purpose of the present study was to further investigate the protective effect of GDNF, as well as the possible protective effects of several other trophic factors, against METH-induced reductions in striatal DA content.

MATERIALS AND METHODS

Animals

Male Fischer-344 rats (Harlan Sprague Dawley, Indianapolis, IN) weighing 250–344 g were used for all experiments. They were housed in groups of two under a 12-h light–dark cycle with food and water freely available. All animal use procedures were in strict accordance with the NIH *Guide for the Care and Use of Laboratory Animals* and were approved by the Animal Care and Use Committee at the University of Kentucky.

Trophic Factor Administration

Animals were anesthetized with isoflurane (2.0–2.5% as needed) and positioned in a stereotaxic frame. All surgery was performed using sterile instruments and aseptic conditions. The skull was exposed and a small hole drilled in the skull over the right striatum. Trophic factors or vehicle (PBS) were injected over 10–15 min into the right striatum (1.0–1.2 mm anterior to bregma, 2.5 mm lateral from midline, and 4.5 mm below the surface of the cortex). The total volume injected was 2–5 μL per trophic factor. The needle was left in place for five additional minutes and then slowly withdrawn. For some animals 5 μg GDNF (or vehicle) was injected into the right substantia nigra (5.4 mm posterior to bregma, 2.2 mm lateral from midline, 7.0 mm below the surface of the cortex). All factors were human recombinant factors and were obtained from the following sources: GDNF, neurturin, artemin, brain-derived neurotrophic factor (BDNF), neurotrophin-3 (NT-3), acidic fibroblast growth factor (aFGF), basic fibroblast growth factor (bFGF), and ciliary neurotrophic factor (CNTF) were from PeproTech, Inc. (Rocky Hill, NJ); transforming growth factor-α (TGF-α) was from Sigma-Aldrich, Inc. (St. Louis, MO); heregulin-β1 (HRG-β1) and amphiregulin (AR) were from R&D Systems, Inc. (Minneapolis, MN).

METH Treatment

METH or saline treatments were given 24 h after intracerebral administration of trophic factor or vehicle. The rats were injected subcutaneously with 5 mg/kg METH-hydrochloride (Sigma-Aldrich, Inc.) in saline (1 mL/kg), or saline alone (1 mL/kg), four times in one day at 2-h intervals. Animals were housed individually during the injections. Room temperature during the treatments was 22–23°C.

Tissue Collection and High-Performance Liquid Chromatography (HPLC)

Seven days after the METH or saline treatments the animals were anesthetized with carbon dioxide and killed by decapitation. The brains were rapidly removed, chilled, and a coronal slice of brain 2 mm thick was made at the level of the striatum using a chilled brain mold. The striatum was then dissected from both sides of the slice. The tissue pieces were frozen and stored at −80°C until assayed for DA using HPLC coupled with electrochemical detection.[28]

Data Analysis

DA levels were analyzed statistically using two-factor analysis of variance (ANOVA) (side of brain as a within factor and trophic factor group as a between factor) followed by Newman Keuls *post hoc* comparisons, or paired *t*-tests, as indicated in the results.

RESULTS AND DISCUSSION

GDNF Family of Trophic Factors

The first experiment examined whether the site of GDNF administration, dopaminergic cell bodies or terminals, influenced the ability of GDNF to protect against the neurotoxic effects of METH. Rats were given an intranigral or intrastriatal injection of GDNF (5 μg) or vehicle followed the next day by treatment with saline or neurotoxic doses of METH. Striatal DA levels were determined 7 days after saline or METH treatment. In animals treated with intranigral vehicle or intranigral GDNF the METH treatment led to decreases in striatal DA of 43–52% on both sides of the brain compared to intranigral

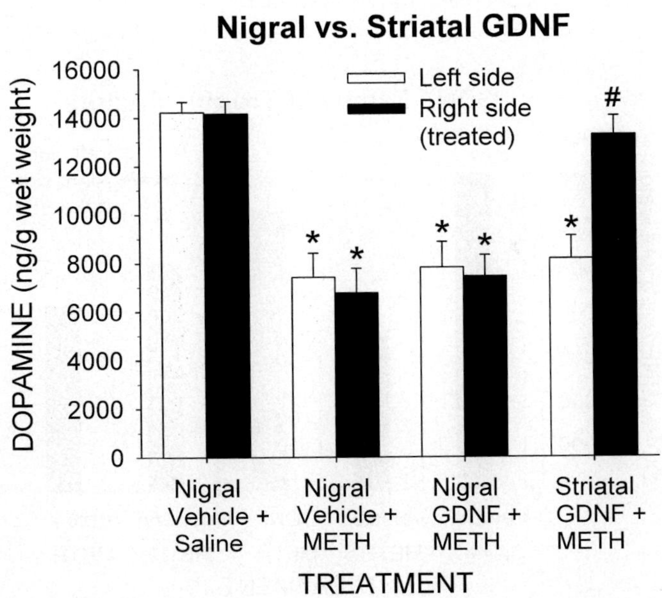

FIGURE 1. Protective effects of intranigral versus intrastriatal GDNF on striatal DA levels. Rats were given an intranigral or intrastriatal injection of GDNF (5 μg) or vehicle followed the next day by treatment with saline or neurotoxic doses of METH. Striatal levels of DA were determined 7 days after the saline or METH treatments. The data shown are mean values ± SEM for 6–8 animals per group.$^{*}P < 0.01$ versus the respective side of the vehicle + saline control group; $^{\#}P < 0.001$ versus left side of the same group (two-factor ANOVA with side of brain as a within factor and treatment group as a between factor; followed by Newman Keuls *post hoc* comparisons).

vehicle + saline-treated control animals (FIG. 1). In contrast, in animals treated with intrastriatal GDNF and METH, DA levels were significantly decreased by 43% in the nontreated striatum, but by only 6% on the GDNF-injected side. Thus, intrastriatal GDNF, but not intranigral GDNF, was protective. In most studies the neurotoxic effects of METH on nigrostriatal DA neurons are confined to striatal DA terminals with little to no effect on DA cell bodies. These results suggest that within the parameters examined (a single injection of GDNF 24 h before METH) the GDNF needs to be administered directly into the region damaged by the METH in order to have protective effects.

We next examined three members of the GDNF family of trophic factors for their ability to attenuate METH-induced striatal DA depletion. GDNF, neurturin, and artemin were all administered into the striatum at a dose of 2 μg. The METH treatments led to a reduction of striatal DA content of 51–58% on both sides of the vehicle + METH-treated animals, and on the nontreated side of the trophic factor-treated animals (FIG. 2). All three factors provided significant protection at the 2 μg dose examined. GDNF provided the greatest degree of protection (12% decrease in DA levels) while artemin provided the least protection (41% decrease in DA content).

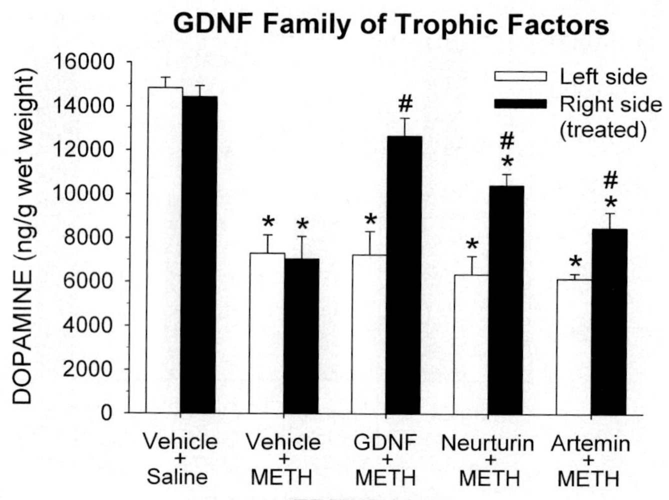

FIGURE 2. Protective effects GDNF, neurturin, and artemin on striatal DA levels. Rats were given an intrastriatal injection of trophic factor (2 μg) or vehicle followed the next day by treatment with saline or neurotoxic doses of METH. Striatal levels of DA were determined 7 days after the saline or METH treatments. The data shown are mean values ± SEM for 6–8 animals per group. $^{*}P < 0.05$ versus the respective side of the vehicle + saline control group; $^{\#}P < 0.01$ versus left side of the same group (two-factor ANOVA with side of brain as a within factor and treatment group as a between factor; followed by Newman Keuls *post hoc* comparisons).

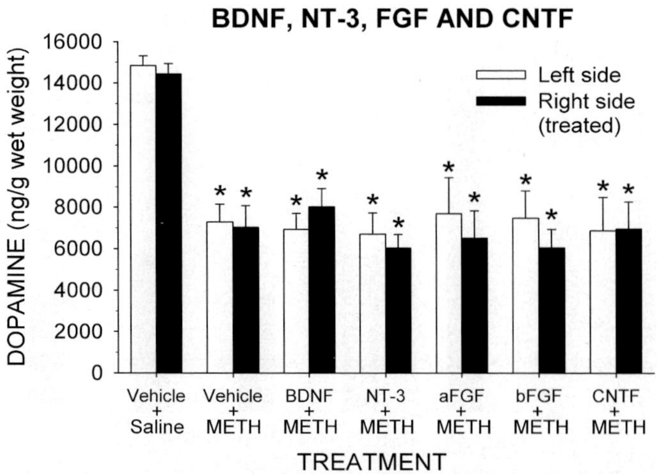

FIGURE 3. Effects BDNF (2 μg), NT-3 (2 μg), aFGF (10 μg), bFGF (10 μg), and CNTF (5 μg) on striatal DA levels. Rats were given an intrastriatal injection of trophic factor or vehicle followed the next day by treatment with saline or neurotoxic doses of METH. Striatal levels of DA were determined 7 days after the saline or METH treatments. The data shown are mean values ± SEM for 4–8 animals per group. $^{*}P < 0.01$ versus the respective side of the vehicle + saline control group (two-factor ANOVA with side of brain as a within factor and treatment group as a between factor; followed by Newman Keuls *post hoc* comparisons).

BDNF, NT-3, FGF, and CNTF

The neurotrophins BDNF (2 μg) and NT-3 (2 μg), as well as aFGF (10 μg), bFGF (10 μg), and CNTF (5 μg), provided no significant protection at the doses examined against METH-induced reductions in striatal DA content (FIG. 3). Striatal DA levels on both sides of the brain were decreased by 44–58% in all METH-treated groups.

TGF-α, HRG-β1, and AR

We next examined TGF-α, HRG-β1, and AR, three members of the epidermal growth factor-like family of trophic factors.[25] All three factors were administered into the striatum at a dose of 10 μg. However, none of these factors provided significant protection against the DA-depleting effects of METH (FIG. 4). In fact, these factors tended to lead to a further decrease in DA levels on the injected side. One factor, AR, led to a significant decrease on the injected side (DA was 35% lower on the injected side compared to the contralateral side). This made it appear that AR was augmenting the effects of the METH. However, in a separate experiment when AR was injected into the striatum of

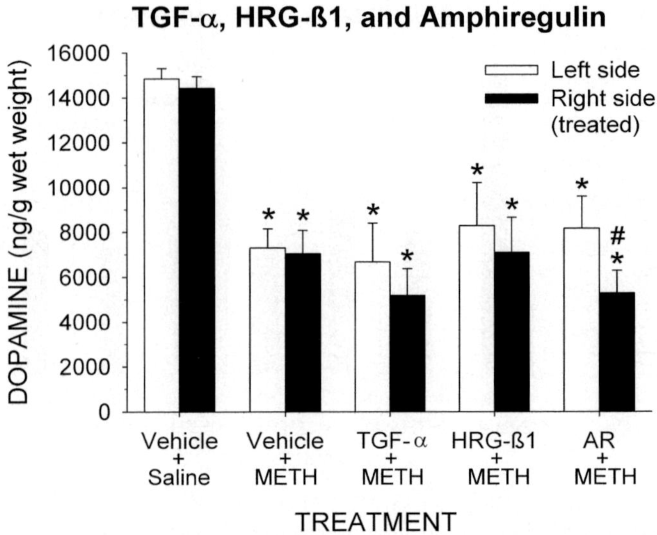

FIGURE 4. Effects TGF-α, HRG-β1, and AR on striatal DA levels. Rats were given an intrastriatal injection of trophic factor (10 μg) or vehicle followed the next day by treatment with saline or neurotoxic doses of METH. Striatal levels of DA were determined 7 days after the saline or METH treatments. The data shown are mean values ± SEM for 4–6 animals per group. $^{*}P < 0.05$ versus the respective side of the vehicle + saline control group; $^{\#}P < 0.01$ versus left side of the same group (two-factor ANOVA with side of brain as a within factor and treatment group as a between factor; followed by Newman Keuls *post hoc* comparisons).

normal animals (i.e., the animals were not treated with METH) there was still a 22% decrease in DA on the injected side compared to the contralateral side 7 days later (DA levels in ng/g wet weight of tissue: AR injected side, 10,830 ± 717; contralateral side, 13,935 ± 548; $n = 9$, $P < 0.01$, paired *t*-test). Thus, AR by itself is causing a reduction in striatal DA levels, by a presently unknown mechanism, and is not necessarily further enhancing the effects of the METH.

GENERAL DISCUSSION

Of the trophic factors examined in this study, only members of the GDNF family provided significant protection against the DA-depleting effects of neurotoxic doses of METH. However, it is possible that some of the other trophic factors may also provide protection under different conditions. For example, using higher doses or a different timing (or even continuous delivery) of trophic factor administration may have increased their protective properties. Along these lines, the BDNF results are based on seven animals. However, if only the four best responders are analyzed, then the BDNF did provide a significant degree of protection (+32% compared to the contralateral side). Thus, it is possible that the 2 μg dose of BDNF examined is at the threshold for providing protection. Other variables that may have influenced the present results are the ability of the trophic factors to diffuse through the striatum and the relative density and cellular localization of the receptors for the individual trophic factors with the striatum.

Although the mechanism for the protective effects of the GDNF family was not examined in the present study, one possibility is a reduction in METH-induced free radicals. Increased production of reactive oxygen and nitrogen species are likely involved with the neurotoxic effects of METH.[3,4,29–31] GDNF has been shown to increase activity of antioxidant enzyme systems in the striatum *in vivo*[32] and suppress accumulation of free radicals *in vitro*.[33] In addition, we have recently observed that GDNF reduces oxidative damage produced in the striatum following intrastriatal administration of 6-OHDA (manuscript in preparation). Thus, it is reasonable to speculate that some of the protective effects of GDNF may be due to reducing or preventing accumulation of free radicals. Further studies will be needed to determine the mechanisms responsible for the protective effects of GDNF.

ACKNOWLEDGMENTS

This work was supported in part by USPHS Grants DA10115 and NS39128.

REFERENCES

1. Seiden, L.S. & G.A. Ricaurte. 1987. Neurotoxicity of methamphetamine and related drugs. *In* Psychopharmacology: The Third Generation of Progress. H.Y. Meltzer, Ed.: 359–366. Raven Press. New York.
2. Gibb, J.W., G.R. Hanson & M. Johnson. 1994. Neurochemical mechanisms of toxicity. *In* Amphetamine and its Analogs: psychopharmacology, Toxicology, and Abuse. A.K. Cho & D.S. Segal, Eds.: 269–295. Academic Press. San Diego, CA.
3. Cadet, J.L., S. Jayanthi & X. Deng. 2003. Speed kills: cellular and molecular bases of methamphetamine-induced nerve terminal degeneration and neuronal apoptosis. FASEB J. **17:** 1775–1788.
4. Kita, T., G.C. Wagner & T. Nakashima. 2003. Current research on methamphetamine-induced neurotoxicity: animal models of monoamine disruption. J. Pharmacol. Sci. **92:** 178–195.
5. Cass, W.A. 1997. Decreases in evoked overflow of dopamine in rat striatum following neurotoxic doses of methamphetamine. J. Pharmacol. Exp. Ther. **280:** 105–113.

6. WALLACE, T.L., G.A. GUDELSKY & C.V. VORHEES. 1999. Methamphetamine-induced neurotoxicity alters locomotor activity, stereotypic behavior, and stimulated dopamine release in the rat. J. Neurosci. **19:** 9141–9148.
7. WOOLVERTON, W.L., G.A. RICAURTE, L.S. FORNO, *et al.* 1989. Long-term effects of chronic methamphetamine administration in rhesus monkeys. Brain Res. **486:** 73–78.
8. MELEGA, W.P., M.J. RALEIGH, D.B. STOUT, *et al.* 1997. Recovery of striatal dopamine function after acute amphetamine- and methamphetamine-induced neurotoxicity in the vervet monkey. Brain Res. **766:** 113–120.
9. FRIEDMAN, S.D., E. CASTAÑEDA & G.K. HODGE. 1998. Long-term monoamine depletion, differential recovery, and subtle behavioral impairment following methamphetamine-induced neurotoxicity. Pharmacol. Biochem. Behav. **61:** 35–44.
10. CASS, W.A. & M.W. MANNING. 1999. Recovery of presynaptic dopaminergic functioning in rats treated with neurotoxic doses of methamphetamine. J. Neurosci. **19:** 7653–7660.
11. WILSON, J.M., K.S. KALASINSKY, A.I. LEVEY, *et al.* 1996. Striatal dopamine nerve terminal markers in human, chronic methamphetamine users. Nature Med. **2:** 699–703.
12. MCCANN, U.D., D.F. WONG, F. YOKOI, *et al.* 1998. Reduced striatal dopamine transporter density in abstinent methamphetamine and methcathinone users: evidence from positron emission tomography studies with [^{11}C]WIN-35,428. J. Neurosci. **18:** 8417–8422.
13. ERNST, T., L. CHANG, M. LEONIDO-YEE, *et al.* 2000. Evidence for long-term neuro-toxicity associated with methamphetamine abuse. Neurology **54:** 1344–1349.
14. SEKINE, Y., M. IYO, Y. OUCHI, *et al.* 2001. Methamphetamine-related psychiatric symptoms and reduced brain dopamine transporters studied with PET. Am. J. Psychiatry **158:** 1206–1214.
15. VOLKOW, N.D., L. CHANG, G.-J. WANG, *et al.* 2001. Association of dopamine transporter reduction with psychomotor impairment in methamphetamine abusers. Am. J. Psychiatry **158:** 377–382.
16. LIN, L.-F.H., D.H. DOHERTY, J.D. LILE, *et al.* 1993. GDNF: a glial cell line-derived neurotrophic factor for midbrain dopaminergic neurons. Science **260:** 1130–1132.
17. CASS, W.A., C.M. KEARNS & D.M. GASH. 1998. Protective and regenerative properties of GDNF in the central nervous system. *In* Neuroprotective Signal Transduction. M.P. Mattson, Ed.: 145–161. Humana Press. Totowa, NJ.
18. WINKLER, C., H. SAUER, C.S. LEE, *et al.* 1996. Short-term GDNF treatment provides long-term rescue of lesioned nigral dopaminergic neurons in a rat model of Parkinson's disease. J. Neurosci. **16:** 7206–7215.
19. ROSENBLAD, C., A. MARTINEZ-SERRANO & A. BJÖRKLUND. 1998. Intrastriatal glial cell line-derived neurotrophic factor promotes sprouting of spared nigrostriatal dopaminergic afferents and induces recovery of function in a rat model of Parkinson's disease. Neuroscience **82:** 129–137.
20. CASS, W.A. & M.W. MANNING. 1999. GDNF protection against 6-OHDA-induced reductions in potassium-evoked overflow of striatal dopamine. J. Neurosci. **19:** 1416–1423.
21. TOMAC, A., E. LINDQVIST, L.-F.H. LIN, *et al.* 1995. Protection and repair of the nigrostriatal dopaminergic system by GDNF in vivo. Nature **373:** 335–339.

22. GASH, D.M., Z. ZHANG, A. OVADIA, *et al.* 1996. Functional recovery in GDNF-treated parkinsonian monkeys. Nature **380:** 252–255.
23. CASS, W.A. 1996. GDNF selectively protects dopamine neurons over serotonin neurons against the neurotoxic effects of methamphetamine. J. Neurosci. **16:** 8132–8139.
24. MELEGA, W.P., G. LACAN, A.A.F. DESALLES, *et al.* 2000. Long-term methamphetamine-induced decreases of [^{11}C]WIN 35,428 binding in striatum are reduced by GDNF: PET studies in the vervet monkey. Synapse **35:** 243–249.
25. YUREK, D.M. & K.B. SEROOGY. 2001. Neurotrophic factor protection of dopaminergic neurons. *In* Neurobiology of the Neurotrophins. I. Mocchetti, Ed.: 355–397. FP Graham. Johnson City, TN.
26. HORGER, B.A., M.C. NISHIMURA, M.P. ARMANINI, *et al.* 1998. Neurturin exerts potent actions on survival and function of midbrain dopamine neurons. J. Neurosci. **18:** 4929–4937.
27. ROSENBLAD, C., M. GRONBORG, C. HANSEN, *et al.* 2000. *In vivo* protection of nigral dopamine neurons by lentiviral gene transfer of the novel GDNF-family member neublastin/artemin. Mol. Cell. Neurosci. **15:** 199–214.
28. CASS, W.A., M.E. HARNED, L.E. PETERS, *et al.* 2003. HIV-1 protein Tat potentiation of methamphetamine-induced decreases in evoked overflow of dopamine in the striatum of the rat. Brain Res. **984:** 133–142.
29. IMAM, S.Z., J. EL-YAZAL, G.D. NEWPORT, *et al.* 2001. Methamphetamine-induced dopaminergic neurotoxicity: role of peroxynitrite and neuroprotective role of antioxidants and peroxynitrite decomposition catalysts. Ann. N.Y. Acad. Sci. **939:** 366–380.
30. DAVIDSON, C., A.J. GOW, T.H. LEE, *et al.* 2001. Methamphetamine neurotoxicity: necrotic and apoptotic mechanisms and relevance to human abuse and treatment. Brain Res. Rev. **36:** 1–22.
31. BROWN, J.M. & B.K. YAMAMOTO. 2003. Effects of amphetamines on mitochondrial function: role of free radicals and oxidative stress. Pharmacol. Ther. **99:** 45–53.
32. CHAO, C.C. & E.H.Y. LEE. 1999. Neuroprotective mechanism of glial cell line-derived neurotrophic factor on dopamine neurons: role of antioxidation. Neuropharmacology **38:** 913–916.
33. SAWADA, H., M. IBI, T. KIHARA, *et al.* 2000. Neuroprotective mechanism of glial cell line-derived neurotrophic factor in mesencephalic neurons. J. Neurochem. **74:** 1175–1184.

Estrogen, Testosterone, and Methamphetamine Toxicity

DEAN E. DLUZEN AND JANET L. MCDERMOTT

Department of Anatomy Northeastern Ohio Universities College of Medicine (NEOUCOM), Rootstown, Ohio 44272, USA

ABSTRACT: The gonadal steroid hormone, estrogen, can diminish the degree of striatal dopamine depletion resulting from methamphetamine. In this article, we describe the conditions of this estrogen neuroprotection as well as the potential for estrogen and testosterone to enhance methamphetamine-induced neurodegeneration of the nigrostriatal dopaminergic system. When administered prior to a neurotoxic regimen of methamphetamine, estrogen significantly decreases the amount of striatal dopamine depletion in intact or gonadectomized female, but not male, mice. This capacity for estrogen to function as a neuroprotectant can occur quite rapidly, at 30 min prior to methamphetamine administration, and with relatively low doses of estrogen (1 μg estradiol benzoate). Estrogen remains an effective neuroprotectant in neonatally gonadectomized female mice treated with testosterone, but not in female mice that were gonadectomized prior to puberty. Nor does estrogen demonstrate any beneficial effects when administered after methamphetamine. Recent data have indicated some conditions where gonadal steroids can increase the extent of striatal neurodegeneration in response to methamphetamine. Specifically, when some existing perturbation is present in the nigrostriatal dopaminergic system, treatment with estrogen enhances the extent of striatal dopamine depletion to methamphetamine. Similarly, increased striatal dopamine depletion to methamphetamine is observed in gonadectomized male mice treated with testosterone.

KEYWORDS: neurotoxicity; neurodegeneration; neuroprotection; nigrostriatal; sex differences; gonadal steroids; striatum

INTRODUCTION

It has been over 10 years since Wagner and colleagues[1] reported that the amount of dopamine (DA) remaining in the striatum of female mice was significantly greater than that of males when treated with equivalent neurotoxic

Address for correspondence: Dean Dluzen, Department of Anatomy, Northeastern Ohio Universities College of Medicine (NEOUCOM), 4209 State Route 44, PO Box 95, Rootstown, OH 44272-0095. Voice: 330-325-6300; fax: 330-325-5913.
e-mail: ded@neoucom.edu

Ann. N.Y. Acad. Sci. 1074: 282–294 (2006).
doi: 10.1196/annals.1369.025

regimens of methamphetamine (METH). These authors speculated that estrogen (E) might represent an important variable contributing to the sex differences obtained in response to METH. However, it was several years later before this hypothesis was formally tested. The data from these subsequent studies support this speculation as striatal DA concentrations of gonadectomized female mice treated with E were significantly greater than non-E-treated females following METH administration.[2,3] Given that E can diminish METH-induced neurodegeneration of striatal DA, within the present article we review some of the salient conditions in which E displays, positive, negative, or no effects upon neuroprotection of striatal DA concentrations. In addition, we report some initial findings on the influence of the predominantly male gonadal steroid hormone, testosterone, in METH-induced neurodegeneration of striatal DA.

Estrogen—Positive/Neuroprotective Effects

A variety of positive or neuroprotective effects of E upon METH-induced neurodegeneration of striatal DA have been related. As noted above, E preserves striatal DA concentrations within gonadectomized female mice.[2,3] A similar neuroprotective response was also observed within E-treated intact female mice (FIG. 1).[4] It had been reported that endogenous increases in

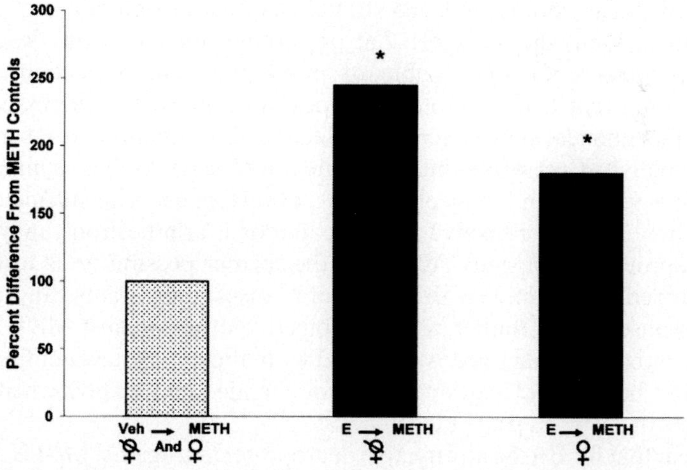

FIGURE 1. Percent difference in striatal DA concentrations in response to METH (20 mg/kg × 4 @ 2h) of E-treated (0.1 mg estrogen pellet, 21 day release) female mice relative to that of gonadectomized and intact female mice not receiving E (Veh→METH). Both gonadectomized and intact female mice treated with E prior to METH (E→METH) showed significantly increased (∗) striatal DA concentrations as compared with that of controls receiving the vehicle for E. (Data generated from Refs. 2–4.)

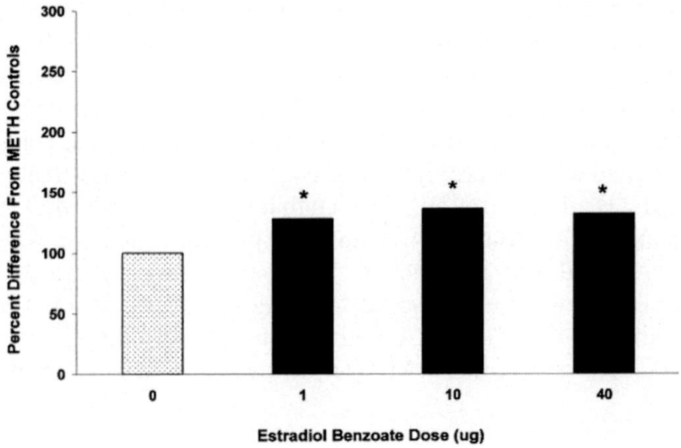

FIGURE 2. Percent difference in striatal DA concentrations in response to METH (40 mg/kg × 1) of gonadectomized female mice treated with varying doses of E (estradiol benzoate in oil, subcutaneously [s.c.]) at 24 h prior to METH administration. All doses of E tested resulted in significantly increased (∗) striatal DA concentrations as compared with that of controls receiving no estradiol benzoate (0 μg). (Data generated from Ref. 7.)

E, as occur around the proestrous period of the mouse estrous cycle, offers neuroprotection against METH[5] as well as to the neurotoxic agent, 6-hydroxydopamine within the rat.[6] The estrous cycle variations in METH- (and 6-hydroxydopamine) induced striatal DA neurotoxicity have two salient implications. First, they suggest that physiological/endogenous levels in E (and/or progesterone) are capable of producing neuroprotection, thereby demonstrating that E neuroprotection does not represent a pharmacological effect of this gonadal steroid hormone. Second, the findings that E can exert a neuroprotective effect within intact female mice, suggests that supplementing endogenous levels with E may provide diestrous females with sufficient levels of E to show a neuroprotective response and/or E at proestrous, may further the neuroprotective capacity. We favor the former possibility as testing gonadectomized female mice with a range of E doses, fails to show any apparent dose–response effect. Rather, a neuroprotective effect against METH within gonadectomized female mice is observed with a relatively low administration of estradiol benzoate (1 μg) and does not change significantly when treated with doses of 10 or 40 μg (FIG. 2).[7]

It is clear that for E to be an effective neuroprotectant against METH-induced striatal DA depletion, it is necessary to administer the E prior to METH. Interestingly, E can be administered as early as 30 min prior to METH to show an indication of neuroprotection which becomes more robust at 12 and 24 h prior to METH (FIG. 3).[8] Such findings suggest the potential for both a rapid, non-genomic and/or a more gradual or delayed, genomic mechanism of action for this E neuroprotection.

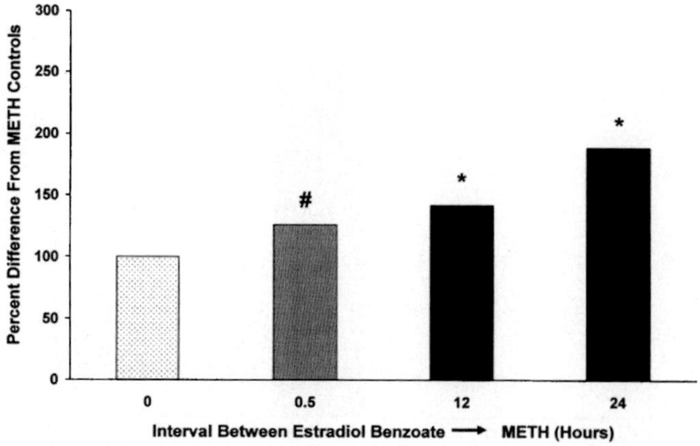

FIGURE 3. Percent difference in striatal DA concentrations in response to METH (40 mg/kg × 1) of gonadectomized female mice treated with 10 μg estradiol benzoate (s.c.) at varying times prior to METH administration. Treatment with estradiol benzoate at 12 and 24 h prior to METH resulted in significantly increased (∗) striatal DA concentrations as compared with controls receiving no estradiol benzoate (0 h). Striatal DA concentrations of mice receiving estradiol benzoate at 0.5 h prior to METH were increased, albeit not significantly, however DOPAC/DA ratios of these mice were significantly decreased compared with the 0 h controls (#). (Data generated from Ref. 8.)

Gonadal steroid hormones exert organizational as well as activational effects within the central nervous system. Activational represent transient effects of an impermanent nature, with the physiological and behavioral changes that occur over the estrous cycle being an example of an activational effect. The neuroprotectant properties of E upon METH-induced neurotoxicity represent activational effects. By contrast, organizational actions involve manipulations of gonadal steroids at critical embryonic and/or neonatal periods of development.[9,10] Such manipulations can produce a permanent change in central nervous system functioning. The reproductive phenotype of the female can be masculinized when treated with testosterone, and males feminized when gonadectomized at the early postnatal period. We have examined the effect of reproductively masculinizing the female mouse, through neonatal (2–5 days of age) gonadectomy combined with testosterone propionate (1.25 mg) treatment, to assess whether E would remain effective as a neuroprotectant when these females were tested as adults. Interestingly, these reproductively masculinized females retain their capacity to display a neuroprotectant response against METH when treated with E as an adult (FIG. 4).[11] The inability for neonatal testosterone treatment to alter E neuroprotection within these female mice can be contrasted with other functions of the nigrostriatal dopaminergic system which can be masculinized by early postnatal testosterone treatment in the female rat.[12] Conclusions from these findings include the possibility that genetic factors appear critical for the sexually dimorphic neuroprotectant

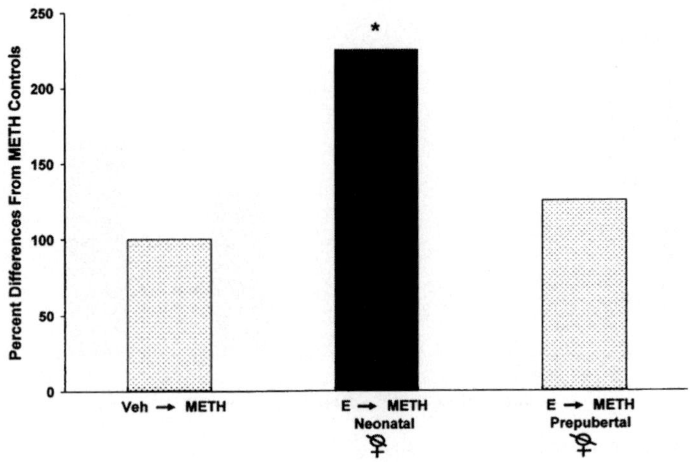

FIGURE 4. Percent difference in striatal DA concentrations in response to METH (20 mg/kg × 4 @ 2 h) of female mice that were either gonadectomized during the neonatal period (2–5 days of age) and treated with testosterone propionate or gonadectomized at the pre-pubertal period (25 days of age). As adults (55 days of age) both groups were treated with E (0.1 mg estrogen pellet, 21 day release) and at 62 days of age with METH. Striatal DA concentrations of mice gonadectomized and treated with testosterone neonatally were significantly increased (∗) when treated with E as adults, while those gonadectomized at the pre-pubertal period failed to show a significant increase in striatal DA concentrations when treated with E as adults. (Data generated from Ref. 11.)

response to E and/or the possibility that sexual differentiation of the nigrostriatal dopaminergic system may be present prior to birth. In support of this latter conjecture are data which show that sex differences in the dopaminergic system may be present prior to birth.[13] Moreover, it would seem that different components of the nigrostriatal dopaminergic system can differentially respond to the masculinizing effects of postnatal testosterone treatment.

Estrogen—No Effects

There are a number of circumstances where E fails to demonstrate any neuroprotectant effects against METH. As noted above, E neuroprotection of striatal DA to METH is sexually dimorphic. Accordingly, we have yet to observe any indication for neuroprotection by E against METH within male mice. These include studies with intact males,[4] males gonadectomized as adults[14] or prepubertally[11] and males reproductively feminized at birth, through neonatal gonadectomy (FIG. 5).[11] In this way, E neuroprotection against METH is clearly absent within males and the findings that neonatal manipulations fail to alter this response suggest either a genetic basis for this differential response between males and females (FIG. 4 versus FIG. 5) and/or the presence

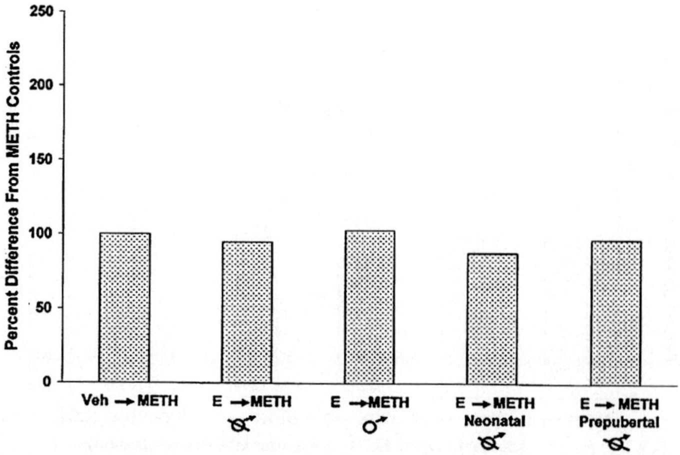

FIGURE 5. Percent difference in striatal DA concentrations in response to METH (20 mg/kg × 4 @ 2 h) of male mice treated with E (0.1 mg estrogen pellet, 21 day release) as adults. Male mice were either gonadectomized as adults, remained intact, gonadectomized during the neonatal period (2–5 days of age) or gonadectomized during the pre-pubertal period (25 days of age). Under none of these conditions were striatal DA concentrations significantly altered when these male mice were treated with E at 55 days of age followed by METH at 62 days of age. (Data generated from Refs. 4, 11 and14.)

of embryonic sexual differentiation.[13] It is interesting to note that in contrast to this sexually dimorphic response to E-METH, E-l-methyl-4-phenyl-1,2,3,6 tetrahydropyridine (MPTP) neuroprotection effects are observed in both male and female mice.[15,16] Whether the differences between these two studies can be attributable to the neurotoxins (METH versus MPTP) and/or strain of mice (CD-1 versus C57/BL) remains to be determined.

There are also circumstances where E fails to show any neuroprotection against METH-induced neurotoxicity of striatal DA concentrations within females. E must be administered prior to METH in order for any neuroprotective effects to be realized. When tested at 0.25, 0.5, 1 or 2 h[8] or at 1 week[3] post-METH (FIG. 6), no indication for E neuroprotection within gonadectomized female mice was present. This lack of an E effect when administered post-METH can be contrasted with the beneficial effects of E when administered in post-ischemia models of central nervous system degeneration.[17]

Finally, if female mice are gonadectomized prior to puberty and subsequently tested as adults, there is no evidence for E neuroprotection.[11,18] These findings represent an interesting contrast with that of the neonatally gonadectomized/testosterone-treated female mice which retain an E neuroprotectant response to METH (FIG. 4). In this way, there appears to be a critical interaction between development and a change/presence of E that is required for E neuroprotection within the adult.

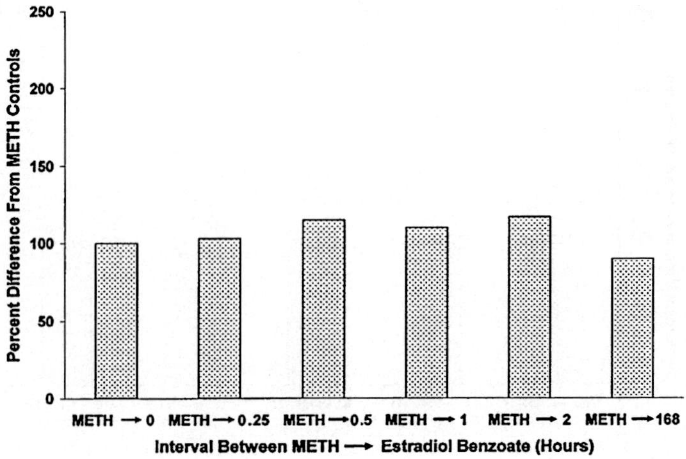

FIGURE 6. Percent difference in striatal DA concentrations in response to METH (40 mg/kg × 1) of gonadectomized female mice treated with 10 μg estradiol benzoate (s.c.) at varying times after METH administration. At none of the time periods sampled were striatal DA concentrations significantly altered when E was administered subsequent to the METH treatment. (Data generated from Refs. 3 and 8.)

Estrogen—Negative/Neurodegenerative Effects

As indicated above, an extensive amount of data are available in support of the hypothesis that E can function as a neuroprotectant against METH-induced neurodegeneration of the striatal dopaminergic system. We have also reviewed conditions where there is an absence of any E neuroprotection within this model. Recently, we have observed a situation where E appears to increase the degree of nigrostriatal dopaminergic neurodegeneration in response to METH. When gonadectomized female mice were treated initially with METH to induce a perturbation of nigrostriatal dopaminergic function, followed by E and a second treatment with METH, those mice receiving the E treatment showed a greater depletion of striatal DA concentrations than controls receiving the oil vehicle (FIG. 7).[19] Therefore, when there is an initial impairment or perturbation in the nigrostriatal dopaminergic system, subsequent treatment with E not only lacks the ability to show neuroprotection, but contrarily, seems to enhance the degree of neurodegeneration to a second insult with METH. There exists considerable controversy with regard to the effects of E treatment in nigrostriatal dopaminergic neurodegeneration conditions, such as Parkinson's disease, with positive,[20,21] negative[22,23] or no[24] effects being reported. The present data might aid in understanding such seemingly inconsistent findings as they imply that E has the capability of exerting neuroprotectant or neurodegenerative effects depending upon the existing condition of the nigrostriatal dopaminergic system.

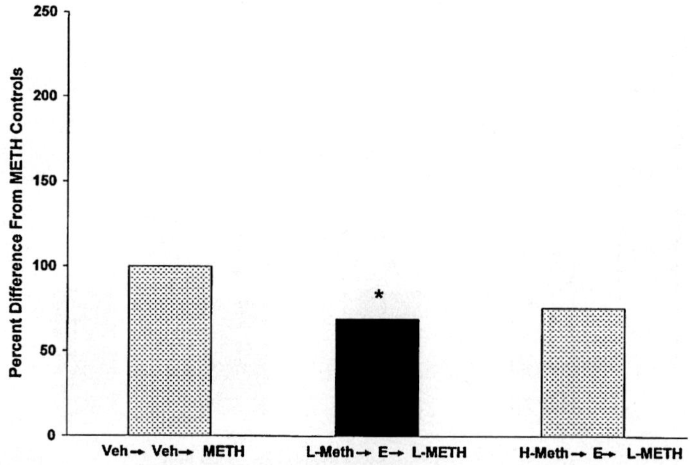

FIGURE 7. Percent difference in striatal DA concentrations in response to two administrations of METH to gonadectomized female mice treated with 10 μg estradiol benzoate (s.c.). The mice received either an initial low-METH (L-METH: 20 mg/kg × 2 @ 2 h) or high-METH (H-METH: 20 mg/kg × 4 @ 2 h) treatment. At 7 days after this initial METH treatment, mice received estrogen (or vehicle) followed 24 h later with a L-METH treatment. Striatal DA concentrations of these estrogen-treated mice were decreased with a statistically significant (∗) reduction obtained in the L-METH-treated mice. (Data generated from Ref. 19.)

Testosterone Effect

There exists a very limited amount of information on the potential role of testosterone in METH-induced neurotoxicity of striatal DA. When gonadectomized male mice were treated with a testosterone pellet followed 1 week later with METH, the amount of striatal DA depletion was decreased (83%), although not significantly, compared with that observed in non-testosterone-treated controls.[14] These results were similar to that of reports showing a lack of testosterone neuroprotection against MPTP-induced striatal DA depletion.[25,26] Taken together, it seems clear that, unlike E, the predominantly male gonadal steroid hormone, testosterone, offers no protection against neurotoxins which target striatal DA. Since our testosterone-METH results suggested that testosterone might actually increase the degree of striatal DA depletion to METH, we designed an experiment to examine this possibility. In this experiment, gonadectomized male mice received a single injection of testosterone propionate at 0 (control) 5, 50, or 500 μg followed 24 h later with METH (40 mg/kg). When compared with the 0 μg controls, all testosterone-treated mice showed significantly greater depletions of striatal DA with levels ranging from 71% to 78% that of controls. No statistically significant differences were obtained among the three doses of testosterone tested (FIG. 8).[27] These results

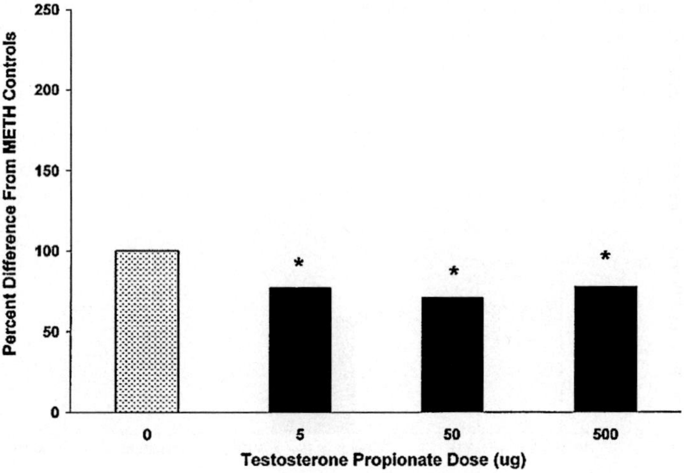

FIGURE 8. Percent difference in striatal DA concentrations in response to methamphetamine (METH−40 mg/kg × 1) treatment of gonadectomized male mice receiving varying doses of testosterone propionate at 24 h prior to METH administration. Striatal DA concentrations of the testosterone-treated mice were significantly decreased (∗) as compared with METH-treated controls (0 μg). (Data generated from Ref. 27.)

suggest that testosterone might not simply lack a neuroprotective effect, but actually increase the extent of neurotoxicity induced by METH. In support of this hypothesis are data which indicate that testosterone increases striatal DA neurotoxicity to MPTP in mice[28] and 6-hydroxydopamine in rats.[29] Accordingly, the sex differences in striatal DA depletion to METH[1,5,30] (and to MPTP and 6-hydroxydopamine) might result from a combination of neuroprotectant properties of estrogen within females and neurodegenerative effects of testosterone within males.

Summary and Conclusions

In this brief article, we have considered the various conditions under which the gonadal steroid hormones, E and testosterone, can affect METH-induced neurotoxicity of the striatal DA system. A summary of the positive/neuroprotective, negative/neurodegenerative and absence/no effects exerted by E and testosterone is displayed in TABLE 1.

A salient characteristic of the positive/neuroprotective actions of E upon METH-induced striatal DA depletion is that it is limited to females. An increase in E concentrations prior to METH treatment as can be achieved with exogenous E administration to gonadectomized (adult) or intact female mice, or as can occur endogenously during the natural estrous cycle of the mouse, diminishes the degree of METH-induced striatal DA depletion. The female mice

TABLE 1. Summary of conditions under which the gonadal steroid hormones, E and testosterone, produce positive/neuroprotective effects (+), no effects (0), or negative/neurodegenerative effects (−) upon METH- induced depletion of striatal dopamine concentrations

	+	0	−
Sex	♀	♂̸ (TP-Pellet)	♂̸ (5-500 ug TP)
Gonadal Condition	♀̸ & ♀	♂̸ & ♂	
Dose	1-40 ug EB 0.1 mg EB Pellet		
Timing			
Pre-METH	0.5 h – 1 Week		
Post-METH		0.25 – 1 Week	
Developmental			
Neonatal	Testosterone ♀̸	♂̸	
Pubertal		♀̸ & ♂̸	
Impaired NSDA System			Meth → E → Meth

are quite sensitive to this effect of E as neuroprotective effects can be obtained with relatively low amounts of E replacement in gonadectomized females (1 μg of estradiol benzoate) and within the limited range of changes that are present across the estrous cycle. On the bases of data which show that sexually dimorphic neuroprotection to E remains in phenotypically altered reproductively masculinized females, and remains absent in reproductively feminized male mice the potential exists that this sexual dimorphism in E's ability to function as a neuroprotectant might have a genetic basis. However, a sexual differentiation of the nigrostriatal dopaminergic system might occur at embryological stages of development. Interestingly, it appears critical for the female to proceed through a normal pubertal development in order to demonstrate this E neuroprotection as pre-pubertal gonadectomy abolished this response in the female mouse. In marked contrast to the plethora of conditions in which E can function as a neuroprotectant within the female, we have been unable to identify a situation where E can serve as a neuroprotectant against METH in the male.

A critical feature of E neuroprotection is the necessity for this gonadal steroid hormone to be present prior to METH exposure. Such findings might indicate an important component for understanding these E effects. There exist a number of potential mechanisms through which E can work to produce neuroprotection of striatal DA concentrations.[31] Some of the proposed mechanisms described for E neuroprotection of the central nervous system include processes involving anti-apoptosis, nitric oxide, antioxidants, neurotrophins, blood flow, CREB, and thermoregulation. This list highlights the complexity and multifarious nature of the E neuroprotection mechanisms. The necessity for E's presence prior to METH suggests that E might exert its neuroprotection through affecting the initial stages of METH neurotoxicity. To this end, we have considered the incipient interactions between E and METH as one approach to examine E's neuroprotective effects. With regard to such initial interactions are data which show that E can inhibit the amount of DA evoked by METH infusion.[32] One interpretation of this result is that E may be inhibiting the uptake of METH, and there are data which indicate that DA transporter function can be inhibited by E.[33–35] Accordingly, this inhibition of DA transporter function might represent an important mechanism that can contribute to the E neuroprotection against METH-induced neurotoxicity of the nigrostriatal dopaminergic system.

The observation of negative or neurodegenerative effects of gonadal steroid hormones, as observed with E in the impaired/perturbed nigrostriatal dopaminergic system of the female and testosterone in the male, represent some equally intriguing findings. An important implication of the increased neurotoxicity with testosterone in the male is that sex/gender differences to METH might not simply be attributable to neuroprotection by E. Rather, this sex/gender disparity in METH-induced neurotoxicity may involve a combination of increased neurotoxicity due to the presence of testosterone within males along with decreased neurotoxicity due to E within females. Equally significant are the results which indicate that E can actually increase METH-induced neurotoxicity within specific conditions in the female. Such findings reveal that E neuroprotection is not ubiquitous. Of greater potential significance is the implication that the specific existing condition of the nigrostriatal dopaminergic system exerts a significant influence on the direction that E can produce in response to METH. In this way, under conditions of long-term or repeated METH use, which can produce an impaired or perturbed nigrostriatal dopaminergic system, the presence of E within females may now result in an increased risk for METH-induced neurodegeneration. In addition, some of the conflicting clinical literature regarding the effects of E on the nigrostriatal neurodegenerative condition of Parkinson's disease may be better understood since this animal model data reveal that E can result in increased or decreased neurodegeneration depending upon the current state of the nigrostriatal dopaminergic system.

REFERENCES

1. WAGNER, G.C., T.L. TEKIRIAN & C.T. CHEO. 1993. Sexual differences in sensitivity to methamphetamine toxicity. J. Neural Transm. Gen. Sect. **93**: 67–70.

2. DLUZEN, D.E. & J.L. MCDERMOTT. 2000. Neuroprotective role of estrogen upon methamphetamine and related neurotoxins within the nigrostriatal dopaminergic system. Ann. N. Y. Acad. Sci. **914**: 112–126.
3. GAO, X. & D.E. DLUZEN. 2001. Tamoxifen abolishes estrogen's neuroprotective effect upon methamphetamine neurotoxicity of the nigrostriatal dopaminergic system. Neuroscience **103**: 385–394.
4. DLUZEN, D.E., L.I. ANDERSON & C.F. PILATI. 2002. Methamphetamine-gonadal steroid interactions: effects upon acute toxicity and striatal dopamine concentrations. Neurotox. Teratol. **24**: 267–273.
5. YU, L. & P.-C. LIAO. 2000. Sexual differences and estrous cycle in methamphetamine-induced dopamine and serotonin depletions in the striatum of mice. J. Neural Transm. **107**: 419–427.
6. DATLA, K.P., H.E. MURRAY, A.V. PILLAI, *et al.* 2003. Differences in dopaminergic neuroprotective effects of estrogen during estrous cycle. Neuroreport **14**: 47–50.
7. MICKLEY, K.R. & D.E. DLUZEN. 2004. Dose–response effects of estrogen and tamoxifen upon methamphetamine-induced behavioral responses and neurotoxicity of the nigrostriatal dopaminergic system in female mice. Neuroendocrinology **79**: 305–316.
8. GAJJAR, T.M., L.I. ANDERSON & D.E. DLUZEN. 2003. Acute effects of estrogen upon methamphetamine induced neurotoxicity of the nigrostriatal dopaminergic system. J. Neural. Transm. **110**: 1215–1224.
9. BEYER, C. 1999. Estrogen and the developing mammalian brain. Anat. Embryol. **199**: 379–390.
10. GORSKI, R.A. 1980. Sexual differentiation of the brain. *In* Neuroendocrinology. D.T. Kreiger & J.C. Hughes, Eds.: pp. 215–222 Sinauer Associates Inc. Sunderland, MA.
11. ANDERSON, L.I., R.E. LEIPHEIMER & D.E. DLUZEN. 2005. Effects of neonatal and prepubertal hormonal manipulations upon estrogen neuroprotection of the nigrostriatal dopaminergic system within female and male mice. Neuroscience **130**: 369–382.
12. VELISKOVA, J. & S.L. MOSHE. 2001. Sexual dimorphism and developmental regulation of substantia nigra function. Ann. Neurol. **50**: 596–601.
13. SIBUG, R., E. KUPPERS, C. BEYER, *et al.* 1996. Genotype-dependent sex differentiation of dopaminergic neurons in primary cultures of embryonic mouse brain. Dev. Brain Res. **93**: 136–142.
14. GAO, X. & D.E. DLUZEN. 2001. The effect of testosterone upon methamphetamine neurotoxicity of the nigrostriatal dopaminergic system. Brain Res. **892**: 63–69.
15. DLUZEN, D.E., J.L. MCDERMOTT & B. LIU. 1996. Estrogen as a neuroprotectant against MPTP-induced neurotoxicity in C57/Bl mice. Neurotox. Teratol. **18**: 603–606.
16. CALLIER, S., M. MORISSETTE, M. GRANDBOIS & T. DI PAOLO. 2000. Stereospecific prevention by 17beta-estradiol of MPTP-induced dopamine depletion in mice. Synapse **37**: 245–251.
17. YANG, S.H., J. SHI, A.L. DAY & J.W. SIMPKINS. 2000. Estradiol exerts neuroprotective effects when administered after ischemic insult. Stroke **31**: 745–755.
18. YU, L., Y. KUO, C.G. CHENG, *et al.* 2002. Ovarian hormones do not attenuate methamphetamine-induced dopaminergic neurotoxicity in mice gonadectomized at 4 weeks postpartum. Neuroendocrinology **75**: 282–287.

19. LIU, B. & D.E. DLUZEN. 2006. Effect of estrogen upon methamphetamine-induced neurotoxicity within the impaired nigrostriatal dopaminergic system. Synapse **60:** In press.
20. SAUNDERS-PULLMAN, R., J. GORDON-ELLIOTT, M. PARIDES, *et al.* 1999. The effect of estrogen replacement on early Parkinson's disease. Neurology **52**: 1417–1421.
21. RAVINA, B.M., S.C. FAGAN, R.G. HART, *et al.* 2003. Neuroprotective agents for clinical trials in Parkinson's disease: a systematic assessment. Neurology **60**: 1234–1240.
22. BEDARD, P., P. LANGELIER & A. VILLENEUVE. 1977. Oestrogens and extrapyramidal system. Lancet **2**: 1367–1368.
23. SHULMAN, L.M., A. MINAGAR & W.J. WEINER. 2000. The effect of pregnancy in Parkinson's disease. Mov. Disord. **15**: 132–135.
24. STRIJKS, E.J., A. KREMER & M.W.I.M. HORSTINK. 1999. Effects of female sex steroids on Parkinson's disease in post-menopausal women. Clin. Neuropharmacol. **22**: 93–97.
25. DLUZEN, D.E. 1996. Effects of testosterone upon MPTP-induced neurotoxicity of the nigrostriatal dopaminergic system of C57/Bl mice. Brain Res. **715**: 113–118.
26. EKUE, A., J.F. BOULANGER, M. MORISSETTE & T. DI PAOLO. 2002. Lack of effect of testosterone and dihydrotestosterone compared to 17beta-oestradiol in 1-methyl-4-phenyl-1,2,3,6-tetrahydropyridine-mice. J. Neuroendocrinol **19**: 731–736.
27. LEWIS, C.M. & D.E. DLUZEN. 2004. Effect of testosterone upon methamphetamine-induced neurotoxicity of striatal dopamine within male and female mice. Soc. Neurosci. 34th Mtg., Abst # 345.4.
28. DLUZEN, D.E., R. JIAN & L.I. ANDERSON. 1994. Modulatory effects of testosterone on 1-methyl-4-phenyl-1,2,3,6-tetrahydropyridine-induced neurotoxicity. J. Neurochem. **64**: 94–101.
29. MURRAY, H.E., A.V. PILLAI, S.R. MCARTHUR, *et al.* 2003. Dose- and sex-dependent effects of the neurotoxin 6-hydroxydopamine on the nigrostriatal dopaminergic pathways of adult rats: differences in action of estrogen in males and females. Neuroscience **116**: 213–222.
30. DLUZEN, D.E., C. TWEED, L.I. ANDERSON & N.J. LAPING. 2003. Gender differences in methamphetamine-induced mRNA associated with neurodegeneration in the mouse nigrostriatal dopaminergic system. Neuroendocrinology **77**: 232–238.
31. DLUZEN, D.E. & J.L. MCDERMOTT. 2002. Estrogen, anti-estrogen, and gender differences in methamphetamine neurotoxicity. Ann. N. Y. Acad. Sci. **965**: 136–156.
32. MYERS, R.E., L.I. ANDERSON & D.E. DLUZEN. 2003. Estrogen, but not testosterone, attenuates methamphetamine-evoked dopamine output from superfused striatal tissue of female and male mice. Neuropharmacology **44**: 624–632.
33. DISSHON, K.A., J.W. BOJA & D.E. DLUZEN. 1998. Inhibition of striatal dopamine transporter activity by 17ß-estradiol. Eur. J. Pharmacol. **345**: 207–211.
34. THOMPSON, T.L. 1999. Attenuation of dopamine uptake in vivo following priming with estradiol benzoate. Brain Res. **834**: 164–167.
35. THOMPSON, T.L. & M.E. CERTAIN. 2005. Estrogen mediated inhibition of dopamine transport in the striatum: regulation by $Ga_{i/o}$. Eur. J. Pharmacol. **511**: 121–126.

Fluoxetine as a Potential Pharmacotherapy for Methamphetamine Dependence

Studies in Mice

YUKIO TAKAMATSU,[a] HIDEKO YAMAMOTO,[a] YASUKAZU OGAI,[a] YOKO HAGINO,[a] ATHINA MARKOU,[b] AND KAZUTAKA IKEDA[a]

[a]*Division of Psychobiology, Tokyo Institute of Psychiatry, Tokyo 156-8585, Japan*

[b]*Department of Molecular and Integrative Neuroscience, The Scripps Research Institute, La Jolla, California 92037, USA*

ABSTRACT: The monoamine transporters are the main targets of psychostimulant drugs, including methamphetamine (METH) and cocaine. Interestingly, the rewarding effects of cocaine are retained in dopamine transporter (DAT) knockout (KO) mice, while serotonin transporter (SERT) and DAT double KO mice do not exhibit conditioned place preference (CPP) to cocaine. These data suggest that SERT inhibition decreases the rewarding effects of psychostimulants. To further test this hypothesis, in the present study, we investigated the effects of intraperitoneal (i.p.) injections of 20 mg/kg fluoxetine, a selective serotonin reuptake inhibitor (SSRI), on 2 mg/kg METH (i.p.) CPP and locomotor sensitization to 1 mg/kg METH (i.p.) in C57BL/6J mice. Fluoxetine treatment before both the conditioning and preference tests abolished METH CPP. A two-way analysis of variance (ANOVA) revealed that METH CPP tended to be lower in mice pretreated with fluoxetine before the preference test than in control mice pretreated with saline before the preference test. Furthermore, pretreatment with fluoxetine had inhibitory effects on METH-induced locomotor sensitization. These results suggest that fluoxetine, a widely used medication for depression, may be also a useful tool for treating METH dependence.

KEYWORDS: methamphetamine; fluoxetine; conditioned place preference; locomotor activity; sensitization; mice

Address for correspondence: Kazutaka Ikeda, Division of Psychobiology, Tokyo Institute of Psychiatry, 2-1-8 Kamikitazawa, Setagaya-ku, Tokyo 156-8585, Japan. Voice: +81-3-3304-5701, ext. 508; fax: +81-3-3329-8035.
e-mail: ikedak@prit.go.jp

**Ann. N.Y. Acad. Sci. 1074: 295–302 (2006). © 2006 New York Academy of Sciences.
doi: 10.1196/annals.1369.026**

INTRODUCTION

Methamphetamine (METH) is widely abused in the world.[1] Especially in Japan, the number of people arrested for METH possession or use is approximately 100 times more than those arrested for cocaine or cannabis. Further, METH frequently induces psychotic states with symptoms similar to those seen in schizophrenia of the paranoid type.[2] Such psychotic states are mainly treated in hospitals resulting in large medical costs. Thus, there is great need for the discovery of new medications for METH abuse,[3] as the current treatments are primarily oriented toward the treatment of psychosis with no treatments available to prevent relapse to METH abuse.

Dopamine transporters (DAT) are the main targets for METH and cocaine. However, mice lacking the DAT show preference for cocaine[4] and self-administer cocaine.[5] Interestingly, heterozygous and homozygous serotonin transporter (SERT) knockout (KO) mice that also have a homozygous KO of the DAT do not exhibit cocaine place preference.[6] Further, findings indicated that extracellular dopamine concentration increases after cocaine administration in the striatum of DAT KO mice but not of DAT/SERT double KO mice.[7] Taken together, these reports suggest that SERT inhibition may decrease METH and cocaine place preference.

In the present study, we tested this hypothesis by assessing whether fluoxetine, a selective serotonin reuptake inhibitor (SSRI) with the trade name of Prozac, reduces METH place preference and sensitization to the locomotor activating effects of METH.

MATERIALS AND METHODS

Male C57BL/6J mice (8–10 weeks old) were purchased from CLEA Japan, Inc. (Tokyo, Japan) and were housed for 1–2 weeks before the experiments were begun in an animal facility maintained at $24 \pm 1°C$ and 50% relative humidity under a 12/12 h light/dark cycle with lights on at 8:00 AM and off at 8:00 PM. Food and water were available *ad libitum*. The experimental procedures and housing conditions were approved by the Institutional Animal Care and Use Committee of the Tokyo Institute of Psychiatry, and all animals were cared for and treated humanely in accordance with our institutional animal experimentation guidelines.

Conditioned Place Preference (CPP) Test

The conditioned place preference (CPP) test was carried out according to the method of Hoffman and Beninger[8] with some modifications. For this test, we used a two-compartment Plexiglas chamber (Neuroscience Inc., Osaka, Japan), one compartment was black with a smooth floor and the other was of the same dimensions, but white with a textured floor. This two-compartment chamber was placed in a sound- and light-attenuated box under conditions of dim illumination (about 40 lx). There was no significant difference between time spent in the black compartment and time spent in the white compartment on day 2 of testing (see below), indicating that there was no preference for either side under the present conditions before conditioning. As described previously,[9] we selected a counterbalanced protocol in order to nullify each mouse's initial compartment preference.

On day 1, the mice ($n = 15{\sim}16$ per group) were allowed to freely explore the two compartments for 15 min. On day 2, again the mice were allowed to explore the two compartments freely for 15 min, and the time spent in each compartment and the number of transitions between compartments were measured. Then, conditioning sessions were conducted once daily for 4 consecutive days (days 5–8). Mice were intraperitoneally (i.p.) injected with METH (2 mg/kg) and immediately confined to the black or white compartment for 50 min on day 5. On day 6, the mice were injected with saline and immediately confined to the opposite compartment for 50 min. On days 7 and 8, the same conditioning as on days 5 and 6 was repeated. Fluoxetine (20 mg/kg i.p.) or saline was injected 60 min before METH or saline treatment. On day 9, the mice were pretreated with saline or fluoxetine (20 mg/kg). Sixty minutes later, the mice were allowed to freely explore the two compartments for 15 min without METH injection, and the time spent in each compartment and the number of transitions between compartments were measured (see FIG. 1 for a diagram of the experimental design). The CPP score was designated as the time spent

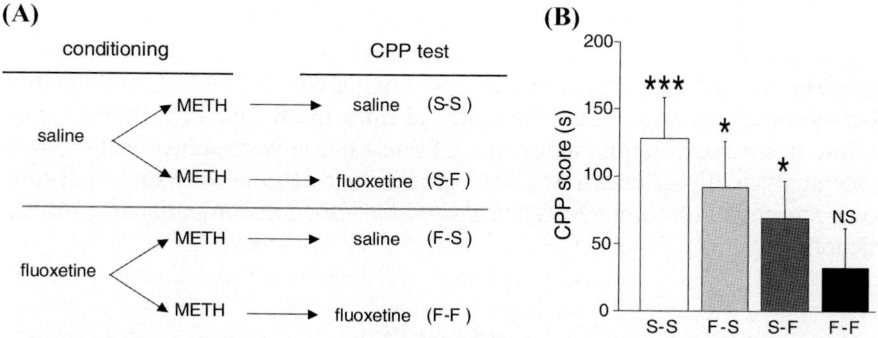

FIGURE 1. **(A)** Depiction of the experimental design. Four mouse groups were treated with saline or fluoxetine during the conditioning phase and the CPP test phase. **(B)** Abolishment of METH CPP by fluoxetine pretreatment. The CPP score was designated as the time spent in the METH-paired compartment minus the time in the same compartment in the preconditioning phase. There was significant CPP in the S-S, F-S, and S-F groups, but not when fluoxetine was administered before both the conditioning phase and the CPP test phase (F-F) (within-group paired *t*-tests, $^{***}P < 0.001$, $^{*}P < 0.05$, NS: not significant [$P > 0.05$]). The CPP scores were expressed as means ± the standard error of the mean (SEM).

in the METH-paired compartment on day 9 minus the time spent in the same compartment in the preconditioning phase on day 2.

Locomotor Activity

METH-induced locomotor activity was examined in mice ($n = 15{\sim}16$ per group) injected with METH (1 mg/kg i.p.) seven times every other day, for a total of seven injections over 13 consecutive days. Mice were placed at the center of the test chamber (250 mm in diameter and 270 mm in height; Muromachi Kikai Co., Tokyo, Japan) and allowed to freely explore the chamber for 120 min. Then, fluoxetine (20 mg/kg) or saline was injected i.p. and the mice were placed in the locomotor activity chamber immediately afterwards. Sixty minutes later, METH was injected i.p. and locomotor activity was assessed for 60 min after the METH administration by using an infrared activity monitor.

Drugs

Methamphetamine hydrochloride was purchased from Dainippon Pharmaceutical (Osaka, Japan), and fluoxetine hydrochloride was purchased from Sigma (St. Louis, MO, USA). All drugs were dissolved in saline. Drugs and vehicle were administered (i.p.) in a volume of 0.1 mL/10 g of body weight.

Statistical Analyses

For the CPP data, the time that the mice spent in the METH-paired compartment before and after conditioning were compared with within-group paired *t*-tests for each group. The CPP scores of mice pretreated with fluoxetine or saline in the conditioning phase and CPP test phase were subjected to a two-way analysis of variance (ANOVA). Locomotor activity was subjected to a two-way mixed-design ANOVA followed by *post hoc* comparisons with the Scheffe test.

RESULTS

Effects of Fluoxetine on the METH CPP

Mice pretreated with saline in the conditioning phase and the CPP test phase (S-S) spent significantly longer time in the METH-paired compartment after conditioning than before conditioning ($df = 14$, $t = -4.262$, $P = 0.0008$) (FIG. 1). The mice pretreated with fluoxetine (20 mg/kg) in the conditioning phase or the CPP test phase (F-S and S-F) also showed significant METH

CPP ($df = 14, t = -2.739, P = 0.0160$; $df = 14, t = -2.400, P = 0.0309$, respectively), although the CPP scores were lower than that of S-S group. Mice pretreated with fluoxetine (20 mg/kg) in the conditioning phase and the CPP test phase (F-F) did not show METH-CPP ($df = 14, t = -1.073, P = 0.3015$). Furthermore, the two-way ANOVA revealed that fluoxetine pretreatment in the CPP test phase resulted in a trend toward a decrease of the CPP score when compared to mice treated with saline before the CPP test phase ($F_{1,56} = 3.857, P = 0.0545$). There was no statistically significant interaction between the factors fluoxetine/saline for the conditioning phase and CPP test phase ($F_{1,56} < 0.0001, P = 0.9972$). Fluoxetine pretreatment had no significant effects on number of transitions between the compartments (data not shown).

Effects of Fluoxetine on METH-Induced Locomotor Sensitization

Fluoxetine (20 mg/kg) or saline was injected 60 min before METH (1 mg/kg) administration every other day when METH was administered. We selected this fluoxetine dose because the number of transitions between compartments in the CPP test was not altered by this dose of fluoxetine, indicating no significant influence of fluoxetine itself on locomotor activity at this dose. Locomotor activity during the 60-min period immediately after METH administration was analyzed using a two-way mixed-design ANOVA (FIG. 2). The administration of METH led to sensitization to the locomotor activating effects of METH as

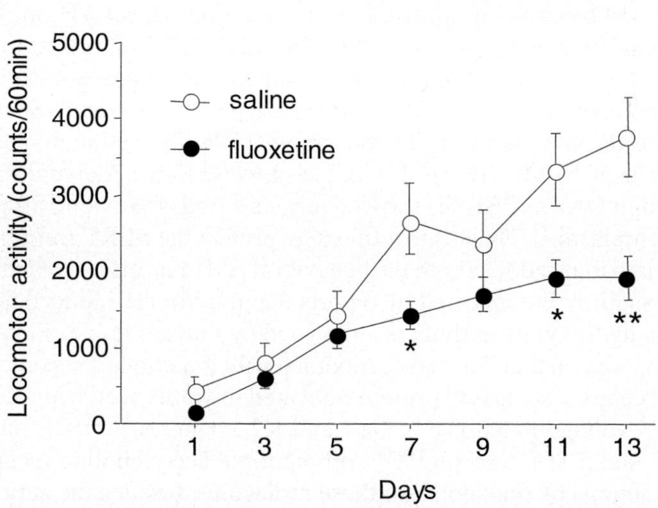

FIGURE 2. Locomotor activity after METH injection in mice pretreated with either fluoxetine or saline. Locomotor activity was measured by infrared activity counters. Locomotor activity of mice pretreated with fluoxetine was significantly lower than that of mice pretreated with saline. The locomotor activity counts were expressed as mean ± SEM $^{*}P < 0.05$, $^{**}P < 0.01$.

reflected by a main effect of Day ($F_{6,29} = 41.542$, $P < 0.0001$). Further, there was a main effect of fluoxetine indicating that fluoxetine inhibited locomotor activity ($F_{1,29} = 6.696$, $P = 0.0149$) at this test. Finally, there was also a statistically significant interaction effect reflecting the fact that pretreatment with fluoxetine had inhibitory effects on locomotor sensitization (interaction between the factor METH and the factor pretreatment; $F_{6,29} = 4.851$, $P = 0.0001$). The *post hoc* comparisons revealed that the locomotor activity of mice pretreated with fluoxetine was significantly lower than that of mice pretreated with saline on days 7, 11, and 13.

DISCUSSION

Fluoxetine abolished METH CPP and significantly reduced sensitization to the locomotor activating effects of METH in the present study. The abolishment of METH CPP by fluoxetine pretreatment suggests that fluoxetine reduces preference for contextual stimuli previously associated with METH, while the inhibition of sensitization to METH-induced locomotor activation by fluoxetine indicates that fluoxetine may be a useful tool for preventing sensitization to some of the effects of METH, such as psychosis that is often seen after repeated use of high METH doses.

There are three candidate mechanisms possibly mediating the inhibitory effects of fluoxetine on behaviors relating to METH dependence: (a) increase of basal extracellular serotonin concentration due to inhibition of SERT by fluoxetine, (b) blockade by fluoxetine of the actions of METH on SERT, and (c) actions of fluoxetine on molecules other than SERT. The first mechanism is supported by a report that inhibition of monoamine oxydase A, a major serotonin metabolizer, reduces METH-induced hyperlocomotion.[10] Secondly, the blockade of the actions of METH on the SERT by fluoxetine may reduce the toxicity induced by METH. METH induces reverse flow of dopamine and serotonin through DAT and SERT, respectively, and leads to toxicity after entering into the cytoplasm.[11] Thus, fluoxetine may protect the SERT from the actions of METH and thus reduces both the behavioral and toxic effects of METH. This second possibility is supported by reports that the METH-induced decrease in tryptophan hydroxylase activity is attenuated by fluoxetine.[12,13] Finally, recent studies have shown that fluoxetine modulates the function of several ion channels and receptors, such as G protein-activated inwardly rectifying K^+ (GIRK) channels,[14] voltage-gated Ca^{2+}, Na^+ and K^+ channels,[15–21] Cl^- channels,[22] 5-HT2C[23] and 5-HT3 receptors,[24] and nicotinic acetylcholine receptors.[25,26] Thus, the actions of fluoxetine on these molecules, besides the actions on the SERT, may mediate the inhibitory effects of fluoxetine on METH dependence. Reduced cocaine self-administration in mice lacking the GIRK2 or GIRK3 subunit[27] supports this third possibility that fluoxetine inhibits METH dependence through inhibition of the GIRK channels.

In conclusion, we found that fluoxetine, a widely used medication for depression, inhibited both METH CPP and sensitization to METH-induced locomotor activation in mice. Although further preclinical studies are needed to elucidate the mechanisms underlying these inhibitory effects of fluoxetine on processed relating to METH dependence, it appears worthwhile to investigate the clinical effects of fluoxetine on METH abuse.

ACKNOWLEDGMENTS

We are grateful to Dr. Keiko Matsuoka for animal care, and Kazuya Tawara and Akira Sato for technical assistance. This work was supported by a research grant (17025054) from the MEXT of Japan, and by grants (H17-pharmaco-001, H16-iyaku-029, H15-kou-3–03) from the MHLW of Japan. AM was supported by a USA National Institute on Drug Abuse grant (R01 DA11946).

REFERENCES

1. United Nations Office for Drug Control and Crime Prevention Ed. 2005. World Drug Report 2005. Oxford University Press. New York, NY.
2. Ujike, H. 2002. Stimulant-induced psychosis and schizophrenia: the role of sensitization. Curr. Psychiatry Rep. **4:** 177–184.
3. National Institute on Drug Abuse (NIDA) Ed. 2002. Research Report Series: Methamphetamine Abuse and Addiction. National Institutes of Health. Maryland, MA.
4. Sora, I. *et al.* 1998. Cocaine reward models: conditioned place preference can be established in dopamine- and in serotonin-transporter knockout mice. Proc. Natl. Acad. Sci. USA **95:** 7699–7704.
5. Rocha, B.A. *et al.* 1998. Cocaine self-administration in dopamine-transporter knockout mice. Nat. Neurosci. **1:** 132–137.
6. Sora, I. *et al.* 2001. Molecular mechanisms of cocaine reward: combined dopamine and serotonin transporter knockouts eliminate cocaine place preference. Proc. Natl. Acad. Sci. USA **98:** 5300–5305.
7. Shen, H.-W. *et al.* 2004. Regional differences in extracellular dopamine and serotonin assessed by in vivo microdialysis in mice lacking dopamine and/or serotonin transporters. Neuropsychopharmacology **29:** 1790–1799.
8. Hoffman, D.C. & R.J. Beninger. 1989. Preferential stimulation of D1 or D2 receptors disrupts food-rewarded operant responding in rats. Pharmacol. Biochem. Behav. **34:** 923–925.
9. Ide, S. *et al.* 2004. Buprenorphine antinociception is abolished, but naloxone-sensitive reward is retained, in mu-opioid receptor knockout mice. Neuropsychopharmacology **29:** 1656–1663.
10. Kitanaka, N. *et al.* 2005. Inhibition of methamphetamine-induced hyperlocomotion in mice by clorgyline, a monoamine oxidase-A inhibitor, through alteration of the 5-hydroxytriptamine turnover in the striatum. Neuroscience **130:** 295–308.
11. Sulzer, D. *et al.* 1995. Amphetamine redistributes dopamine from synaptic vesicles to the cytosol and promotes reverse transport. J. Neurosci. **15:** 4102–4108.

12. HOTCHKISS, A.J. & J.W. GIBB. 1980. Long-term effects of multiple doses of methamphetamine on tryptophan hydroxylase and tyrosine hydroxylase activity in rat brain. J. Pharmacol. Exp. Ther. **214:** 257–262.
13. FLECKENSTEIN, A.E. *et al.* 1997. Methamphetamine-induced decrease in tryptophan hydroxylase activity: role of 5-hydroxytryptaminergic transporters. Eur. J. Pharmacol. **324:** 179–186.
14. KOBAYASHI, T. *et al.* 2003. Inhibition of G protein-activated inwardly rectifying K^+ channels by fluoxetine (Prozac). Br. J. Pharmacol. **138:** 1119–1128.
15. PANCRAZIO, J.J. *et al.* 1998. Inhibition of neuronal Na^+ channels by antidepressant drugs. J. Pharmacol. Exp. Ther. **284:** 208–214.
16. CHOI, J.-S. *et al.* 1999. Mechanism of fluoxetine block of cloned voltage-activated potassium channel Kv1.3. J. Pharmacol. Exp. Ther. **291:** 1–6.
17. YEUNG, S.Y. *et al.* 1999. Inhibition of neuronal KV potassium currents by the antidepressant drug, fluoxetine. Br. J. Pharmacol. **128:** 1609–1615.
18. DEÁK, F.B. *et al.* 2000. Inhibition of voltage-gated calcium channels by fluoxetine in rat hippocampal pyramidal cells. Neuropharmacology **39:** 1029–1036.
19. CHOI, B.H. *et al.* 2001. Effects of norfluoxetine, the major metabolite of fluoxetine, on the cloned neuronal potassium channel Kv3.1. Neuropharmacology **41:** 443–453.
20. PERCHENET, L. *et al.* 2001. Effects of anorexinogen agents on cloned voltage-gated K^+ channel hKv1.5. J. Pharmacol. Exp. Ther. **298:** 1108–1119.
21. THOMAS, D. *et al.* 2002. The antidepressant drug fluoxetine is an inhibitor of human ether-a-go-go-related gene (HERG) potassium channels. J. Pharmacol. Exp. Ther. **300:** 543–548.
22. MAERTENS, C. *et al.* 1999. Block by fluoxetine of volume-regulated anion channels. Br. J. Pharmacol. **126:** 508–514.
23. NI, Y.G. & R. MILEDI. 1997. Blockage of 5HT2C serotonin receptors by fluoxetine (Prozac). Proc. Natl. Acad. Sci. USA **94:** 2036–2040.
24. FAN, P. 1994. Effects of antidepressants on the inward current mediated by 5-HT3 receptors in rat nodose ganglion neurones. Br. J. Pharmacol. **112:** 741–744.
25. GARCÍA-COLUNGA *et al.* 1997. Blockage of muscle and neuronal nicotinic acetylcholine receptors by fluoxetine (Prozac). Proc. Natl. Acad. Sci. USA **94:** 2041–2044.
26. MAGGI, L. *et al.* 1998. Effects of fluoxetine on wild and mutant neuronal alpha 7 nicotinic receptors. Mol. Psychiatry **3:** 350–355.
27. MORGAN, A.D. *et al.* 2003. Decreased cocaine self-administration in Kir3 potassium channel subunit knockout mice. Neuropsychopharmacology **28:** 932–938.

Links between Nutrition, Drug Abuse, and the Metabolic Syndrome

ASHRAF VIRMANI,[a] ZBIGNIEW BINIENDA,[b] SYED ALI,[c] AND FRANCO GAETANI[a]

[a]*Research and Development, Sigma tau-HealthScience, Pomezia 00040, Italy*

[b]*Neurophysiology Laboratory, Division of Neurotoxicology, National Center for Toxicological Research, Food and Drug Administration, Jefferson, Arkansas 72079, USA*

[c]*Neurochemistry Laboratory, Division of Neurotoxicology, National Center for Toxicological Research, Food and Drug Administration, Jefferson, Arkansas 72079, USA*

ABSTRACT: Nutritional deficiency in combination with drug abuse may increase risk of developing the metabolic syndrome by augmenting cell damage, excitotoxicity, reducing energy production, and lowering the antioxidant potential of the cells. We have reviewed here the following points: effects of drugs of abuse on nutrition and brain metabolism; effects of nutrition on actions of the drugs of abuse; drug abuse and probability of developing metabolic syndrome; role of genetic vulnerability in nutrition/drug abuse and brain damage; and the role of neuroprotective supplements in drug abuse. Nutrition education is an essential component of substance abuse treatment programs and can enhance substance abuse treatment outcomes. The strategies available, in particular the nutritional approach to protect the drug abusers from the metabolic syndrome and other diseases are discussed.

KEYWORDS: nutrition; drug abuse; metabolic syndrome; L-carnitine; acetyl-L-carnitine; creatine; selenium; cocaine; ecstasy; methamphetamine; alcohol; brain; liver; metabolic compromise; metabolic modifier; glycolysis; free radicals; reactive oxygen species (ROS); vitamins; minerals; zinc; thiamine; supplements; diabetes; metabolic compensation

INTRODUCTION

The role of nutrition as a risk factor during drug abuse in provoking disease pathogenesis, e.g., alcohol abuse associated with liver injury, is well known. Nutritional deficiency may increase potential for cell damage by augmenting

Address for correspondence: Dr. Ashraf Virmani, Sigma tau-HealthScience, Via Treviso 4, Pomezia, 00040, Italy. Voice: + 39-06-916-19721; fax: + 39-06-916-12631.
e-mail: ashraf.virmani@st-hs.it

**Ann. N.Y. Acad. Sci. 1074: 303–314 (2006). © 2006 New York Academy of Sciences.
doi: 10.1196/annals.1369.027**

excitotoxicity, reducing energy production, and lowering the antioxidant potential of the cells. One of the risk factors for brain developmental disorders is nutritional deficiency.[1] Role of nutrition in drug abuse is well studied for alcohol abuse but not for other drugs of abuse.

Alcohol abuse is generally associated with steatohepatitis but already in the early 1980s it was recognized that there was a population subgroup that developed this condition despite not using alcohol (non-alcoholic steatohepatitis).[2–4] This subgroup typically suffered from insulin resistance syndrome, synonymous with the metabolic syndrome (syndrome X, dysmetabolic syndrome), which is characterized by obesity, diabetes, hyperlipidemia, and hypertension.[5] The triggers of the non-alcoholic steatohepatitis include drugs, such as tamoxifen, and certain industrial toxins together with steatosis associated with inflammation, fibrosis, or necrosis. It is the interactions of nutritional abnormalities, cytokines, oxidative stress, and mitochondrial dysfunction that may underlie the induction of steatohepatitis, both alcoholic and non-alcoholic in origin.[2]

Although designer drugs, such as the amphetamine and its analogs, are popular and considered safe by the abusers, a variety of adverse effects have been associated with their use, such as the serotonin syndrome, hepatotoxicity, neurotoxicity, and psychopathology.[6] In this article, we examine the possibility that there is an increased probability of developing the metabolic syndrome in drug-abuse subjects. Treatment with antipsychotics has been associated with increased risk of developing diabetes and ketoacidosis.[7–9]

The role of nutrition together with other risk factors such as level of education, poverty, heredity, and environmental factors must be taken into account in assessing whether a drug abuser will develop the metabolic syndrome. The strategies available, in particular, the nutritional approach to protect the drug abusers from the metabolic syndrome and other diseases are discussed.

Effects of Drug Abuse on Nutrition

Abused drugs have adverse effects on the mind and on the body itself. They weaken the immune system and affect nutrition.[10] The effects on nutrition are related to behavioral changes as well as direct effects on the energy balance-related signaling systems. Alcohol-and drug-dependent subjects have distorted eating behavior that predisposes them to eating disorders (anorexia, bulimia, obesity, habitual eating). Many alcoholics are malnourished since alcohol and its metabolism prevents the body from properly absorbing, digesting, and using those nutrients. These nutritional deficiencies are not as well studied in other types of drug abuse. Drug addicts suffer from calorie and protein malnutrition with over 90% being underweight[11] and 74% of them showing clinical signs of nutrient deficiency with significantly lower hemoglobin and serum total protein levels.[12]

Effects of Drug of Abuse on Brain Metabolism

Drugs of abuse affect brain activity mainly at the level of neurotransmitter signaling and concomitantly brain metabolism in specific regions. Brain energy requirements and in particular glucose metabolism is affected. Metabolism of amino acids and fatty acids may be affected as well. Many of the studies have used positron emission tomography (PET) and an analog of glucose, 2-deoxy-2-[18F]fluoro-D-glucose, to measure regional brain glucose metabolism during drug abuse. These studies show that each drug has its own pattern of brain stimulation, inducing therefore, unique changes in brain metabolism.[13] Thus, psilocybin (hallucinogen) increases cerebral glucose metabolism in distinct right hemispheric frontotemporal cortical regions and decreases it in the thalamus.[14] The widely abused drugs like the analog of "ecstasy," 3,4-methylenedioxyethamphetamine (MDE) and methamphetamine (METH) induce cortical hypometabolism and cerebellar hypermetabolism.[14,15] Abuse of "ecstasy" (3,4-methylenedioxymethamphetamine or MDMA) reduces glucose metabolism globally in the brain but mainly in the striatum.[16] Drugs of abuse cause metabolic changes even in healthy volunteers, for example MDE significantly decreased glucose metabolism in the frontal cortex and increased it in the cerebellum and the right putamen.[17] The action of cocaine on brain is associated with metabolic changes in the prefrontal cortex.[18]

Many studies have also examined the scenario underlying these metabolic changes, such as the neurotransmission changes, i.e., dopamine and other neurotransmitters, as well as associated receptors, transporters, and enzymes.[13] Drug abusers have abnormalities in brain regions implicated in mood disorders. It is interesting to note that in METH users, PET scans of brain metabolic activity have shown that the glucose metabolism is lower in brain regions linked to depressive disorders, depressed mood, and sadness, but higher in brain regions linked to anxiety and drug cravings.[19] Chronic cocaine administration to rats results in upregulation of cytochrome *c* oxidase and therefore metabolic activity in brain reward regions such as the nucleus accumbens.[20] In the case of alcohol abuse, it has been shown by PET studies that the abuse of alcohol produces a global brain depression and that the long-term effects of alcohol abuse require several weeks of abstinence to subside.

Effect of Nutrition on Actions of the Drugs of Abuse

Several environmental factors including the individual's feeding habits will affect the reaction to the abused drug. Studies have shown that chronic food restriction increases the systemic self-administration and locomotor-stimulating effect of abused drugs (FIG. 1).[21] These nutritional effects via metabolic changes are transformed into behavioral changes and may reflect enhanced rewarding potency or a central nervous system (CNS)-based modulatory process. Differences in the amounts of macronutrients in the diet also cause different

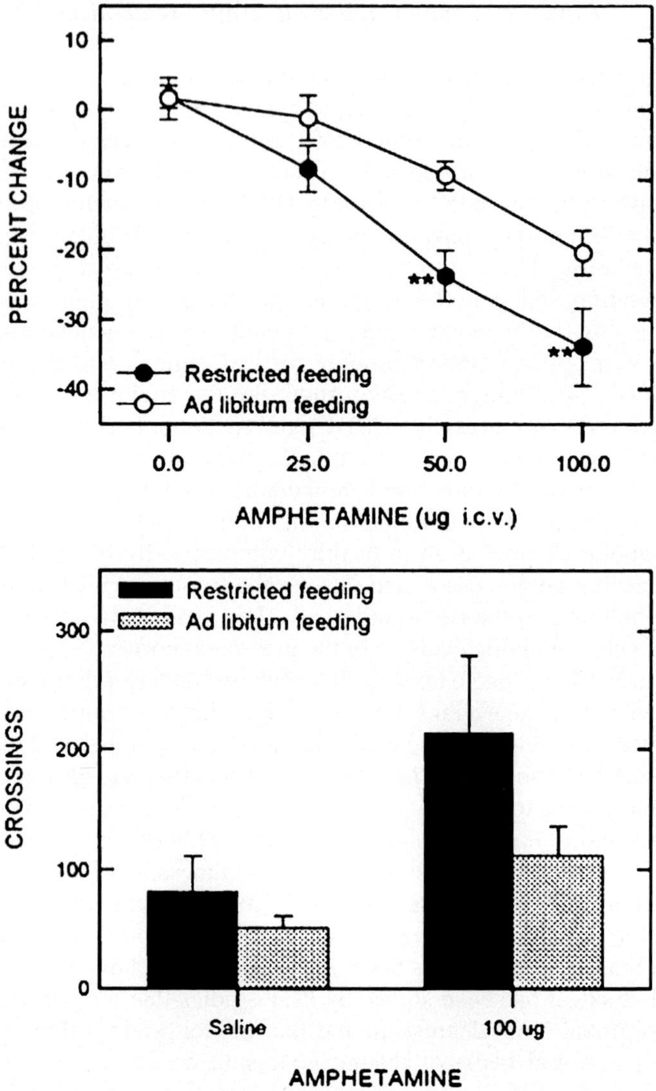

FIGURE 1. Chronic food restriction increases the systemic self-administration and locomotor-stimulating effect of amphetamine. *Top*: percentage of change in reward threshold as a function of D-amphetamine dose for food-restricted (*filled circles*) and *ad libitum* fed (*open circles*) rats. Reward thresholds were derived from lateral hypothalamic self-stimulation (LHSS) rate-frequency curves obtained immediately before and 5 min after intracerebroventricular injection of D-amphetamine. Mean ± SEM. *Bottom*: number of crossings in a shuttle box during two 30 min tests: (*a*) 5 min after intracerebroventricular injection of saline, and (*b*) 5 min after intracerebroventricular injection of 100.0 μg of D-amphetamine. Mean ± SEM. (Reprinted from Cabeza de Vaca and Carr[21] with permission from *The Journal of Neuroscience.*)

TABLE 1. Nutritional deficiency may affect cellular defenses and increase susceptibility to the metabolic syndrome during drug abuse via following pathways

- Decreased energy production
- Decreased cellular antioxidant potential
- Increased excitotoxicity
- Increased genetic susceptibility
- Reduced insulin sensitivity
- Increased susceptibility to inflammation/fibrosis
- Other?

behavioral outcomes. For instance, after cocaine withdrawal, rats were more immobile if fed a high-fat diet and were less immobile if fed a high-protein or high-carbohydrate diet.[22]

Drug Abuse May Increase Probability of Developing Metabolic Syndrome

The metabolic syndrome represents a cluster of interrelated risk factors that identify individuals at increased risk for the development of type-2 diabetes mellitus and cardiovascular events.[23] The metabolic syndrome is triggered by initial imbalances at the cellular level in various metabolic pathways (TABLE 1). These initially small metabolic imbalances cascade with time and lead to the larger problems in body functions and finally to what has been termed the *metabolic syndrome* and is generally characterized by hyperinsulinemia (impaired glucose metabolism), obesity, dyslipidemia, and hypertension.

Are drug abusers at higher risk of metabolic syndrome? The problem as to whether drug abuse is a risk factor for developing the metabolic syndrome has not been well studied but there are some indications that would suggest that drug abuse is linked with the metabolic syndrome.

First, drug-abusing patients have higher rates of diabetes complications. A study in the United Kingdom indicated that street drug use in young adults with diabetes may contribute to poor glycemic control and serious complications of diabetes.[24] The metabolic disturbances such as diabetic ketoacidosis and poor glycemic control may be further exacerbated by MDMA abuse during prolonged exercise.[25]

Second, substance abuse is a significant contributing factor for treatment non-compliance in diabetes and other diseases. A significant number of adults admitted to hospital with diabetic ketoacidosis were found to use cocaine use. Further, these individuals were associated with more frequent omission of insulin therapy in the absence of precipitating systemic illness.[26] In another study, adolescents with diabetes who reported alcohol and drug use or who reported they live in an environment of substance abuse had poorer diabetes control than patients who did not.[27]

Although more studies are needed in this area, it appears that drug abuse is indeed a risk factor for metabolic syndrome. Thus, as part of the strategy aimed at the prevention of drug abuse by drug-naïve adolescents and young adults, the detrimental effects on health and risk of developing metabolic syndrome should also be pointed out. For those drug abusers attempting abstinence and recovery from their addictions, a special treatment strategy to prevent the metabolic syndrome is advisable, possibly focusing on aerobic exercise, weight loss, and adequate nutrition with the right supplements (as discussed below). To tackle the insulin resistance, treatment with insulin sensitizers, such as metformin and thiazolidinediones, may improve both metabolic and hormonal patterns.[28] Stopping drug abuse early and following such a broad approach may delay or prevent the development of the metabolic syndrome.

Role of Genetic Vulnerability in Nutrition/Drug Abuse and Brain Damage

Another risk factor that must be mentioned here is the role of genetic susceptibility, especially in combination with nutrition and drug abuse in the development of the metabolic syndrome. Genetic polymorphism in individuals may contribute in a positive or negative manner depending on the circumstances. From affecting the drug metabolizing enzyme activities, to transport and excretion up to the level of the individual's behavior, the genetic influence should be considerable on the overall effects to the abused drug response/toxicity.[29,30] The presence or absence of certain alleles in the subjects, or the presence of defective alleles, will change drastically the behavior of that subject to the effects of drug abuse. The actual efficacy/toxicity will be affected, for example, by the rate of metabolism of the drug caused by multiple genes or by induction of gene expression.

The individual's susceptibility may already be affected even earlier by the imprinted genes which play key roles in controlling feto–placental nutrient supply and demand and their epigenetic liability in response to nutrients.[31] The maternal nutritional imbalance and resulting metabolic disturbances during critical phases of development may predispose the offspring to the adverse effects of drug abuse and development of the metabolic syndrome and may even be transmitted to the next generation.

Alcohol dependence is associated with specific genetic markers.[32] Chronic alcohol abuse causes well localized damage in the brain, mainly in the superior frontal cortex. The study conducted by Dodd and collaborators in alcoholic versus non-alcoholic subjects, revealed that alcohol dehydrogenase (ADH)3 genotype interacted significantly with NMDA receptor efficacy and affinity in a region-specific manner. Furthermore, the EAAT2 genotype was associated with local $GABA_A$ receptor β subunit mRNA expression, and GABB2 and DRD2B genotypes. They, therefore, concluded that the genotype modulated amino acid transmission locally and influenced neuronal vulnerability.[29]

Role of Neuroprotective Supplements in Drug Abuse

Alcohol abuse is linked with marked steatosis and liver injury, and malnutrition is common associated with vitamin (B1, B2, B6, B12, C, K, A, and D) and mineral deficiencies (selenium, zinc, magnesium, iron, and phosphorus). Many alcoholics suffer from a deficiency of zinc which is necessary for the body to manufacture the enzymes essential for the detoxification of alcohol.[33,34] But the most important and common deficiency in alcoholics is in the B vitamins. Thiamine (B1) deficiency in alcoholics causes neurological damage leading to Wernicke–Korsakoff syndrome.[35] Antioxidants have been proposed to counteract liver damage and vitamin E may decrease damage in cirrhotic livers,[36] but another study reported that vitamin E supplementation (500 IU per day) for 1 year did not influence liver function, survival, or hospitalization rates in people with alcoholic cirrhosis.[37] This could be related to differences in ingested doses, bioavailability, and the ability of the liver to accumulate the various antioxidant compounds.[38] On the basis of the studies reviewed, these authors suggested that lycopene-rich foods should be considered as therapeutic treatment of some liver pathologies.

The amount of alcohol that can injure the liver varies greatly from person to person as well as the gender. Alcohol seems to injure the liver by blocking the normal metabolism of protein, fats, and carbohydrates. Mechanisms involving cellular energy failure and mitochondrial dysfunction have also been implicated.[39]

There is some suggestion that alcohol in moderate amounts may infer cardioprotective effects. The "French Paradox," where diet is high in saturated fat accompanied by regular consumption of red wine is associated with such effects. However, it must be noted that it is probably the antioxidant effect of the grape polyphenols, e.g., resveratrol, found in the wine and not the actual alcohol that provide these benefits.[40] Strategies to limit the processes leading to the induction of alcoholic and non-alcoholic steatohepatitis, such as modulation of insulin resistance, normalizing lipoprotein metabolism, and down regulating inflammatory mediators, have been suggested.[3]

Compounds such as L-carnitine have been shown to protect against the alcohol toxicity. L-carnitine is a naturally occurring quaternary ammonium compound (trimethylamino-β-hydroxybutyrate) and is a vital cofactor for the mitochondrial oxidation of fatty acids, and is an endogenous compound in all mammalian species.[41] L-Carnitine exists in the body primarily in its unesterified form, but also as a number of esters (acylcarnitines) including acetyl-L-carnitine, propionyl-L-carnitine, and palmitoyl-L-carnitine. Humans take in carnitine primarily from diet 75% with the remaining 25% coming from endogenous synthesis. Supplementation with L-carnitine alleviated alcohol-induced liver damage possibly by reducing hepatic concentrations of thiobarbituric acid reactive substances, an indicator of lipid peroxidation.[42] Part of this action of L-carnitine may be related to restoration of normal transport of

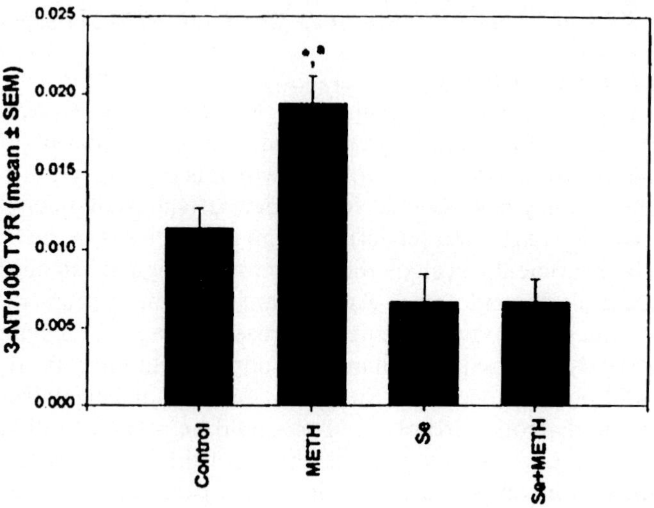

FIGURE 2. Selenium supplementation protects striatum in mouse against METH-toxicity. Effects of METH (4 × 10 mg/kg, i.p.) on 3-nitrotyrosine in the striatum of adult male C57BL/6N mice. Animals received selenium for 1 week before the first injection of METH and 1 week after the last injection of METH. Each value is mean and SEM from eight animals per group. $^*P < 0.05$ significantly different from control. $^aP < 0.05$ significantly different from Se and Se + METH groups. (Reprinted from Imam and Ali[47] with permission from Elsevier.)

fatty acids from the liver. It helps us to reduce free fatty acid load produced by ingestion of alcohol, and it also reduces elevated triglycerides and liver enzymes.[43,44] The administration of its ester, acetyl-L-carnitine has been reported to reduce cognitive deficits in chronic alcoholics.[45] A protective action of L-carnitine against METH neurotoxicity has also been found.[46]

Other supplements such as selenium also protect against METH toxicity in CNS (FIG. 2)[47] as well as against cocaine-induced myocardial oxidative stress.[48] Selenium is a well-known antioxidant that is also an essential component of several major metabolic pathways, which include not only the antioxidant defense systems but also thyroid hormone metabolism and immune function. Selenium is necessary for glutathione peroxidase action; this enzyme functions synergistically with the other antioxidants, e.g., vitamin E. Selenium deficiency has been linked to neurodegenerative and cardiovascular diseases.[49]

A number of other compounds could also be helpful against the damage induced by drug abuse. For example, creatine has been reported to have neuroprotective actions.[1,50] Creatine is a natural nutrient found in animal foods, and is commonly used as a nutritional ergogenic aid to enhance exercise performance. The creatine and its related creatine kinase enzymes are found in tissues with high-energy demand and energy production mainly muscle, where creatine readily combines with phosphate to form creatine phosphate (PCr), a high-energy phosphagen.[51] Creatine deficiency syndromes manifesting as inborn errors of metabolism have been recently described.[52] These syndromes are characterized by a lack of creatine/phosphocreatine in the brain. Clinically, most of the patients develop a variable mental retardation and a severe speech delay associated with epilepsy, extra-pyramidal syndrome, and behavior disturbances. In animal experiments, the supplementation with creatine was reported recently to protect against the dopamine depleting effects of neurotoxic doses of METH.[53] They found that rats fed with 1% creatine in normal diet had greater striatal dopamine after 1 week of METH treatment. They also found that the indices of oxidative damage were reduced in the creatine fed compared to the animals on normal diet.

CONCLUSION

Apart from the compounds mentioned above, a number of dietary antioxidants, such as coenzyme Q10, lipoic acid, resveratrol, melatonin, polyphenols (green tea, curcumin), and flavonoids (quercetin, isoflanones, and catechins), as well as other compounds, such as omega 3 fatty acids, may also be useful in drug abuse and in the prevention of the metabolic syndrome; however, further studies are necessary.

There is a delicate balance between the metabolic systems producing energy and the intrinsic cellular protective mechanisms. Drug abuse can be detrimental to that balance. This may explain the higher risk of developing the metabolic syndrome in drug abuse condition. Such a link with the metabolic syndrome has also been found for antipsychotic medicines and tobacco.[54,55]

The correction of metabolism as well as the mineral, vitamin, specific metabolic cofactors, and supplemental compounds may reinforce the balance. Nutrition education is an essential component of substance abuse treatment programs and can enhance substance abuse treatment outcome.[56]

REFERENCES

1. Virmani, A., F. Gaetani & Z., Binienda. 2005. Effects of metabolic modifiers such as carnitines, coenzyme Q10, and PUFAs against different dorms of neurotoxic insults: metabolic inhibitors, MPTP, and methamphetamine. Ann. N. Y. Acad. Sci. **1053**: 183–191.
2. McLain, C.J. *et al.* 2004. Mechanisms of non-alcoholic steatohepatitis. Alcohol **34**: 67–79.
3. Medina, J. *et al.* 2004. Approach to the pathogenesis and treatment of nonalcoholic steatohepatitis. Diabetes Care **27**: 2057–2066.
4. Hanley, A.J. *et al.* 2005. Liver markers and development of the metabolic syndrome: the insulin resistance atherosclerosis study. Diabetes **54**: 3140–3147.

5. BOEHM, B.O. & S. CLAUDI-BOEHM. 2005. The metabolic syndrome. Scand. J. Clin. Lab. Invest. Suppl. **240**: 3–13.
6. MAURER, H.H. 2004. Chemistry, pharmacology, toxicology, and hepatic metabolism of designer drugs of the amphetamine (ecstasy), piperazine, and pyrrolidinophenone types: a synopsis. Ther. Drug Monit. **26**: 127–131.
7. HENDERSON, D.C. *et al.* 2000. Clozapine, diabetes mellitus, weight gain, and lipid abnormalities: a five-year naturalistic study. Am. J. Psych. **157**: 975–981.
8. TIMAR, O., F. SESTIER & E. LEVY. 2000. Metabolic syndrome X: a review. Can. J. Cardiol. **16**: 779–789.
9. KOHEN, D. 2004. Diabetes mellitus and schizophrenia: historical perspective. Br, J. Psych. Suppl. **47**: S64–S66.
10. DANIEL, E.L. 1991. Nutritional implications in recovery from substance abuse. Empl. Assist. Q. **7**: 1–7.
11. SANTOLARIA-FERNANDEZ, F.J. *et al.* 1995. Nutritional assessment of drug addicts. Drug. Alcohol. Depend. **38**: 11–18.
12. NAZRUL ISLAM, S.K. *et al.* 2001. Serum vitamin E, C and A status of the drug addicts undergoing detoxification: influence of drug habit, sexual practice and lifestyle factors. Eur. J. Clin. Nutr. **55**: 1022–1027.
13. VOLKOW, N.D., J.S. FOWLER & G.J. WANG. 2003. The addicted human brain: insights from imaging studies. J. Clin. Invest. **111**: 1444–1451.
14. GOUZOULIS-MAYFRANK, *et al.* 1999. Neurometabolic effects of psilocybin, 3,4-methylenedioxyethylamphetamine (MDE) and D-methamphetamine in healthy volunteers: a double-blind, placebo-controlled PET study with [18F]FDG. Neuropsychopharmacology **20**: 565–581.
15. VOLLENWEIDER, F.X. *et al.* 1997. Positron emission tomography and fluorodeoxyglucose studies of metabolic hyperfrontality and psychopathology in the psilocybin model of psychosis. Neuropsychopharmacology **16**: 357–372.
16. BUCHERT, R. *et al.* 2001. Long-term effects of 'ecstasy' abuse on the human brain studied by FDG PET. Nucl. Med. Commun. **22**: 889–897.
17. SCHRECKENBERGER, M. *et al.* 1998. Investigations on the effect of "ecstasy" on cerebral glucose metabolism: an 18-FDG PET study. Nuklearmedizin **37**: 262–267.
18. GOLDSTEIN, R.Z. *et al.* 2004. Severity of neuropsychological impairment in cocaine and alcohol addiction: association with metabolism in the prefrontal cortex. Neuropsychologia **42**: 1447–1458.
19. LONDON, E.D. *et al.* 2004. Mood disturbances and regional cerebral metabolic abnormalities in recently abstinent methamphetamine abusers. Arch. Gen. Psych. **61**: 73–84.
20. WALKER, J.R. & K.A. SEVARINO. 1995. Regulation of cytochrome *c* oxidase subunit mRNA and enzyme activity in rat brain reward regions during withdrawal from chronic cocaine. J. Neurochem. **64**: 497–502.
21. CABEZA DE VACA, S. & K.D. CARR. 1998. Food restriction enhances the central rewarding effect of abused drugs. J. Neurosci. **15**: 7502–7510.
22. LOEBENS, M. & H.M. BARROS. 2003. Diet influences cocaine withdrawal behaviors in the forced swimming test. Pharmacol. Biochem. Behav. **74**: 259–267.
23. LOVE, A. & D. OLDFORD. 2005. Metabolic syndrome. Can. J. Cardiovasc. Nurs. **15**: 6–8.
24. NG, R.S., D.A. DARKO & R.M. HILLSON. 2004. Street drug use among young patients with type 1 diabetes in the UK. Diabetes Med. **21**: 295–296.

25. Seymour, H.R., D. Gilman & J.D. Quin. 1996. Severe ketoacidosis complicated by 'ecstasy' ingestion and prolonged exercise. Diabetes Med. **13**: 908–909.
26. Warner, E.A. *et al.* 1998. Diabetic ketoacidosis associated with cocaine use. Arch. Intern Med. **158**: 1799–1802.
27. Glasgow, A.M. *et al.* 1991. Alcohol and drug use in teenagers with diabetes mellitus. J. Adolesc. Health **12**: 11–14.
28. Fowler, S.B., M. Moussouttas & B. Mancini. 2005. Metabolic syndrome: contributing factors and treatment strategies. J. Neurosci. Nurs. **37**: 220–223.
29. Dodd, P.R. *et al.* 2004. Genes and gene expression in the brain of the alcoholic. Addict Behav. **29**: 1295–1309.
30. Kreek, M.J. *et al.* 2005. Genetic influences on impulsivity, risk taking, stress responsivity and vulnerability to drug abuse and addiction. Nat. Neurosci. **8**: 1450–1457.
31. Gallou-Kabani, C. & C. Junien. 2005. Nutritional epigenomics of metabolic syndrome: new perspective against the epidemic. Diabetes **54**: 1899–1906.
32. Lewohl, J.M. *et al.* 2005. Expression of MBP, PLP, MAG, CNP, and GFAP in the human alcoholic brain. Alcohol Clin. Exp. Res. **29**: 1698–1705.
33. Scholmerich, J. *et al.* 1983. Zinc and vitamin A deficiency in liver cirrhosis. Hepatogastroenterology **30**: 119–125.
34. Taniguchi, S., K. Kaneto & T. Hamada. 1995. Acquired zinc deficiency associated with alcoholic liver cirrhosis. Int. J. Dermatol. **34**: 651–652.
35. Thomson, A.D. 2000. Mechanisms of vitamin deficiency in chronic alcohol misusers and the development of the Wernicke–Korsakoff syndrome. Alcohol Alcohol. Suppl. **35**: 2–7.
36. Ferro, D. *et al.* 1999. Vitamin E reduces monocyte tissue factor expression in cirrhotic patients. Blood **93**: 2945–2950.
37. de la Maza, M.P. *et al.* 1995. Effects of long-term vitamin E supplementation in alcoholic cirrhotics. J. Am. Coll. Nutr. **14**: 192–196.
38. Vitaglione, P. *et al.* 2004. Dietary antioxidant compounds and liver health. Crit. Rev. Food Sci. Nutr. **44**: 575–586.
39. Desjardins, P. & R.F. Butterworth. 2005. Role of mitochondrial dysfunction and oxidative stress in the pathogenesis of selective neuronal loss in Wernicke's encephalopathy. Mol. Neurobiol. **31**: 17–26.
40. Zern, T.L. & M.L. Fernandez. 2005. Cardioprotective effects of dietary polyphenols. J. Nutr. **135**: 2291–2294.
41. Virmani, A. & Z. Binienda. 2004. Role of carnitine esters in brain neuropathology. Mol. Aspects Med. **25**: 533–549.
42. Bykov, I., H. Jarvelainen & K. Lindros. 2003. L-carnitine alleviates alcohol-induced liver damage in rats: role of tumor necrosis factor-alpha. Alcohol Alcohol. **38**: 400–406.
43. Sachan, D.L., T.H. Rhew & R.A. Ruark. 1984. Ameliorating effects of carnitine and its precursors on alcohol-induced fatty liver. Am. J. Clin. Nutr. **39**: 738–744.
44. Dayanandan, A., P. Kumar & C. Panneerselvam. 2001. Protective role of L-carnitine on liver and heart lipid peroxidation in atherosclerotic rats. J. Nutr. Biochem **12**: 254–257.
45. Tempesta, E. *et al.* 1990. Role of acetyl-L-carnitine in the treatment of cognitive deficit in chronic alcoholism. Int. J. Clin. Pharmacol. Res. **10**: 101–107.
46. Virmani, A. *et al.* 2002. The protective role of L-carnitine against neurotoxicity evoked by drug of abuse, methamphetamine, could be related to mitochondrial dysfunction. Ann. N. Y. Acad. Sci. **965**: 225–232.

47. IMAM, S.Z. & S.F. ALI. 2000. Selenium, an antioxidant, attenuates methamphetamine-induced dopaminergic toxicity and peroxynitrite generation. Brain Res. **855**: 186–191.
48. KIM, H. *et al.* 2000. Selenium deficiency potentiates methamphetamine-induced nigral neuronal loss: comparison with MPTP model. Brain Res. **17**: 247–252.
49. BRENNEISEN, P. *et al.* 2005. Selenium, oxidative stress, and health aspects. Mol. Aspects Med. **26**: 256–267.
50. BEAL, M.F. 2003. Bioenergetic approaches for neuroprotection in Parkinson's disease. Ann. Neurol. **53**: S39–47.
51. MCLEISH, M. & G. KENYON. 2005. Relating structure to mechanism in creatine kinase. Crit. Rev. Biochem. Mol. Biol. **40**: 1–20.
52. CHEILLAN, D. *et al.* 2005. Creatine deficiency syndromes. Rev. Neurol. (Paris) **161**: 284–289.
53. CASS, W.A., M.P. SMITH & L.E. PETERS. 2005. Protection against the dopamine depleting effects of neurotoxic doses of methamphetamine. ISN/ESN Satellite Meeting, Abst. # 11: 39.
54. CITROME, L. *et al.* 2005. Metabolic issues in patients with severe mental illness. South Med. J. **98**: 714–720.
55. WEITZMAN, M. *et al.* 2005. Tobacco smoke exposure is associated with the metabolic syndrome in adolescents. Circulation **112**: 862–869.
56. GRANT, L.P., B. HAUGHTON & D.S. SACHAN. 2004. Nutrition education is positively associated with substance abuse treatment program outcomes. J. Am. Diet. Assoc. **104**: 604–610.

Inclusion Dynamics in PC12 is Comparable Between Amphetamines and MPTP

MARCO GESI,[a] GLORIA LAZZERI,[a] MICHELA FERRUCCI,[a] ANTONIO PELLEGRINI,[a] PAOLA LENZI,[a] STEFANO RUGGIERI,[b] FRANCESCO FORNAI,[a,b] AND ANTONIO PAPARELLI[a]

[a] *Department of Human Morphology and Applied Biology, University of Pisa, I-56126 Pisa, Italy*

[b] *Laboratory of Neurobiology of the Movement Disorders, I.R.C.C.S. I.N.M. Neuromed, 86077 Pozzilli (IS), Italy*

ABSTRACT: In previous studies it was demonstrated that amphetamine derivatives and 1-methyl article-4-phenylpyridinium produce neuronal cell bodies. In the present work, we compared the fine ultrastructure of the intracellular inclusions induced by these different neurotoxic treatments. In particular, we compared the dynamical changes occurring when a mild toxic stimulus acts for different time intervals. For this purpose, we exposed catecholamine-synthesizing PC12 cells to different amphetamine derivatives (methamphetamine and 3,4-methylenedioxymethamphetamine), or 1-methyl-4-phenylpyridinium ion, which represents the active metabolite of the neurotoxin 1-methyl-4-phenyl-1,3,4,6-tetrahydropyridine. Despite inclusions that are elicited by different mechanisms depending on the specific neurotoxin, their ultrastructural features are similar and there is a high parallelism in their temporal evolution. This suggests that formation of inclusions is a multi-step process that might be elicited by different stimuli and, once triggered, leads to the same final effect.

KEYWORDS: amphetamine derivatives; 1,4-methylphenylpyridinium; catecholamine cells; morphological analysis

INTRODUCTION

A number of neurodegenerative diseases are characterized by the presence of intracellular inclusions that can affect distinct populations of neuronal and/or

Address for correspondence: Francesco Fornai, M.D., Department of Human Morphology and Applied Biology, University of Pisa, Via Roma, 55, I-56126 Pisa, Italy. Voice: +39-50-221-8611; fax: +39-50-221-8606.
e-mail: f.fornai@med.unipi.it

**Ann. N.Y. Acad. Sci. 1074: 315–319 (2006). © 2006 New York Academy of Sciences.
doi: 10.1196/annals.1369.028**

glial cells. Among these, Lewy bodies (LB) are neuronal inclusions originally found in the central nervous system of Parkinsonian patients,[1] and are considered a pathological hallmark of Parkinson's disease (PD).[1,2]

LB are classically described as pale eosinophilic cytoplasmic inclusions, within catecholamine neurons of various brain areas. Despite the general description, LB exhibit a large variety of morphological features, differing in size, shape, and ultrastructure, as well. This heterogeneity might depend on the brain area involved, allowing description of two types of LB, called classic and cortical.[3,4]

Despite the occurrence of a wide range of different morphological features, LB share a common immunologic profile. In fact, in the last years increasing evidence showed that LB, and other types of intracellular inclusions, contain proteins that are components or substrates of the ubiquitin–proteasome (UP) system, a multi-enzymatic proteolytic complex, which degrades mutant, misfolded, or exceeding cellular proteins.[5] In fact, recent progress in clinical and experimental studies demonstrated that impairment of the UP activity is critical to initiating the progressive accumulation of altered proteins.[6,7] Intracellular inclusions consist of dynamic structures, and this might lead to variation in their morphology.

In the present article, we investigated the fine ultrastructure of intracellular inclusions produced by various neurotoxins in rat pheochromocytome cell cultures (PC12) at different time intervals. The use of a simple cellular model allowed us to compare the morphology and maturation of these inclusions as a simple function of time.

DIFFERENT NEUROTOXIC MECHANISMS CONVERGE IN PRODUCING SIMILAR INTRACELLULAR INCLUSIONS IN A TIME-DEPENDENT MANNER

PC12 cell cultures were exposed to the following neurotoxins: amphetamine derivatives methamphetamine (METH) or 3,4-methylenedioxymethamphetamine (MDMA); and 1-methyl-4-phenylpyridinium (MPP^+), which represents the active metabolite of the neurotoxin 1-methyl-2-phenyl-1,3,4,6-tetrahydropyridine (MPTP).

The dose of each compound was established in pilot experiments in order to induce intracellular inclusions in the absence of cell death.

METH and MDMA (1 μM and 100 μM, respectively), and MPP^+ (50 μM) were diluted in the culture medium up to 168 h, whereas subgroups of cells were examined at intermediate time intervals corresponding to 4, 12, 24, and 72 h of exposure. At the end of each exposure, cell pellets were processed for plane transmission electron microscope (TEM).

Ultrastructural analysis showed that morphological features of these inclusions underwent significant changes in a time-dependent way (FIG. 1). In

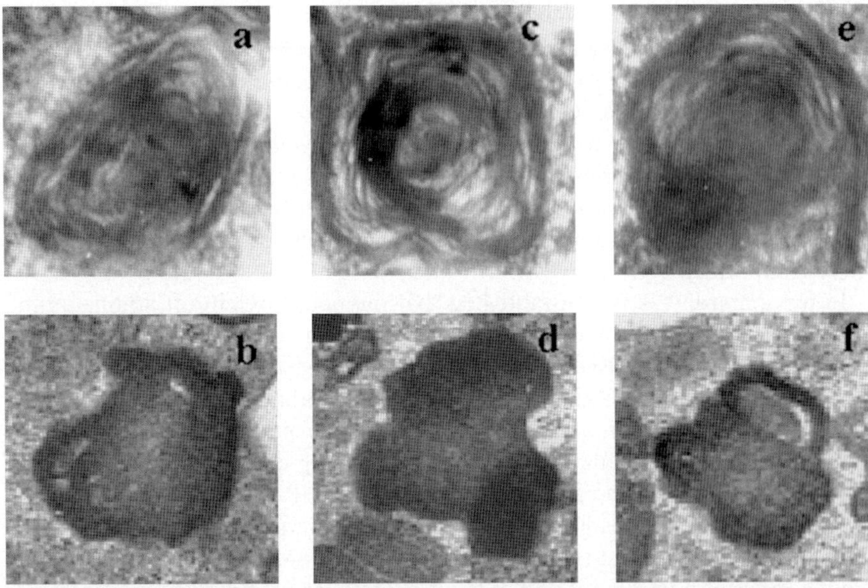

FIGURE 1. Ultrastructure of cytosolic inclusions observed in PC12 cells after exposure to different neurotoxins. Similar morphological maturation of intracellular inclusions produced by exposure of PC12 cell cultures to either **(a,b)** METH, **(c,d)** MDMA, or **(e,f)** MPP^+, and featuring as membrane-like structures at early time of exposure (**a,c,e**) which change into highly condensed and electron-dense structures after prolonged exposure (**b,d,f**). Magnification = ×16,500 (**a,c,e**); ×15,000 (**b,d,f**).

particular, we found that increasing the time of exposure produced a progressive maturation of the cellular inclusions, which from membrane-like limited structures, observed at early time of exposure, change to highly condensed structures, with an electron-dense central core, for prolonged exposure. No differences in the ultrastructural features of the inclusions were found following different neurotoxins, whereas the kinetics of inclusion formation and maturation was specific for each compound.

SUMMARY AND CONCLUSION

The present data compare for the first time at ultrastructural level the dynamical changes of intracellular inclusions induced by exposure to different neurotoxins. Analysis of the morphological features of these inclusions carried out at TEM confirmed that these inclusions are dynamic structures, which modify their shape time dependently. In particular, the morphology of the inclusions produced by exposure to amphetamine derivatives (METH or MDMA) or MPP^+ undergo a progressive maturation that was elicited by increasing the time of exposure to each compound. This consists of a fusion of the external membranes and condensation of the inner material, which we observed in early structures, leading to a progressive more electron-dense core, in which it is not possible to distinguish a defined structure.

The homogeneity of the final structures achieved by inclusions obtained following different neurotoxic treatments suggests that formation of intracellular inclusions is a multi-step process in which different initial mechanisms converge to trigger the same final biological response and thereby produce the same final effect.

In this regard, it is well established that the neurotoxicity of amphetamine derivatives and MPP^+ on dopamine (DA) cells is mediated by oxidative stress and production of reactive oxygen species (ROS),[8–11] both enhanced by endogenous DA itself.[7,8] Oxidative stress and ROS production are also involved in causing the formation of intracellular inclusions, perhaps by causing oxidative damage to the cellular proteins and producing excess amount of altered proteins that engulf the catalytic activity of the UP system.[12–14] Persistence of the toxic stimulus leads to the progressive accumulation of damaged proteins within the cell that segregate in a restricted portion of the cell volume, thereby promoting precipitation of these proteinaceous aggregates as intracellular inclusions.[8,14] In addition, inhibition of the complex I of the mitochondrial respiratory chain and the consequent decrease in ATP availability caused by MPP^+, is demonstrated as playing a seminal role in affecting the activity of the proteasome and determining the formation of cell inclusions.[15] Interestingly, the same mechanisms that can provoke cell death are able to trigger within the cell the metabolic pathways that lead to the formation of intracellular inclusions, allowing the cell to arrange a protective response against the initial insult without impairing cell viability. The ridge between the two opposite fates, death and inclusion formation, is represented by the intensity and/or the persistence of these toxic stimuli. This is a crucial aspect that we investigated in depth in previous studies, where we demonstrated that cell death may occur as a late event in the time course analysis, when a mild stimulus is allowed to act continuously.

REFERENCES

1. LEWY, F.H. 1912. In Handbuch der Neurologie. M. LEWANDOWSKY Ed.: 920–933. Springer. Berlin.
2. GREENFIELD, I.G. & F.D. BOSANQUET. 1953. The brain-stem lesions in Parkinsonism. J. Neurol. Neurosurg. Psychiatry **16:** 213–226.
3. OHAMA, E. & F. IKUTA. 1976. Parkinson's disease: distribution of Lewy bodies and monoamine neuron system. Acta Neuropathol. (Berl.) **34:** 311–319.
4. ZWEIG, R.M. *et al.* 1989. Linkage to the Huntington's disease locus in a family with unusual clinical and pathological features. Ann. Neurol. **26:** 78–84.

5. CIECHANOVER, A. 1998. The ubiquitin-proteasome pathway: on protein death and cell life. EMBO J. **17:** 7151–7160.
6. MCNAUGHT, K.S. & P. JENNER. 2001. Proteasomal function is impaired in substantia nigra in Parkinson's disease. Neurosci. Lett. **297:** 191–194.
7. FORNAI, F. *et al.* 2003. Fine structure and biochemical mechanisms underlying nigrostriatal inclusions and cell death after proteasome inhibition. J. Neurosci. **23:** 8955–8966.
8. FORNAI, F. *et al.* 2004. Methamphetamine produces neuronal inclusions in the nigrostriatal system and in PC12 cells. J. Neurochem. **88:** 114–123.
9. LANGSTON, J.W. & P. BALLARD. 1984. Parkinsonism induced by 1-methyl-4-phenyl-1,2,3,6-tetrahydropyridine (MPTP): implications for treatment and the pathogenesis of Parkinson's disease. Can. J. Neurol. Sci. **11**(1 Suppl): 160–165.
10. SONSALLA, P.K. *et al.* 1992. Characteristics of dopaminergic neurotoxicity produced by MPTP and methamphetamine. Ann. N. Y. Acad. Sci. **648:** 229–238.
11. LAMBERT, C.E. & S.C. BONDY. 1989. Effects of MPTP, MPP^+ and paraquat on mitochondrial potential and oxidative stress. Life Sci. **44:** 1277–1284.
12. CUBELLS, J.F. *et al.* 1994. Methamphetamine neurotoxicity involves vacuolation of endocytic organelles and dopamine-dependent intracellular oxidative stress. J. Neurosci. **14:** 2260–2271.
13. LARSEN, K.E. *et al.* 2002. Methamphetamine-induced degeneration of dopaminergic neurons involves autophagy and upregulation of dopamine synthesis. J. Neurosci. **22:** 8951–8960.
14. FORNAI, F. *et al.* 2005. Parkinson-like syndrome induced by continuous MPTP infusion: convergent roles of the ubiquitin-proteasome system and alpha-synuclein. Proc. Natl. Acad. Sci. USA **102:** 3413–3418.
15. HOGLINGER, G.U. *et al.* 2003. Dysfunction of mitochondrial complex I and the proteasome: interactions between two biochemical deficits in a cellular model of Parkinson's disease. J. Neurochem. **86:** 1297–1307.

On the Effects of Psychostimulants, Antidepressants, and the Antiparkinsonian Drug Levodopa on Dopamine Neurons

RAFFAELLA GERACITANO,[a] MAURO FEDERICI,[a] GIORGIO BERNARDI,[a,b] AND NICOLA B. MERCURI[a,b]

[a]*Experimental Neurology Laboratory C.E.R.C.- Fondazione S. Lucia I.R.C.C.S., 65-00143 Rome, Italy*

[b]*University of Rome "Tor Vergata," 00133 Rome, Italy*

ABSTRACT: The dopaminergic system constitutes the principal target of many psychostimulants, antidepressant, and antiparkinsonian drugs. The effects caused by these compounds are partly associated with an increased dopamine (DA) levels within the terminal areas of DA neurons and in the ventral midbrain. Therefore, several substances of abuse, antidepressants, and endogenous compounds (levodopa and trace amines [TAs]) regulate the activity of DA cells by activating D2 autoreceptors located on the terminals, soma, and dendrites. Considering our past and recent experimental studies on this issue, here we will briefly reexamine the mechanisms of action of several psychoactive drugs on DA neurons. In particular, we propose three different modalities by which the mesencephalic DA neurons can be regulated by drugs: amphetamine/TAs-like, cocaine-like, and levodopa-like. We, therefore, discuss the potential therapeutic and addictive properties of the psychoactive substances.

KEYWORDS: amineptine; amphetamine; cocaine; dopamine; ecstasy; levodopa; methylphenidate; nomifensine; trace amines

INTRODUCTION

There is a general consensus that the dopaminergic system is linked to many processes controlling reward, movement, and cognition.[1] Remarkably, its improper activity is also involved in pathological states, such as drug addiction, schizophrenia, depression, attention-deficit/hyperactivity disorder (ADHD), and Parkinson's disease.[2–4]

Address for correspondence: Nicola B. Mercuri, Experimental Neurology, Laboratory - C.E.R.C.-Fondazione S. Lucia I.R.C.C.S., Via del Fosso di Fiorano, 65-00143 Rome, Italy. Voice: 0039-06501703317; fax: 0039-06501703307.
e-mail: mercurin@med.uniroma2.it

**Ann. N.Y. Acad. Sci. 1074: 320–329 (2006). © 2006 New York Academy of Sciences.
doi: 10.1196/annals.1369.029**

Another important topic concerning the dopaminergic system is that it is a main site of action for psychostimulants/addictive drugs (amphetamine, cocaine, ecstasy, methylphenidate [MPH]) and therapeutic agents for depression, ADHD, and Parkinson's disease (amineptine, amphetamine, nomifensine, MPH, levodopa).[3–6] Moreover, endogenous substances present in the central nervous system at low concentrations, trace amines (TAs) (tyramine, β-phenylalanine), are able to modulate the dopaminergic system.[7,8]

Therefore, it emerges that there are at least three important aspects in the pharmacology of drugs affecting the dopaminergic system: (*a*) the same psychostimulant can be in some cases a therapeutic and an abused drug in others, depending upon the context in which it is administered (see amphetamine or MPH); (*b*) different drugs, used for various purposes (addiction, depression, ADHD), share the same mechanism of action at cellular level (cocaine, ecstasy, MPH, and antidepressants binding to the dopamine transporter [DAT]); and (*c*) substances known to be precursors in dopamine (DA) synthesis (levodopa) or resulting anyhow, from catecholamines' synthetic/degrading pathways (TAs) also affect DA tone in the brain.

Based on these considerations, we believe that the dopaminergic system can be modulated through different mechanisms that are classified as follow: (*a*) enhancement of DA release (amphetamine/TAs-like mechanisms)[7,9,10]; (*b*) blockade of DAT (cocaine-like mechanism)[8,10–13]; and (*c*) increase of DA synthesis (levodopa-like mechanism).[14–16]

In this article, we present an overview of our main results examining the electrophysiological effects of several psychoactive drugs on DA neurons.

DAT AND INTRACELLULAR DA: TARGETS FOR DISEASES THERAPY AND DRUG ADDICTION

Numerous psychostimulants that are characterized by their high-abuse potential, as well as therapeutic agents in specific pathophysiological conditions, such as depression and ADHD, affect the dopaminergic transmission by a modification of the extracellular and/or intracellular level of DA. Their effects result from specific mechanisms of action that involve the DAT and/or DA intracellular storage and metabolic processes.

The DAT is a plasmalemmal protein that uses energy stored in the Na-Cl ionic gradients to reuptake released DA into the cytosol.[17–19]

However, several studies have also described that this protein is not only involved in the normal uptake of DA but also in a reversed transport, leading to nonexocytotic DA release.[20,21] Moreover, DAT also plays an electrogenic role as an ion channel.[20,21]

On the basis of our results, the mechanism of action of pharmacological agents affecting the function of DAT on native DA neurons can be essentially classified as: cocaine-like, amphetamine-like, and levodopa-like.

Cocaine-Like Substances and DAT Blockade

Cocaine acts as a reuptake inhibitor that binds to the transporter protein, DAT, but is not itself transported into the cells. Therefore, it mainly elevates extracellular DA in the synapses.[22]

Amineptine, ecstasy, MPH, and nomifensine have been grouped as cocaine-like substances due to the fact that all of them work through the same mechanism used by cocaine.

In line with this, electrophysiological studies carried out in brain slices, have shown that amineptine, cocaine, ecstasy, MPH, and nomifensine reduce the spontaneous firing rate of midbrain DA neurons by hyperpolarizing the cell membrane.[10–13]

In particular, the reduction in the firing rate caused by 1–10 μM cocaine is concentration-dependent and depends from a hyperpolarization. In neurons voltage clamped at −60 mV, cocaine causes an outward current.[11]

Similarly, bath application of 30 μM MHP hyperpolarizes the DA neurons and abolishes their spontaneous activity. Under voltage clamp conditions at −60 mV, MPH causes an outward current.[13]

Furthermore, amineptine (1–30 μM) and nomifensine (1–30 μM) also decrease the spontaneous firing in a concentration-dependent manner and these effects are associated with a hyperpolarization of the cells. Under voltage clamp conditions, both substances produce outward membrane currents.[10,12] A comparable inhibitory action caused by a hyperpolarization of the membrane has been recently observed on DA neurons exposed to ecstasy (3–30 μM) (our unpublished results).

In all cases, the reduction in firing rate and/or the development of the outward current, caused by the agents presented above, are due to an inhibition of the DAT that determines a rise in the extracellular concentration of endogenous DA and a subsequent activation of D2 somatodendritic autoreceptors. In fact, the cellular responses of all these drugs are reversed by the DA-antagonist, sulpiride, suggesting the activation of D2-like autoreceptors. The actions of cocaine-like compounds are resistant to TTX but are abolished in Ca^{++}-free solutions confirming the involvement of the DAT protein to increase the extracellular concentration of synaptically released DA. Remarkably, in accordance with an effect on DAT, all these substances potentiate the cellular response to exogenously applied DA.

Finally, in support to the contention that cocaine-like substances have the same mechanism of action, is the example obtained with amineptine, whose potentiation of DA responses is occluded in the presence of saturating concentrations of cocaine.[10]

An interesting feature that characterizes some of the cocaine-like compounds affecting the DAT is the possibility that they also affect the noradrenergic and the serotoninergic transmission. In fact, cocaine is a blocker of all three aminergic uptake membrane proteins (DAT, noradrenalin reuptake system [NET], and 5-HT transporter [SERT]). For this reason cocaine has effects on DA neurons, which are not only attributable to an increased level of extracellular DA but also 5-hydroxytryptamine (5-HT).

Thus, the blockade of the SERT induced by cocaine, causes a disinhibition of DA cells that is due to reduced amplitude of the GABAB inhibitory potential. In fact, the increase in serotonin concentration caused by cocaine, leads to an activation of presynaptic 5-HT1B receptors located on GABAergic terminals, which in turn depress the release of GABA on DA cells.[23,24]

A similar disinhibition, 5-HT mediated, has been recently observed when ecstasy is superfused on DA neurons of the rat midbrain maintained *in vitro*. These data suggest that ecstasy, as well as cocaine, increases the extracellular levels of DA and 5-HT in the brain by blocking DAT and SERT, respectively. On the contrary MPH does not affect the GABAB IPSP evoked on DA cell and this is consistent with the hypothesis that MPH blocks DAT but does not inhibit SERT.[13]

Finally, amineptine and nomifensine are two antidepressants that besides blocking DAT also affect the NET having no affect on SERT. Thus, their subjective effects are mediated by DA and NA and should not be attributed to an increase of the synaptic concentration of 5-HT.[25]

Amphetamine-Like Substances and Modulation of DA Release

An amphetamine-like substance acts as "substrate-type releaser" that binds to transporter proteins, and is subsequently carried into the cytoplasm of nerve terminals. Regarding the dopaminergic system, it elevates extracellular DA concentration by two mechanisms: (*a*) it promotes DA efflux by a process dependent on DAT-mediated exchange and (*b*) increases cytoplasmic DA level by disrupting its storage into vesicles.[26] This latter action might increase the pool of DA available for release by transporter-dependent and -independent exchange.

Amphetamine (3–100 μM), applied on DA neurons, inhibits the action potential discharge by hyperpolarizing the cells. Under voltage clamp recordings, it produces an outward current. These effects are blocked by sulpiride suggesting the involvement of D2 autoreceptors. In addition, the effects of amphetamine are eliminated after a treatment with the dopa-decarboxylase enzyme inhibitor carbidopa, suggesting an indirect drug action.

Interestingly, responses to exogenously applied DA are left unaffected by amphetamine but potentiated by cocaine. Taken together, these evidences suggest that the inhibition of DA neurons by amphetamine is mainly due to the release of endogenous DA and not due to the blockade of DAT.[9] Because amphetamine-like drugs must be transported into nerve terminals by DAT to promote a subsequent transmitter release, the role of DAT in amphetamine's actions is not marginal and reuptake inhibitors can reduce the effects of the DA releasers.[27] Accordingly, we have confirmed that the outward current induced by amphetamine in DA cells is attenuated by the DAT blockers (cocaine and nomifensine). This inhibition of the amphetamine-induced outward current is very likely due to a reduction of the efflux of endogenous DA from the somatodendritic regions of DA neurons and not, to nonspecific depressant effects of the DAT blockers on the mechanisms generating the outward current. In fact, cocaine potentiates the outward current caused by the exogenous application of DA, while reduces the current caused by the endogenous release of DA stimulated by amphetamine.[28]

In spite of the fact that 3,4-methylenedioxymethamphetamine (ecstasy) is generally considered an amphetamine-like DA releaser, our recent results suggest that the pharmacological profile of this drug is more similar to cocaine rather than amphetamine.

Levodopa, TAs, and Modulation of the Endogenous Release of DA

Levodopa (3–100 μM), inhibits substantia nigra pars compacta neurons in a concentration-dependent manner by hyperpolarizing the membrane. It also produces an outward current under voltage clamp conditions. The depression of the neuronal activity results from the stimulation of D2 autoreceptors by DA neosynthesized from levodopa via the endogenous aromatic amino acid decarboxylase enzyme. In support to this point, we have shown that sulpiride reverses the effects of levodopa, which are also depressed by carbidopa, confirming the indirect nature of levodopa interaction with DA receptors. An interesting difference between the effects of levodopa and DA is in the intensity of the neuronal responses to these agents. Although levodopa induces less ample effects than those caused by DA, they are more sustained.[14,16]

TAs are endogenous compounds that are detected in the mammalian nervous system in low amounts. Nevertheless, it appears that they do not have a minor role in brain functioning. In fact, a dysregulation of TAs activity has been linked to several diseases, such as schizophrenia, depression, migraine, ADHD, drug addiction, and eating disorders.[29]

Recently, we have examined the effects of two TAs, tyramine (TYR) and β-phenylethylamine (β-PEA) on the dopaminergic system. Both β-PEA (3–100 μM) and TYR (3–100 μM) inhibit the DA cells of the ventral mesencephalon. The effects of these two amines are indirect and are mediated via an increased extracellular level of endogenous DA.

Thus, the functional effects of both amines disappear in the presence of the D2-selective antagonist sulpiride and when an inhibition of DA synthesis is obtained with carbidopa. Furthermore, our electrophysiological experiments cannot simply classify TYR and β-PEA as amphetamine- or cocaine-like substances. Indeed, a block of DAT, as observed for cocaine-like substances,[28,30] is unlikely because TAs do not potentiate the inhibitory response to exogenously applied DA. On the other hand, since their electrophysiological effects are not reduced by cocaine, it is still possible that TAs, as amphetamine, also release newly synthesized DA in the extracellular space by a DAT-independent mechanism.[31,32]

DISCUSSION

In this article, we have briefly described the electrophysiological effects of some psychoactive drugs on midbrain DA neurons. Interestingly, all the substances, we have examined so far, are active on DA neurons and continue to represent new challenges to basic researchers and clinicians.

The psychostimulants are a fascinating group of compounds that produce a spectrum of effects in humans that include elevated mood and motor activation. Some of these drugs are useful medications, whereas others are highly addictive substances.

With regard to the abuse liability, it is recognized that some psychostimulants, as well as, antidepressants mainly act on DAT or augment extracellular DA levels by modifying DA synthetic/degrading pathways. Thus, a common feature of the psychoactive substances, examined in this article, is their ability to increase the extracellular content of DA. Interestingly, a different balance of action on DAT and SERT could partly account for their different utilizations. There is also a difference in the functional responses caused by cocaine-like respect to those caused by amphetamine/levodopa/TAs-like agents at a cellular level. (*a*) The cocaine-like (DAT blockers) substances should cause a potentiation of the signals mediated by synaptically released DA. (*b*) The amphetamine-like substances (TAs and levodopa) cause more generalized DA responses by increasing the dopaminergic tone in the extracellular space. Thus, a synaptic dopaminergic signal might be augmented in the presence of cocaine but left indistinct in the presence of amphetamine, TAs, and levodopa that instead indiscriminately raise extracellular DA levels. This could explain some differences in the subjective effects caused by drugs and side effects related to a long-term use.

Apart from the considerations exposed above on the dynamics and pattern of neuronal responses to psychoactive drugs, a central issue is why they are going to be used therapeutically or abused?

It is recognized that DA clearly plays a central role in the reinforcing effects of psychostimulants. However, several studies have also implicated serotonin and norepinephrine in the generation of an addictive profile, suggesting for example, that the interaction of cocaine with SERT, and possibly NET, may be necessary to initiate, maintain cocaine reward, and to regulate abstinence.[33,34]

An additional concern is the neurotoxic potential of amphetamines as revealed in animal studies. For instance, dopaminergic neurotoxicity induced by amphetamines is associated with a decrease in the vesicular DA uptake capacity and the level of VMAT2 immunoreactivity in a striatal synaptosomal vesicular fraction.[35] On the other hand, ecstasy mainly induces neurotoxicity within the terminal field of serotoninergic neurons.[36]

At this point the main question is why there is a different use of stimulating drugs if their basic modalities of actions in the brain are more or less similar? Perhaps the difference does not reside in the drug itself but in the features of the receiver. Certainly, there is an individual susceptibility to drug abuse that is often genetically determined.[37,38] Conversely, the normal or altered functioning of the brain could be important to induce addiction or to treat diseases with psychostimulants. Thus, a pathological condition, such as DA deficiency in Parkinson's disease would mainly recognize levodopa as a therapeutic agent rather than a stimulant. In spite of this, an addictive intake of levodopa has been also reported in parkinsonian patients and in nonaffected individuals.[39,40] Similarly, a pathological state, such as depression has been cured with amineptine and nomifensine. However, these substances have abuse potentials in animals and humans.[41] The state of brain maturation is also another important factor.[42] The paradoxical calming effects of amphetamines and MPH in children with ADHD with respect to the hyperactivity induced in adults is a specific individual characteristic that goes beyond the basic properties of the drugs.

In spite of this, we do not want to underscore the sociocultural factors and the contextual aspects associated with drug intake that anyway contribute to modify the properties of the person but not those of the psychostimulants.[43–45]

Therefore, in a broader sense, both environmental and internal states modulate the individual response induced by psychoactive agents.

CONCLUSIONS

In this article we have delineated the basic characteristics of actions of psychostimulants on DA neurons. We have also compared electrophysiological differences and similarities between classes of psychoactive drugs. We conclude that in spite of the pharmacological and physiological properties of each drug, inner and external individual factors should contribute to determine their fate either as therapeutic or abused substances.

ACKNOWLEDGMENTS

This work was supported by grants from Ministero della Salute and della Ricerca Scientifica to N.B.M.

REFERENCES

1. Giros, B. & M.G. Caron. 1993. Molecular characterization of the dopamine transporter. Trends Pharmacol. Sci. **14:** 43–49.
2. Di Chiara, G. & A. Imperato. 1988. Drugs abused by humans preferentially increase synaptic dopamine concentrations in the mesolimbic system of freely moving rats. Proc. Natl. Acad. Sci. USA. **85:** 5274–5278.
3. Seeman, P. & H.B. Niznik. 1990. Dopamine receptors and transporters in Parkinson's disease and schizophrenia. FASEB J. **4:** 2737–2744.
4. Mercuri, N.B., P. Calabresi & G. Bernardi. 1992. The electrophysiological actions of dopamine and dopaminergic drugs on neurons of the substantia nigra pars compacta and ventral tegmental area. Life Sci. **51:** 711–718.
5. Hunt, R.D. *et al.* 1984. Possible change in noradrenergic receptor sensitivity following methylphenidate treatment: growth hormone and MHPG response to clonidine challenge in children with attention deficit disorder and hyperactivity. Life Sci. **35:** 885–897.
6. Koob, G.F. & E.J. Nestler. 1997. The neurobiology of drug addiction. J. Neuropsychiatry Clin. Neurosci. **9:** 482–497.
7. Geracitano, R. *et al.* 2004. Inhibitory effects of trace amines on rat midbrain dopaminergic neurons. Neuropharmacology **46:** 807–814.
8. Skerritt, J.H. *et al.* 2000. Development of immunoassays for tyramine and tryptamine toxins of Phalaris aquatica L. J. Agric. Food Chem. **48:** 27–32.
9. Mercuri, N.B., P. Calabresi & G. Bernardi. 1989. The mechanism of amphetamine-induced inhibition of rat substantia nigra compacta neurones investigated with intracellular recording in vitro. Br. J. Pharmacol. **98:** 127–134.
10. Mercuri, N.B. *et al.* 1991. Electrophysiological effects of amineptine on neurones of the rat substantia nigra pars compacta: evidence for an inhibition of the dopamine uptake system. Br. J. Pharmacol. **104:** 700–704.
11. Lacey, M.G., N.B. Mercuri & R.A. North. 1990. Actions of cocaine on rat dopaminergic neurones in vitro. Br. J. Pharmacol. **99:** 731–735.
12. Mercuri, N.B. *et al.* 1991. Nomifensine but not amantadine increases dopamine-induced responses on rat substantia nigra zona compacta neurons. Neurosci. Lett. **131:** 145–148.
13. Federici, M. *et al.* 2005. Actions of methylphenidate on dopaminergic neurons of the ventral midbrain. Biol. Psychiatry **57:** 361–365.
14. Mercuri, N.B., P. Calabresi & G. Bernardi. 1990. Responses of rat substantia nigra compacta neurones to L-DOPA. Br. J. Pharmacol. **100:** 257–260.
15. Mercuri, N.B., P. Calabresi & G. Bernardi. 1991. Dopamine uptake inhibition potentiates the effects of L-DOPA on rat substantia nigra zona compacta neurons. Neurosci. Lett. **126:** 79–82.
16. Mercuri, N.B. & G. Bernardi. 2005. The 'magic' of L-dopa: why is it the gold standard Parkinson's disease therapy? Trends Pharmacol. Sci. **26:** 341–344.
17. Iversen, L.L. 1971. Role of transmitter uptake mechanisms in synaptic neurotransmission. Br. J. Pharmacol. **41:** 571–591.
18. Amara, S.G. *et al.* 1998. Molecular physiology and regulation of catecholamine transporters. Adv. Pharmacol. **42:** 164–168.
19. Amara, S.G. & M.S. Sonders. 1998. Neurotransmitter transporters as molecular targets for addictive drugs. Drug Alcohol Depend. **51:** 87–96.

20. INGRAM, S.L., B.M. PRASAD & S.G. AMARA. 2002. Dopamine transporter-mediated conductances increase excitability of midbrain dopamine neurons. Nat. Neurosci. **5:** 971–978.
21. SULZER, D. & A. GALLI. 2003. Dopamine transport currents are promoted from curiosity to physiology. Trends Neurosci. **26:** 173–176.
22. SOTNIKOVA, T.D. *et al.* 2006. Molecular biology, pharmacology and functional role of the plasma membrane dopamine transporter. CNS Neurol. Disord. Drug Targets **5:** 45–56.
23. CAMERON, D.L. & J.T. WILLIAMS. 1994. Cocaine inhibits GABA release in the VTA through endogenous 5-HT. J. Neurosci. **14:** 6763–6767.
24. JOHNSON, S.W., N.B. MERCURI & R.A. NORTH. 1992. 5-hydroxytryptamine1B receptors block the GABAB synaptic potential in rat dopamine neurons. J. Neurosci. **12:** 2000–2006.
25. TALBOT, P.S. & M. LARUELLE. 2002. The role of in vivo molecular imaging with PET and SPECT in the elucidation of psychiatric drug action and new drug development. Eur. Neuropsychopharmacol. **12:** 503–511.
26. RUDNICK, G. & J. CLARK. 1993. From synapse to vesicle: the reuptake and storage of biogenic amine neurotransmitters. Biochim. Biophys. Acta **1144:** 249–263.
27. RAITERI, M. *et al.* 1979. Dopamine can be released by two mechanisms differentially affected by the dopamine transport inhibitor nomifensine. J. Pharmacol. Exp. Ther. **208:** 195–202.
28. SCARPONI, M., G. BERNARDI & N.B. MERCURI. 1999. Electrophysiological evidence for a reciprocal interaction between amphetamine and cocaine-related drugs on rat midbrain dopaminergic neurons. Eur. J. Neurosci. **11:** 593–598.
29. LINDEMANN, L. & M.C. HOENER. 2005. A renaissance in trace amines inspired by a novel GPCR family. Trends Pharmacol. Sci. **26:** 274–281.
30. PALADINI, C.A. *et al.* 2001. Amphetamine selectively blocks inhibitory glutamate transmission in dopamine neurons. Nat. Neurosci. **4:** 275–281.
31. MUNDORF, M.L., S.E. HOCHSTETLER & R.M. WIGHTMAN. 1999. Amine weak bases disrupt vesicular storage and promote exocytosis in chromaffin cells. J. Neurochem. **73:** 2397–2405.
32. JANSSEN, P.A. *et al.* 1999. Does phenylethylamine act as an endogenous amphetamine in some patients? Int. J. Neuropsychopharmacol. **2:** 229–240.
33. SORA, I. *et al.* 2001. Molecular mechanisms of cocaine reward: combined dopamine and serotonin transporter knockouts eliminate cocaine place preference. Proc. Natl. Acad. Sci. USA **98:** 5300–5305.
34. HARRIS, G.C., K. ALTOMARE & G. ASTON-JONES. 2001. Preference for a cocaine-associated environment is attenuated by augmented accumbal serotonin in cocaine withdrawn rats. Psychopharmacology (Berl). **156:** 14–22.
35. FLECKENSTEIN, A.E. & G.R. HANSON. 2003. Impact of psychostimulants on vesicular monoamine transporter function. Eur. J. Pharmacol. **479:** 283–289.
36. GREEN, A.R. *et al.* 2003. The pharmacology and clinical pharmacology of 3,4-methylenedioxymethamphetamine (MDMA, "ecstasy"). Pharmacol. Rev. **55:** 463–508.
37. GOLDMAN, D., G. OROSZI & F. DUCCI. 2005. The genetics of addictions: uncovering the genes. Nat. Rev. Genet. **6:** 521–532.
38. VOLKOW, N.D. *et al.* 1999. Methylphenidate and cocaine have a similar in vivo potency to block dopamine transporters in the human brain. Life Sci. **65:** PL7–PL12.

39. STEINER, I. & I. WIRGUIN. 2003. Levodopa addiction in non-parkinsonian patients. Neurology **61:** 1451–1453.
40. MERIMS, D., R. GALILI-MOSBERG & E. MELAMED. 2000. Is there addiction to levodopa in patients with Parkinson's disease?. Mov. Disord. **15:** 1014–1016.
41. HADDAD, P. 1999. Do antidepressants have any potential to cause addiction? J. Psychopharmacol. **13:** 300–307.
42. STANSFIELD, K.H. & C.L. KIRSTEIN. 2005. Neurochemical effects of cocaine in adolescence compared to adulthood. Brain Res. Dev. Brain Res. **159:** 119–125.
43. KELLEY, A.E., C.A. SCHILTZ & C.F. LANDRY. 2005. Neural systems recruited by drug- and food-related cues: studies of gene activation in corticolimbic regions. Physiol. Behav. **86:** 11–14.
44. WESTERMEYER, J. 1999. The role of cultural and social factors in the cause of addictive disorders. Psychiatr. Clin. North Am. **22:** 253–273.
45. ROBINSON, T.E. & K.C. BERRIDGE. 2000. The psychology and neurobiology of addiction: an incentive-sensitization view. Addiction **95**(Suppl 2): S91–S117.

Effect of Oxidative Stress Induced by L-Dopa on Endogenous Antioxidants in PC-12 Cells

GOVIND T. VATASSERY, W. ED SMITH, AND HUNG T. QUACH

Research Service and GRECC, VA Medical Center, Minneapolis, Minnesota 55417 and Department of Psychiatry and the Graduate Program in Neuroscience, University of Minnesota, Minneapolis, Minnesota 55455, USA

ABSTRACT: The mechanism of action of many drugs of abuse involves the dopaminergic pathway. One method of increasing dopamine in brain is by ingestion of L-dopa (3,4-dihydroxy-L-phenylalanine). Interestingly, both dopamine and L-dopa cause oxidative stress which is also a factor in drug-induced damage. Oxidative stress can be reduced by the antioxidant activities of vitamins C (ascorbate) and E (tocopherols). However, the interactions between L-dopa and tocopherols and ascorbate are not well understood. In this article, PC-12 cells (as models of neurons) were cultured for 21 hours with ascorbate (400 μM) and/or alpha tocopherol (25 μM) and in the presence or absence of L-dopa (250 μM). After incubation, cells were harvested and analyzed for the various biochemical components by HPLC. As expected, the addition of L-dopa resulted in an almost threefold increase in cellular dopamine content. Addition of alpha tocopherol resulted in marked increase in cellular tocopherol. Similarly, addition of ascorbate substantially increased its cellular concentration. These increases were strongly attenuated by the presence of L-dopa in the medium. The data indicate that: (*a*) the uptake systems for ascorbate and tocopherols in these cells are inhibited by L-dopa and/or (*b*) L-dopa treatment causes an increase in the rate of utilization of the two nutrients. Thus L-dopa modulates the cellular dynamics of ascorbate and tocopherol altering cellular antioxidant protection.

KEYWORDS: vitamin E; vitamin C; antioxidants; L-dopa; dopamine

INTRODUCTION

The use of L-dopa for Parkinson's disease (PD) is associated with toxic manifestations characterized by motor fluctuations and dyskinesia; whether L-dopa itself is the cause of such toxicity has been an area of controversy.[1] L-dopa

Address for correspondence: Dr. Govind T. Vatassery, Research Service (151), VA Medical Center, Minneapolis, MN 55417. Voice: 612-467-2910; fax: 612-725-2084.
e-mail: vatas001@umn.edu

Ann. N.Y. Acad. Sci. 1074: 330–336 (2006). © 2006 New York Academy of Sciences.
doi: 10.1196/annals.1369.030

ingestion is also known to be associated with behavioral alterations. One example is a report that a few patients with PD take increasing amounts of dopamine replacement therapy far in excess of the amounts required to control their motor disabilities.[2] In fact, these authors have characterized the compulsive use of dopamine replacement therapy as reward systems gone awry.[3] Thus even though use of L-dopa could not be considered as a substance abuse problem, it is likely that the compound does alter the reward system. In addition, Fornai *et al.*[4] observed the presence of inclusion bodies like Lewy bodies in neurons of substantia nigra pars compacta in rats treated with methamphetamine, another link between drug use and potential PD-like pathology.

Studies have also suggested that both dopamine and L-dopa can cause biological oxidative stress[5,6] as is the case with many drugs. The potential interaction between 3,4-methylenedioxymethamphetamine (MDMA) and the antioxidant nutrients, vitamins C and E, has also been reported. Johnson *et al.*[7] found that subcutaneous injections of MDMA reduced the concentrations of vitamin E, total antioxidant reserve, and protein thiols in mice brains. They also found that vitamin E deficiency increased the susceptibility of the animals to MDMA-induced neurotoxicity. Shankaran *et al.*[8] found that intraperitoneal injections of MDMA resulted in decreases in vitamin E and ascorbate in the striatum and hippocampus of rats. The depletion of serotonin found with MDMA was attenuated by treatment with ascorbate.

The above reports suggest that oxidative stress may be involved in the biologic effects of a number of drugs including L-dopa. In this article, we sought to examine the effect of L-dopa upon endogenous antioxidants in a catecholaminergic cell using PC-12 cells as a model.

MATERIALS AND METHODS

Cell Culturing and Protocols for Incubation

PC-12 cells were obtained from American Type Culture Collection (ATCC; Manassas, VA) and cultured on matrigel-coated plates as recommended. After culturing for 1 day, the media was replaced with new media containing alpha tocopherol, ascorbate, combination of both, or none of these compounds. At the same time, 250 μM L-dopa was added to some of the flasks. Culturing was continued for 21 h. The media was removed and cells were recovered by trypsinization. The cells were washed three times with Krebs buffer and then processed for different assays.

Biochemical Assays:

1. Assays for catecholamines: An HPLC procedure involving electrochemical detection recommended by ESA Inc. (Chelmsford, MA) was followed.

2. Determination of ascorbate: The samples for assays were stabilized with metaphosphoric acid and ascorbate levels were determined by HPLC according to the method of Margolis.[9]
3. Determination of alpha tocopherol: Alpha tocopherol was determined by HPLC with electrochemical detection as described previously.[10]
4. Analysis of glutathione: The samples were treated with 5% trichloroacetic acid and 0.5 mM EDTA (final). The glutathione in the acid extract was derivatized with 7-fluor-2,1,3-benzoxazole-4-sulfonamide (SBDF) and analyzed by reverse phase HPLC with fluorescent detection.
5. Other biochemical assays: Concentration of total protein was determined by the Lowry technique as modified by Markwell *et al.*[11]

RESULTS

Several reports in the literature have examined the effect of L-dopa upon cell viability under a number of conditions. The incubation times with L-dopa used in this study were relatively short compared with those in most of the previous reports. Upon microscopic examination, the cells were relatively intact. The protein levels in the flasks declined by 20% when the cells were incubated with 250 μM L-dopa. This loss may be the result of lack of adherence and/or cell death. Cell viability was assayed using [3-(4,5-dimethylthiazol-2-yl)-2,5-diphenyl tetrazolium bromide] (MTT) and we found that 80% of cells were viable cells. Thus, there was loss of cells at the higher concentration of L-dopa. This cell loss has been taken into account in all our calculations.

Catecholamines were produced efficiently by the PC-12 cells used in this study. The percent conversion of L-dopa to catecholamines and metabolites was calculated to be 36.5% under basal conditions as well as in the presence of alpha tocopherol. However, this conversion rate increased to 47.8% in the presence of ascorbate.

There is considerable evidence to indicate that L-dopa can induce oxidative stress under *in vitro* conditions. Hence, experiments were designed to examine the effect of incubations of PC-12 cells upon the endogenous antioxidants: vitamins C and E. In the first study, we analyzed the cells for alpha tocopherol in PC-12 cells, which had been incubated with 25 μM alpha tocopherol that was added to the medium at the same time as L-dopa. The results are shown in FIGURE 1.

We added 25 μM alpha tocopherol into the medium since this concentration is within the range of normal human plasma in adults. The most important finding is that L-dopa treatment resulted in a lower concentration of alpha tocopherol within the cells. We have also measured the levels of alpha tocopherol in the medium after the incubation and found that nearly all of the alpha tocopherol added to the medium can be recovered in the cell pellet plus the medium. Thus L-dopa treatment did not cause oxidation of alpha

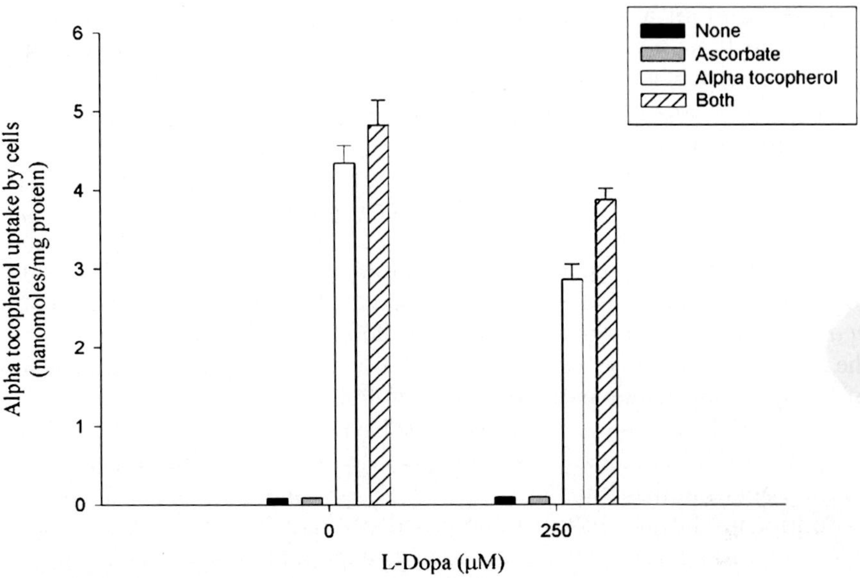

FIGURE 1. Effect of incubations with L-dopa upon alpha tocopherol concentrations in PC-12 cells. PC-12 cells were cultured under standard conditions in the presence of alpha tocopherol, ascorbate, or a combination of both with or without the addition of 250 μM L-dopa into the medium. Cells were isolated and alpha tocopherol concentrations determined by HPLC.

tocopherol in the cells or medium. It is also interesting to note that levels of cellular tocopherol were higher when the incubation media also contained ascorbate. This is due to the well-known sparing of vitamin E by vitamin C.

Next, we examined the effect of L-dopa on ascorbate concentrations after incubation of PC-12 cells with L-dopa and 400 μM ascorbate. The concentration of ascorbate used is higher than that present in normal human serum and is closer to that in cerebrospinal fluid. Since brain has one of the highest levels of ascorbate, we decided to use this higher concentration. L-dopa incubations resulted in reductions in levels of ascorbate very similar to that seen with alpha tocopherol. Thus, the levels of both tocopherol and ascorbate within the cells were reduced by L-dopa treatment. The data suggest the presence of oxidative stress when cells are exposed to L-dopa.

DISCUSSION

The experiments reported in this study were designed to investigate the impact of L-dopa on endogenous antioxidants using a prototype cell capable of synthesizing and secreting catecholamines. Our results show that PC-12 cells are good models for studies on catecholamine synthesis in cells. The effect of L-dopa on PC-12 cells can be divided into two categories. The first is the effect of the antioxidants on the synthesis of dopamine and its turnover after incubations in the presence of L-dopa. The results of these experiments are not presented here. The second is the effect of L-dopa on the antioxidants and their interactions with one another; selected results from these experiments are reported here.

General Effects of L-Dopa

In this study, we used L-dopa concentrations that are higher than those found in human plasma after human subjects are treated with L-dopa. Nyholm *et al.*[12] studied the pharmacokinetics of L-dopa in PD patients and found that the serum concentration was as high as 70 μM in one subject taking 1100 mg of L-dopa along with a catechol-O-methyl transferase inhibitor even though the usual levels were smaller than this. We have used 250 μM L-dopa in these experiments. Most of the studies dealing with toxicity of L-dopa have employed concentrations in this range.

Rodriguez-Martin *et al.*[13] have proposed an interesting explanation for neurotoxicity and neurotrophism induced by L-dopa. This group has shown both effects with different cell types and different conditions of growth. They conclude that toxicity or protection is controlled by the redox environment of the cell. Glial-conditioned medium containing antioxidants, such as glutathione and ascorbate as well as other bioactive molecules, enhanced the neuroprotective effects of L-dopa.

Effects of Ascorbic Acid

Brain, spinal cord, and adrenals have the highest levels of ascorbic acid[14] and the latter is a true co-substrate for dopamine beta monooxygenase (3,4-dihydroxyphenethylamine, ascorbate:oxygen oxidoreductase EC 1.14.17.1). The concentration of ascorbate in the extracellular environment of the brain is controlled by glutamate-ascorbate heteroexchange. Ascorbate can modulate synaptic activity of dopamine and glutamate (see review[15]). It is released from the glutamatergic neurons as glutamate is taken up. This takes place also in glial cells. Both D1 and D2 dopamine receptors are involved in this process in the neuron. Amphetamine, apomorphine, and D1 and D2 agonists increase release of ascorbate from glutamatergic terminals in the neostriatum. Therefore, the decreases in ascorbate upon incubations with L-dopa that we have observed could have functional impact upon dopamine and glutamate transmission in the brain. More work *in vivo* on the impact of L-dopa upon catecholaminergic cells in the presence and absence of ascorbate needs to be performed.

In addition to its role as a neuromodulator, ascorbate may also have beneficial antioxidant effects. L-dopa toxicity was studied in adrenal chromaffin cells by Corona-Morales *et al.*[16] who found that ascorbic acid protected against toxicity from L-dopa. The influence of several antioxidants upon oxidative stress and toxicity induced by dopamine was studied in PC12 cells by Offen *et al.*[5] who found that both vitamins C and E were protective against toxicity. These data also support our postulate that antioxidants may have a role in modulating the toxicity induced by L-dopa.

Effects of Alpha Tocopherol

Unlike ascorbate, few specific effects of tocopherol on neural transmitters have been reported. Our results show that both alpha tocopherol and ascorbate levels are reduced upon treatment with L-dopa. As expected, ascorbate stabilized the concentrations of alpha tocopherol. Since the latter is the most effective lipid-soluble antioxidant present in membranes, it is quite likely that one of the functions of ascorbate may indeed be to stabilize the membrane by regenerating alpha tocopherol. Using radiolabeled alpha tocopherol, we have observed that the uptake of tocopherol is reduced by the presence of L-dopa in the medium (data not shown). This supports the idea that L-dopa treatment is associated with membrane damage. Antioxidant protection may be able to alleviate or retard such membrane abnormalities.

CONCLUSIONS

Treatment with L-dopa at a concentration of 250 μM resulted in a decrease in both tocopherol and ascorbate in PC-12 cells. These findings indicate that L-dopa treatment is associated with changes in cellular redox status. It is well known that cells possess interacting mechanisms for stabilizing the redox status via redox cycles involving these antioxidants (see review by Winkler *et al.*[17]). We propose that vitamins C, E, and/or other redox-active agents, such as glutathione or combinations of these compounds, could be used as effective agents to ameliorate oxidative stress in cells that produce catecholamines from ingested L-dopa. Further work on the mechanisms involved in the changes in antioxidants caused by L-dopa treatment would help understand the biology of this phenomenon and assist in the selection of the appropriate agent(s) for clinical use in PD during L-dopa treatment.

ACKNOWLEDGMENTS

These investigations were supported by Medical Research Funds from the Department of Veterans Affairs, Washington DC, USA.

REFERENCES

1. HACHINSKI, V. 2000. Levodopa toxicity. Arch. Neurol. **57:** 410.
2. EVANS, A.H. & A.J. LEES. 2004. Dopamine dysregulation syndrome in Parkinson's disease. Curr. Opin. Neurol. **17:** 393–398.

3. Lawrence, A.D., A.H. Evans & A.J. Lees. 2003. Compulsive use of dopamine replacement therapy in Parkinson's disease: reward systems gone awry. Lancet Neurol. **2:** 595–604.
4. Fornai, F., P. Lenzi, M. Gesi, *et al.* 2004. Methamphetamine produces neuronal inclusions in the nigrostriatal system and in PC12 cells. J. Neurochem. **88:** 114–123.
5. Offen, D., A. Hochman, S. Gorodin, *et al.* 1999. Oxidative stress and neuroprotection in Parkinson's disease: implications from studies on dopamine-induced apoptosis. Adv. Neurol. **80:** 265–269.
6. Asanuma, M., I. Miyazaki, F.J. Diaz-Corrales & N. Ogawa. 2004. Quinone formation as dopaminergic neuron-specific oxidative stress in the pathogenesis of sporadic Parkinon's disease and neurotoxin-induced Parkinsonism. Acta Med. Okayama **58:** 221–233.
7. Johnson, E.A., A.A. Shvedova, E. Kisin, *et al.* 2002. d-MDMA during vitamin E deficiency: effects on dopaminergic neurotoxicity and hepatotoxicity. Brain Res. **933:** 150–163.
8. Shankaran, M., Y. Yamamoto & G.A. Gudelsky. 2001. Ascorbic acid prevents 3,4-methylenedioxymethamphetamine (MDMA)-induced hydroxyl radical formation and the behavioral and neurochemical consequences of the depletion of brain 5-HT. Synapse **40:** 55–64.
9. Margolis, S.A. 1988. Stabilization of ascorbic acid in plasma, and its liquid chromatographic determination. Clin. Chem. **34:** 2217–2223.
10. Vatassery, G.T., W.E. Smith & H.T. Quach. 1993. A liquid chromatographic method for the simultaneous determination of alpha tocopherol and tocopherolquinone in human red blood cells and other biological samples where tocopherol is easily oxidized during sample treatment. Anal. Biochem. **214:** 426–430.
11. Markwell, M.A.K., S.M. Haas, L.L. Bieber & N.E. Tolbert. 1978. A modification of the Lowry procedure to simplify protein determination in membrane and lipoprotein samples. Anal. Biochem. **87:** 206–210.
12. Nyholm, D., H. Lennernas, C. Gomes-Trolin & S.M. Aquilonius. 2002. Levodopa pharmacokinetics and motor performance during activities of daily living in patients with Parkinson's disease on individual drug combinations. Clin. Neuropharmacol **25:** 89–96.
13. Rodriguez-Martin, E., S. Canals, M.J. Casarejos, *et al.* 2001. L-Dopa and glia-conditioned medium have additive effects on tyrosine hydroxylase expression in human catecholamine-rich neuroblastoma NB69 cells. J. Neurochem. **78:** 535–545.
14. Rice, M.E. 2000. Ascorbate regulation and its neuroprotective role in the brain. Trends Neurosci. **23:** 209–216.
15. Rebec, G.V. & C. Pierce. 1994. A vitamin as a modulator: ascorbate release into the extracellular fluid of the brain regulates dopaminergic and glutamatergic transmission. Prog. Neurobiol. **43:** 537–565.
16. Corona-Morales, A.A., A. Castell, A. Escobar, *et al.* 2003. Fullerene C60 and ascorbic acid protect cultured chromaffin cells against levodopa toxicity. J. Neurosci. Res. **71:** 121–126.
17. Winkler, B.S., S.M. Orsell & T.S. Rex. 1994. The redox couple between glutathione and ascrobic acid: a chemical and physiological perspective. Free Rad. Biol. Med. **17:** 333–349.

Dopamine Stimulation via Infusion in the Lateral Ventricle

FRANCESCA BIAGIONI,[a,b] CARLA L. BUSCETI,[a] GEMMA MOLINARO,[a] GIUSEPPE BATTAGLIA,[a] FILIPPO S. GIORGI,[c] STEFANO RUGGIERI,[a,d] AND FRANCESCO FORNAI[a,b]

[a]*I.R.C.C.S., I.N.M., Neuromed, 86077 Pozzilli, Italy*

[b]*Department of Human Morphology and Applied Biology, University of Pisa, I-56126 Pisa, Italy*

[c]*Department of Neuroscience, University of Pisa, I-56127 Pisa, Italy*

[d]*Department of Neurological Sciences, University of Rome "La Sapienza," 00185 Rome, Italy*

ABSTRACT: **Continuous dopamine (DA) stimulation is a therapeutic approach that applies to the treatment of motor fluctuations due to pulsatile DA stimulation in Parkinson's disease (PD), to cure the abuse of drugs, such as cocaine or amphetamine (which produce short-lasting peaks of extracellular DA), and as a safe therapeutic approach to avoid hedonistic homeostatic dysregulation (which sometime develops as an abuse pattern in PD patients receiving a pulsatile DA replacement therapy). However, systemic continuous delivery of DA agonists leads to a variety of side effects. In search for an alterative approach, in the present study we evaluated the possibility of delivering intracerebroventricularly (i.c.v.), a DA agonist: lisuride that was already shown to be effective when administered continuously subcutaneously (s.c.). In particular, we were interested in examining whether lisuride infused within the lateral ventricle was still able to stimulate DA receptor by inducing contralateral turning behavior in hemiparkinsonian rats. We found that lisuride, when infused in the lateral ventricle was effective in reducing the threshold for stimulating DA receptors. These results offer a more reliable and safe therapeutic approach to deliver continuous DA selectively in the brain.**

KEYWORDS: **lisuride; dopamine stimulation; cocaine; amphetamines; intracerebroventricular; hedonistic homeostatic dysregulation; Parkinson's disease; dyskinesia**

Address for correspondence: Francesco Fornai, M.D., Department of Human Morphology and Applied Biology, University of Pisa, Via Roma, 55, I-56126 Pisa, Italy. Voice: +39-50-2218611; fax: +39-50-2218606.
e-mail: f.fornai@med.unipi.it

Ann. N.Y. Acad. Sci. 1074: 337–343 (2006).
doi: 10.1196/annals.1369.031

INTRODUCTION

Pulsatile dopamine (DA) stimulation produces deleterious effects that are evident as motor fluctuation both in the long-term treatment of Parkinson's disease (PD) and during the chronic abuse of short-acting DA-releasing drugs. In line with this, even in parkinsonian patients treated with DA agonists following a pulsatile pattern, a clinical syndrome called hedonistic homeostatic dysregulation, reminiscent of drug dependence can be described.[1–4] On the other hand, specific drugs of abuse, such as cocaine or amphetamines, produce a massive DA release, which is critical in sustaining rewarding effects and addiction.[5,6] In a recent study, Giovannoni *et al.*,[7] found that a major trigger to initiate the hedonistic homeostatic dysregulation is the intermittent administration of a short-acting DA agonist. On the other hand, continuous administration of a DA agonist seems to be the best approach to prevent the onset of drug dependence when curing parkinsonian subject.[7] In keeping with this, moving beyond parkinsonian patients, toward cocaine- or amphetamine-abusing subject, continuous DA stimulation, achieved via long-acting DA uptake blockers has been suggested as a novel approach in the treatment of drug abuse.[8–10] In fact, the transient and robust increase in extracellular DA levels is a common effect, which sustains the rewarding properties of drugs of abuse. Similarly, the onset of hedonistic homeostatic dysregulation in neurological patients is related to pulsatile DA replacement therapy. In both cases the critical issue concerns the short duration and the amount of the DA stimulation. Interestingly, the same features apply to the onset of abnormal involuntary movements (AIMs) that develops following DA replacement therapy. These symptoms resemble the neurological counterpart of the psychiatric consequence of a brief and intense DA stimulation. Continuous DA stimulation is useful both for the treatment of motor fluctuations due to pulsatile DA stimulation in PD[11–14] and to cure the abuse of drugs, such as cocaine or amphetamine, which produce short-lasting peaks of extracellular DA. Nonetheless, when continuous DA stimulation is applied through subcutaneous (s.c.) pump, it might produce severe local side effects. Again, as a drug delivered systemically, this is associated with a variety of peripheral effects that might also be severe. Finally, the delivery of the drug might be erratic and produce variability in the penetration through the central nervous system (CNS) where it is required to produce its effects.

Therefore, in the present study carried out in rats we evaluated the efficacy of a DA agonist (lisuride) to stimulate central DA receptors when infused intracerebroventricularly (i.c.v.) in the lateral ventricle. In order to assess the motor response we injected lisuride to hemiparkinsonian rats previously infused with 6-hydroxydopamine (6-OHDA). The effects of i.c.v. infusions were compared with those obtained through s.c. injections in particular, for various doses we compared the time of onset, the duration and the intensity of the DA stimulation, as well as the plateau of the response.

MATERIALS AND METHODS

Male Wistar rats (Charles River, Calco, Italy) weighing 150–160 g were used in all experiments. Animals were housed individually at 20–22°C on a 12-h light/dark cycle with free access to food and water. All experimental protocols used were in compliance with the guideline of the Italian Minister of Health. Drugs: 6-hydroxydopamine hydrochloride (Sigma Chemical Co., St. Louis, MO, USA); apomorphine chloridrate (Chiesi Farmaceutici S.p.A, Parma, Italy); lisuride (Lisuridhydrogenmaleat/AMP, Schering Plough, Berlin).

To obtain unilateral nigrostriatal lesions, Wistar rats, were anesthetized with 50 mg/kg of thiopental sodium intraperitoneally (i.p.), and placed in a small animal stereotaxic apparatus (David Kopf Instruments, Tujunga, CA) to be unilaterally injected with 6-OHDA (8 μg/4μl dissolved in saline containing 0.1% ascorbic acid) by a Hamilton Syringe (flow rate of 2 μl/min) rostral to the substantia nigra using the following stereotaxic coordinates: 4.4 mm posterior to the bregma, 1.2 mm lateral to the midline, and 7.8 mm ventral from the skull surface (Paxinos and Watson, 1986).

Fifteen days later, the rats were challenged with apomorphine (0.05 mg/kg s.c). and contralateral turns in 1 h were used to monitor the outcome of the unilateral parkinsonism. Only those rats that turned under apomorphine (at least 400 turn/h) were selected for further experimental steps.

Rats were treated either s.c. or i.c.v with various doses of the DA agonist, lisuride (200, 100, 50, 33.3, 16.6, 3.3 μg/kg, $N = 4$–6 for each dose). The i.c.v. administration was carried out by implanting rats with guide cannulas (external diameter = 0.71 mm), which were stereotaxically implanted through a hole drilled in the skull and secured with an anchor screw and dental acrylic. Thus the guide cannula was placed in the lateral ventricle at the following stereotaxic coordinates: 0.8 mm posterior to the bregma, 1.4 mm lateral to the midline, and 3.5 mm ventral from the skull surface (Paxinos and Watson, 1986). Rats were allowed to recover for at least 2 days after surgery.

Lisuride was delivered through an injection cannula (external diameter 0.36 mm) that extended 2 mm below the tip of the guide cannula and it was connected with a polyethylene tubing to a 10 μl Hamilton Syringe driven by a Sage infusion pump. Intracerebroventricular injections were carried for a period of 1 min at the flow rate of 2 μl/min in freely moving animals. After this treatment rats were observed for 1 h to measure turning behavior by an automated rotometer mounted on a hemispherical perspex bowls. We measured the number, the duration, and the latency of rotation.

The outcome of the unilateral striatal denervation was confirmed by the massive loss of tyrosine hydroxylase (TH) immunostaining in the striatum and within neurons of the substantia nigra pars compacta. This was confirmed by measuring striatal DA levels by high-performance liquid chromatography (HPLC) with electrochemical detection. Brains were dissected out and immediately frozen and stored at $-80°C$. Ten millimeter sections were incubated overnight with monoclonal antibodies (1:2000; Sigma), for the detection of TH and then for 1h with secondary antibodies. For the detection of TH (ABC elite kit, Vector Laboratories, Burlingame, CA, USA) 3,3′-diaminobenzidine tetrachloride (DAB) immunostaining was used. Control staining was performed without the primary antibody. Analysis data: Statistical analysis was performed by using one-way analysis of variance (ANOVA) + Dunnet test , $* = P < 0.05$).

RESULTS

We found that administration of lisurde in the lateral ventricle was effective at low doses in stimulating DA receptors.

Latency

s.c.: Lisuride when administered s.c. elicited turning behavior with a time latency, which was dose-dependent. In particular, we found that at the dose of 200 μg/kg the mean of the onset of motor response was <2 min. This latency increased while decreasing the dose of lisuride down to 16.6 μg/kg, which produced a latency of about 20 min before the motor response was induced. When the dose was further reduced to 3.3 μg/Kg we failed to detect any motor activity during 1 h of observation.

i.c.v.: At the dose of 200 μg/kg the average of latency was comparable with s.c. injection (<2 min), however, we did not observe the dramatic delay in the onset of motor response by decreasing the dose. For instance, reducing the dose of lisuride to 100 μg/kg led to a latency of 2.5 min, which did not further increase also decreasing the dose of lisuride at 3.3 μg/kg.

Intensity

s.c.: The administration of lisuride s.c. at the dose of 200 μg/kg led to the highest number of rotation (980/h). This response decreased dose-dependently at 100 and 50 μg/kg down to no rotation at 33.3, 16.6, and 3.3 μg/kg.

i.c.v.: When lisuride was administered i.c.v., it led to a plateau of intensity in the motor response for the dose of 100 μg/kg (same effect as s.c. but obtained with half dose) and we could detect a response that decreased dose-dependently (Number of rotation, FIG. 1).

Duration s.c.: After s.c. administration the duration of turning reached 1 h for the dose of 200 μg/kg. This effect corresponded to the maximal response since the plateau of the duration was reached already for 50 μg/kg, while it decreased dose-dependently down to 0 for the dose of 3.3 μg/kg.

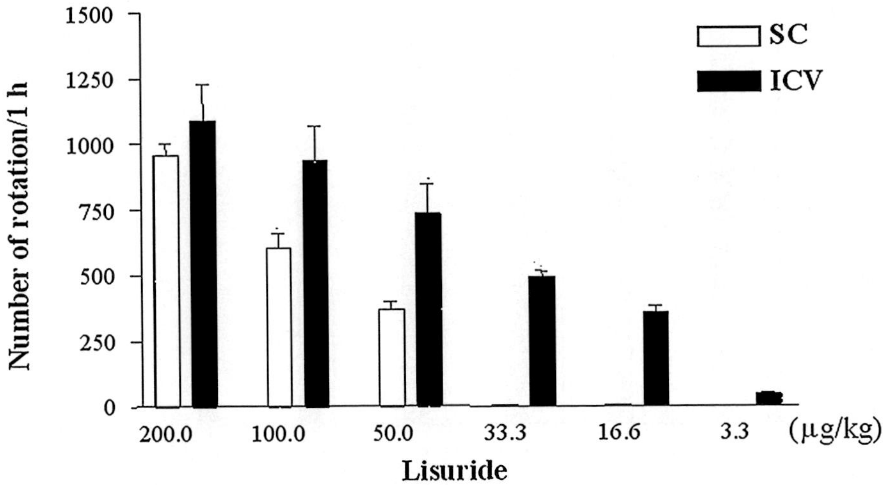

FIGURE 1. Effects of various doses of lisuride s.c. or i.c.v. infusion on the intensity of the motor response (number of rotation in 1 h).

i.c.v.: The effects of i.c.v. injections were most evident in the duration compared with all other motor features: as usual the maximal response was reached with lower doses compared with s.c., but, most remarkably, we could detect a widening of the response window. In fact, the s.c. route did not further increase the duration even for doses up to fourfold. In contrast, the i.c.v. infusion even for low doses led to a duration of the motor response which was double of the maximal effect induced following the s.c. This long-lasting motor activity following i.c.v. administration was already present following the dose of 33.3 μg/kg. (FIG. 2).

DISCUSSION

The present data demonstrate that lisuride can be administered i.c.v. where it is able to stimulate the CNS leading to an effect that is significantly stronger compared with s.c. injections. In particular, when looking at the time of onset and the intensity of the motor response we found that the i.c.v. administration was able to reach the same effect as the s.c. injection but with an average of half dose. This result, important for drug development, was expected in light of the absence of the blood–brain barrier affecting the penetration of the drug. Unexpectedly, though, when examining the duration of the motor response this was beyond the result of any dose of lisuride administered s.c. In fact, when lisuride was administered i.c.v we found a plateau effect (around 200 min of rotation) that was not possible to achieve with any dose of lisuride administered s.c. Namely, s.c. lisuride led to a plateau in the duration of the

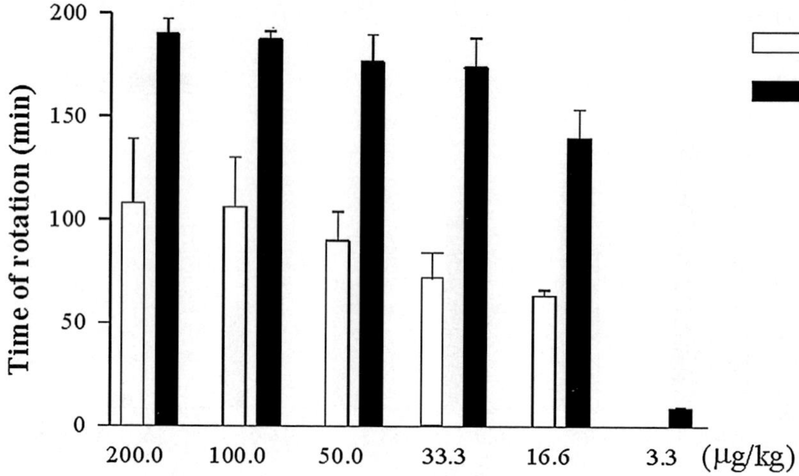

FIGURE 2. Effects of various doses of lisuride s.c. or i.c.v. infusion on the duration of the motor response (time of rotation).

motor response (around 100 min), which did not further increase even when the dose was increased fourfold. These latter data remain difficult to explain and suggest that when administered i.c.v., lisuride leads to an effect that is more powerful. This seems to involve different mechanisms that cannot be recruited by any dose of lisuride when it is administered s.c. In other words, while the latency and the intensity of the motor response are merely dose-dependent, the duration of the motor response is both dose- and route-dependent, since it cannot be replicated by any dose of lisuride using the s.c. route. One point that is worth investigating concerns the recruitment of other brain areas critical for the persistence of motor activity, which might be difficult or impossible to reach by the DA agonist coming from outside the blood–brain barrier. Alternatively, one might hypothesize that only following the i.c.v. route of administration a sort of short-term potentiation is elicited leading to a self-sustaining motor activity.

These data lend substance to the future development of i.c.v. injections as a novel route of administration of DA agonists allowing lower dosages and more reliable steady-state levels for continuous infusions. Continuous stimulation of DA receptor is a valid tool to reduce the onset of dyskinesia, to ameliorate the withdrawal from cocaine and amphetamines, and to prevent the onset of hedonistic homeostatic dysregulation. This can been carried out via s.c. pumps; however, this therapeutic approach is limited by local side effects as well as peripheral side effects in order to produce an efficacious stimulation of the DA receptors in the CNS. This preliminary study provides evidence for the efficacy of continuous low dosage i.c.v. DA stimulation as a safer and reliable therapeutic approach, which discloses intriguing effects concerning the duration of the motor response.

ACKNOWLEDGMENT

NeuroBiotec GmbH Tegeler Strasse 6 D-13353 Berlin is gratefully acknowledged for supporting this study.

REFERENCES

1. KOOB, G.F. & M. LE MOAL. 1997. Drug abuse: hedonic homeostatic dysregulation. Science **278:** 52–68.
2. BEARN, J., A. EVANS, M. KELLEHER, *et al.* 2004. Recognition of a dopamine replacement therapy dependence syndrome in Parkinson's disease: a pilot study. Drug Alcohol Depend. **76:** 305–310.
3. GROSSET, K. & D. GROSSET. 2005. Hedonistic homeostatic dysregulation in Parkinson's disease and excess dopamine replacement therapy. Mov. Disord. **20:** 1230–1231.
4. PEZZELLA, F.R., C. COLOSIMO, N. VANACORE, *et al.* 2005. Prevalence and clinical features of hedonistic homeostatic dysregulation in Parkinson's disease. Mov. Disord. **20:** 77–81.
5. HANSON, G.R., L.A. MATSUDA & J.W. GIBB. 1987. Effects of cocaine on methamphetamine-induced neurochemical changes: characterization of cocaine as a monoamine uptake blocker. J. Pharmacol. Exp. Ther. **242:** 507–513.
6. WEISS, F. & G.F. KOOB. 2001. Drug addiction: functional neurotoxicity of the brain reward systems. Neurotox. Res. **3:** 145–156.
7. GIOVANNONI, G., J.D. O'SULLIVAN, *et al.* 2000. Hedonistic homeostatic dysregulation in patients with Parkinson's disease on dopamine replacement therapies. J. Neurol. Neurosurg. Psychiatry **68:** 423–428.
8. BAUMANN, M.H., J.M. PHILLIPS, M.A. AYESTAS, *et al.* 2002. Preclinical evaluation of GBR12909 decanoate as a long-acting medication for methamphetamine dependence. Ann. N.Y. Acad. Sci. **965:** 92–108.
9. BAUMANN, M.H., M.A. AYESTAS, L.G., SHARPE, *et al.* 2002. Persistent antagonism of methamphetamine-induced dopamine release in rats pretreated with GBR12909 decanoate. J. Pharmacol. Exp. Ther. **301:** 1190–1197.
10. HSIN, L.W., C.M. DERSCH, M.H. BAUMANN, *et al.* 2002. Development of long-acting dopamine transporter ligands as potential cocaine-abuse therapeutic agents: chiral hydroxyl-containing derivatives of 1-[2-[bis(4-fluorophenyl) methoxy]ethyl]-4-(3-phenylpropyl)piperazine and 1-[2-(diphenylmethoxy) ethyl]-4-(3-phenylpropyl)piperazine. J. Med. Chem. **45:** 1321–1329.
11. HOROWSKI, R., C.D. MARSDEN & J.A. OBESO. 1988. Continuous dopaminergic stimulation: state of the art and outlook. J. Neural Transm. Suppl. **27:** 249–252.
12. SCHELOSKY, L. & W. POEWE. 1993. Current strategies in the drug treatment of advanced Parkinson's disease-new modes of dopamine substitution. Acta Neurol. Scand. Suppl. **146:** 46–49.
13. STOCCHI, F., S. RUGGIERI, L. VACCA & C.W. OLANOW. 2002. Prospective randomized trial of lisuride infusion versus oral levodopa in patients with Parkinson's disease. Brain **125:** 2058–2066.
14. KATZENSCHLAGER, R., A. HUGHES, A. EVANS, *et al.* 2005. Continuous subcutaneous apomorphine therapy improves dyskinesias in Parkinson's disease: a prospective study using single-dose challenges. Mov. Disord. **20:** 151–157.

Nigrostriatal Damage with 6-OHDA

Validation of Routinely Applied Procedures

FEDERICA FULCERI,[a] FRANCESCA BIAGIONI,[b] PAOLA LENZI,[a] ALESSANDRA FALLENI,[a] MARCO GESI,[a] STEFANO RUGGIERI,[b] AND FRANCESCO FORNAI[a,b]

[a]*Department of Human Morphology and Applied Biology, University of Pisa, 56126 Pisa, Italy*

[b]*Laboratory of Neurobiology of Movement Disorders, I.R.C.C.S I.N.M. Neuromed, 86077 Pozzilli, Isernia, Italy*

ABSTRACT: The 6-hydroxydopamine (6-OHDA) model of Parkinson's disease in the rat represents a fundamental tool for investigating the pathophysiology of dopamine denervation. Nevertheless, 6-OHDA can induce also noradrenergic lesions; therefore desmethylimipramine (DMI) is co-administrated as a selective inhibitor of noradrenergic reuptake to protect noradrenaline (NA) fibers neighboring DA neurons and/or axons. The neurotoxin 6-OHDA must be microinfused selectively into the substantia nigra pars compacta (SNpc) or into the medial forebrain bundle (MFB) to determine the nigrostriatal lesion. However, this experimental procedure is invasive and always produces a certain amount of mechanical damage that cannot be prevented by pharmacological approaches. For this reason, we have compared two types of experimental design in which we tested critical steps of the procedures, such as the flow rate. We microinfused rats in MFB with 8 μL of total volume of a solution containing the neurotoxin (infusion rate 2 μL/min in 4 min) according with general practice, and rats microinfused with an amount of 2μL of total volume with a slower rate (0.2 μL/min in 10 min) of infusion. Rats infused with a higher flow rate of infusion underwent striatal NA loss in spite of the administration of DMI. On the contrary, rats infused with a slow infusion flow rate had spared NA axons following DMI. These results suggest that the flow rate and the volume of 6-OHDA infusion are critical to prevent the occurrence of nonspecific mechanical effects.

KEYWORDS: Parkinson's disease; nigrostriatal pathway; 6-hydroxydopamine

Address for correspondence: Francesco Fornai, M.D., Ph.D., Department of Human Morphology and Applied Biology, University of Pisa, Via Roma 55, 56126 Pisa, Italy. Voice: +39-0502218611; fax: +39-0502218606.
e-mail: f.fornai@med.unipi.it

**Ann. N.Y. Acad. Sci. 1074: 344–348 (2006). © 2006 New York Academy of Sciences.
doi: 10.1196/annals.1369.032**

INTRODUCTION

Parkinson's disease (PD) is a neurodegenerative disorder characterized by the loss of nigrostriatal dopaminergic neurons[1] and noradrenergic neurons of locus coeruleus (LC).[2,3] However, the pathogenesis of PD is not completely understood.

Therefore, to understand the pathophysiology of PD and to develop novel therapies to improve movement disorders, it is important to have an animal model that reproduces parkinsonian motor deficits and selective of dopamine (DA) neurons. Since its first description,[4] the 6-hydroxydopamine (6-OHDA) model of PD in the rat represents an important tool to study the loss of catecholamine neurons of the nigrostriatal pathway.[5]

The chemical structure of 6-OHDA is analogous to those of catecholaminergic neurotransmitters, in fact the membrane uptake systems of catecholaminergic neurons can transport 6-OHDA into these cells.[6] Then 6-OHDA is very rapidly oxidized producing free radicals and hydrogen peroxidase, which affect proteins, membrane lipids, and DNA. The neurotoxin needs to be microinfused selectively into the substantia nigra pars compacta (SNpc) or into the medial forebrain bundle (MFB) to determine the nigrostriatal lesion.

Recent experimental and clinical studies pointed out the importance of the LC in modulating PD,[3] so to understand the role of noradrenaline (NA) input in the progression of this disease, it is necessary, during experimental conditions, to reduce the damage of NA fibers.

Since 6-OHDA damages both DA and NA axons in the MFB, investigators use desmethylimipramine (DMI)[7] to prevent the damage to NA neurons (or benztropine to protect DA neurons).[8] However, this experimental procedure is invasive and the flow rate and the volume of 6-OHDA infusion are critical to prevent the occurrence of nonspecific mechanical effects. In fact, when a strong mechanical damage is produced, this cannot be prevented by pharmacological approaches.

For this purpose, under controlled experimental conditions we compared different protocols varying the flow rate and the volume of infusion from those which are applied routinely[9,10] to slower and smaller deliveries.

METHODS AND RESULTS

Male Wistar rats (weight 180 g) were used. Rats were divided into three groups, ten rats each. Two groups were microinfused with 6-OHDA. Only one group was microinfused with saline. Rats were deeply anesthetized with chloral hydrate 8% (400 μL/hg, i.p.) and placed in a stereotaxic apparatus; an injection cannula (0.36 mm external diameter, 17 mm long) was inserted through a hole drilled in the skull, in the right MFB using the following coordinates (in mm): anteroposterior (AP) −4.4; mediolateral (ML) ±1.2; dorsoventral (DV)

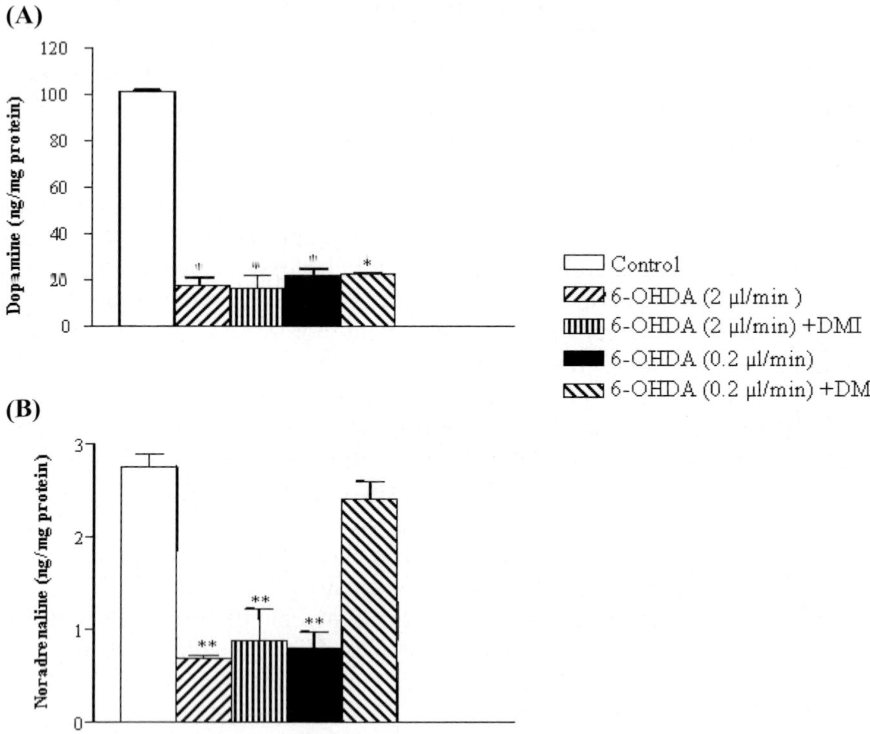

FIGURE 1. Striatal effect of 6-OHDA microinfusion in MFB. **(A)** Biochemical analysis of striatum shows a significant loss of DA terminal after 6-OHDA infusion (infusion rate 2 μL/mL and 0.2 μL/mL). **(B)** DMI injection has protected NE fibers in striatum only when 6-OHDA was infused without mechanic damage. $^{*}P < 0.05$ versus control, $^{**}P < 0.05$ versus control and 6-OHDA (0.2 μL/min) + DMI.

−7.8.[11] The cannula was connected by a polyethylene tubing to a Hamilton (Sigma-Aldrich St. Louis, MO) 10 mL syringe driven by a microinfusion pump. The 6-OHDA was dissolved in 0.01% ascorbic acid (to avoid the toxin was metabolized before being taken up into the cells) at a concentration of 8 μg. We have choice two different volume of infusion: one group was infused with 8 μL of total volume, according to common practice, at a rate of 2μL/min in 4 min, and the other one with 2 μL of total volume, at a slower rate of 0.2 μL/min in 10 min to avoid mechanic damage.

Five rats of each group were treated with DMI (25 mg/kg) 15 min before the microinfusion with 6-OHDA to protect the NA fibers present in MFB.

One month after the surgery, the rats were sacrificed and the striatum processed for HPLC analysis to assess catecholaminergic content.

We found that a slower rate and a smaller volume of infusion protect from mechanical damage, in fact the striatal NA content remains unchanged following

DMI administration in these rats (2.5 ± 0.14 ng/mg protein) while it was reduced without DMI (0.75 ng/mg protein) (FIG. 1).

However, when rats were microinfused with a volume of 8 μL at a faster rate (2 μL/min), we could not detect any protective effects of DMI on striatal NE levels (0.8 ng/mg protein for DMI pretreated rats compared with 0.65 ± 0.25 ng/mg protein for rats which did not receive DMI, respectively) (FIG. 1).

SUMMARY AND CONCLUSION

In this study, we investigated the degeneration of catecholaminergic fibers in MFB after injection of 6-OHDA toxin. The aim was to assess the more appropriate parameters for a selective lesion of DA neurons, with a protection of close NA axons. The use of a lower volume and a slower rate of infusion compared with those applied routinely reduce the mechanical damage and allow to prevent the NA damage by pharmacological tools (DMI).

These data call for more careful injection procedures when interpreting the data obtained through stereotaxic infusions of 6-OHDA, with a special emphasis to the efficacy of real protective effects for NA fibers of co-administration of DMI. In fact in most cases, NA levels are not controlled.

REFERENCES

1. FORNO, L.S. 1992. Neuropathological features of Parkinson's, Huntington's Alzheimer's diseases. Ann. N. Y. Acad. Sci. **648:** 6–16.
2. GESI, M. *et al.* 2000. The role of the locus coeruleus in the development of Parkinson's disease. Neurosci. Biobehav. Rev. **24:** 655–668.
3. ZAROW, C. *et al.* 2003. Neuronal loss is greater in the Locus Coeruleus than nucleus basalis and substantia nigra in Alzheimer and Parkinson disease. Arch. Neurol. **60:** 337–341.
4. UNGERSTEDT, U. 1968. 6-Hydroxydopamine-induced degeneration of central monoamine neurons. Eur. J. Pharmacol. **5:** 107–110.
5. SCHARTING, R.K.W. & J.P. HUSTON. 1996. The unilateral 6-hydroxydopamine lesion model in behavioural brain research. Analysis of functional deficits, recovery and treatments. Prog. Neurobiol. **50:** 275–331.
6. SCHARTING, R.K.W. & J.P. HUSTON. 1996. Unilateral 6-OHDA lesions model of meso-striatal dopamine neurons and their physiological sequelae. Prog. Neurobiol. **49:** 215–266.
7. TAGHZOUTI, K. *et al.* 1991. Suppression of noradrenergic innervation compensates for behavioural deficits induced by lesion dopaminergic terminals in the lateral septum. Brain Res. **552:** 124–128.
8. HERNANDEZ, L. & B.G. HOEBEL. 1982. Overeating after midbrain 6-hydroxydopamine: prevention by central injection of selective catecholamine reuptake blockers. Brain Res. **245:** 333–343.

9. DELFINO, M.A. *et al.* 2004. Behavioural sensitization to different dopamine agonists in a parkinsonian rodent model of drug-induced dyskinesia. Behav. Brain Res. **152:** 297–306.
10. ARAI, A. *et al.* 2003. Amantidine increases L-DOPA-derived extracellular dopamine in the striatum of 6-hydroxydopamine-lesioned rats. Brain Res. **972:** 229–234.
11. PAXINOS, G. & C. WATSON. 1986. The Rat Brain in Stereotaxic Coordinates. Academic. San Diego.

Calpain Activation in Apoptosis of Motoneurons in Cell Culture Models of Experimental Parkinsonism

SUPRITI SAMANTARAY,[a] SWAPAN K. RAY,[a] SYED F. ALI,[b] AND NAREN L. BANIK[a]

[a]*Department of Neurosciences, Division of Neurology, Medical University of South Carolina, Charleston, South Carolina 29425, USA*

[b]*Neurochemistry Laboratory, Division of Neurotoxicology, National Center for Toxicological Research-FDA, Jefferson, Arkansas 72079, USA*

ABSTRACT: Parkinson's disease (PD) is a movement disorder characterized by progressive degeneration of primarily the dopaminergic neurons in the substantia nigra (SN). The present study briefly describes our findings to support the hypothesis that there is a possibility of degeneration of spinal cord (SC) motoneurons in course of parkinsonism. In cell culture models of experimental parkinsonism, we examined the degeneration of ventral SC motoneuron cell line (VSC4.1) following exposure to two different toxins, such as 1-methyl-4-phenyl-1,2,3,6-tetrahydropyridine (MPTP) and rotenone. Our studies suggested calpain activation in the apoptosis of VSC4.1 motoneurons due to exposure to these parkinsonian toxins. Furthermore, our study showed the toxic effects of the dopaminergic toxin methamphetamine (METH) on VSC4.1 cells. The results strongly implicated a possible role for calpain in the mechanism of motoneuron apoptosis during parkinsonian degeneration, at large. Hence, we examined the neuroprotective efficacy of calpeptin, a specific inhibitor of calpain, in cell culture model of experimental parkinsonism.

KEYWORDS: apoptosis; calpain; parkinsonism; METH; MPTP; motoneurons; rotenone; VSC4.1 cells

INTRODUCTION

Parkinson's disease (PD) is the second most common neurodegenerative disorder, primarily associated with progressive loss of dopaminergic neurons

Address for correspondence: Naren L. Banik, Ph.D., Department of Neurosciences, Division of Neurology, Medical University of South Carolina, 96 Jonathan Lucas Street, Charleston, SC 29425. Voice: 843-792-7594; fax: 843-792-8626.
e-mail: baniknl@musc.edu

Ann. N.Y. Acad. Sci. 1074: 349–356 (2006). © 2006 New York Academy of Sciences.
doi: 10.1196/annals.1369.034

in the substantia nigra (SN).[1] It leads to development of motor disorder symptoms, such as tremor, rigidity, bradykinesia, and postural instability.[2] Existing therapeutic modalities are largely symptomatic, which does not halt the disease progression; hence, development of newer therapies is warranted. During progession of PD, motoneurons of the spinal cord (SC), which is the final motor co-ordinator, may also be dying. We hypothesize a possibility of motoneuron degeneration, in addition to SN in brain, in course of this disease. There are a few discrete bodies of evidences from clinical studies showing SC degeneration in PD patients, such as presence of Lewy bodies in intermedio-lateral and -medial nuclei as well as in anterior horn,[3] and degenerated mono-aminergic pathways in lumbar SC.[4] Furthermore, modified excitability of spinal interneuronal pathways in PD patients has been reported.[5] However, relevant experimental studies are lacking to delineate the neurodegeneration in SC and to understand the activation of proteolytic mechanism in SC in addition to the brain nuclei in parkinsonism. Our present study was aimed at testing our hypothesis in two different models of experimental parkinsonism induced by the neurotoxin MPTP and the environmental toxin rotenone. We also compared our findings with the effect of the drug methamphetamine (METH), which is known to exhibit dopaminergic toxicity.[6] Use of calpeptin, an inhibitor of calpain, provided neuroprotection to VSC4.1 motoneurons exposed to the toxins.

EXPERIMENTAL PARKINSONISM

The pathophysiology of PD can be experimentally induced in cell culture and animal models, often referred as experimental parkinsonism. Both MPTP[7] and rotenone[8] can induce characteristic nigrostriatal degeneration and behavioral anomalies akin to clinical PD in a range of laboratory animals. However, the models differ greatly in features, such as being acute or chronic and progressive; dopamine transporter-mediated or independent; presence or absence of the α-synnuclein containing inclusion bodies; selective or systemic inhibition of the mitochondrial complex-I, as well as others.[9–11] Thus, we have conceived the idea of testing the hypothesis of degeneration of SC motoneurons in PD by investigating our concept currently in motoneuron cell culture models using different toxins that are also known to be detrimental to dopaminergic neurons. The findings from motoneuron degeneration with MPTP, rotenone, and METH may eventually help us validate the concept in animal models of experimental parkinsonism.

INVOLVEMENT OF CALPAIN ACTIVITY IN SC DEGENERATION IN ANIMAL MODELS OF PD

Calpain, a Ca^{2+} activated neutral protease has been implicated in various models of neurodegeneration.[12] A total of 15 ubiquitous and tissue-specific calpains have been identified to date.[12] Of the ubiquitous forms, the two major isoforms are micro-calpain (μ-calpain) and milli-calpain (m-calpain), which require μM and mM concentrations for activation, respectively. Each calpain is formed by an 80-kDa catalytic subunit and a 30-kDa regulatory subunit, and regulation is controlled by calpastatin (endogenous inhibitor), lipids, and an activator protein.[12,13] Calpain cleaves many cytoskeletal proteins (α-spectrin, actin, and NFP) and cell signaling proteins, such as caspase-3.[12]

Calpain-mediated pathophysiology has been suggested in PD patients.[14,15] We previously reported increased calpain expression and cell death in SC from cervical and thoracic region of MPTP administered C57BL/6N mice.[16–18] The marked increase in calpain in neuronal population by day 1 led to significant neuronal cell death by day 7. An accompanying gliosis was evident as there was copious calpain expression in astrocytes and microglia by day 1.[18] We further affirmed increased calpain expression and presence of TUNEL positive cells in the lumbar SC of these animals (our unpublished observations). Thus, our findings substantiate the possibility of a calpain-mediated neurodegeneration in SC in addition to SN in MPTP-treated mice.[18] A putative role for calpain in nigrostriatal degeneration in PD is in agreement with others[14,15,19] and in the present study; we focus on the SC motoneuron degeneration with calpain involvement *in vitro* in experimental parkinsonism.

MPTP model being acute and nonprogressive, we are also currently investigating the SC degeneration in male Lewis rats injected subcutaneously with low doses of rotenone (2.5 mg/kg/day). Significant expression of the active calpain has been observed in cervical SC of these animals. A role for calpain in the mechanism of cell death and degenerative process was investigated in METH (20 mg/kg) administered to male C57Bl/6 mice for different time intervals up to a maximum of 1 day. Significant rise in calpain activity was also observed in METH injected animals by 1 h and 2 h. Thus, neurodegeneration of SC with putative involvement of calpain in the degenerative mechanism was observed with three different dopaminergic toxins.

To substantiate our findings of SC degeneration in experimental animals, we studied the cell death mechanisms in the ventral spinal cord (VSC4.1) motoneuron cell line with these toxins. The VSC4.1 motoneurons used in our study was formed by fusion of dissociated embryonic rat ventral SC neuron with mouse N18TG2 neuroblastoma cell.[20] We recently reported calpain-mediated degeneration in this motoneuron cell line following glutamate exposure.[21]

MATERIALS AND METHODS

VSC4.1 cells were gift from Dr. Stanley H. Appel's laboratory of the Department of Neurology, Baylor College of Medicine, Houston, Texas. The motoneurons were grown in monolayer to subconfluency in poly-L-ornithine coated 75-cm^2 flasks containing 10 mL of DMEM/F12 medium with 15 mM HEPES, pyridoxine, and $NaHCO_3$ (Sigma, St. Louis, MO), supplemented with 2%

(A)

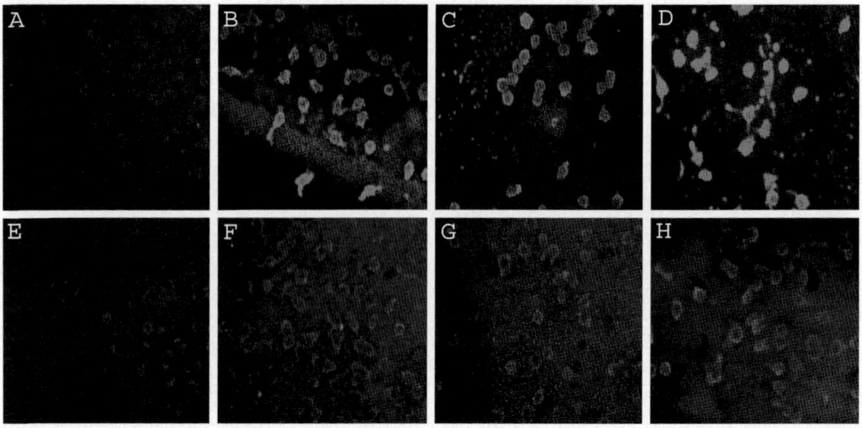

(B)

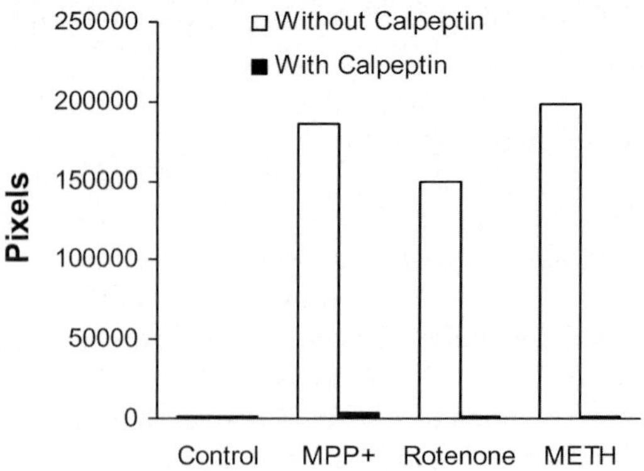

FIGURE 1. **(A)** Increased TUNEL+ cells following exposure of VSC4.1 motoneurons to dopaminergic toxins and calpeptin pretreatment rendered neuroprotection. Immunofluorescent labelings were carried out with monolayers of VSC4.1 cells after TUNEL assay. Cells were treated with MPP^+ (100 μM) (B & F), rotenone (100 nM) (C & G) or METH (500 μM) (D & H) for 12 h. A parallel set of cells were pretreated with 10 mM of calpeptin for 1 h prior to neurotoxin exposure (F-H). No appreciable cell death was observed in control (A) or only calpeptin-treated cells (E). **(B)** Quantitation of pixel values to assess the degeneration of VSC4.1 motoneurons exposed to toxins and neuroprotection with calpain inhibitor.

Sato's components, 1% penicillin and streptomycin (GIBCO-Invitrogen, Grand Island, NY), and 2% heat-inactivated fetal bovine serum (Hyclone, Logan, UT). Cells were incubated in a humidified, water-jacketed incubator at 37°C and with 5% CO_2, and grown upto 60% confluence. This growth medium was replaced with medium containing only 0.5% FBS 24 h before treatment with neurotoxins or calpain inhibitor. This low-serum medium was used both for the dilution of treatment agents and for the remainder of the experiment. Cells were pretreated with 10 μM calpeptin, for 1 h, and the calpeptin-pretreated or untreated cells were subsequently treated with 100 μM MPP^+ or 100 nM rotenone or 500 μM METH for 12 h. After treatments, cells were harvested for evaluation of cell death.

TUNEL ASSAY FOR IDENTIFYING DNA FRAGMENTATION IN APOPTOTIC CELLS

A monolayer of cells was grown on the chamber slide (Nalge Nunc International, Rochester, NY) before actual treatments. Harvested cells in chamber slide after the treatment were spun at low speed and fixed in 95% ethanol for 10 min. Cells were further fixed to the slide by immersing in a freshly prepared 4% methanol-free formaldehyde solution in phosphate buffer solution (PBS), pH 7.4, for 15 min. Slides were washed twice in PBS, before detection of fragmented DNA (high molecular weight or internucleosomal) in the apoptotic cells by incorporating fluorescein-12-dUTP at 3′-OH ends using terminal deoxynucleotidyl transferase (TdT). After TdT-mediated dUTP nick-end labeling (TUNEL) assay with Apoptosis Detection System (Promega, Madison, WI), the cells were visualized directly by fluorescence microscopy, and photographed. The bright red labeling of DNA fragmentation by TUNEL assay indicated cell death.

CALPAIN ACTIVATION DURING VSC4.1 APOPTOSIS

Although the precise physiological functions of calpain remain unclear, it is considered to participate in a number of signaling pathways that are regulated by intracellular Ca^{2+} concentrations.[22,23] Calpain is involved in apoptosis of central nervous system (CNS) cells during injury and in pathological conditions.[12] Apoptotic pathways involve cross-talks between proteins, indicating that calpain and caspases may act together or separately in the mediation of neuronal apoptosis. For instance, calpain has been shown to cleave caspase-3 into active forms.[24] Caspase-3 degrades calpastatin, the endogenous inhibitor of calpain, through proteolysis and further increases calpain activity.[25] Calpain also cleaves capsase-12, which can in turn activate caspase-3-induced apoptosis.[26] We have previously demonstrated a proteolytic role for calpain in apoptosis of neuronal[27] and glial[28] cells.

Whether these neurotoxins, primarily classified as dopaminergic toxin could induce apoptosis in the motoneuron cell line, VSC4.1 was our quest. Furthermore, we wanted to explore if calpain had a role to play as inferred from our observations in animal studies. Hence, we investigated the effects of calpain inhibitor, calpeptin on cell death in VSC4.1 cells exposed to MPP^+, rotenone and METH toxicity in culture. This cell line has so far been used to study the mechanisms in motoneuron disease, amyotrophic lateral sclerosis (ALS) , and SC injury by us and others.[20,21] We wanted to study the effect of parkinsonian toxins on this cell line so as to unravel the SC degeneration in experimental parkinsonism *in vitro*. All the three toxins induced dose-dependent cell death in undifferentiated VSC4.1. Upon differentiation, a much lower dose of the toxins could induce apoptosis. Toxin treatment resulted in a significant upregulation of calpain expression and calpain activity with MPP^+ (100 μM), rotenone (1 μM), and METH (500 μM) by 12 h (FIG. 1). Lower doses of the toxin could induce similar calpain expression when left for longer time period (up to 36 h) thus emphasizing involvement of a calpain-mediated mechanism in subtle and prolonged exposure of these toxins as well. The later sets of experimental design seem to be plausible explanation of parkinsonian degeneration and are currently being tested in differentiated VSC4.1 cells in our laboratory.

CALPAIN INHIBITORS RENDERED NEUROPROTECTION

Calpain inhibition has been shown to render neuroprotection in several acute mode of neurodegeneration by us and others.[21,29–31] Overexpression of the endogenous calpain inhibitor, calpastatin has been reported to render neuroprotection to the nigrostriatal degeneration in MPTP-induced PD.[19] Such protection of neurons by calpain inhibitors has been demonstrated in brain,[29] SC injury,[30] ischemia,[31] and VSC4.1 cells undergoing stress in culture.[21] Inhibition of calpain with calpain inhibitors has been shown to prevent cytoskeletal protein degradation, preserve membrane integrity, and block apoptosis.[12] We studied the neuroprotective efficacy of a specific calpain inhibitor, calpeptin (FIG. 1).[12]

Optimal doses of the neurotoxins MPP^+, rotenone, and METH (Sigma) and calpeptin (Calbiochem, San Diego, CA) were determined for VSC4.1 cells. Cells were treated with toxins with or without calpeptin (10 μM) for 12 h to examine. Cells were harvested at 12 h to study cell death via TUNEL staining. Cells were pretreated for 1 h calpeptin (10 μM) or vehicle then exposed for 12 h with/without MPP^+ (100 μM), rotenone (100 nM) or METH (500 μM). Neurotoxin treatment increased the number of cells staining TUNEL+, compared to control. Calpeptin is a dipeptidyl aldehyde, which is known to be cell permeable and highly specific for inhibition of calpain activity in various cell culture models.[12] Pretreatment of the VSC4.1 cells with calpeptin reduced the number of TUNEL+ cells in all the three groups substantially to the levels similar to control. However, calpeptin alone had no effect on the VSC4.1 cells.

CONCLUSION

Our current studies using the VSC4.1 motoneuron cell line demonstrate the induction of apoptosis by two parkinsonian toxins and one dopaminergic toxin with involvement of calpain. Calpeptin, the specific inhibitor of calpain, could render protection to the motoneurons undergoing apoptosis in culture. The study, though preliminary, scores in favor of our hypothesis of a probable degeneration of the SC motoneuron in experimental parkinsonism and suggests therapeutic potential for calpain inhibitors.

REFERENCES

1. HIRSCH, E.C. *et al.* 1989. Selective vulnerability of pigmented dopaminergic neurons in Parkinson's disease. Acta Neurol. Scand. Suppl. **126:** 19–22.
2. WICHMANN, T. & M.R. DELONG. 1993. Pathophysiology of parkinsonian motor abnormalities. Adv. Neurol. **60:** 53–61.
3. OHAMA, E. & F. IKUTA. 1976. Parkinson's disease: distribution of Lewy bodies and monoamine neuron system. Acta Neuropathol. (Berl.) **34:** 311–319.
4. SCATTON, B. *et al.* 1986. Degeneration of noradrenergic and serotonergic but not dopaminergic neurones in the lumbar spinal cord of parkinsonian patients. Brain Res. **380:** 181–185.
5. DELWAIDE, P.J. *et al.* 1996. From basal ganglia to motoneurons. Probable involvement of pathways relaying in the medulla. Adv. Neurol. **69:** 111–116.
6. IMAM, S.Z. *et al.* 1999. Methamphetamine generates peroxynitrite and produces dopaminergic neurotoxicity in mice: protective effects of peroxynitrite decomposition catalyst. Brain Res. **837:** 15–21.
7. HEIKKILA, R.E. *et al.* 1984. Dopaminergic neurotoxicity of 1-methyl-4-phenyl-1,2,5,6-tetrahydropyridine in mice. Science **224:** 1451–1453.
8. BETARBET, R. *et al.* 2000. Chronic systemic pesticide exposure reproduces features of Parkinson's disease. Nat. Neurosci. **3:** 1301–1306.
9. BETARBET, R. *et al.* 2002. Animal models of Parkinson's disease. Bioessays **24:** 308–318.
10. HIRSCH, E.C. *et al.* 2003. Animal models of Parkinson's disease in rodents induced by toxins: an update. J. Neural. Transm. Suppl. **65:** 89–100.
11. UVERSKY, V.N. 2004. Neurotoxicant-induced animal models of Parkinson's disease: understanding the role of rotenone, maneb and paraquat in neurodegeneration. Cell Tissue Res. **318:** 225–241.
12. RAY, S.K. & N.L. BANIK. 2003. Calpain and its involvement in the pathophysiology of CNS injuries and diseases: therapeutic potential of calpain inhibitors for prevention of neurodegeneration. Curr. Drug Targets CNS Neurol. Disord. **2:** 173–189.
13. MURACHI, T. 1984. Calcium-dependent proteinases and specific inhibitors: calpain and calpastatin. Biochem. Soc. Symp. **49:** 149–167.
14. MOUATT-PRIGENT, A. *et al.* 1996. Increased m-calpain expression in the mesencephalon of patients with Parkinson's disease but not in other neurodegenerative disorders involving the mesencephalon: a role in nerve cell death? Neuroscience **73:** 979–987.
15. MOUATT-PRIGENT, A. *et al.* 2000. Calpastatin immunoreactivity in the monkey and human brain of control subjects and patients with Parkinson's disease. J. Comp. Neurol. **419:** 175–192.

16. RAY, S.K. *et al.* 2000. Calpain upregulation in spinal cords of mice with 1-methyl-4-phenyl-1,2,3,6-tetrahydropyridine (MPTP)-induced Parkinson's disease. Ann. N. Y. Acad. Sci. **914:** 275–283.
17. CHERA, B. *et al.* 2002. Calpain upregulation and neuron death in spinal cord of MPTP-induced parkinsonism in mice. Ann. N. Y. Acad. Sci. **965:** 274–280.
18. CHERA, B. *et al.* 2004. Immunofluorescent labeling of increased calpain expression and neuronal death in the spinal cord of 1-methyl-4-phenyl-1,2,3,6-tetrahydropyridine-treated mice. Brain Res. **1006:** 150–156.
19. CROCKER, S.J. *et al.* 2003. Inhibition of calpains prevents neuronal and behavioral deficits in an MPTP mouse model of Parkinson's disease. J. Neurosci. **23:** 4081–4091.
20. SMITH, R.G. *et al.* 1994. Cytotoxicity of immunoglobulins from amyotrophic lateral sclerosis patients on a hybrid motoneuron cell line. Proc. Natl. Acad. Sci. USA **91:** 3393–3397.
21. DAS, A. *et al.* 2005. Calpain activation in apoptosis of ventral spinal cord 4.1 (VSC4.1) motoneurons exposed to glutamate: calpain inhibition provides functional neuroprotection. J. Neurosci. Res. **81:** 551–562.
22. SORIMACHI, H. *et al.* 1997. Structure and physiological function of calpains. Biochem. J. **328:** 721–732.
23. CARAFOLI, E. & M. MOLINARI. 1998. Calpain: a protease in search of a function? Biochem. Biophys. Res. Commun. **247:** 193–203.
24. BLOMGREN, K. *et al.* 2001. Synergistic activation of caspase-3 by m-calpain after neonatal hypoxia-ischemia: a mechanism of "pathological apoptosis"? J. Biol. Chem. **276:** 10191–10198.
25. WANG, K.K. *et al.* 1998. Caspase-mediated fragmentation of calpain inhibitor protein calpastatin during apoptosis. Arch. Biochem. Biophys. **356:** 187–196.
26. NAKAGAWA, T. & J. YUAN. 2000. Cross-talk between two cysteine protease families. Activation of caspase-12 by calpain in apoptosis. J. Cell Biol. **150:** 887–894.
27. RAY, S.K. *et al.* 2000. Oxidative stress and Ca^{2+} influx upregulate calpain and induce apoptosis in PC12 cells. Brain Res. **852:** 326–334.
28. RAY, S.K. *et al.* 1999. Diverse stimuli induce calpain overexpression and apoptosis in C6 glioma cells. Brain Res. **829:** 18–27.
29. SAATMAN, K.E. *et al.* 1996. Calpain inhibitor AK295 attenuates motor and cognitive deficits following experimental brain injury in the rat. Proc. Natl. Acad. Sci. USA **93:** 3428–3433.
30. RAY, S.K. *et al.* 1999. Calpain activity and translational expression increased in spinal cord injury. Brain Res. **816:** 375–380.
31. BARTUS, R.T. *et al.* 1998. Temporal ordering of pathogenic events following transient global ischemia. Brain Res. **790:** 1–13.

MDMA and Seizures: A Dangerous Liaison?

FILIPPO S. GIORGI,[a,b] GLORIA LAZZERI,[a] GIANFRANCO NATALE,[a] ALFONSO IUDICE,[b] STEFANO RUGGIERI,[c,d] ANTONIO PAPARELLI,[a] LUIGI MURRI,[b] AND FRANCESCO FORNAI[a,d]

[a]*Department of Human Morphology and Applied Biology, University of Pisa, 56126 Pisa, Italy*

[b]*Department of Neurosciences, Section of Neurology, University of Pisa, 56126 Pisa, Italy*

[c]*Department of Neurological Sciences, University of Rome "La Sapienza," 00185 Rome, Italy*

[d]*Laboratory of Neurobiology of Movement Disorders, I.R.C.C.S. I.N.M. Neuromed, 86077 Pozzilli, Isernia, Italy*

ABSTRACT: In the past decades, there was a massive increase in the abuse of methylenedioxymethamphetamine (MDMA) in the Western countries. Seizure onset after MDMA is considered to be related mainly to its acute systemic effects (e.g., hyponatremia and hyperthermia). However, additional mechanisms might concur to it as well. Experiments aimed at disclosing the basis for such an acute effect have the advantage of profiting of controlled conditions and the "pure" compounds, as opposed to the limits of clinical data which are biased by several confounding factors. Amphetamines exert profound effect on different monoaminergic systems, which might participate to lowering of seizure threshold. Chronic effects of MDMA abuse on seizure threshold have not been explored in detail so far. Recent data showed that in mice receiving small, repeated doses of MDMA, a persisting pro-convulsant effect toward limbic seizures and metabolic hyperexcitability can be observed. In the present article, we reviewed these studies and we report our preliminary experimental data documenting the lack of mossy fiber sprouting at short time intervals following MDMA, when seizure susceptibility is already present.

KEYWORDS: MDMA; seizures; serotonin; dopamine; kainate; status epilepticus; limbic system; mossy fiber sprouting

Address for correspondence: Francesco Fornai, M.D. Ph.D., Department of Human Morphology and Applied Biology, University of Pisa, via Roma 55, 56126 Pisa, Italy. Voice: +39-0502218611; fax: +39-0502218606.

e-mail: f.fornai@med.unipi.it

Ann. N.Y. Acad. Sci. 1074: 357–364 (2006).
doi: 10.1196/annals.1369.035

INTRODUCTION

Substituted amphetamines include a variety of compounds, which are abused due to rewarding and socializing effects co-existing with the wrong perception of a safe neurotoxic profile. In the last decade, methylenedioxymethamphetamine (MDMA) has become the most widely abused.[1]

MDMA can produce systemic effects, such as hyperthermia, rhabdomyolysis with acute renal failure, hypertension, seizures, and cerebral hemorrhage, which may lead to lethal cases.[2]

The relative occurrence of these effects after MDMA intake is difficult to be extracted from the existing literature, in light of the kind of papers addressing this problem (mainly anecdotical and case report).

An issue, which is not clear, is the extent of the correlation between MDMA abuse and seizures, and whether MDMA abuse predisposes chronically to spontaneous seizures.

In the following paragraphs, we will address some of the relevant experimental data, which can help to set the point of our current knowledge about such a link between MDMA and seizures.

ACUTE SEIZURES AFTER MDMA INTAKE

Epileptic seizures are the phenotypic manifestation of an excessive and/or hypersyncronous discharge of cortical neurons. Such a discharge can start and remain confined in a circumscribed cortical region or originate/spread from/to the entire cortex. Seizures can be isolated, or recurrent. Epilepsy currently refers to a brain disorder "characterized by an *enduring predisposition* to generate epileptic seizures" and which "requires the occurrence of at least one epileptic seizure" (from the definition proposed by the International League Against Epilepsy in 2005[3]). Seizures can be related to a clear structural cause (e.g., a cortical or extracortical damage) or to non-structural, functional, and often genetic neuronal defects (idiopathic epilepsies). Epileptic seizures can be either unprovoked or provoked by certain stimuli. Among the inducing stimuli, acute metabolic modifications can induce seizures.

The occurrence of seizures in MDMA abusers is commonly attributed to the acute metabolic effects of MDMA. In particular, acute hyponatremia is considered by most researchers the most likely candidate, since it is well known to trigger occasional acute seizures.[4] The pathogenesis of hyponatremia after MDMA consumption has been related to inappropriate secretion of antidiuretic hormone (ADH)[5] associated with increased drinking which occurs frequently in people within hours after MDMA injection.

Concerning MDMA, the most detailed report on the clinical manifestation (including seizures) of such an adverse event in a selected population of patients abusing MDMA is the one provided by Hartung *et al.*[5] The design of the study by itself gives an idea of the difficulties of performing such a study. Data were extrapolated by retrospective reviews of phone inquiries to National Poisons Unit based at Guy's Hospital in London concerning MDMA intoxication. Interestingly, in ~58% of patients in which hyponatremia was confirmed, seizures were part of the early syndrome. It should be noted that all of them were generalized tonic-clonic seizures, although occurrence of previous seizures in those patients was not investigated.

Another potential cause for seizure onset following MDMA is hyperthermia, which is well described[6] despite the lack of solid correlative studies with the onset of seizures.

Finally, a potential link between acute seizure susceptibility and MDMA intake might be related to the well-known effect of MDMA on brain monoamine systems. In fact, several experimental and clinical studies have addressed the role of monoamines in modulating seizure threshold. Such a modulatory role has been documented for serotonin (5-HT) and norepinephrine (NE), while conflicting data exist concerning the role of dopamine (DA).[7,8]

NE is known to play significant role in modulating experimental seizures, since it exerts a general inhibitory role on seizure onset and spreading.[7,9] In the last decades, a lot of data have been produced concerning the role of 5-HT in modulating seizures, and even though the first evidences for such an effect have been produced more than 20 years ago, the relevance of such a role is probably still underestimated. In fact, 5-HT inhibits seizures produced by different models, such as generalized tonic-clonic seizures in genetically epileptic prone rats[7] and focal limbic seizures elicited from the anterior piriform cortex in rats.[10] Moreover, a clear impairment of the brain 5-HT system has been demonstrated to be directly involved in the lower seizure threshold of genetically epileptic prone rats.[11]

The role of DA in modulating seizures is less defined; however, it possesses pro-convulsant effect within specific brain areas.[8]

In light of these data, it should be considered that extracellular monoamines peak within 2 h after MDMA administration in a dose-dependent manner.[12,13] Following this extracellular increase, there is a loss of monoamine transmission in the central nervous system (CNS); thus, seizures might be induced both by early DA release and by the following 5-HT and NE depletion.

Apart from the mechanism underlying seizures in humans abusing MDMA, this effect has been replicated also in animal models. However, only a few studies analyzed the mechanisms of MDMA-induced seizures. In line with this, it is worth to mention a detailed study recently performed in mice[14] which demonstrated that: (*a*) acute seizures induced by MDMA occur quickly; (*b*) behavioral features consist both of running-bouncing/rolling and clonic episodes, thus suggesting a generalized origin; and (*c*) as compared with other stimulants, such as cocaine and methamphetamine, MDMA needs a higher dosage of administration to induce seizures.

POTENTIAL MECHANISMS UNDERLYING DECREASED SEIZURE THRESHOLD IN MDMA ABUSERS

The lack of clinical studies concerning potential chronic lowering of seizure threshold after MDMA is due mainly to two facts: (*a*) previous abuse of psychostimulants is not commonly explored during studies on epilepsy, and (*b*) even in the case that such a connection might be evaluated in clinical studies, the fact that MDMA abusers are often poly-drugs abusers, and the presence of contaminants in the "ecstasy" pills available in the illicit market would significantly bias any findings of these studies.

As a consequence, apart from a very recent investigation[15] (see later), to our knowledge no clinical or experimental studies investigated chronic effects of amphetamine derivatives on seizure threshold.

When looking reports on seizure onset following MDMA, the general interpretation relates to chronic toxicity on monoamine systems. The chronic effects of MDMA on brain monoamines are well established and they depend on the animal species. For instance, MDMA induces chronic depletion of 5-HT in several brain areas in the rat and therefore is used as 5-HT neurotoxin in this species. Conversely, several studies in the last decades have shown that in mice methamphetamine and MDMA produce a chronic depletion of DA in the striatum and cortical areas, much higher than on 5-HT terminals.[16]

Concerning humans, big efforts have been done in the last decades to understand the pattern of monoamine toxicity of methamphetamine and MDMA, by profiting of direct measurements in primates and indirect data collected in humans. In particular, direct measurements have been performed after different routes of administrations and dosages of MDMA in primates. At present, it appears likely that MDMA exerts chronic depleting brain effects mainly on 5-HT terminals, while DA terminals are relatively spared,[17] thus more closely resembling what observed in rats than in mice. Such neurotoxicity presents, however, some differences as compared to what observed in rodents. The dose required in M. Rhesus to induce a significant 5-HT loss is significantly lower than in rats.[17,18] Moreover, the recovery of 5-HT levels is significantly slower than in rodents.[19] In humans, direct evaluations of monoamines and metabolites levels, which are related to the brain content of 5-HT, have been performed in the cerebrospinal fluid (CSF) of MDMA abusers,[20] showing a depletion of 5-HT metabolites, in populations homogeneous for sex and age and where particular care was taken to include patients lacking psychiatric co-morbidities.[20] Thus, at least potentially, the chronic depleting effects of MDMA on brain 5-HT might be relevant in lowering seizure threshold both in experimental animals and humans.

In a very recent study, we profit from controlled experimental conditions to address the chronic alterations induced by MDMA on brain excitability as a potential substrate to explain seizure susceptibility.

With this aim, we developed an experimental protocol to evaluate the persisting effects of MDMA on seizures susceptibility in mice.

CHRONIC SEIZURE SUSCEPTIBILITY AFTER REPEATED "LOW" DOSES OF MDMA IN MICE

Recent data obtained in mice disclosed the occurrence of a persistent hyperexcitability of limbic structures in mice treated with MDMA.[15]

Adult C57 Black mice were injected i.p. with MDMA, 5 mg/kg × 2, 2 h apart, for 1, 2, or 3 consecutive days. Mice were administered with i.p. injections of kainic acid (KA) 2 weeks after MDMA administration. Such a time interval between MDMA injection and the challenge with KA was selected to rule out any potential interference of MDMA itself, or its metabolites, on seizures. The dosage of KA selected (5 and 10 mg/kg) were way subthreshold for eliciting seizures in control mice used in this study (C57 Black), which are "resistant" to limbic seizures.[21] Interestingly, all of the mice administered with the intermediate (5 mg/kg × 4) and highest (5 mg/kg × 6) dose of MDMA, and even a few of those injected with 5 mg/kg × 2, exhibited seizures. However, only the highest dose of MDMA (5 mg/kg × 6) induced a significant 5-HT loss in selected brain areas (hippocampus and striatum), while in mice administered with lower doses (5 mg/kg × 2 and 5 mg/kg × 4) 5-HT levels were similar to controls in all of the areas examined. This suggests that 5-HT loss may be not the specific mechanism by which seizure threshold is modified in this experimental setting. Similarly, DA loss was non-related to seizures[15] and NE loss does not occur.[22] Of course, repeated release of these monoamines might have contributed to altered brain excitability despite the absence of monoamine terminals damage.

THE AIM OF THE PRESENT STUDY: TO CORRELATE SEIZURES SUSCEPTIBILITY WITH MOSSY FIBERS SPROUTING

In mice, it has been shown that dosages, which are able to induce status epilepticus (SE), are usually associated with a high mortality[21] and to high seizure score. Interestingly, MDMA pre-treated mice, which experience seizures after KA, never showed generalized tonic-clonic seizures of the four limbs, and this was the case also in the few animals which developed status epilepticus (i.e., seizures lasting more than 30 min without interruption),[15] this suggesting a specific hyperexcitability in limbic structures. Finally, the mortality due to KA in MDMA pre-treated mice, including also mice which developed SE, was similar to controls. Experimental data collected in animal models of limbic seizures/SE have documented an association between a persistent lowering of threshold to limbic seizures, and specific structural changes occurring at the level of the hippocampus. In particular, it has been observed that a persistent excitability is associated to "mossy fiber sprouting" (MFS).[23] MFS consists in the formation of abnormal recurrent collaterals from the glutamatergic mossy fibers originating from the granule cells of the dentate gyrus.[24] Due to the selective presence of zinc in mossy fiber terminals, mossy fibers (and MFS) can be selective stained by Timm staining, a histochemical technique which selectively stains zinc-containing fibers.[25] In the present study, we evaluated whether hippocampal MFS could be one of the effects of a previous MDMA injection to C57Black mice. Therefore, we injected mice with 5 mg/kg × 2 for either 2 or 3 days and we sacrificed the animals 2 weeks later. Furthermore, we performed Timm staining in mice, which had been injected with MDMA 5 mg/kg × 2 for 3 days, underwent seizures following KA (10 mg/kg) 2 weeks later, and were sacrificed 4 weeks after seizures. We could not observe the occurrence of MFS in any of the animals treated with MDMA alone. Moreover, even in animals which had been previously injected with MDMA and undergoing SE by KA injection 2 weeks later, no MFS could be detected at 4 weeks after seizure induction (FIG. 1).

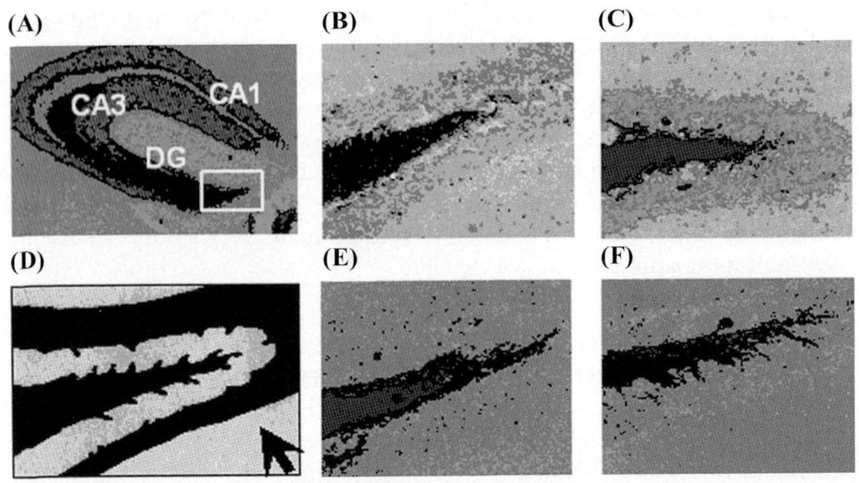

FIGURE 1. Lack of an effect of MDMA by itself and KA-induced seizures in MDMA pre-treated mice on MFS. Timm staining reveals, in black, the distribution of mossy fibers in the hilus of the hippocampus in a control mouse (**A** and **B**, which is a detail of **A** at higher magnification). In a representative mouse pre-treated with MDMA 5 mg/kg, i.p. × 2, for 3 consecutive days, no MFS toward the dentate gyrus molecular layer can be observed 2 weeks after injection (**C**). In panel **D**, there is a schematic drawing of the distribution of mossy fiber terminals in the inner molecular layer of the dentate gyrus in the presence of MFS (arrow), as it can be found chronically after KA-induced SE in rats. In control mice injected with KA (10 mg/kg, i.p.) (panel **E**) or in mice pre-treated with MDMA (5 mg/kg, i.p. × 2, for 3 consecutive days) (panel **F**), and experiencing seizures 2 weeks later after kainic acid injection (10 mg/kg, i.p.), no MFS was observed at 4 weeks after KA.

MFS is considered to occur at its highest degree several weeks after an initial SE. We evaluated its occurrence at 2 weeks after MDMA injection, since this is the time interval when we observed a reduced threshold to KA in MDMA pre-treated mice[15]: further studies are in progress at longer time interval. Moreover, the critical role of MFS in limbic hyperexcitability has been questioned.[26] Therefore, evaluation of MFS represents just one of several experimental approaches we are undertaking to document a correlation between epileptogenesis due to brain hyperexcitability induced by MDMA and neuronal plasticity. An evaluation of MFS occurrence at longer time points after MDMA alone or MDMA+KA is required to clarify the role, if any, of this phenomenon in the chronic effects of a previous MDMA administration on KA seizures.

REFERENCES

1. LANDRY, M.J. 2002. MDMA: a review of epidemiologic data. J. Psychoactive Drugs **34:** 163–169.
2. BURGESS, C. *et al.* 2000. Agony and ecstasy: a review of MDMA effects and toxicity. Eur. Psychiatry **15:** 287–294.
3. FISHER, R.S. *et al.* 2005. Epileptic seizures and epilepsy: definitions proposed by the International League Against Epilepsy (ILAE) and the International Bureau for Epilepsy (IBE). Epilepsia **46:** 470–472.
4. LEVINSKY, N.G. 1994. Fluids and electrolytes. *In* Harrison's Principles of Internal Medicine, 13th ed. K.J. Isselbacher, *et al.*, Eds.: 101–118 Mc Graw-Hill. New York.
5. HARTUNG, T.K. *et al.* 2002. Hyponatraemic states following 3,4-methylenedioxymethamphetamine (MDMA, 'ecstasy') injestion. Q. J. Med. **95:** 431–437.
6. DAFTERS, R.I. 1994. Effect of ambient temperature on hyperthermia and hyperkinesis induced by 3,4-methylenedioxymethamphetamine (MDMA or "ecstasy") in rats. Psychopharmacology **114:** 505–508.
7. JOBE, P.C. & R.A. BROWNING. 2005. The serotonergic and noradrenergic effects of antidepressant drugs are anticonvulsant, not proconvulsant. Epilepsy Behav. **7:** 602–619.
8. STARR, M.S. 1996. The role of dopamine in epilepsy. Synapse **22:** 159–194.
9. GIORGI, F.S. *et al.* 2004. The role of norepinephrine in epilepsy: from the bench to the bedside. Neurosci. Biobehav. Rev. **28:** 507–524.
10. PRENDIVILLE, S. & K. GALE. 1993. Anticonvulsant effect of systemic fluoxetine on focally-evoked limbic motor seizure in rats. Epilepsia **34:** 381–384.
11. DAILEY, J.W. *et al.* 1992. Effects of fluoxetine on convulsions and brain serotonin as detected by microdialysis in genetically epilepsy-prone rats. J. Pharmacol. Exp. Ther. **260:** 533–540.
12. SCHMIDT, C.J. *et al.* 1994. Blockade of striatal 5-hydroxytryptamine 2 receptors reduces the increase in extracellular concentrations of dopamine produced by the amphetamine analogue 3,4-methylenedioxymethamphetamine. J. Neurochem. **62:** 1382–1389.
13. GUDELSKY, G.A. & J.F. NASH. 1996. Carrier-mediated release of serotonin by 3,4,-methylenedioxymethamphetamine: implications for serotonin-dopamine interactions. J. Neurochem. **66:** 243–249.

14. HANSON, G.R. *et al.* 1999. Distinct features of seizures induced by cocaine and amphetamine analogs. Eur. J. Pharmacol. **377:** 167–173.
15. GIORGI, F.S. *et al.* 2005. Previous exposure to (±) 3,4-methylenedioxymethamphetamine produces long-lasting alteration in limbic brain excitability measured by electroencephalogram spectrum analysis, brain metabolism and seizure susceptibility. Neuroscience **136:** 43–53.
16. COLADO, M.I. *et al.* 2001. A study of the mechanisms involved in the neurotoxic effects of 3,4 methylenedioxymethamphetamine (MDMA, ecstasy) on dopamine neurons in mouse brain. Br. J. Pharmacol. **134:** 1711–1723.
17. ALI, S.F. *et al.* 1993. Oral administration of 3,4-methylenedioxymethamphetamine (MDMA) produces selective serotonergic depletion in the nonhuman primate. Neurotoxicol. Teratol. **15:** 91–96.
18. RICAURTE, G.A. *et al.* 1988. (±)3,4-Methylenedioxymethamphetamine selectevely damages central serotonergic neurons in nonhuman primates. JAMA **260:** 51–56.
19. RICAURTE, G.A. *et al.* 1992. Lasting effects of (±)3,4-methylenedioxymethamphetamine (MDMA) on central serotoninergic neurons in nonhuman primates: neurochemical observations. J. Pharmacol. Exp. Ther. **261:** 616–622.
20. MCCANN, U.D. *et al.* 1994. Serotonin neurotoxicity after (±)3,4-methylenedioxymethamphetamine (MDMA; "Ecstasy"): a controlled study in humans. Neuropsychopharmacology **10:** 129–138.
21. MCKHANN, G.M. *et al.* 2003. Mouse strain differences in kainic acid sensitivity, seizure behaviour, mortality, and hippocampal pathology. Neuroscience **122:** 551–561.
22. FORNAI, F. *et al.* 2001. Biochemical effects of the monoamine neurotoxins DSP-4 and MDMA in specific brain regions of MAO-B-deficient mice. Synapse **39:** 213–221.
23. TAUCK, D.L. & J.V. NADLER. 1985. Evidence of functional mossy fiber sprouting in hippocampal formation of kainic acid-treated rats. J. Neurosci. **5:** 1016–1022.
24. NADLER, J.V. *et al.* 1980. Selective reinnervation of hippocampal area CA1 and the fascia dentata after destruction of CA3-CA4 afferents with kainic acid. Brain Res. **182:** 1–9.
25. DANSCHER, G. 1981. Histochemical demonstration of heavy metals: a revised version of the sulphide silver method suitable for both light and electronmicroscopy. Histochemistry **71:** 1–16.
26. LONGO, B.M. & L.E. MELLO. 1998. Supragranular mossy fiber sprouting is not necessary for spontaneous seizures in the intrahippocampal kainate model of epilepsy in the rat. Epilepsy Res. **32:** 172–182.

Neural Effects of MDMA as Determined by Functional Magnetic Resonance Imaging and Magnetic Resonance Spectroscopy in Awake Marmoset Monkeys

JERROLD S. MEYER,[a,b] MATTHEW E. BREVARD,[c] BRIAN J. PIPER,[b] SYED F. ALI,[d] AND CRAIG F. FERRIS[c]

[a]*Department of Psychology, University of Massachusetts, Amherst, Massachusetts 01003, USA*

[b]*Neuroscience and Behavior Program, University of Massachusetts, Amherst, Massachusetts 01003, USA*

[c]*Center for Comparative Neuroimaging, University of Massachusetts Medical School, Worcester, Massachusetts 01655, USA*

[d]*Division of Neurotoxicology, National Center for Toxicological Research, Food and Drug Administration, Jefferson, Arkansas 72079, USA*

ABSTRACT: We used functional magnetic resonance imaging (fMRI) to investigate the acute effects of a recreational dose (1 mg/kg p.o.) of 3,4-methylenedioxymethamphetamine (MDMA) on regional brain activity in awake, restrained marmoset monkeys. In a second study, magnetic resonance spectroscopy (MRS) and postmortem measurements of serotonin transporter (SERT) binding and serotonin (5-HT) concentrations were used to determine the neurotoxic effects of low (4 × 1 mg/kg p.o.) and high (4 × 10 mg/kg i.m.) doses of MDMA. Several brain areas were significantly activated by the low oral dose of MDMA, including the midbrain raphe nuclei, hippocampus, hypothalamus, amygdala, and the corticostriatal circuit composed of the dorsal thalamus, sensory motor cortex, and basal ganglia. MDMA activated the primary visual cortex under baseline conditions and also enhanced the visual cortical response to photic stimulation. The onset of brain activation correlated well with the rise in plasma MDMA concentrations measured in separate monkeys given the same drug treatment. In the second study, the ratio of *N*-acetylaspartate (NAA; a putative neuronal marker) to creatine was significantly reduced in the hypothalamus following either MDMA treatment regimen, suggesting a particular vulnerability of this structure to MDMA-induced damage. Monkeys given the high-dose regimen also

Address for correspondence: Dr. Jerrold S. Meyer, Department of Psychology, 135 Hicks Way, University of Massachusetts, Amherst, MA 01003. Voice: 413-545-2168; fax: 413-545-0996. e-mail: jmeyer@psych.umass.edu

Ann. N.Y. Acad. Sci. 1074: 365–376 (2006).
doi: 10.1196/annals.1369.036

showed prolonged hyperthermia and reductions in 5-HT and SERT in a number of brain areas. These results are the first to identify the pattern of MDMA-induced brain activation in a nonhuman primate model, and they further suggest that even recreational doses of MDMA may have adverse consequences as indicated by the reduced hypothalamic NAA/creatine ratio.

KEYWORDS: magnetic resonance imaging; magnetic resonance spectroscopy; BOLD; 3,4-methylenedioxymethamphetamine; visual cortex; serotonin; common marmoset

INTRODUCTION

Recreational use of 3,4-methylenedioxymethamphetamine (MDMA, or "Ecstasy") increased dramatically among adolescents and young adults during the late 1990s.[1,2] The subjective effects of this compound include elevated mood, increased closeness to others, and enhanced sensitivity to sensory stimuli.[3] Although Ecstasy is generally considered to be a relatively benign drug by users, a number of animal studies have shown that high doses of MDMA can damage serotonergic fibers in the forebrain.[4] Moreover, neurochemical, neuroendocrine, and neuropsychological studies of Ecstasy users suggest that repeated exposure to MDMA may also cause serotonergic neurotoxicity in humans.[4,5]

Several laboratories have used neuroimaging to characterize the influence of Ecstasy use on neuronal integrity, particularly as applied to the serotonergic system. For example, studies using either positron emission tomography (PET) or single-photon emission computed tomography (SPECT) have found that radioligand binding to the serotonin transporter (SERT, a marker for serotonergic fibers) in the neocortex and various subcortical areas is reduced in current or recent Ecstasy users.[6–8] These results raise the possibility that serotonergic axons and terminals may be pruned in Ecstasy users, similar to the findings obtained in laboratory animals. Interestingly, a SPECT study using the selective 5-HT_{2A} receptor antagonist [^{123}I]R91150 found evidence for decreased cortical 5-HT_{2A} receptor density in recent Ecstasy users compared to nonusers, whereas exusers (no use within the previous 2 months) showed elevated receptor density in the occipital cortex.[9] The authors argued that these effects reflect time-dependent changes in serotonergic transmission associated with repeated MDMA exposure (i.e., an initial enhancement of transmission followed by a subsequent deficit). Researchers have also used proton magnetic resonance spectroscopy (^{1}H MRS) to assess overall neuronal integrity in Ecstasy users compared to controls. One group of investigators found that Ecstasy use was associated with a significantly reduced ratio of the putative neuronal marker *N*-acetylaspartate (NAA) to both creatine and choline in the frontal cortex,[10] as well as a significant correlation between prefrontal NAA/creatine and delayed recall memory in Ecstasy users (i.e., a lower ratio predicted poorer memory function).[11] However, other investigators found no significant relationship between Ecstasy use and changes in NAA[12], but rather an increase in the putative glial marker *myo*inositol.[13] Finally, a number of functional magnetic resonance imaging (fMRI) studies have examined brain activation patterns in Ecstasy users and nonusers during working memory/retrieval tasks. Group differences were reported for several cortical and subcortical areas, notably the hippocampus.[14–19] Such findings suggest abnormal information processing in Ecstasy users that may or may not be related to the serotonergic deficits mentioned earlier.[8,20]

Despite the growing application of neuroimaging techniques in comparing Ecstasy-using with nonusing populations, there has been relatively little use of these techniques to investigate the acute effects of MDMA on regional neural activity or physiology. PET imaging studies with radiolabeled H_2O found complex MDMA-related changes in regional cerebral flow (CBF) in pigs and humans.[21,22] One rat study examined the effects of MDMA on CBF and glucose utilization (CMRglu) by means of autoradiographic techniques.[23] However, we are unaware of any other studies mapping brain activation patterns either in human subjects or in laboratory animals under the influence of MDMA.

The present study used fMRI and ^{1}H MRS to determine the influence of various doses of MDMA on neural activity and neuronal integrity in common marmosets (*Callithrix jacchus*). This species is an excellent model for investigating the neurobiological and behavioral effects of abused drugs. Marmosets are relatively small primates (300–400 g), are easily handled, and breed well in captivity. The females usually give birth to dizygotic twins that are raised in family groups that include fathers and older siblings. These features can be exploited in longitudinal studies of drug effects on offspring development and social interactions within the familial group. Various learning and memory tasks are available for studying marmoset cognitive function and the long-term effects of drug exposure on such function. Most importantly, these animals are adaptable to conscious restraint and thus can be used for imaging regional brain activity without the need for anesthesia.[24–26] Here we present the results of an fMRI study investigating changes in brain activity following a single "recreational" dose of MDMA given orally to marmosets during a scanning session. We also report preliminary findings from a second study using ^{1}H MRS to assess overall neuronal integrity as well as specific neurochemical markers for the serotonergic system to determine the neurotoxic effects of low and high MDMA dosing regimens in this species.

METHODS

Experiment 1

Methodological details for the first experiment may be found in Brevard *et al.*[27] Briefly, we used six adult marmoset monkeys (4 male and 2 female),

4–7 years old and weighing 350–410 g. On the day of testing, the animals were lightly anesthetized with a mixture of medetomidine and ketamine, secured in an MR-compatible restraining device with built-in imaging coils (see FIG. 1), and positioned within the bore of the magnet. Anesthesia was reversed with atipamizole after placement in the restrainer and prior to the onset of testing. During the imaging session, heart rate, respiration, and expired CO_2 were monitored by means of pulse oximetry and capnography. For drug dosing, a line of PE-10 tubing ending at the back of the animal's tongue was used to deliver a single dose of 1 mg/kg (±)MDMA HCl in 0.1 mL of water. This dose is equivalent to a 70-kg user consuming a single "Ecstasy" tablet containing 70 mg of MDMA (a typical single recreational dose[28]). All animals had previously been acclimated to the restraint device and imaging procedure. Acclimation involved placing the restrained animal into a black opaque tube that served as a "mock scanner" and playing a tape-recording of an MRI pulse sequence for 90 min to simulate the bore of the magnet and an imaging protocol.[24] This procedure was repeated every other day for 3–4 days.

Imaging was conducted in a 4.7T/40cm imager (Bruker Biospec, Billerica, MA) with a 12 cm diameter, 22 G/cm gradient insert. We first collected a set of high-resolution anatomical images, after which we ran a functional (i.e., blood oxygen level-dependent; BOLD) imaging sequence using a visual stimulation paradigm consisting of 4–6 epochs of 60s off, 60s on, with a blinking LED array. Following this visual stimulation experiment, additional sets of functional images were collected before and after oral administration of water vehicle and of MDMA. Thus, the overall design of the drug component of the study was as follows: 5 min of base line, administration of 0.1 mL water vehicle, 5 min postvehicle, administration of MDMA, and 35 min post-MDMA for a total scan time of 45 min. The imaging session concluded with a second visual stimulation experiment identical to the first. MRI data were analyzed using the Stimulate software package.[29] Details of the anatomical and functional imaging protocols are presented in Brevard *et al.*[27]

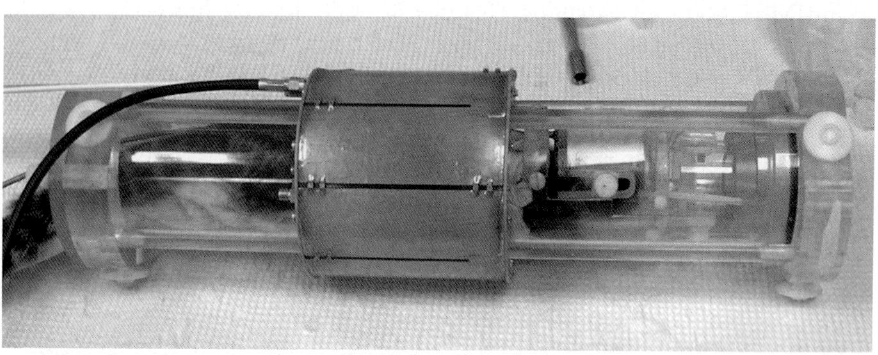

FIGURE 1. Commercially available restraint device for high-resolution fMRI of awake marmoset monkeys.

Administration of the water vehicle did not affect the BOLD signal compared to the previous 5-min baseline period. Consequently, the pre- and postvehicle periods were combined into a single 10-min control period of 300 data time points prior to MDMA administration. This base line was compared to the 35 min MDMA period of 700 data time points. Data for each animal were analyzed by two-tailed *t*-tests using a 95% confidence level and heteroscedastic variance assumptions. Anatomical regions of interest (ROIs) were defined on the basis of a standard marmoset brain atlas.[30]

To determine the relationship between the temporal pattern of brain activation and the time course of plasma levels of MDMA, a separate group of four marmosets (2 male and 2 female) was administered the same oral dose of MDMA used in the imaging study, and serial blood samples were collected 12, 24, and 35 min later. Plasma was stored and subsequently analyzed for MDMA-like immunoreactivity by means of a sensitive and selective enzyme-linked immunosorbent assay (Neogen, Lexington, KY).

Experiment 2

The second experiment obtained preliminary data concerning the effects of either a low- or high-dose regimen of repeated MDMA administration. Adult marmosets were given either vehicle ($N = 2$) or MDMA twice daily over 2 days using either a recreational (1 mg/kg p.o.; $N = 5$) or a neurotoxic (10 mg/kg i.m.; $N = 3$) dosing regimen. For animals given the high dose of MDMA, core body temperature was measured prior to drug administration and then again 24 and 36 h following the last dose. The same imaging system as in Experiment 1 was used to obtain ^{1}H MRS measurements of regional NAA/creatine ratios before and 1 week after MDMA exposure. Vehicle-treated and high-dose MDMA subjects were subsequently sacrificed and brain tissues were analyzed for regional SERT binding as well as 5-HT and 5-HIAA levels. Binding studies were performed with a single concentration of [^{3}H]citalopram as described in Piper *et al.*[31] except for two methodological differences. First, we used a radioligand concentration of 4.0 nM that is the apparent Kd for [^{3}H]citalopram binding to marmoset brain SERT (Piper & Meyer, unpublished observations). Second, to occlude any possible binding of the radiolabeled citalopram to σ_1 receptors,[32] all incubations were carried out in the presence of 10 μM haloperidol. High-performance liquid chromatography with electrochemical detection determined the 5-HT and 5-HIAA levels.[33]

RESULTS

Experiment 1

Low-dose oral MDMA administration had no effect on heart rate, respiration rate, or expired CO_2 compared to the baseline period. In contrast, the drug produced substantial increases in BOLD signal intensity in multiple brain areas. As detailed activational maps and time course plots of these changes are provided in Brevard *et al.*,[27] we will only summarize the effects here. BOLD signal intensity in a number of brain areas began rising soon after drug administration, generally reaching increases of at least 1% over base line by 5 min. Peak increases of 3–4% were reached by 25–35 min, depending on the area. Brain regions activated by acute MDMA treatment included the hypothalamus, midbrain raphe nuclei, and limbic system structures, such as the hippocampus and amygdala. A temporally coherent activation pattern was also observed in the corticostriatal circuit consisting of the substantia nigra, basal ganglia (caudate, putamen, and globus pallidus), thalamus, and sensory motor cortex. MDMA activated the lateral geniculate nucleus and the primary visual cortex in parallel, and it also enhanced the effect of photic stimulation on visual cortical activity. Several of the brain areas examined were not activated by acute MDMA administration, including the nucleus accumbens, superior colliculus, and the prefrontal, orbitofrontal, frontal, anterior cingulated, and temporal cortices.

When a separate group of marmosets was given the same dose of oral MDMA, plasma MDMA-like immunoreactivity rose rapidly and reached peak levels of approximately 200 ng/mL.[27] There was a close relationship between the temporal course of plasma MDMA and the observed increases in regional brain activation as determined by BOLD signal intensity.

Experiment 2

The high-dose regimen of MDMA led to a significant hyperthermic response (mean temperature elevation of approximately 3°C) that persisted for at least 36 h after the last dose. For technical reasons, only a few brain areas yielded reliable NAA/creatine data for all animals within a given treatment group. These results, which are shown in FIGURE 2, reveal that the NAA/creatine ratio was significantly reduced in the hypothalamus in both the low-dose (4×1 mg/kg p.o.) and high-dose (4×10 mg/kg i.m.) MDMA groups when the postdrug values were compared to those obtained before the treatment. Because there were only two marmosets in the saline control group for this preliminary study, no comparisons to the MDMA-treated animals will be made until the sample size has been increased. Measurements of SERT binding as well as 5-HT and 5-HIAA levels in the high-dose MDMA group revealed decreases in these serotonergic markers in most cortical areas studied as well as the striatum, hypothalamus, thalamus, and brain stem (data not shown). For SERT binding, such decreases reached statistical significance in the temporal and occipital cortex, striatum, and thalamus.

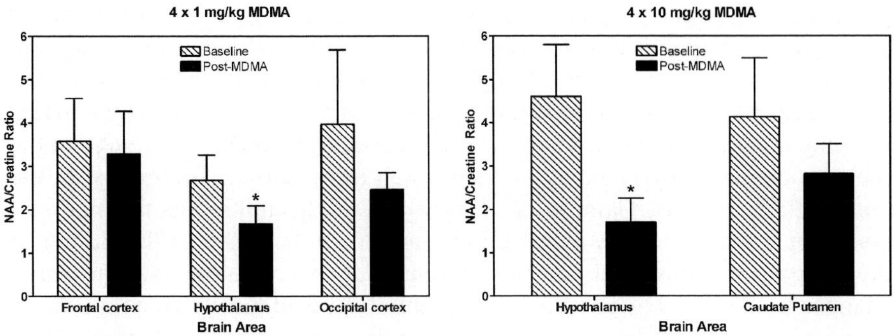

FIGURE 2. Effects of low- and high-dose MDMA treatment regimens on regional NAA/creatine ratios. * $P < 0.05$ compared to baseline value.

DISCUSSION

This is the first study using MRI and MRS in animals to investigate regional hemodynamic and biochemical changes in the brain following a single or multiple doses of MDMA. In the first experiment, awake marmosets were administered a single, oral dose of MDMA that produced plasma levels of MDMA-like immunoreactivity comparable to those found in humans given a recreational dose of this compound.[34] Under these conditions, we observed a significant drug-induced activation of the midbrain raphe nuclei and substantia nigra, major origins of ascending serotonergic and dopaminergic projections, respectively. Other areas that were activated include the hippocampus, amygdala, hypothalamus, primary visual cortex, and the corticostriatal circuit consisting of the sensory motor cortex, caudate, putamen, globus pallidus, and dorsal thalamus.

Although the acute effects of MDMA on regional brain activity have not previously been studied with BOLD fMRI, other approaches have been used to investigate MDMA-induced changes in brain activity. For example, Gamma and colleagues[22] reported complex effects of a single oral dose of 1.7 mg/kg of MDMA on regional CBF by [$H_2{}^{15}O$]-PET in previously drug-naïve humans. Specifically, blood flow was increased bilaterally in several cortical areas (e.g., ventromedial prefrontal, ventral anterior cingulate, inferior temporal, and medial occipital) as well as the cerebellum, whereas bilateral decreases in blood flow were observed in several other cortical areas as well as the thalamus. No changes were found in the hippocampus, hypothalamus, caudate, putamen, or globus pallidus. In a more recent study, Quate and co-workers[23] used quantitative autoradiography for [^{14}C]2-deoxyglucose to investigate local CMRglu changes in response to 15 mg/kg of MDMA injected intraperitoneally (i.p). in Dark Agouti rats. Out of 50 brain areas examined, 23 showed significant increases in CMRglu. These included the sensorimotor cortex, striatum, globus pallidus, substantia nigra, hippocampal CA1, lateral amygdala, septal nucleus, and nucleus accumbens. Most other brain areas showed either no change or, in a few cases, decreases in CMRglu. Although there are several important differences between the present results and those found in MDMA-treated rats (notably an activational effect in the nucleus accumbens but no change in the raphe nuclei), the two studies yielded much more similar findings than the human PET study of Gamma *et al.* One potentially important factor to account for the disparate results from the human study concerns the timing of the imaging measurements. In the present study, we continuously measured changes in the BOLD signal from the point of drug administration until these changes appeared to plateau around 30–35 min later. In contrast, Gamma *et al.* did not begin imaging their subjects until 75 min after drug ingestion, an interval chosen based on the peak subjective effects of MDMA in humans after oral dosing.[35] This difference raises the interesting possibility that MDMA may elicit a biphasic response consisting of an early activation of neural pathways involved in the onset of drug action followed by a deactivation of these pathways as drug effects reach their peak.

Unlike the dorsal striatum, the nucleus accumbens failed to show activation following MDMA administration to marmosets. This was unexpected in view of the prominent role of accumbens dopamine (DA) in mechanisms of drug reward[36] as well as the results of imaging studies in rats showing accumbens activation in response to either MDMA[23] or cocaine administration.[37,38] We cannot exclude the possibility of a species difference in accumbens response patterns between marmosets and rats. However, a more likely explanation for the lack of accumbens activation in the present study concerns the drug dose and route of administration. The other cited studies used higher doses and/or intracerebroventricular or intravenous treatment paradigms, all of which would be expected to cause greater increases in extracellular DA levels in the nucleus accumbens than may have occurred in our animals.

The use of MRI to monitor regional hemodynamic changes in response to a pharmacological challenge, sometimes termed *pharmacological MRI* (phMRI),[39] is a powerful new tool for exploring changes in neurotransmitter activity produced by psychoactive drugs. For example, several phMRI studies have shown an important role for DA in the hemodynamic responses to cocaine or amphetamine in rats and monkeys.[38,40,41] Although we did not directly investigate the neurotransmitter mediation of the BOLD signal responses observed in MDMA-treated marmosets, this compound is known to acutely stimulate the release of 5-HT[4] and, to a lesser extent, DA and norepinephrine. Consequently, we hypothesized that areas of the marmoset brain high in serotonergic nerve terminals would be most affected by acute oral MDMA. Central 5-HT originates from the brain stem raphe nuclei, with the dorsal raphe containing the largest and most dense population of serotonergic neurons in marmosets.[42] In turn, the rostrally located raphe groups (including the dorsal raphe) innervate virtually all forebrain areas, including the basal ganglia, limbic systems structures, such as the hippocampus and amygdala, hypothalamus, neocortex, and the substantia nigra. Our study found that all of the aforementioned subcortical structures were activated by MDMA, whereas most cortical areas were not except for the sensory motor and primary visual cortices. Thus, the BOLD response to MDMA appears to be mediated in a more complex manner than can be attributed simply to 5-HT release (see Ref. 27 for more discussion). Interestingly, the visual cortex was one of the few brain areas activated in both marmosets and humans[22] given an oral dose of MDMA. These findings along with others that show various effects of MDMA exposure on the visual or occipital cortex[9,43] suggest that this brain region is particularly sensitive to MDMA, and they may also account at least partially for the heightened visual sensations and (at high doses) visual hallucinations that occur with human Ecstasy use.[44,45]

In previous animal work, MDMA-induced neurotoxicity to the 5-HT system has been inferred from long-term reductions in various serotonergic markers.[4] A few studies have also found evidence for toxic effects of MDMA on non-serotonergic neurons both *in vivo*[46] and *in vitro*.[47] However, almost all of these studies used relatively high doses of MDMA that may not be clinically relevant for typical recreational users. It is therefore noteworthy that in our second experiment, significant reductions in the NAA/creatine ratio were observed in the hypothalamus not only after a severe MDMA dosing regimen that was expected to produce neurotoxic effects, but also following several low oral doses of MDMA. These results are preliminary and require confirmation with a larger sample size. Nevertheless, they raise the possibility that repeated MDMA exposure, even at typical recreational levels, could produce adverse consequences for neuronal function.

In summary, we used BOLD imaging of awake marmoset monkeys to investigate the regional pattern of brain activation following a single low dose of MDMA administered orally. The results indicate profound activational effects of the drug in many subcortical structures as well as a few cortical areas. These hemodynamic changes closely follow the time course of plasma MDMA-like immunoreactivity, and they are likely mediated by the combined effects of MDMA on the release of 5-HT along with other monoamine neurotransmitters. A second, preliminary, experiment using ^{1}H MRS found evidence for a reduced NAA/creatine ratio in the hypothalamus following repeated MDMA exposure under two different dosing regimens. Further work is warranted to determine whether chronic MDMA could cause damage to non-serotonergic neurons in the hypothalamus and possibly other brain regions as well.

ACKNOWLEDGMENTS

The authors would like to acknowledge the NIDA Drug Supply Program for their generous donation of MDMA and Drs. Nancy Shultz-Darken and Toni

Ziegler, Wisconsin Primate Center, Madison, for their technical assistance in blood collection. This work was supported by NIDA grants R01 DA013517 and R01 DA019158 to CFF.

REFERENCES

1. BANKEN, J.A. 2004. Drug abuse trends among youth in the United States. Ann. N. Y. Acad. Sci. **1025:** 465–471.
2. LANDRY, M.J. 2002. MDMA: a review of epidemiologic data. J. Psychoactive Drugs **34:** 163–169.
3. VOLLENWEIDER, F.X., M.E. LIECHTI, A. GAMMA, *et al.* 2002. Acute psychological and neurophysiological effects of MDMA in humans. J. Psychoactive Drugs **34:** 171–184.
4. GREEN, A.R, A.O. MECHAN, J.M. ELLIOTT, *et al.* 2003. The pharmacology and clinical pharmacology of 3,4-methylenedioxymethamphetamine (MDMA, "ecstasy"). Pharmacol. Rev. **55:** 463–508.
5. MORGAN, M.J. 2000. Ecstasy (MDMA): a review of its possible persistent psychological effects. Psychopharmacology **152:** 230–248.
6. BUCHERT, R., R. THOMASIUS, F. WILKE, *et al.* 2004. A voxel-based PET investigation of the long-term effects of "Ecstasy" consumption on brain serotonin transporters. Am. J. Psychiatry **161:** 1181–1189.
7. MCCANN, U.D., Z. SZABO, E. SECKIN, *et al.* 2005. Quantitative PET studies of the serotonin transporter in MDMA users and controls using [^{11}C]McN5652 and [^{11}C]DASB. Neuropsychopharmacology **30:** 1741–1750.
8. RENEMAN, L., J. LAVALAYE, B. SCHMAND, *et al.* 2001. Cortical serotonin transporter density and verbal memory in individuals who stopped using 3,4-methylenedioxymethamphetamine (MDMA or "Ecstasy"). Arch. Gen. Psychiatry **58:** 901–906.
9. RENEMAN, L., E. ENDERT, K. DE BRUIN, *et al.* 2002. The acute and chronic effects of MDMA ("Ecstasy") on cortical 5-HT_{2A} receptors in rat and human brain. Neuropsychopharmacology **26:** 387–396.
10. RENEMAN, L., C.B. MAJOIE, H. FLICK & G.J. DEN HEETEN. 2002. Reduced *N*-acetylaspartate levels in the frontal cortex of 3,4-methylenedioxymethamphetamine (Ecstasy) users: preliminary results. Am. J. Neuroradiol. **23:** 231–237.
11. RENEMAN, L., C.B.L.M. MAJOIE, B. SCHMAND, *et al.* 2001. Prefrontal *N*-acetylaspartate is strongly associated with memory performance in (abstinent) Ecstasy users: preliminary report. Biol. Psychiatry **50:** 550–554.
12. DAUMANN, J., T. FISCHERMANN, U. PILATUS, *et al.* 2004. Proton magnetic resonance spectroscopy in ecstasy (MDMA) users. Neurosci. Lett. **362:** 113–116.
13. CHANG, L., T. ERNST, C.S. GROB & R.E. POLAND. 1999. Cerebral ^{1}H MRS alterations in recreational 3,4-methylenedioxymethamphetamine (MDMA, "Ecstasy") users. J. Magn. Reson. Imaging **10:** 521–526.
14. DAUMANN, J., B. FIMM, K. WILLMES, *et al.* 2003. Cerebral activation in abstinent ecstasy (MDMA) users during a working memory task: a functional magnetic resonance imaging (fMRI) study. Cogn. Brain Res. **16:** 479–487.
15. DAUMANN, J., T. FISCHERMANN, K. HEEKEREN, *et al.* 2005. Memory-related hippocampal dysfunction in poly-drug ecstasy (3,4-methylenedioxymethamphetamine) users. Psychopharmacology **180:** 607–611.

16. DAUMANN, J., T. FISCHERMANN, K. HEEKEREN, *et al.* 2004. Neural mechanisms of working memory in ecstasy (MDMA) users who continue or discontinue ecstasy and amphetamine use: evidence from an 18-month longitudinal functional magnetic resonance imaging study. Biol. Psychiatry **56:** 349–355.
17. DAUMANN, J., R. SCHNITKER, J. WEIDEMANN, *et al.* 2003. Neural correlates of working memory in pure and polyvalent ecstasy (MDMA) users. Neuroreport 14: 1983–1987.
18. JACOBSEN, L.K., W.E. MENCI, K.R. PUGH, *et al.* Preliminary evidence of hippocampal dysfunction in adolescent MDMA ("ecstasy") users: possible relationship to neurotoxic effects. Psychopharmacology **173:** 383–390.
19. MOELLER, F.G., J.L. STEINBERG, D.M. DOUGHERTY, *et al.* 2004. Functional MRI study of working memory in MDMA users. Psychopharmacology **177:** 185–194.
20. RENEMAN, L. J. BOOIJ, B. SCHMAND, *et al.* 2000. Memory disturbances in "Ecstasy" users are correlated with an altered brain serotonin neurotransmission. Psychopharmacology **148:** 322–324.
21. ROSA-NETO, P., A.K. OLSEN, A. GJEDDE, *et al.* 2004. MDMA-evoked changes in cerebral blood flow in living porcine brain: correlation with hyperthermia. Synapse **53:** 214–221.
22. GAMMA, A., A. BUCK, T. BERTHOLD, *et al.* 2000. 3,4-Methylenedioxymethamphetamine (MDMA) modulates cortical and limbic brain activity as measured by $[H_2{}^{15}O]$-PET in healthy humans. Neuropsychopharmacology **23:** 388–395.
23. QUATE, L., D.E. MCBEAN, I.M. RITCHIE, *et al.* 2004. Acute methylenedioxymethamphetamine administration: effects on local cerebral blood flow and glucose utilization in the dark agouti rat. Psychopharmacology **173:** 287–295.
24. FERRIS, C.F. & C.T. SNOWDON. 2005. Methods and applications for functional magnetic resonance imaging in conscious marmoset monkeys. *In* The Laboratory Primate (Handbook of Experimental Animals). S. Wolfe-Coote, Ed.: 351–369. Academic Press. London.
25. FERRIS, C.F., C.T. SNOWDON, J.A. KING, *et al.* 2004. Activation of neural pathways associated with sexual arousal in non-human primates. J. Magn. Reson. Imaging **19:** 168–175.
26. TENNEY, J.R., P.C. MARSHALL, J.A. KING & C.F. FERRIS. 2004. fMRI of generalized absence status epilepticus in conscious marmoset monkeys reveals corticothalamic activation. Epilepsia **45:** 1240–1247.
27. BREVARD, M.E., J.S. MEYER, J.A. HARDER & C.F. FERRIS. 2006. Imaging brain activity in conscious monkeys following oral MDMA ("Ecstasy"). J. Magn. Res. Imaging In Press.
28. PARROTT, A.C. 2004. Is ecstasy MDMA? A review of the proportion of ecstasy tablets containing MDMA, their dosage levels, and the changing perceptions of purity. Psychopharmacology **173:** 234–241.
29. STRUPP, J.P. 1996. Stimulate: a GUI based fMRI analysis software package. Neuroimage **3:** S607.
30. SAAVEDRA, J.P. & A.L. MAZZUCHELLI. 1969. A stereotaxic atlas of the brain of the marmoset (*Hapale jacchus*). J. Hirnforsch. **11:** 105–122.
31. PIPER, B.J., J.B. FRAIMAN & J.S. MEYER. 2005. Repeated MDMA ("Ecstasy") exposure in adolescent male rats alters temperature regulation, spontaneous motor activity, attention, and serotonin transporter binding. Dev. Psychobiol. **47:** 145–157.

32. NARITA, N., K. HASHIMOTO, S.-I. TOMITAKA & Y. MINABE. 1996. Interactions of selective serotonin reuptake inhibitors with subtypes of σ receptors in rat brain. Eur. J. Pharmacol. **307:** 117–119.
33. ALI, S.F., G.D. NEWPORT, R.R. HOLSON, *et al.* 1994. Low environmental temperatures or pharmacologic agents that produce hypothermia decrease methamphetamine neurotoxicity in mice. Brain Res. **658:** 33–38.
34. SAMYN, N., G. DE BROECK, M. WOOD, *et al.* 2002. Plasma, oral fluid and sweat wipe ecstasy concentrations in controlled and real life conditions. Forensic Sci. Int. **128:** 90–97.
35. VOLLENWEIDER, F.X., A. GAMMA, M. LIECHTI & T. HUBER. 1998. Psychological and cardiovascular effects and short-term sequelae of MDMA (Ecstasy) in healthy volunteers. Neuropsychopharmacology **19:** 241–251.
36. CARDINAL, R.N. & B.J. EVERITT. 2004. Neural and psychological mechanisms underlying appetitive learning: links to drug addiction. Curr. Opin. Neurobiol. **14:** 156–162.
37. FEBO, M., A.C. SEGARRA, J.R. TENNEY, *et al.* 2004. Imaging cocaine-induced changes in the mesocorticolimbic dopaminergic system of conscious rats. J. Neurosci. Method. **139:** 167–176.
38. MAROTA, J.J.A., J.B. MANDEVILLE, R.M. WEISSKOFF, *et al.* 2000. Cocaine activation discriminates dopaminergic projections by temporal response: an fMRI study in rat. Neuroimage **11:** 13–23.
39. JENKINS, B.G., Y.-C.I. CHEN & J.B. MANDEVILLE. 2003. Pharmacological magnetic resonance imaging (phMRI). *In* Biomedical Imaging in Experimental Neuroscience. N. van Bruggen & T. Roberts, Eds.: 155–209. CRC Press. New York.
40. DIXON, A.L., M. PRIOR, P.M. MORRIS, *et al.* 2005. Dopamine antagonist modulation of amphetamine response as detected using pharmacological MRI. Neuropharmacology **48:** 236–245.
41. JENKINS, B.G., R. SANCHEZ-PERNAUTE, A.-L. BROWNELL, *et al.* 2004. Mapping dopamine function in primates using pharmacologic magnetic resonance imaging. J. Neurosci. **27:** 9553–9560.
42. HORNUNG, J.P & J.M. FRITSCHY. 1988. Serotoninergic system in the brainstem of the marmoset: a combined immunocytochemical and three-dimensional reconstruction study. J. Comp. Neurol. **270:** 471–487.
43. OLIVERI, M. & G. CALVO. 2003. Increased visual cortical excitability in ecstasy users: a transcranial magnetic stimulation study. J. Neurol. Neurosurg. Psychiatry **74:** 1136–1138.
44. DAVISON, D. & A.C. PARROTT. 1997. Ecstasy (MDMA) in recreational users: self-reported psychological and physiological effects. Hum. Psychopharmacol. **12:** 221–226.
45. PEROUTKA, S.J., H. NEWMAN & H. HARRIS. 1988. Subjective effects of 3,4-methylenedioxymethamphetamine in recreational users. Neuropsychopharmacology **1:** 273–277.
46. SCHMUED, L.C. 2003. Demonstration and localization of neuronal degeneration in the rat forebrain following a single exposure to MDMA. Brain Res. **974:** 127–133.
47. JIMENEZ, A., E.G. JORDA, E. VERDAGUER, *et al.* 2004. Neurotoxicity of amphetamine derivatives is mediated by caspase pathway activation in rat cerebellar granule cells. Toxicol. Appl. Pharmacol. **196:** 223–234.

MDMA Induces Caspase-3 Activation in the Limbic System but not in Striatum

ILARIA TAMBURINI,[a] FABIO BLANDINI,[b] MARCO GESI,[a] GIADA FRENZILLI,[a] MARCO NIGRO,[a] MARIO GIUSIANI,[c] ANTONIO PAPARELLI,[a] AND FRANCESCO FORNAI[a,d]

[a]*Department of Human Morphology and Applied Biology, University of Pisa, 56126 Pisa, Italy*

[b]*I.R.C.C.S. I.N.M. "C. Mondino," 27100 Pavia, Italy*

[c]*Department of Public Health, University of Pisa, 56126 Pisa, Italy*

[d]*Laboratory of Neurobiology of Movement Disorders, I.R.C.C.S. I.N.M. Neuromed, Pozzilli, Isernia, Italy*

ABSTRACT: Several studies, carried out in chronic (+/−) 3,4-methylenedioxymethamphetamine (MDMA) abusers, have shown memory loss and cognitive impairment, as well as persistent electroencephalographic changes. This suggests that, at least in humans, forebrain areas, including the limbic system, might be altered by MDMA. Consistently, recent experimental evidences suggest that, in rodents, MDMA, besides effects on the basal ganglia, produces alterations in the hippocampus. Therefore, the aim of the present article was to investigate whether treatment with MDMA produces activation of the caspase-3 enzyme, which is part of an enzymatic pathway involved in cell death, within limbic areas (i.e., hippocampus, amygdala, and piriform cortex) and striatum. A marked induction of caspase-3 activity was demonstrated in the amygdala and hippocampus, although MDMA did not affect caspase-3 activity neither in the striatum nor in the frontal cortex. These data indicate that limbic structures possess a high sensitivity to MDMA with respect to the activation of at least one step in the apoptotic pathway. Potential implications and pitfalls of such an experimental observation are reported.

KEYWORDS: MDMA; caspase; limbic areas; striatum

INTRODUCTION

3,4-Methylenedioxymethamphetamine (MDMA, ecstasy) is widely abused in the western world, where a large number of young subjects takes the drug in

Address for correspondence: Francesco Fornai, M.D., Ph.D., Department of Human Morphology and Applied Biology, Univerity of Pisa, Via Roma 55, 56126 Pisa, Italy. Voice: +39-0502218611; fax: +39-0502218606.
e-mail: f.fornai@med.unipi.it

**Ann. N.Y. Acad. Sci. 1074: 377–381 (2006). © 2006 New York Academy of Sciences.
doi: 10.1196/annals.1369.037**

a recreational context.[1] It is widely established that, early after MDMA administration, there is a marked increase in free radicals and oxidative species.[2–4] Interestingly, oxidative stress and increase in free radicals were recently reported in human MDMA abusers.[5] A frequent effect, which is described in chronic MDMA abusers, consist in memory and cognitive impairment which was attributed to a deficit in monoamine innervation in limbic/cortical areas.[6] However, studies on MDMA focused much more on deleterious effects on the basal ganglia compared with limbic regions. Again, only a few *in vitro* studies led to the hypothesis that MDMA administration might lead to cell death, making it critical to evaluate whether MDMA might produce neuronal loss within those forebrain/limbic regions which are important for learning and memory, such as the hippocampus and the amygdala. In the present article, as a preliminary approach to address these points, we explored the effects of MDMA on caspase-3 activity in selected neocortical, subcortical, and limbic regions. Caspase-3 belongs to the "caspases" family and it is involved in the process of the apoptotic cascade (together with caspase-2 and -7). We focused on this specific enzymatic activity, in light of recent data showing its pivotal role in apoptosis in a variety of tissues.[7]

MATERIALS AND METHODS

Male C57 Black mice (C57BL/6J) ($n = 5$, 9–10 weeks) were used for the experiments. Animals were housed individually in a temperature- ($22 \pm 2°C$) and light-controlled environment, with free access to food and water. The day of the experiment, mice received an i.p. injection of MDMA (5 mg/kg, $\times$ 3, 2 h apart) or saline (controls). Seven days later, animals were killed by cervical dislocation, brains were rapidly removed and placed on an ice-cold plate. The frontal cortex, striatum, hippocampus, amygdala, and piriform cortex were dissected out and frozen immediately at $-80°C$. The day of the analysis, brain samples were homogenized by ultrasounds (Vibra Cell, Sonics & Materials, Inc., Newtown, CT) in phosphate-buffered saline, pH 7.4 (Sigma, St. Louis, MO). Homogenates were centrifuged at 18,000 *g* for 8 min at 4°C and supernatants were used for the biochemical assays. A fluorometric assay, based on proteolytic cleavage of the 7-amino-4-methylcoumarin (AMC)-derived substrate Z-DEVD-AMC (where Z represents a benzyloxycarbonyl group), was used for determination of caspase-3 activity (Molecular Probes, Paisley, UK). The substrate, which is weakly fluorescent in the UV spectral range (excitation/emission maxima ~330/390 nm), yields the bright-blue-fluorescent product AMC, which has excitation/emission maxima of 342/441 nm, upon proteolytic cleavage. Readings were performed on a fluorometric microplate reader (Spectramax Gemini XS, Molecular Devices, Sunnyvale, CA). Protein content of brain samples was estimated using a commercially available kit (Bio-Rad, Hercules, CA), after dissolving the precipitates in 0.5 N NaOH. The results

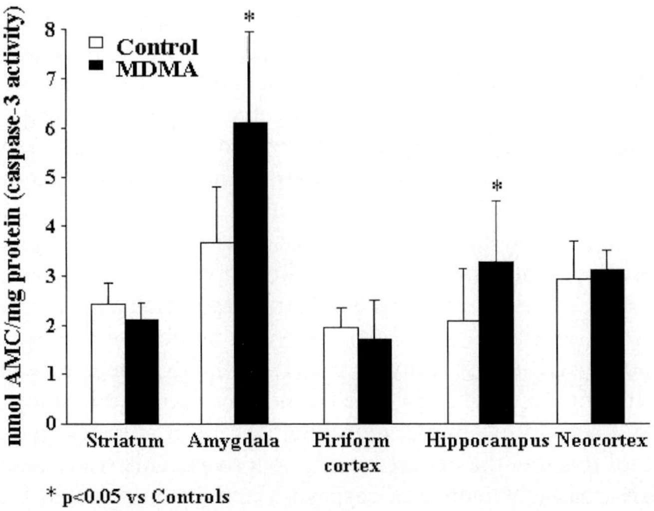

FIGURE 1. Effects of systemic administration of MDMA (5 mg/kg, i.p., repeated thrice with 2 h of interval), after 7 days from the last administration, on the caspase-3 activity in striatum, limbic areas, and neocortex. $^* = P < 0.05$ (as compared to control values).

from control and treated mice were expressed as the mean ± SD for each group and were compared using one-way analysis of variance (ANOVA) with Sheffè's *post hoc* analysis.

RESULTS

Systemic administration of MDMA (5 mg/kg, i.p., × 3, 2 h apart) produced, 7 days later, a significant increase in the caspase-3 activity in selected limbic areas. In particular, there was an increase in the amygdala and the hippocampus. Conversely, MDMA did not modify caspase-3 activity in the striatum, frontal, and piriform cortex (FIG. 1).

DISCUSSION

In this study, we found a significant increase in the caspase-3 activity in selected limbic areas, such as amygdala and hippocampus, 7 days after systemic administration of MDMA (5 mg/kg, i.p., × 3, 2 h apart). Caspases are a class of cysteine proteases, consisting of at least 14 members subdivided on the basis of structural homology, substrate preference, or biological function. They are involved in the complex biochemical events associated with apoptosis; for example, several caspases have been shown to be important contributors to the inflammatory response by processing cytokines (caspase-1, -4, -5, and -13), whereas others are activated either as an early step in the initiation of apoptosis (caspase-6, -8, -9, and -10) or in the execution of the apoptotic response (caspase-2, -3, and -7). Caspase-3 has received particular attention from a therapeutic perspective, because it is expressed in almost all tissues and at relatively high levels (versus other caspases) and has high catalytic activity compared with the other executioner caspases. Furthermore, genetic knockout studies have shown that caspase-3 plays a critical role in apoptosis during neuronal development, whereas other studies support a role in neurodegenerative diseases. Caspase-3, that has a substrate specificity for the amino acid sequence Asp-Glu-Val-Asp (DEVD), cleaves a number of different proteins, including poly (ADP-ribose) polymerase (PARP), DNA-dependent protein kinase, protein kinase C, and actin. The method we used in this study for assaying caspase-3 activity is simple, reproducible, and it is generally considered a reliable tool to show the occurrence of apoptosis. This study demonstrated that MDMA treatment increases caspase-3 activity in selected brain areas: in particular, such an increase was at level of amygdala and hippocampus, whereas caspase-3 activity in striatum and neocortex was not affected. Despite most of the studies performed in rodents to evaluate MDMA-induced neurotoxicity focused on the effects on monoaminergic terminals, the possibility that amphetamine derivatives might exert a neurotoxic effect also on cell bodies of classes of neurons other than monoaminergic is suggested by the present findings. In line with this, there is evidence in rodents that MDMA produces degenerating neurons within limbic areas.[8] These data call for in-depth studies aimed at documenting neuronal death induced by MDMA in limbic structures.

REFERENCES

1. Parrott, A.C. *et al.* 2001. Recreational ecstasy/MDMA and other drug users from the U.K. and Italy: psychiatric symptoms and psychobiological problems. Psychopharmacology (Berl.) **159**: 77–82.
2. Colado, M.I. & A.R. Green. 1995. The spin trap reagent α-phenyl-N-tert-butyl nitrone prevents "ecstasy"-induced neurodegeneration of 5-hydroxytryptamine neurones. Eur. J. Pharmacol. **280**: 343–346.
3. Colado, M.I. *et al.* 1995. The hyperthermic and neurotoxic effects of "ecstasy" (MDMA) and 3,4-methyl-enedioxyamphetamine (MDA) in the Dark Agouti (DA) rat, a model of the CYTP2D6 poor metaboliser phenotype. Br. J. Pharmacol. **115**: 1281–1289.
4. Colado, M.I. *et al.* 1997. In vivo evidence for free radical involvement in the degeneration of rat brain 5-HT following administration of MDMA ("ecstasy") and p-chloroamphetamine but not the degeneration following fenfluramine. Br. J. Pharmacol. **121**: 889–900.

5. ZHOU, J.F. *et al.* 2003. 3,4-Methylenedioxymethamphetamine (MDMA) abuse may cause oxidative stress and potential free radical damage. Free Radic. Res. **37**: 491–497.
6. MCCANN, U.D. *et al.* 1999. Cognitive performance in (±) 3,4-methylenedioxymethamphetamine (MDMA, "ecstasy") users: a controlled study. Psychopharmacology (Berl.) **143**: 417–425.
7. SCOTT, C.W. *et al.* 2003. Novel small molecule inhibitors of caspase-3 block cellular and biochemical features of apoptosis. J. Pharmacol. Exp. Ther. **304**: 433–440.
8. SCHMUED, L.C. 2003. Demonstration and localization of neuronal degeneration in the rat forebrain following a single exposure to MDMA. Brain Res. **974**: 127–133.

Induction by Cocaine of the Serotonergic 5-HT$_3$ Receptor in Rat Cerebellum

MARIE-PIERRE ARPIN-BOTT,[a] JEAN-BERNARD DIETRICH,[a] SYLVIE DIRRIG-GROSCH,[b] DOMINIQUE AUNIS,[a] AND JEAN ZWILLER[a]

[a]*INSERM, Unité 575, Centre de Neurochimie, 5 rue Pascal, 67084 Strasbourg, France*

[b]*IFR037, Centre de Neurochimie, 5 rue Pascal, 67084 Strasbourg, France*

ABSTRACT: The expression of the 5-HT$_3$ receptor, a member of the serotonin receptor family, was examined in rat cerebellum of saline- or cocaine-treated rats. Both immunohistochemistry and Western blot analysis were used. We found that the expression of this serotonin receptor subtype was increased in the cerebellum of rats injected either acutely or repeatedly (1 injection/day for 10 days) with cocaine. The stimulation was more pronounced after a single injection than after a series of 10 injections. Surprisingly, the expression of the 5-HT$_3$ receptor was mainly localized in Bergmann glial cells, as assessed from the co-localization of the receptor with the glial cell marker glial fibrillary acidic protein (GFAP). Our data emphasize the importance of the 5-HT$_3$ receptor induction in the cerebellum as part of the neuroadaptations taking place in rat brain in response to the psychostimulant cocaine.

KEYWORDS: cocaine; serotonin 5-HT$_3$ receptor; Bergmann glial cells; rat cerebellum

INTRODUCTION

Several reports have indicated that the serotonergic 5-HT$_3$ receptor is involved in the mode of action of drugs of abuse.[1,2] For instance, cocaine-induced expression of the immediate early genes *c-fos* and *egr-1* was found to be reduced in dopaminergic brain areas by the prior treatment of rats with the 5-HT$_3$ receptor antagonist tropisetron.[3] Conversely, the 5-HT$_3$ receptor agonist 2-methyl-serotonin induced the early gene expression in the same structures. A gene profiling analysis has shown that the 5-HT$_3$ receptor gene was among the genes transcriptionally activated in rat cortex in response to MDMA (3,4-methylenedioxy-methamphetamine).[4] Modulating 5-HT$_3$ receptor activity was

Address for correspondence: Jean Zwiller, INSERM, Unité U575, Centre de Neurochimie, 5 rue Blaise Pascal, 67084 Strasbourg Cedex, France. Voice: 33-3-88-45-67-27; fax: 33-3-88-60-08-06. e-mail: zwiller@neurochem.u-strasbg.fr

Ann. N.Y. Acad. Sci. 1074: 382–389 (2006).
doi: 10.1196/annals.1369.038

also found to modify behavioral parameters induced by psychostimulants. 5-HT$_3$ receptor antagonists are among the few classes of compounds that are able to inhibit cocaine-induced conditioned place preference, a method believed capable of measuring the affective properties of psychoactive drugs.[5] The antagonists tropisetron and zacopride were reported to block the locomotor elevating effects of cocaine.[6,7] Long-term blockade of the expression of cocaine sensitization by ondansetron has also been reported.[8] On the other hand, evidence for the involvement of the 5-HT$_3$ receptor in cocaine self-administration within the posterior ventral tegmental area has been reported, suggesting that the reinforcing effects of cocaine are mediated by activation of 5-HT$_3$ receptors.[9] Ethanol is also a positive modulator at the 5-HT$_3$ receptor, which has been implicated in alcohol drinking, anxiety, and aggression.[10] The receptor has emerged as a potential therapeutic target in the treatment of alcohol abuse and dependence, because selective pharmacological antagonists reduce alcohol consumption in preclinical and clinical models.[11]

The 5-HT$_3$ receptor is the only member of the serotonergic family of receptors that is characterized as a ionotropic receptor. It is constituted of five co-assembled subunits surrounding a centrally ligand-gated cation channel.[12] Two main subunits, named 5-HT$_{3A}$ and 5-HT$_{3B}$, have been found to be expressed in the human and rodent nervous system.[13,14] It is noteworthy that the 5-HT$_{3A}$ receptor subunit is required for antagonist-induced reduction in alcohol drinking[11] and that co-expression of both subunits is required for reducing alcohol sensitivity.[15]

Whereas the effects of cocaine have been extensively studied in dopaminergic brain areas such as the prefrontal cortex and the striatum, only few studies have documented effects in the cerebellum, despite the fact that spontaneous and glutamate-evoked firing of Purkinje cells as well as γ-aminobutyric acid (GABA)-induced discharges were shown to be reduced in this structure by cocaine.[16] Given the function of the cerebellum in behavior and cognition, we have analyzed the effects of acute and repeated cocaine treatment on the expression of the 5-HT$_3$ receptor in rat cerebellum.

MATERIALS AND METHODS

Animals and Tissue Preparation

Male Wistar rats (180–230 g) were housed with a fixed 12-h light-dark cycle and free access to food and water. All experiments were conducted in conformity with the European Community Council guidelines. Rats were injected intraperitoneally (i.p.) with either 20 mg/kg cocaine hydrochloride (Sigma, St. Louis, MO) or an equivalent volume of saline (NaCl 0.9%). For chronic treatments, rats were treated for 10 days (1 injection/ day). Animals were sacrificed 15 h after injection (or after the last injection in the case of repeated treatment) by an overdose of pentobarbital (100 mg/kg, i.p.) and perfused transcardially with 50 mL saline followed by 4% paraformaldehyde in phosphate-buffered saline (pH 7.2; 250 mL). The brains were kept overnight at 4°C in 15% sucrose, frozen in isopentane at −40°C, and then stored at −80°C. Parasagittal tissue sections (30 μm) were prepared using a Leica VT 1000S vibratome (Leica Microsystems GmBH, Wetzlar, Germany) and stored in Watson cryoprotective medium containing 30% sucrose, 1% polyvinylpyrrolidone, 30% ethyleneglycol, 0.9% NaCl in 0.1 M phosphate buffer; pH 7.2 .

Antibodies

Goat polyclonal anti-5-HT_3 receptor antibodies from Santa Cruz Biotechnology (Santa Cruz, CA) and from Abcam (Cambridge, UK) were used for immunohistochemistry and for Western blotting, respectively . Anti-GFAP (glial fibrillary acidic protein) mouse monoclonal antibody was obtained from Chemicon (Temecula, CA). Secondary antibodies were Cy3-conjugated donkey anti-goat IgG (Molecular Probes, Eugene, OR), donkey anti-goat peroxidase-conjugated IgG (Jackson Lab., West Grove, PA), and goat anti-mouse Alexa Fluor 488-conjugated IgG (Molecular Probes).

Immunohistochemistry

Free-floating sections were washed in 50 mM Tris-buffered saline, pH 7.4 (TBS) and blocked with 600 μL of TBS supplemented with 5% bovine serumalbumin and 0.5% (v/v) Triton X-100 (Euromedex, Souffelweyersheim, France). Sections were incubated overnight in primary anti-5-HT_3 receptor antibody diluted 1:200. After several washes, sections were incubated with Cy3-conjugated donkey anti-goat IgG diluted 1:200 for 2 h. After extensive washing in TBS, the sections were mounted onto glass slides using Vectashield (Vector Lab., Burlingame, CA). Immunofluorescence staining was monitored with a laser scanning microscope (LSM 510, Carl Zeiss, Thornwood, NY) equipped with a Plan-Apochromat 63x oil immersion lens . Cy3 was excited using the 543-nm line of the helium/neon laser and emission signals were filtered with an LP560 filter.

Immunoblotting

Identical amounts of protein (20 μg) from cerebellar homogenates were subjected to SDS-PAGE (10%), using the BioRad MiniProtean System (Bio-Rad, Richmond, CA). The separated proteins were transferred onto nitrocellulose membranes. The resulting blots were treated with blocking buffer containing 0.05% (v/v) Tween-20 (ICN Biomedicals, Aurora, OH) for 1 h at room temperature under agitation, followed by overnight incubation at 4°C with primary polyclonal goat anti-5-HT_3 antibody diluted 1:200. Blots were washed in 0.05% Tween-20 in TBS and then incubated with agitation in

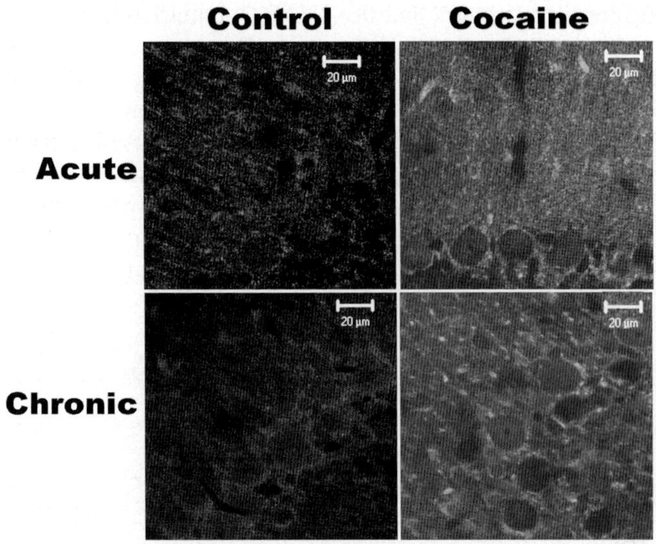

FIGURE 1. Single labeling for 5-HT$_3$ receptor in rat cerebellum. Immunofluorescence confocal micrographs of cerebellum sagittal sections from rats treated acutely or repeatedly for 10 days with 20 mg/kg cocaine are shown as indicated. Sections were incubated with polyclonal antibody against 5-HT$_3$, followed by secondary Cy3-conjugated donkey-anti-goat antibody. Scale bars: 20 μm.

secondary donkey anti-goat peroxidase-conjugated antibody diluted 1:25,000 for 1 h at room temperature. Antibody binding was detected by chemiluminescence (Pierce, Rockford, IL) with 5- to 10-min exposure on Kodak Biomax autoradiographic film (Eastman Kodak, Rochester, NY). SeeBlue Plus prestained protein standards were obtained from Invitrogen (Carlsbad, CA).

RESULTS

Using immunohistochemistry, we first studied the expression of the 5-HT$_3$ receptor in the cerebellum of rats treated either acutely or chronically with cocaine. Constitutive expression of the 5-HT$_3$ receptor was detected in control saline-injected animals (FIG. 1, left panels). As shown in FIGURE 1, cocaine was found to elicit a robust induction in the receptor expression in rat cerebellum. This effect was already observed in response to a single cocaine injection, and appeared somewhat attenuated after the chronic treatment. Surprisingly, 5-HT$_3$ receptor immunoreactivity was mainly localized within Bergmann glial cells and in their radial fibers which project into the molecular layer of the cerebellum. Less intense and scattered immunoreactivity was observed throughout the granular layer. No significant labeling was found in the adjacent Purkinje neurons. The glial localization was assessed by double immunofluorescence confocal analysis on rat sagittal sections, using antibodies for 5-HT$_3$

receptor and for the astrocytic marker GFAP. A remarkable co-localization of the two proteins was observed in Bergmann fibers as well as at the periphery of Purkinje cell soma (data not shown), confirming the glial localization of 5-HT$_3$ receptor and the absence of significant expression in neurons. In order to further address the specificity of the antibody we used, we analyzed the localization of 5-HT$_3$ receptor in other rat brain regions. 5-HT$_3$ immunoreactivity was found in the striatum as well as in the hippocampus (data not shown), and the distribution of the receptor in these structures was consistent with the localization previously reported,[17] thus validating the immunological technique we used.

To confirm that cocaine was actually inducing 5-HT$_3$ receptor in the cerebellum, we measured the 5-HT$_3$ receptor expression after cocaine treatment using the Western blot analysis. As shown in FIGURE 2, a strong increase in the receptor expression was observed in the cerebellum after a single cocaine

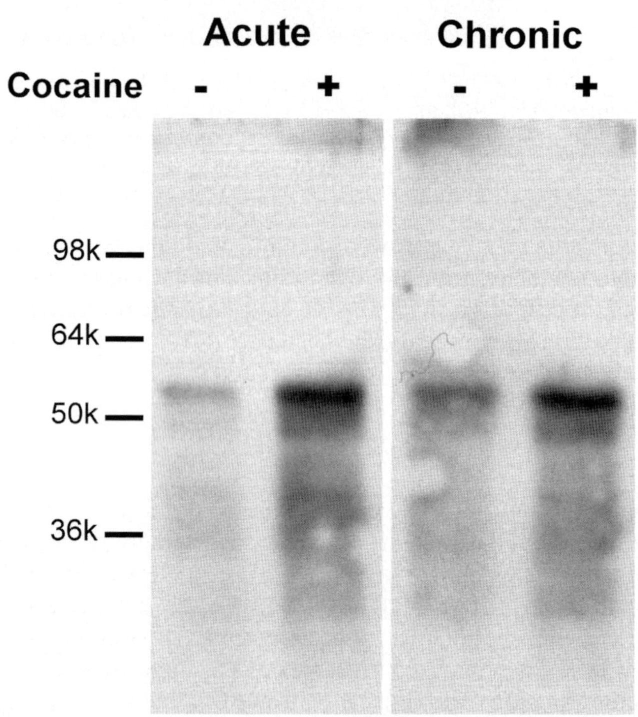

FIGURE 2. Western blot analysis of rat cerebellum homogenate probed with anti-5-HT$_3$ receptor antibody. Proteins in homogenate were separated on a 10% SDS-polyacrylamide gel and transferred onto nitrocellulose membrane, as described in Materials and Methods. Immunostaining was carried out with polyclonal anti-5-HT$_3$ receptor antibody, showing 5-HT$_3$ expression as a major band of Mr approximately 55,000. Molecular weight of prestained protein standards are indicated on the left hand side.

injection to rats, as assessed by the increase in intensity of the major band, which exhibited the expected apparent molecular mass of approximately 55,000.[18] A similar response was obtained after a series of 10 injections. It is noteworthy that the antibody detected a second band located below the major one, which was similarly induced after drug treatment. It is not clear whether the presence of two bands can be attributed to the expression of the two subunits 5-HT$_{3A}$ and 5-HT$_{3B}$ of the receptor.

DISCUSSION

We report here the induction by cocaine of the serotonergic 5-HT$_3$ receptor in rat cerebellum. The receptor was found to be mainly expressed in glial cells, as inferred from the thorough co-localization of 5-HT$_3$ receptor and GFAP. Whereas early studies have indicated a lack of 5-HT$_3$ receptors in the cerebellum,[19] the presence of this receptor has finally been demonstrated immunohistochemically in the molecular and granular layers on varicose fibers sparsely distributed throughout the cerebellum.[20] It has also been shown that 5-HT$_3$ receptor subtype is present in cerebellar synaptosomes, because changes in intracellular calcium concentration were noticed in response to a 5-HT$_3$ agonist.[21] Hence, our data showing a glial localization of the 5-HT$_3$ receptor does not appear consistent with the presence of the receptor in synaptosomes. In fact, the data may be reconciled when considering that Bergmann glial cells are closely related to synapses, as they serve homeostatic functions for the extracellular spaces around synapses such as K^+ clearance.[22] Synaptosomal preparations may therefore contain substantial amounts of 5-HT$_3$ receptors originating from contaminating Bergmann cell membranes. Moreover, Bergmann cells are known to be equipped with a large repertoire of receptors allowing them to sense the activity of synapses.[22] For instance, they express Ca2+-permeable alpha-amino-3-hydroxy-5-methyl-4-isoxazole propionic acid (AMPA) receptors, which are cation-conducting glutamate receptors .[23] It is therefore conceivable that they also express cation-conducting 5-HT$_3$ serotonin receptors.

If the glial ensheathment is viewed as fully participating in the functioning of the synapse, it should be considered as undergoing plastic changes similarly to pre- or postsynaptic regions. In this way of thinking, the enhanced expression of the 5-HT$_3$ receptor in response to cocaine can be viewed as an adaptative response from the cerebellum to the psychostimulant. It has already been shown that cocaine suppresses both spontaneous activity and glutamate-evoked excitation of Purkinje cells,[16] which are known to be associated with Bergmann glia in the adult cerebellum. Modulation of the 5-HT$_3$ receptor synthesis may be a consequence of the abnormal serotonergic system itself. In effect, neonatal cocaine exposure has been shown to affect the serotonergic cerebellar system by increasing its serotonin content.[24] It remains, however, to be demonstrated that cocaine treatment modifies the serotonin level also in adult cerebellum. Extracellular serotonin levels are likely to be increased in the cerebellum which receives significant serotonin projections, because cocaine is known to strongly inhibit the serotonin transporter.[25] In the developing cerebellum, serotonin is known to play a trophic role in the differentiation of neural cells by participating in axonogenesis and synaptogenesis.[26] Similarly, cocaine-induced increase in serotonin synthesis in adult cerebellum may be involved in counterbalancing cell damage that occurs in response to cocaine administration. The effect may be mediated, at least partially, by the enhancement of the 5-HT_3 receptor synthesis we report here.

In summary, treatment with cocaine was found to increase 5-HT_3 receptor expression in rat cerebellum. Modifications by cocaine of normal functioning of the serotonergic system in the cerebellum may be involved in drug-induced alterations in behavior and cognition. The data also highlight the importance of the cerebellum in cocaine mode of action.

REFERENCES

1. Bloom, F.E. & M. Morales. 1998. The central 5-HT3 receptor in CNS disorders. Neurochem. Res. **23:** 653–659.
2. Grant, K.A. 1995. The role of 5-HT3 receptors in drug dependence. Drug Alcohol Depend. **38:** 155–171.
3. Humblot, N. *et al.* 1998. The serotonergic system modulates the cocaine-induced expression of the immediate early genes egr-1 and c-fos in rat brain. Ann. N. Y. Acad. Sci. **844:** 7–20.
4. Thiriet, N. *et al.* 2002. Analysis of ecstasy (MDMA)-induced transcriptional responses in the rat cortex. FASEB J. **16:** 1887–1894.
5. Calcagnetti, D.J. *et al.* 1995. Blockade of cocaine-induced conditioned place preference: relevance to cocaine abuse therapeutics. Life Sci. **56:** 475–483.
6. Reith, M.E. 1990. 5-HT3 receptor antagonists attenuate cocaine-induced locomotion in mice. Eur. J. Pharmacol. **186:** 327–330.
7. Svingos, A.L. & R. Hitzemann. 1992. 5-HT3 receptor antagonists block cocaine-induced locomotion via a PCPA-sensitive mechanism. Pharmacol. Biochem. Behav. **43:** 871–879.
8. King, G.R. *et al.* 2000. Long-term blockade of the expression of cocaine sensitization by ondansetron, a 5-HT(3) receptor antagonist. Eur. J. Pharmacol. **394:** 97–101.
9. Rodd, Z.A. *et al.* 2005. Intracranial self-administration of cocaine within the posterior ventral tegmental area of Wistar rats: evidence for involvement of serotonin-3 receptors and dopamine neurons. J. Pharmacol. Exp. Ther. **313:** 134–145.
10. McKenzie-Quirk, S.D. *et al.* 2005. 5-HT(3) receptors, alcohol and aggressive behavior in mice. Behav. Pharmacol. **16:** 163–169.
11. Hodge, C.W. *et al.* 2004. 5-HT(3A) receptor subunit is required for 5-HT3 antagonist-induced reductions in alcohol drinking. Neuropsychopharmacology **29:** 1807–1813.

12. BOESS, F.G., R. BEROUKHIM & I.L. MARTIN. 1995. Ultrastructure of the 5-hydroxytryptamine3 receptor. J. Neurochem. **64:** 1401–1405.
13. DAVIES, P.A. *et al.* 1999. The 5-HT3B subunit is a major determinant of serotonin-receptor function. Nature **397:** 359–363.
14. HANNA, M.C. *et al.* 2000. Evidence for expression of heteromeric serotonin 5-HT(3) receptors in rodents. J. Neurochem. **75:** 240–247.
15. HAYRAPETYAN, V. *et al.* 2005. Co-expression of the 5-HT(3B) subunit with the 5-HT(3A) receptor reduces alcohol sensitivity. Mol. Brain Res. **142:** 146–150.
16. JIMENEZ-RIVERA, C.A. *et al.* 2000. Effects of intravenous cocaine administration on cerebellar Purkinje cell activity. Eur. J. Pharmacol. **407:** 91–100.
17. MORALES, M., E. BATTENBERG & F.E. BLOOM. 1998. Distribution of neurons expressing immunoreactivity for the 5HT3 receptor subtype in the rat brain and spinal cord. J. Comp. Neurol. **402:** 385–401.
18. MORALES, M. *et al.* 1996. Cellular and subcellular immunolocalization of the type 3 serotonin receptor in the rat central nervous system. Mol. Brain Res. **36:** 251–260.
19. MARICQ, A.V. *et al.* 1991. Primary structure and functional expression of the 5HT3 receptor, a serotonin-gated ion channel. Science **254:** 432–437.
20. GEURTS, F.J., E. DE SCHUTTER & J.P. TIMMERMANS. 2002. Localization of 5-HT2A, 5-HT3, 5-HT5A and 5-HT7 receptor-like immunoreactivity in the rat cerebellum. J. Chem. Neuroanat. **24:** 65–74.
21. NAYAK, S.V. *et al.* 1999. Calcium changes induced by presynaptic 5-hydroxytryptamine-3 serotonin receptors on isolated terminals from various regions of the rat brain. Neuroscience **91:** 107–117.
22. MULLER, T. & H. KETTENMANN. 1995. Physiology of Bergmann glial cells. Int. Rev. Neurobiol. **38:** 341–359.
23. SUZUKI, T. *et al.* 2003. Recent advances in the study of AMPA receptors. Nippon Yakurigaku Zasshi **122:** 515–526.
24. SUMMAVIELLE, T. *et al.* 2004. Abnormal immunoreactivity to serotonin in cerebellar Purkinje cells after neonatal cocaine exposure. Ann. N. Y. Acad. Sci. **1025:** 630–637.
25. RITZ, M.C., E.J. CONE & M.J. KUHAR. 1990. Cocaine inhibition of ligand binding at dopamine, norepinephrine and serotonin transporters: a structure-activity study. Life Sci. **46:** 635–645.
26. LAUDER, J.M. & H. KREBS. 1978. Serotonin as a differentiation signal in early neurogenesis. Dev. Neurosci. **1:** 15–30.

Alpha-Noradrenergic Receptors Modulate the Development and Expression of Cocaine Sensitization

CARLOS A. JIMÉNEZ-RIVERA,[a] MONICA FELIU-MOJER,[b] AND RAFAEL VÁZQUEZ-TORRES[a]

[a] *Department of Physiology, University of Puerto Rico, School of Medicine, San Juan, Puerto Rico, 00936-5067*

[b] *Department of Physiology, Universidad Central del Caribe, Bayamón, Puerto Rico, 00956*

ABSTRACT: The increased activity and stereotyped behaviors that result from repeated administration of cocaine is called cocaine sensitization. This sensitized response has been postulated as one of the basic pathophysiological mechanisms in drug addiction. Recent evidence indicates that noradrenergic neurotransmission might be implicated in some of the behavioral effects of cocaine. The present article examined the role of alpha-adrenergic receptor agonists and antagonists in the development and expression of cocaine sensitization. Rats were injected once per day, for 7 consecutive days, with the alpha-1 receptor antagonist prazosin (0.5 mg/kg, i.p.) 15 min before cocaine administration (15 mg/kg, i.p.). After 8 days, animals received a cocaine challenge (15 mg/kg, i.p.) and were tested for locomotion. Following a 7-day withdrawal period rats received a second cocaine challenge. One day after the last challenge, rats were reinstated to the initial protocol for 1 day. In another set of experiments, rats were injected twice per day with the alpha-2 receptor antagonists yohimbine (5 mg/kg, i.p.), idazoxan (0.25 mg/kg, i.p.), or with the alpha-2 agonist clonidine (0.025 mg/kg, i.p.), followed by cocaine injections (15 mg/kg, i.p.), for 7 consecutive days. Thereafter, the protocol was similar to that following prazosin administration. The results demonstrated that the alpha-1 receptor antagonist prazosin blocked the development and expression of cocaine sensitization. On the other hand, both alpha-2 antagonists failed to inhibit the development or the expression of cocaine sensitization. Instead, they produced an increase in locomotor activity during the first day of experimentation. The alpha-2 agonist clonidine attenuated the acute response to cocaine on day 1 and retarded the increased locomotor activity on the following 2 days. There was a dramatic increase in the level of sensitization after the first cocaine challenge.

Address for correspondence: C.A. Jimenez-Rivera, Department of Physiology, University of Puerto Rico, School of Medicine, Main Building , Room A-688, Medical Sciences Campus, San Juan, Puerto Rico, 00936-5067. Voice: 787-758-2525; ext.: 1676; fax: 787-753-0120.
e-mail: cajimenez@rcm.upr.edu

Ann. N.Y. Acad. Sci. 1074: 390–402 (2006).
doi: 10.1196/annals.1369.039

However, it inhibited the expression of cocaine sensitization during the reinstatement protocol. These results suggest that alpha adrenoreceptors play an important role in modulating different stages of cocaine sensitization and probably cocaine addiction.

KEYWORDS: cocaine; norepinephrine; alpha-1 receptors; alpha-2 receptors; clonidine; yohimbine; prazosin; idazoxan

INTRODUCTION

Cocaine sensitization refers to the increased activity and stereotyped behaviors that result from repeated cocaine administration.[1] This sensitized response can persist for weeks or months following the cessation of drug treatment and has been postulated as one of the basic pathological mechanisms involved in drug addiction.[2–4]

Cocaine-induced sensitization results from neural adaptations in the brain-reward system.[5] One of the most important brain-reward circuits involves dopamine (DA) neurons of the ventral tegmental area (VTA) and its projections to mesolimbic/mesocortical.[6,7] Although extensive evidence indicates that the processes of enhanced locomotion and cocaine sensitization are intimately related with DA transmission, there is compelling data suggesting an important noradrenergic modulatory role in this phenomenon.

The majority of the available data on the role of norepinephrine (NE) in cocaine sensitization deals with alpha-noradrenergic receptors. Recent investigations show that prazosin, an alpha-1 adrenergic receptor antagonist, reduced the acute locomotor effects and blocked behavioral sensitization to both cocaine and amphetamine injections.[8] Additional studies have indicated that stimulation of alpha-1 and alpha-2 adrenergic receptors amplified the DA-mediated locomotor hyperactivity in rats and mice.[9] Furthermore, it was demonstrated that the development of cocaine sensitization was dramatically increased in mice lacking the adrenergic receptor subtype alpha-1b.[10]

In contrast with the aforementioned studies, there are other investigations that suggest that the noradrenergic transmission is not critically involved in the development of cocaine sensitization.[11,12] Therefore, the role of NE transmission in the process of cocaine-induced behavioral sensitization is still equivocal.

The present experiments were designed to investigate the role of alpha adrenoceptors in two distinct processes in cocaine sensitization, initiation and expression. Initiation of sensitization are the immediate molecular and/or cellular effects that induce behavioral sensitization.[13,14] Expression indicates the long-term consequences of these effects. Numerous studies have shown that the VTA is the site where the processes responsible for the initiation of sensitization occur.[15,16] On the other hand, the nucleus accumbens (NAcc) seems to be the anatomical structure more relevant for the expression of sensitization.[14,16–18]

In terms of behavior, the function of noradrenergic neurotransmission in the initiation and expression of cocaine sensitization has been relatively unexplored. We investigated the role of prazosin (an alpha-1 receptor antagonist), yohimbine and idazoxan (alpha-2 receptor antagonists), and clonidine (an alpha-2 agonist) in the development and expression of cocaine sensitization. The results suggest that alpha-adrenergic receptors modulate different stages of cocaine-induced behavioral sensitization.

METHODS

Animal Housing

A total of 76 male Sprague-Dawley rats (250–300 g) were purchased from Taconic Farms (Germantown, NY). They were maintained on a 12-h light/dark cycle. Food and water were available *ad libitum.* All experiments were performed during the light cycle. All procedures were conducted in accordance with approved Institutional Animal Care and Use Committee.

Experimental Design

Prior to injections, and behavioral testing, animals were acclimated to the test cages (AccuScan Instruments Inc., Columbus,OH) for 4 consecutive days.

Alpha-1 Adrenergic Receptors

Behavioral sensitization was induced by once daily administration of saline (1 cc/kg, i.p.), followed by cocaine (15 mg/kg i.p.) or prazosin (0.5 mg/kg, i.p.) for 7 consecutive days. Controls were injected with prazosin (0.5 mg/kg, i.p.) followed by saline (1 cc/kg, i.p.) or with two consecutive saline injections (1 cc/kg, each i.p.). Locomotor activity (counts/60 min) was recorded for all groups on days 1, 3, 5, and 7 of the sensitization protocol. On day 8 all rats received a cocaine challenge (15 mg/kg, i.p.) and locomotor activity was recorded. A 7-day withdrawal period followed, and on day 16 all animals received a second cocaine challenge (15 mg/kg, i.p.) and locomotor activity was recorded. On day 17 all animals were reinstated to the sensitization protocol described above and locomotor activity was measured.

Alpha-2 Adrenergic Receptors

Behavioral sensitization was induced by twice daily administration of saline (1 cc/kg, i.p.), followed by cocaine (15 mg/kg, i.p.) or yohimbine (5 mg/kg, i.p.) for 7 consecutive days. Controls were injected with yohimbine (5 mg/kg, i.p.)

followed by saline (1 cc/kg, i.p.) or with two consecutive saline injections (1 cc/kg each, i.p.) Locomotor activity (counts/60 min) was recorded for all groups on days 1–7 of the sensitization protocol. On day 8 all rats received a cocaine challenge (15 mg/kg, i.p.) and locomotor activity was recorded. A 7-day withdrawal period followed, and on day 16 all animals received a second cocaine challenge (15 mg/kg, i.p.) and locomotor activity was measured. On day 17 all animals were reinstated to the sensitization protocol described above and locomotor activity was measured. The same protocol was used with idazoxan (0.25 mg/kg, i.p.) and clonidine (0.025 mg/kg, i.p.)

Data Analysis

One-way ANOVA followed by the Newman-Kuel's *post hoc* tests were used to analyze the data. A significant level of $P < 0.05$ was employed.

RESULTS

FIGURE 1 illustrates the effects of the alpha-1 receptor antagonist prazosin on the development and expression of cocaine sensitization. Animals pretreated

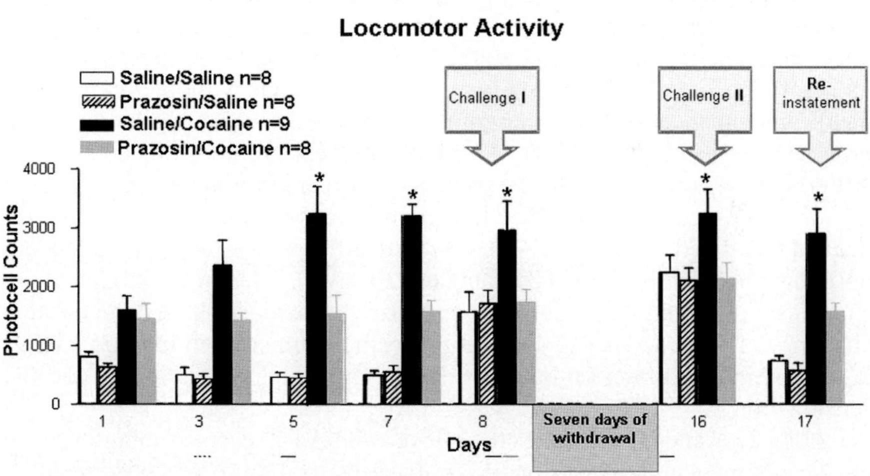

FIGURE 1. The figure illustrates the effects of the alpha-1 receptor antagonist prazosin on the development and expression of cocaine sensitization. Rats that received cocaine alone (saline/cocaine group) were fully sensitized as evidence by their response to a cocaine challenge or a reinstatement protocol (saline/cocaine; $^*P < 0.05$, one-way ANOVA followed by Newman-Kuel's test between first day and days 5, 7, 8,16, and 17 of saline/cocaine group). Although there was an enhanced locomotor response after the first cocaine injection (acute response) no significant changes were observed in the prazosin-injected group thereafter. These results demonstrate that the alpha-1 antagonist prazosin blocks the development and expression of cocaine-induced behavioral sensitization. For details see text.

with saline (1 cc/kg, i.p. injections) followed 15 min later by cocaine administration (15 mg/kg, i.p.) (saline/cocaine group) were already sensitized at days 5 (one-way ANOVA, $F_{3,28} = 12.61$, $P < 0.0001$; Newman-Kuel's $q = 6.40$, $P < 0.001$, day 5 versus 1) and 7 ($q = 6.24$, $P < 0.001$). The level of sensitization remained the same after the first (day 8, $q = 5.31$, $P < 0.01$) and second (day 16, $q = 6.45$, $P < 0.001$) cocaine challenge and following a reinstatement protocol (day 17, $q = 5.10$, $P < 0.05$). On the contrary, animals that were pretreated with prazosin (0.5 mg/kg, i.p.) 15 min before cocaine administration (prazosin/cocaine) demonstrated an inhibition in the development of cocaine sensitization. On day 1, rats in the prazosin/cocaine group had an increased locomotor response similar to the one present in the saline/cocaine group (acute response). This response remained at the same level with subsequent injections and after the first cocaine challenge. This indicates that no sensitized response was developed ($q = 4.61$, $P < 0.05$ for prazosin/cocaine on day 8 versus saline/cocaine). On the other hand, no changes in locomotion were observed between the saline/saline and prazosin/saline groups throughout the initial 7 days demonstrating that prazosin by itself does not produce any alteration in normal locomotor behavior. After a 7-day withdrawal period, on day 16 (second cocaine challenge) there was no expression of behavioral sensitization in the prazosin/cocaine group ($P > 0.05$ compared to day 1). On the other hand, all three groups (saline/saline, saline/prazosin, and prazosin/saline) demonstrated a similar slight increase in locomotion (although not significant) when compared to the first cocaine challenge. Because at this moment all groups had received two cocaine injections without any pretreatment, this enhancement in locomotion could be due to the beginning of the process of sensitization. On day 17 a reinstatement protocol was introduced. All groups were reinstated to the original sensitization protocol given during the initial 7 days. It was observed that animals in the saline/cocaine group remained sensitized ($q = 5.10$, $P < 0.05$) whereas the prazosin/cocaine group did not show sensitization ($P > 0.05$ compared to day 1). There was a small but not significant diminution in locomotor response compared to the second cocaine challenge. These results suggest that prazosin administration induces a long-lasting inhibitory effect on both the development and expression of cocaine sensitization.

FIGURE 2 (A and B) illustrates the effects of alpha-2 receptor antagonists on the development and expression of cocaine sensitization. It was observed that animals that were administered saline 15 min before cocaine (saline/cocaine group) developed an enhanced locomotor response already on day 2 of experimentation (one-way ANOVA $F_{3,40} = 10.96$, $P < 0.0001$; $q = 5.63$, $P < 0.01$ compared to day 1). The increased locomotion remained at the same level for the rest of the experiment with the exception of day 6 ($P > 0.05$ compared to day 1). This enhanced rate of sensitization could be due to the fact that a protocol of two injections per day was employed. As shown in FIGURE 2 A,

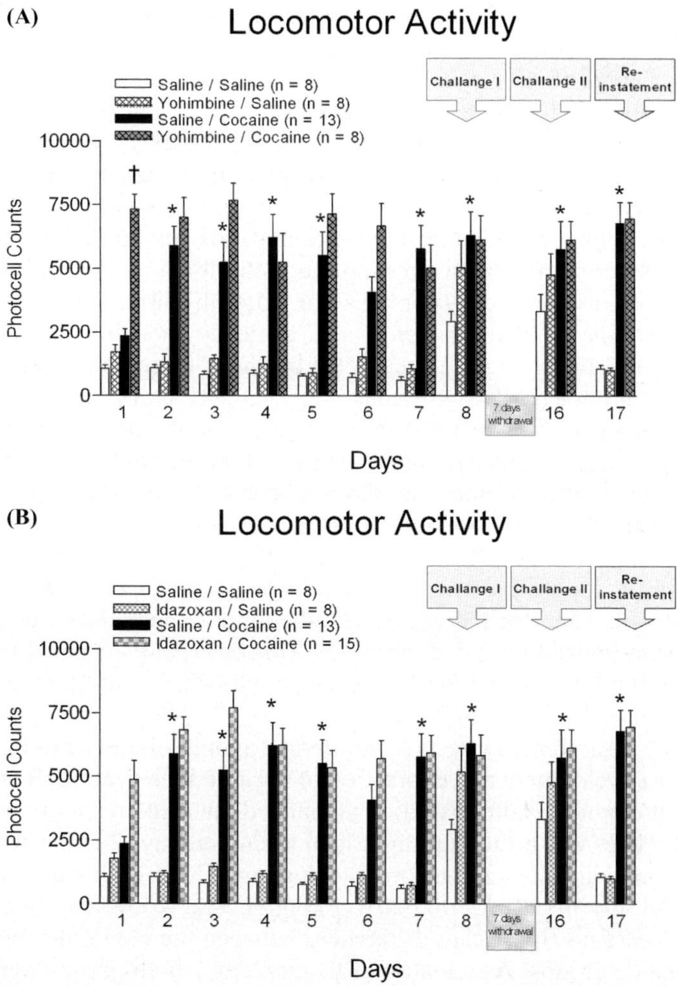

FIGURE 2. The figure (**A** and **B**) illustrates the effects of alpha-2 receptor antagonists on the development and expression of cocaine sensitization. (**A**) Rats that received cocaine (saline/cocaine group) were fully sensitized as evidenced by their response to a cocaine challenge or a reinstatement protocol. Yohimbine (5 mg/kg, i.p.) induced a robust increase in total locomotor activity on day 1 (yohimbine/cocaine; $+P < 0.001$ compared to the saline/cocaine group on day 1, one-way ANOVA followed by Newman-Kuel's test). However, yohimbine administration did not block the development or expression of cocaine-induced sensitization because no significant differences were observed between the yohimbine/cocaine and saline/cocaine groups after a cocaine challenge or a reinstatement protocol. (**B**) The same protocol was used with idazoxan (0.25 mg/kg, i.p.) and similar effects as yohimbine were seen but in lower magnitude. Asterisks denote significant differences ($P < 0.05$, one-way ANOVA followed by Newman-Kuel's test) between the first day and days 2, 3, 4, 5, 7, 8, 16, and 17 of saline/cocaine groups.

animals pretreated with the alpha-2 antagonist yohimbine (5 mg/kg, i.p.), showed a dramatic increase in the acute response to cocaine on day 1 ($q = 6.90$, $P < 0.001$ between saline/cocaine and yohimbine/cocaine groups). There were no significant differences between the yohimbine/cocaine and saline/cocaine groups thereafter. No significant differences were observed within the yohimbine/cocaine group on day 1 versus any other day, including cocaine challenges and the reinstatement period. In addition, no significant changes were seen between the saline/saline and saline/yohimbine groups throughout the initial 7 days of experimentation suggesting that yohimbine by itself did not have any effects on normal locomotor behavior. After the first (day 8) and second (day 16) cocaine challenges there was a tendency for the saline/yohimbine group to show an increase in locomotor behavior when compared to day 1, although it did not reach significance. FIGURE 2 B shows the effects of the alpha-2 antagonist's idazoxan (0.25 mg/kg, i.p.) on the development and expression of cocaine sensitization. It can be observed that on day 1, similar to yohimbine administration, the idaxozan/cocaine group had a tendency to show an increased acute locomotor response, although in this case, it did not reach significance ($P > 0.05$). No differences were observed at any other days, including the two cocaine challenges and during the reinstatement protocol. Therefore, it seems that the alpha-2 antagonists enhance the locomotor response to cocaine during the first day (acute response) of experimentation but failed to inhibit the development or the expression of cocaine sensitization.

FIGURE 3 illustrates the effects of the alpha-2 agonist clonidine (0.025 mg/kg, i.p.) on the development and expression of cocaine sensitization. It can be observed that clonidine administration attenuated the acute response to cocaine on day 1. There was a diminution in locomotion on days 2 and 3 when compared to the saline/cocaine group reaching significance on day 3 (one-way ANOVA $F_{3,40} = 15.11$, $P < 0.0001$; $q = 4.99$, $P < 0.05$). However for days 4–7 there were no significant differences between the clonidine/cocaine and saline/cocaine groups. As a matter of fact, on day 7 both groups were behaviorally sensitized in comparison to their respective day 1 ($q = 6.48$, $P < 0.01$ for clonidine/cocaine and $q = 6.21$, $P < 0.01$ for saline/cocaine). At the time of the first challenge the clonidine/cocaine group demonstrated a dramatic increase in the level of sensitization when compared to the response of the saline/cocaine group ($q = 9.19$, $P < 0.001$). Following the withdrawal period, the clonidine/cocaine group showed an enhanced behavioral response ($q = 8.35$, $P < 0.001$ compared to day 1) during the second cocaine challenge although it was greatly diminished compared to the sensitization demonstrated during the first challenge ($q = 6.12$, $P < 0.001$ for clonidine/cocaine day 16 versus day 8). Clonidine was able to block the expression of cocaine sensitization during the reinstatement protocol ($q = 7.67$, $P < 0.001$ for clonidine/cocaine at day 17 compared to saline/cocaine day 17).

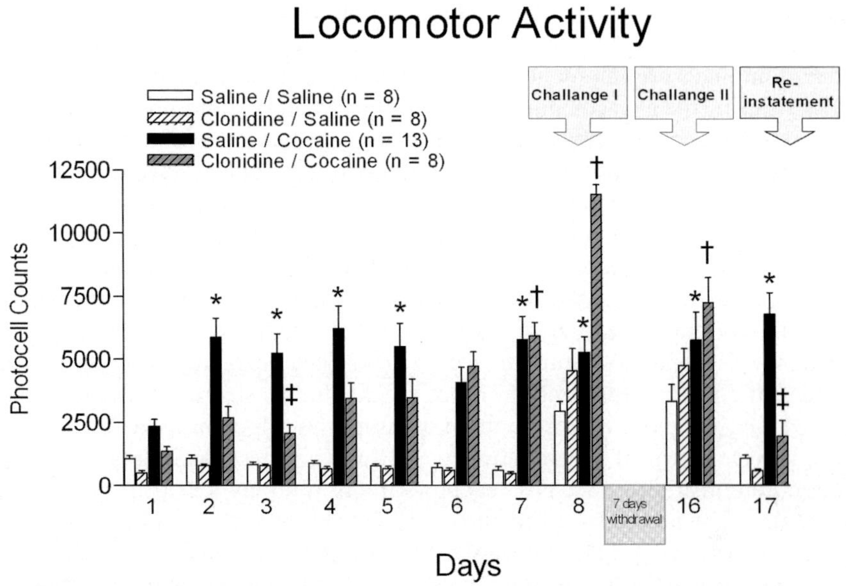

FIGURE 3. The figure illustrates the effects of the alpha-2 agonist clonidine (0.025 mg/kg, i.p.) on the development and expression of cocaine sensitization. Rats that received cocaine alone (saline/cocaine group) were fully sensitized as evidence by their response to a cocaine challenge or a reinstatement protocol. Clonidine attenuated the acute response of cocaine on day 1 and retarded the increase in locomotor activity on the following 2 days (clonidine/cocaine; ‡$P < 0.05$ compared to saline/cocaine on days 3 and 17 one-way ANOVA followed by Newman-Kuel's test) but did not block the development of cocaine sensitization during day 7, or challenges I and II. Clonidine was able to block the expression of cocaine sensitization during the reinstatement protocol (clonidine/cocaine; ‡$P < 0.001$ compared to saline/cocaine on reinstatement protocol, one-way ANOVA, Newman-Kuel's test). Asterisks denote significant differences ($P < 0.05$, one-way ANOVA, Newman-Kuel's test) between the first day and days 2, 3, 4, 5, 7, 8, 16, and 17 of saline/cocaine groups. †denotes a significant difference ($P < 0.05$, one-way ANOVA and Newman-Kuel's test) between first day and days 7, 8, and 16 of clonidine/cocaine groups.

DISCUSSION

The goal of the present experiment was to investigate the role of the alpha-adrenergic receptors in the initiation and expression of cocaine sensitization. The results revealed that the pretreatment with the alpha-1 antagonist prazosin blocked not only the initiation but also the expression of cocaine-induced behavioral sensitization. On the contrary, both alpha-2 antagonists' yohimbine and idazoxan, seemed to affect only the acute response to cocaine by increasing it during the first day of treatment. The administration of clonidine, an alpha-2 receptor agonist, attenuated the acute response to cocaine on experimental day 1 and retarded the increased locomotor activity on the following 2 days. However, it was unable to fully block the development of cocaine sensitization. After clonidine's pretreatment there was a dramatic enhancement of locomotor activity during the first cocaine challenge. Nevertheless, clonidine inhibited the expression of cocaine sensitization during the reinstatement protocol. The data is consistent with the notion that alpha-adrenergic receptors have the capacity to modulate the initiation and expression of cocaine-induced behavioral sensitization. The results also suggest that NE transmission could be an important factor in the development and expression of cocaine sensitization.

Initial studies on the induction of sensitization have implicated alterations in the functioning of DA neurons in the VTA. Changes in D2 autoreceptor sensitivity[19–21] and DA neuronal firing[19] have been correlated with the development of cocaine sensitization. More recent studies suggest that alterations in VTA D1 receptors might be the most important dopaminergic adaptation in the development of sensitization.[22–24] However, there is contrasting information demonstrating that DA receptors might not play a critical role in the induction of behavioral sensitization.[25,26] On the other hand, changes in the spontaneous activity of DA neurons and D_1 receptor-mediated augmentation of γ-aminobutyric acid (GABA) $_B$- mediated inhibitory postsynaptic potentials have been shown to occur with the expression of cocaine sensitization.[27]

It is well known that the VTA and NAcc receive innervation from other catecholaminergic nuclei that release NE and serotonin onto them.[28–30] Because the reuptake mechanisms of these neurotransmitter systems are equally affected by cocaine,[31,32] their role in the initiation and expression of behavioral sensitization should not be overlooked.

Previous behavioral studies have demonstrated that the alpha-1 receptor antagonist prazosin exerted a powerful inhibitory effect on the development of cocaine sensitization.[8] Our results are in agreement with the major finding of the inhibition of the development of cocaine sensitization after prazosin pretreatment. However, we did not find, as the above authors, that prazosin blocked the acute response to cocaine. In our case the acute response remained intact and only the enhanced locomotion, after repeated cocaine administration, was affected. This difference could be due to the cocaine dose of 5 mg/kg, i.p. used in the previous study versus the 15 mg/kg, i.p. employed in our investigation to induce behavioral sensitization. Similar to the above-mentioned study[8] our experiments demonstrated that prazosin administration inhibited the expression of cocaine sensitization. In addition, our results tend to indicate that prazosin might have long-lasting effects on sensitization because the inhibitory actions were clearly present on the reinstatement protocol. However, further studies should be conducted to assess whether prazosin has any effects on the expression of sensitization once it has been developed.

Additional corroboration of the importance of the alpha-1 receptors in the initiation of cocaine sensitization has been demonstrated using alpha-1 receptor knockout mice.[10,33] It was shown that alpha-1b receptors exerted a powerful inhibitory action of the acute and sensitized response to cocaine administration. The reason why other investigations[11,12] have failed to demonstrate that prazosin had any effects on the development or expression of cocaine sensitization could be related to the different environments or doses used for animal testing. For example, in our experiments as well as in those of Drouin *et al.*[8,10] rats were monitored in the test environment (context dependent) and not in the home cages.

Other experiments have demonstrated that prazosin administration significantly reduce the cocaine-induced hypophagia and hyperlocomotion in rats.[34] Prazosin pretreatment was also revealed to significantly reduce the locomotor hyperactivity and striatal Fos expression induced by amphetamine injections.[35] More recently, it was shown that prazosin administration attenuated the cocaine-induced reinstatement of drug-seeking behavior.[36] Therefore, the majority of the recent evidence demonstrates an important role of alpha-adrenergic receptors in long-term behavioral adaptations including psychostimulant-induced behavioral sensitization.

Additional studies have shown that stimulation of alpha-1 and alpha-2 receptors amplified the DA-mediated locomotor activity in rats and mice. An important role of postsynaptic alpha-2 receptors in the induction of locomotor hyperactivity was suggested.[9] Other studies demonstrated that alpha-2 receptor antagonists, like idazoxan and efaroxan, enhanced the circling behavior induced by either methylphenidate or apomorphine.[37] Our studies provide support to this notion because it was demonstrated that with alpha-2 receptor blockers the acute response to cocaine was enhanced whereas with an alpha-2 agonist it was attenuated. As no changes were observed with yohimbine alone, the antagonist-induced enhanced locomotion can not be attributed to the yohimbine's anxiogenic effects or the production of behavioral sensitization with this drug reported by others.[38]

The present investigation demonstrated that alpha-2 receptor blockade was not sufficient to prevent the development or the expression of cocaine sensitization. To our knowledge, studies looking at the role of alpha-2 receptor antagonists on cocaine sensitization are lacking. Other studies have indicated that pharmacological inhibition of alpha-2 receptors triggers a reinstatement of cocaine-seeking behavior in squirrel monkeys.[39] Priming injections of yohimbine or RS-79948 produced a dose-related reinstatement of cocaine-seeking behavior.

On the other hand, the results with the alpha-2 receptor agonist clonidine tend to indicate that alpha-2 receptors can modulate cocaine sensitization. The administration of clonidine was able to retard the development of cocaine sensitization although it was not capable to fully block this process. Again, the differences observed with other studies[11] could be attributed to the doses and variations in protocols used. An interesting finding observed with clonidine administration was the enhanced level of sensitization reached after the first cocaine challenge. It has been demonstrated that repeated cocaine administration alters the sensitivity of alpha-2 receptors in different brain areas.[40,41] It is possible that after prolonged agonist-induced activation of alpha-2 receptors there is a downregulation of this receptor type. Therefore, this apparent enhanced sensitization observed after the first cocaine challenge could be due to a combined effect of a decreased sensitivity and downregulation of alpha-2 receptors. However, whatever the mechanism is present, it is not permanent because this enhanced sensitization returned to normal levels after a withdrawal period. Moreover, clonidine was able to affect the expression of sensitization during the reinstatement protocol suggesting that the receptor regains functionality after a prolonged withdrawal episode. Further studies should investigate if a downregulation of alpha-2 receptors occurs after cocaine sensitization and for how long can clonidine modulate the expression of behavioral sensitization.

Finally, a clear notion of the function of alpha receptors in cocaine sensitization will further add to our knowledge of the specific mechanism of the noradrenergic system in cocaine addictive processes. In addition, it might suggest possible avenues for therapeutic pharmacological interventions.

ACKNOWLEDGMENTS

This work was supported by the NINDS and NCRR SNRP # NS39408 and GM-50695 to C.A. Jiménez-Rivera. The authors thank Dr. Guido Santacana for proofreading and Dr. Priscilla Sanabria for figure preparation of the manuscript.

REFERENCES

1. Robinson, T.E. & K.C. Berridge. 1993. The neural basis of drug craving: an incentive-sensitization theory of addiction. Brain Res. Brain Res. Rev. **18**: 247–291.
2. Koob, G.F. & M. Le Moal. 1997. Drug abuse: hedonic homeostatic dysregulation. Science **278**: 52–58.
3. Robinson, T.E. & K.C. Berridge. 2000. The psychology and neurobiology of addiction: an incentive-sensitization view. Addiction **95**(Suppl. 2): S91–S117.
4. Robinson, T.E. & K.C. Berridge. 2003. Addiction. Annu. Rev. Psychol. **54**: 25–53.
5. White, F.J. & P.W. Kalivas. 1998. Neuroad aptations involved in amphetamine and cocaine addiction [review]. Drug Alcohol Depend. **51**: 141–53.
6. Bjorklund, A. & O. Lindvall. 1984. Dopamine-containing systems in the CNS. *In* Handbook of Chemical Neuroanatomy, Vol. 2. Classical Transmitters in the CNS, Part 1. Bjorklund, A., Hokfelt, T., Eds.: 55–122. Elsevier. Amsterdam.
7. Wise, R.A. & P.P. Rompre. 1989. Brain dopamine and reward. Annu. Rev. Psychol. **40**: 191–225.
8. Drouin, C., G. Blanc, A.S. Villegier, *et al.* 2002. Critical role of alpha1-adrenergic receptors in acute and sensitized locomotor effects of D-amphetamine, cocaine, and GBR 12783: influence of preexposure conditions and pharmacological characteristics. Synapse **43**: 51–61.
9. Villegier, A.S., C. Drouin, J.C. Bizot, *et al.* 2003. Stimulation of postsynaptic alpha1b- and alpha2-adrenergic receptors amplifies dopamine-mediated locomotor activity in both rats and mice. Synapse **50**: 277–284.

10. Drouin, C., L. Darracq, F. Trovero, *et al.* 2002. Alpha1b-adrenergic receptors control locomotor and rewarding effects of psychostimulants and opiates. J. Neurosci. **22**: 2873–2884.
11. Vanderschuren, L.J., P. Beemster & A.N. Schoffelmeer. 2003. On the role of noradrenaline in psychostimulant-induced psychomotor activity and sensitization. Psychopharmacology (Berl.) **169**: 176–185.
12. Filip, M., E. Nowak & I. Papla. 2001. On the role of serotonin2A/2C receptors in the sensitization to cocaine. J. Physiol. Pharmacol. **52**:471–81.
13. Kalivas, P.W. 1995. Interactions between dopamine and excitatory amino acids in behavioral sensitization to psychostimulants [review]. Drug Alcohol Depend. **37**: 95–100.
14. Kalivas, P.W. 1995. Neuronal basis of behavioral sensitization to cocaine. *In* The Neurobiology of Cocaine; Cellular and Molecular Mechanisms. R.P. Hammer, Jr., Ed.: 81–98. CRC Press, Inc. Boca Raton, FL.
15. Kalivas, P.W. & J. Stewart. 1991. Dopamine transmission in the initiation and expression of drug- and stress-induced sensitization of motor activity. [review]. Brain Res. Brain Res. Rev. **16**: 223–244.
16. Vanderschuren, L.J. & P.W. Kalivas. 2000. Alterations in dopaminergic and glutamatergic transmission in the induction and expression of behavioral sensitization: a critical review of preclinical studies. Psychopharmacology (Berl.) **151**: 99–120.
17. Cador, M., Y. Bjijou & L. Stinus. 1995. Evidence of a complete independence of the neurobiological substrates for the induction and expression of behavioral sensitization to amphetamine. Neuroscience **65**: 385–395.
18. Wang, X.B., M. Funada, Y. Imai, *et al.* 1997. rGbeta1: a psychostimulant-regulated gene essential for establishing cocaine sensitization. J. Neurosci. **17**: 5993–6000.
19. Henry, D.J., M.A. Greene & F.J. White. 1989. Electrophysiological effects of cocaine in the mesoaccumbens dopamine system: repeated administration. J. Pharmacol. Exp. Ther. **251**: 833–839.
20. Ackerman, J.M. & F.J. White. 1990. A10 somatodendritic dopamine autoreceptor sensitivity following withdrawal from repeated cocaine treatment. Neurosci. Lett. **117**: 181–187.
21. Wolf, M.E., F.J. White, R. Nassar, *et al.* 1993. Differential development of autoreceptor subsensitivity and enhanced dopamine release during amphetamine sensitization. J. Pharmacol. Exp. Ther. **264**: 249–255.
22. Pierce, R.C., B. Born, M. Adams & P.W. Kalivas. 1996. Repeated intra-ventral tegmental area administration of SKF- 38393 induces behavioral and neurochemical sensitization to a subsequent cocaine challenge. J. Pharmacol. Exp. Ther. **278**: 384–392.
23. Bjijou, Y., L. Stinus, M. Le Moal & M. Cador. 1996. Evidence for selective involvement of dopamine D1 receptors of the ventral tegmental area in the behavioral sensitization induced by intra ventral tegmental area injections of D-amphetamine. J. Pharmacol. Exp. Ther. **277**: 1177–1187.
24. Vezina, P. 1996. D1 dopamine receptor activation is necessary for the induction of sensitization by amphetamine in the ventral tegmental area. J. Neurosci. **16**: 2411–2420.
25. Mattingly, B.A., T.C. Hart, K. Lim & C. Perkins. 1994. Selective antagonism of dopamine D1 and D2 receptors does not block the development of behavioral sensitization to cocaine. Psychopharmacology (Berl.) **114**: 239–242.

26. WHITE, F.J., A. JOSHI, T.E. KOELTZOW & X.T. HU 1998. Dopamine receptor antagonists fail to prevent induction of cocaine sensitization. Neuropsychopharmacology **18**: 26–40.
27. WHITE, F.J. & P.W. KALIVAS. 1998. Neuroadaptations involved in amphetamine and cocaine addiction. Drug Alcohol Depend. **51**:141–153
28. OADES, R.D. & G.M. HALLIDAY. 1987. Ventral tegmental (A10) system: neurobiology. 1. Anatomy and connectivity [review]. Brain Res. **434**: 117–165.
29. DELFS, J.M., Y. ZHU, J.P. DRUHAN & G.S. ASTON-JONES. 1998. Origin of noradrenergic afferents to the shell subregion of the nucleus accumbens: anterograde and retrograde tract-tracing studies in the rat. Brain Res. **806**: 127–140.
30. MEJIAS-APONTE, C.A., F. GEORGES, C.A. JIMENEZ-RIVERA & G. ASTON-JONES. Interactions between VTA Dopaminergic and A2 Noradrenergic Neurons. Program No. 113.3. *2003 Abstract Viewer/Itinerary Planner*. Washington, DC: Society for Neuroscience, 2003. Online www.sfn.org
31. RITZ, M.C., R.J. LAMB, S.R. GOLDBERG & M.J. KUHAR. 1987. Cocaine receptors on dopamine transporters are related to self- administration of cocaine. Science **237**: 1219–1223.
32. KOE, B.K. 1976. Molecular geometry of inhibitors of the uptake of catecholamines and serotonin in synaptosomal preparations of rat brain. J. Pharmacol. Exp. Ther. **199**: 649–661.
33. AUCLAIR, A., C. DROUIN, S. COTECCHIA, *et al.* 2004. 5-HT and alpha1b-adrenergic receptors entirely mediate dopamine release, locomotor response and behavioural sensitization to opiates and psychostimulants. Eur. J. Neurosc. **20**: 3073–3084.
34. WELLMAN, P., D. HO, A. CEPEDA-BENITO, *et al.* 2002. Cocaine-induced hypophagia and hyperlocomotion in rats are attenuated by prazosin. Eur. J. Pharmacol. **455**: 117–126.
35. MUNOZ, A., A. LOPEZ-REAL, J.L. LABANDEIRA-GARCIA & M.J. GUERRA. 2003. Interaction between the noradrenergic and serotonergic systems in locomotor hyperactivity and striatal expression of Fos induced by amphetamine in rats. Exp. Brain Res. **153**: 92–99.
36. ZHANG, X.Y. & T.A. KOSTEN. 2005. Prazosin, an alpha-1 adrenergic antagonist, reduces cocaine-induced reinstatement of drug-seeking. Biol. Psychiatry **57**: 1202–1204.
37. CHOPIN, P., F.C. COLPAERT & M. MARIEN. 1999. Effects of alpha-2 adrenoceptor agonists and antagonists on circling behavior in rats with unilateral 6-hydroxydopamine lesions of the nigrostriatal pathway. J. Pharmacol. Exp. Ther. **288**: 798–804.
38. SCHROEDER, B.E., C.A. SCHILTZ & A.E. KELLEY. 2003. Neural activation profile elicited by cues associated with the anxiogenic drug yohimbine differs from that observed for reward-paired cues. Neuropsychopharmacology **28**: 14–21.
39. LEE, B., S. TIEFENBACHERS, D.M. PLATT & R.D. SPEALMAN. 2004. Pharmacological blockade of alpha-2 adrenoceptors induces reinstatement of cocaine-seeking behavior in squirrel monkeys. Neuropsychopharmacology **29**: 686–93.
40. BAUMANN, M.H., A.B. MILCHANOWSKI & R.B. ROTHMAN. 2004. Evidence for alterations in alpha-2 adrenergic receptor sensitivity in rats exposed to repeated cocaine administration. Neuroscience **125**: 683–90.
41. JIMENEZ-RIVERA, C.A., D. BLOOM, R. CASTRO, *et al.* Decreased Functionality of Alpha-2 Receptors in VTA DA cells after cocaine sensitization. Program No. 688.20. *2004 Abstract Viewer/Itinerary Planner*. Washington, DC: Society for Neuroscience, 2004. Online. www.sfn.org

AMPA and NMDA Receptors in P2 Fractions of Cocaine and Cocaine–Prazosin-Treated Rats

J.G. ORTIZ,[a] S. GONZÁLEZ-CABRERA,[a] M. RUBIO-DÁVILA,[a]
A. TIRADO-COSTACAMPS,[a] R. VÁZQUEZ-TORRES,[b]
N. BERRÍOS-CARTAGENA,[a] W.I. SILVA,[c]
AND C.A. JIMÉNEZ-RIVERA[b]

[a]*Department of Pharmacology and Toxicology School of Medicine, University of Puerto Rico, San Juan, Puerto Rico 00936*

[b]*Department of Physiology, Universidad Central del Caribe, Bayamón, Puerto Rico 00960*

[c]*Department of Physiology, School of Medicine, University of Puerto Rico, San Juan, Puerto Rico 00936*

ABSTRACT: Cocaine sensitization results in the development of increased locomotion and stereotypy. It is accompanied by changes in glutamatergic trasmission that appear to be region-specific. The purpose of this article was to determine the effect(s) of cocaine and prazosin plus cocaine treatments on ionotropic glutamate receptors in rat cerebral cortex (CTX) and prefrontal cortex (PFC). Cocaine-sensitized rats (15 mg/kg, i.p. once for 5 days), withdrawn (7 days) and later challenged with a single cocaine dose, showed region-specific in NMDA-2A and Glu-R2 in the CTX and PFC membranes in cocaine- and prazosin-treated rats when compared to the saline controls. Co-administration of prazosin inhibits sensitization and changes in NMDA 2A and Glu-R2. Furthermore, prazosin inhibits the effect of cocaine in CTX and PFC on [^{3}H]FW (AMPA agonist) binding when compared to controls. In cortex, cocaine treatment causes a marked increase in total binding, while in PFC there is a significant decrease. In both regions, cocaine–prazosin treatment attenuates the effects of cocaine. These results suggest that cocaine affects ionotropic glutamate receptors (NMDA and AMPA) and that prazosin inhibits such effects in a region-specific form in rat brain.

KEYWORDS: AMPA; NMDA; [^{3}H]FW; cocaine; prazosin; PFC

Address for correspondence: Dr. José G. Ortiz, Department of Pharmacology and Toxicology, School of Medicine, University of Puerto Rico, Medical Sciences Campus, P.O. Box 365067, San Juan, Puerto Rico 00936-5067. Voice: 787-758-2525 ext. 1371; fax: 787-282-0568.
e-mail: jg_ortiz@yahoo.com

**Ann. N.Y. Acad. Sci. 1074: 403–410 (2006). © 2006 New York Academy of Sciences.
doi: 10.1196/annals.1369.040**

INTRODUCTION

Cocaine, from *Erythroxylon coca*, causes positive reinforcing (rewarding) effects that depend on the mesocorticolimbic system. [1]This system is involved in both acute and chronic responses to drugs abuse comprising the ventral tegmental area (VTA), nucleus accumbens (NAc), and prefrontal cortex (PFC). The rewarding effects developed in this system are mediated by dopamine neurotransmission enhancement.

Glutamatergic inputs to the VTA and NAc, arising from the PFC, hippocampus, and basolateral amygdala, have been implicated in addiction.[2] In particular, potentiation of glutamatergic synaptic transmission in the VTA may be involved in behavioral sensitization, a phenomenon thought to be important in the development of addiction.[3] Blockage of the N-methyl-D-aspartate (NMDA) receptors with the noncompetitive antagonist MK-801 attenuates the development of behavioral sensitization.[4,5]

Behavioral studies in rats have shown that the administration of cocaine in the medial PFC reinstates cocaine-seeking behavior by increasing AMPA receptor-mediated glutamatergic transmission in the NAc.[6] Electrophysiological studies in mice VTA and hippocampal brain slices have proposed a contribution of AMPA and NMDA receptors to excitatory postsynaptic currents (EPSCs) in dopaminergic cells after a single *in vivo* cocaine exposure. This contribution appears to be region-specific.

Cocaine inhibits DA, NE, and 5-HT uptake[7–9]; thus its effects could be mediated by these mechanisms. Perturbations in NE transmission interfere with cocaine sensitization.[10] Moreover, prazosin, an α_1-antagonist prevents cocaine sensitization (Jiménez-Rivera *et al.*, this volume). We examined NMDA and AMPA receptor changes in cortex and PFC of cocaine-sensitized rats and their cocaine–prazosin-treated counterparts.

MATERIALS AND METHODS

Chemicals

[^{3}H]Fluorowillardiine (FW, 29.08 Ci/mmol) was obtained from American Radiolabeled Chemicals Inc. (ARC, St. Louis, MO). L-glutamate and Trizma Base were obtained from Sigma Chemical Co. (St. Louis, MO). UniverSol scintillation cocktail was obtained from ICN Pharmaceuticals Inc. (Irvine, CA).

Animals

Sprague-Dawley adult male rats (~2 months) were obtained from the Animal Resource Center, Universidad Central del Caribe (Bayamón, Puerto Rico).

One group of rats was injected once daily with cocaine (15 mg/kg, i.p.) for 5 days. The second group of rats was injected once daily with cocaine–prazosin for 5 days and the third group was injected once daily with saline solution. After 5 days, the rats spend 14 days without treatment administration. Then each individual group of rats was injected one time with cocaine. All animals were maintained in a 12-h light:dark cycle and had free access to water and food. The Institutional Animal Care and Use Committee (IACUC) approved all procedures (Jiménez-Rivera *et al.* this volume).

Synaptic Membranes (P2) Fractions

Rats were decapitated and the brain promptly removed. The cortex, hippocampus, and PFC were dissected and homogenized (1:10 w/v) in ice-cold deionized water. The homogenate was centrifuged twice at 2500*g* for 10 min. The resulting supernatant was centrifuged at 12500*g* for 20 min. The pellet was washed twice with ice-cold deionized water (1:10 w/v) and centrifuged at 12,500*g* for 20 min. The pellet (synaptical membrane, P2) was resuspended in deionized ice-cold water and freeze-thawed at least three times before been stored at −80°C until used. Protein concentration was determined using the Bradford assay[11] using bovine serum albumin (BSA) as standard. For Western blot analysis samples were diluted in Laemmli sample buffer solution.

[^{3}H]FW Binding

This assay was performed as described by Hawkins and collaborators.[12] Briefly, 15 nM [^{3}H]FW in TRIS HCl 50 mM/KCl 100 mM buffer, pH 7.4 was incubated with 150 μL protein. Nonspecific binding was determined in the presence of 1 mM unlabeled glutamate. Tubes were incubated at 4°C for 40 min before centrifugation at 13,000*g* for 7 min to separate free radioactivity from bound radioactivity. Pellets were superficially washed with 1 mL Tris-HCl/KCl buffer, resuspended in 400 μL of buffer and three 100 μL replicates of the sample were quantified in a Beckman LS 6000 scintillation counter after addition of scintillation cocktail.

Western Blot Analysis

SDS-PAGE and immunoblot analysis of the P2 fractions was done as described by Silva and collaborators[13] with the following modifications. In brief, equal P2 homogenate amounts (5 μg protein) of rat cortex, hippocampus, and PFC samples plus the molecular weight standards were resuspended in the

Laemmli sample buffer as described above, and separated in 8% SDS polyacrylamide gels (Bio-Rad Laboratories, Hercules, CA). After electrophoresis, the gel was transferred overnight to a PVDF membrane using a Mini Trans-Blot apparatus (Bio-Rad Laboratories) at 4°C. PVDF membranes were stained with India ink to verify transfer efficiency. Subsequently membranes were incubated overnight (at 4°C) with primary polyclonal antibodies against NMDA receptors subunit 2A (1:5000 dilution; Molecular Probes, Eugene, OR) and AMPA receptor subunit 2 (GlU-R2 (N-19) 1:5000 dilution; Santa Cruz Biotechnology, Santa Cruz, CA). After addition of the corresponding secondary antibodies (1:20,000 dilution; Santa Cruz Biotechnology), membranes were processed using the enhanced chemiluminescence assay (SuperSignal® West Dura Extended Duration Substrate; Pierce, Rockford, IL) as described by the manufacturer and exposed to an X-ray film. The molecular weights of the bands reacting with the antibodies were determined according to the migration of kaleidoscope broad range molecular weight standards. The densitometric analysis was performed with Image J Processing and Analysis program (JAVA version 1.32j; National Institutes of Health, Bethesda, MD).

Statistical Analysis

Mean values of data from at least three independent experiments were subsequently calculated and plotted as a percentage compared with untreated controls (which were set to 100%). Standard errors were calculated by one-way analysis of variance (ANOVA) and by Student's paired *t*-test (Student-Newman-Keuls of Instat, v. 2.2, Graph Pad Software Inc., San Diego, CA), using Graph Pad Prism software (Graph Pad Software Inc.).

RESULTS

Western blot analyses of NMDA 2A subunit immunoreactivity (~180 kDa) in P2 fractions under the different treatments are shown in FIGURE 1A. In cortex, the band intensity increases ($P \leq 0.05$) in cocaine-treated rats when compared to the control (saline). In contrast, the band intensity corresponding to cocaine–prazosin-treated rats decreases ($P \leq 0.01$) when compared to cocaine. No significant differences were observed between cocaine–prazosin-treated rats and the control. In PFC, a band of ~180 kDa was also observed in the P2 fraction of saline-treated rats. As in other regions, an increase in the band intensity (~180 kDa) was observed in P2 fractions of cocaine-treated rats when compared to the control (saline). This increase was, however, not statistically significant. In contrast to what was observed in cortical fractions, in cocaine–prazosin-treated rats, the band intensity increases ($P \leq 0.001$) when compared to cocaine-treated rats and control conditions. Similar findings were also observed for NMDA 2B (data not shown).

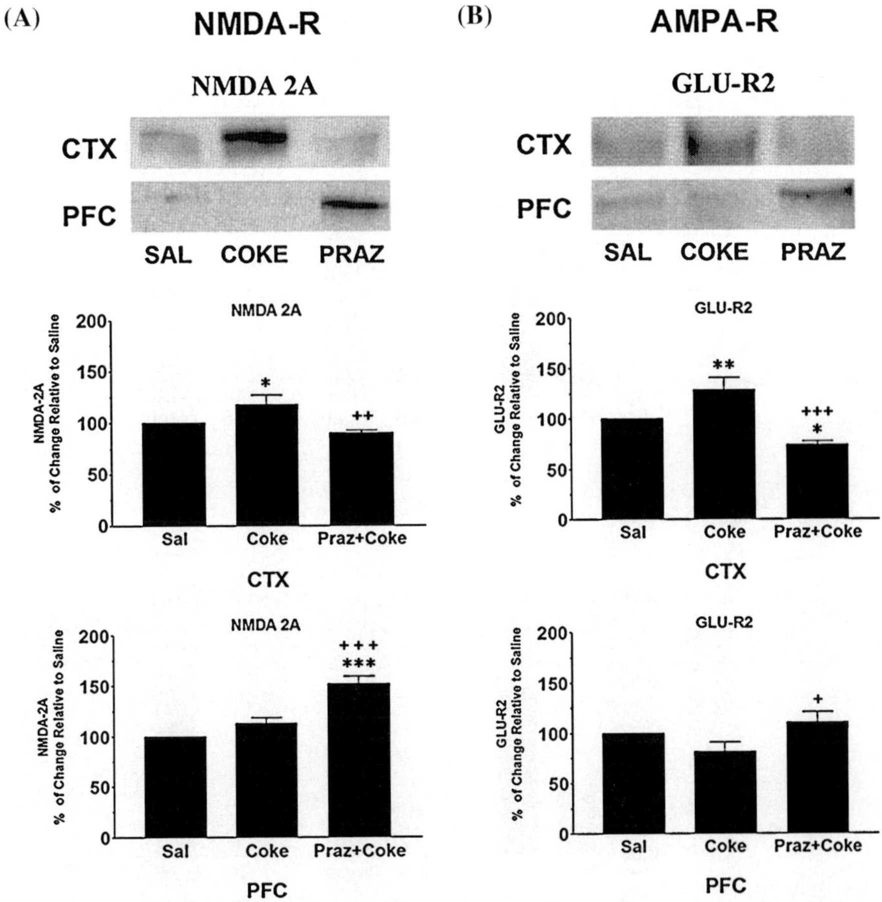

FIGURE 1. NMDA and AMPA immunoblot analysis of NMDA 2A (~180 kDa) and GLU-R2 (~100 kDa) in CTX and PFC P2 fractions of cocaine (Coke) and cocaine–prazosin (Praz)-treated rats. Equal amounts (5 μg) of sample protein were separated by SDS-PAGE. Representative gels are shown. NMDA 2A and GLU-R2 immunoblots and optical density analyses of the specific bands are presented as the percentage change relative to the saline (control) for (**A**) NMDA 2A and (**B**) GLU-R2. Each bar represents the mean ± SD of at least three independent experiments. ($^{+}$coke versus praz-coke, $P < 0.05$; $^{++}P < 0.01$; $^{+++}P < 0.001$; $^{*}P \leq 0.05$; $^{**}P \leq 0.01$; $^{***}P \leq 0.001$).

Western blot analysis was performed with antibodies against AMPA receptors (FIG. 1 B). A single band of ~100 kDA was observed in all regions. The band intensity increases in cortex of cocaine-treated rats ($P \leq 0.01$, versus saline). In prazosin–cocaine-treated rats, however, the band intensity decreases ($P \leq 0.001$; $P \leq 0.05$) when compared to cocaine-treated rats and to the control, respectively. In cocaine-treated rats, the band intensity decreases in PFC, although it is not statistically significant. An increase in band intensity

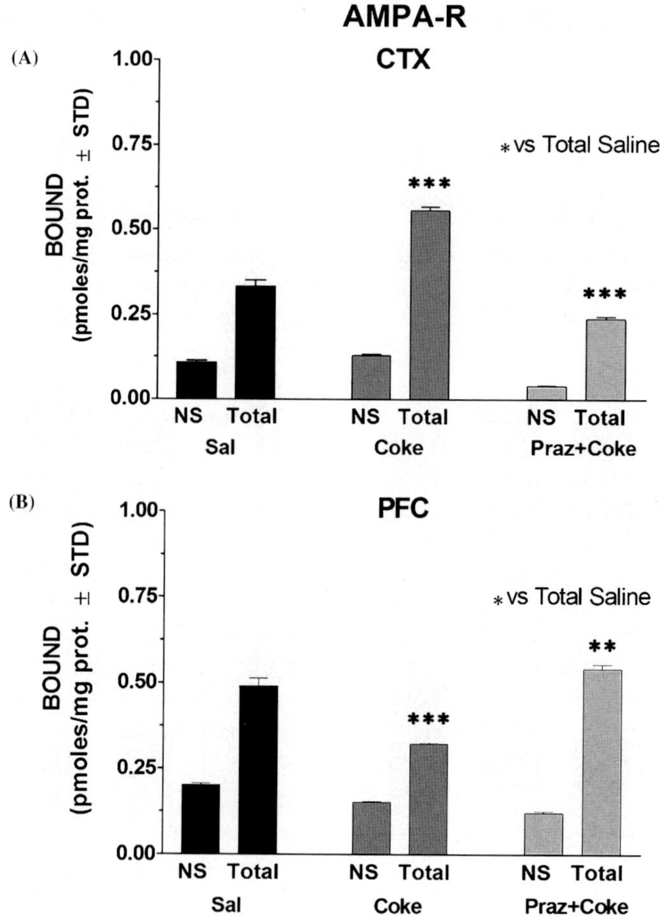

FIGURE 2. **(A)** [^{3}H]FW binding (15 nM) increases in CTX fractions of cocaine-treated (coke) rats ($P \leq 0.001$) when compared to the control (Sal). In contrast, [^{3}H]FW binding decreases ($P \leq 0.001$) cocaine–prazosin (Praz)-treated rats when compared to the saline. **(B)** In PFC, [^{3}H]FW binding ($P \leq 0.001$) decreases in coke-treated rats. However, an increase ($P \leq 0.01$) was observed in PFC cocaine–prazosin-treated rats when compared to control. Data represents values expressed as pmoles/mg protein. Mean ± SD of three independent experiments; $^*P \leq 0.05$; $^{**}P \leq 0.01$; $^{***}P \leq 0.001$.

was observed in cocaine–prazosin-treated rats ($P \leq 0.05$) when compared to cocaine-treated rats.

Cocaine affects [^{3}H]FW binding to AMPA receptors in a region-specific manner (FIG. 2). In rat cerebral cortex (CTX), cocaine treatment causes a marked increase in total binding, while in PFC there is a significant decrease. In both regions, cocaine–prazosin treatment attenuates the effects of cocaine. However, in PFC [^{3}H]FW binding surpasses that of saline. While in cortex,

[^{3}H]FW binding in cocaine–prazosin-treated rats is markedly reduced below that of saline-treated rats.

DISCUSSION

The PFC is part of the circuitry involved in behavioral sensitization, but studies of this region are scarce. In the VTA, single cocaine injections increase the amplitude and frequency of miniature endplate postsynaptic currents (mEPCS) when compared with the controls. These changes are due to changes in receptor number and/or function, but not to changes in the probability in transmitter release.[3]

Studies in the VTA and NAc have shown that AMPA antagonists also prevent behavioral sensitization in rats.[4] The relative contribution of AMPA and NMDA receptors in the brain suggests the that AMPA/NMDA ratio varies in cocaine-treated rats depending on the region studied. Dopamine–noradrenaline interactions have been identified in PFC.[14–16] Furthermore, noradrenaline decreases NMDA and non-NMDA activity.[17]

Our results show that cocaine sensitization is accompanied by region-specific changes in NMDA and AMPA receptors. Prazosin prevents cocaine sensitization as well as the NMDA and AMPA changes. By preventing the effects of cocaine on the ionotropic glutamate receptors, prazosin, an α_1-adrenergic receptor antagonist, could represent a novel therapeutic strategy.

ACKNOWLEDGMENTS

This work was supported by NIH-MBRS-RISE Grant GM61838, and supported in part by NIH SNRP Grant NS 39408-03 and the RCMI Program G12 RR-03051.

REFERENCES

1. SHIMOSATO, K., R.J. MARLEY & T. SAITO. 1995. Differential effects of NMDA receptor and dopamine receptor antagonists on cocaine toxicities. Pharmacol. Biochem. Behav. **51:** 781–788.
2. WHITE, F.J. 2002. A behavioral/systems approach to the neuroscience of drug addiction. J. Neurosci. **22:** 3303–3305.
3. UNGLESS, M.A., J.L. WHISTLER, R.C. MALENKA, *et al.* 2001. Single cocaine exposure *in vivo* induces long term potentiation in dopamine neurons. Nature **411:** 583–587.
4. WOLF, M.E. 1998. The role of excitatory amino acids in behavioral sensitization to psychomotor stimulants. Prog. Neurobiol. **54:** 679–720.

5. ITZHAK, Y. & J.L. MARTIN. 1999. Effects of cocaine, nicotine, dizocipline and alcohol on mice locomotor activity: cocaine-alcohol cross-sensitization involves upregulation of striatal dopamine transporter binding sites. Brain Res. **818:** 204–211.
6. PARK, W.K., A.A. BARI, A.R. JEY, *et al.* 2002. Cocaine administered into the medial prefrontal cortex reinstates cocaine-seeking behavior by increasing AMPA receptor-mediated glutamate transmission in the nucleus accumbens. J. Neurosci. **22**: 2916–2925.
7. KOE, B.K. 1976. Molecular geometry of inhibitors of the uptake of catecholamines and serotonin in synaptosomal preparations of rat brain. J. Pharmacol. Exp. Ther. **199:** 649–661.
8. TAYLOR, D. & B.T. HO. 1978. Comparison of inhibition of monoamine uptake by cocaine, methylphenidate and amphetamine. Res. Commun. Chem. Pathol. Pharmacol. **21:** 67–75.
9. RITZ, M.C., R.J. LAMB, S.R. GOLDBERG, *et al.* 1987. Cocaine receptors on dopamine transporters are related to self-administration of cocaine. Science **237:** 1219–1223.
10. ALMODÓVAR-FÁBREGAS, L.J., O. SEGARRA, N. COLÓN, *et al.* 2002. Effects of cocaine administration on VTA cell activity in response to prefrontal cortex stimulation. Ann. N. Y. Acad. Sci. **965:** 157–171.
11. BRADFORD, M.M. 1976. A rapid and sensitive method for the quantitation of microgram quantities of protein utilizing the principle of protein-dye binding. Anal. Biochem. **72:** 248–254.
12. HAWKINS, L.M., K.M. BEAVER, D.E. JANE, *et al.* 1995. Characterization of the pharmacology and regional distribution of (S)-[^{3}H]5 fluorowillardiine binding in rat brain. Br. J. Pharmacol. **116:** 2033–2039.
13. SILVA, W.I., H.M. MALDONADO, M.P. LISANTI, *et al.* 1999. Identification of caveolae and caveolin in C6 glioma cells. Int. J. Dev. Neurosci. **17:** 705–714.
14. KAWAHARA, H., Y. KAWAHARA & B.H. WESTERING. 2001. The noradrenaline-dopamine interaction in the rat medial prefrontal cortex studied by multi-probe microdialysis. Eur. J. Pharmacol. **418:** 177–186.
15. NASIF, F.J., K. SIDIROPOULOU, X.T. HU, *et al.* 2005. Repeated cocaine administration increases membrane excitability of pyramidal neurons in the rat medial prefrontal cortex. J. Pharmacol. Exp. Ther. **312:** 1305–1313.
16. PAN, W.H., S.Y. YANG & S.K. LIN. 2004. Neurochemical interaction between dopaminergic and noradrenergic neurons in the medial prefrontal cortex. Synapse **53:** 44–52.
17. LAW-THO, D., F. CREPEL, & J.C. HIRSCH. 1993. Noradrenaline decreases transmission of NMDA- and non-NMDA-receptor mediated monosynaptic EPSPs in rat prefrontal neurons *in vitro*. Eur. J. Neurosci. **5:** 494–500.

No Association between CART (Cocaine- and Amphetamine-Regulated Transcript) Gene and Methamphetamine Dependence

A. MORIO,[a] H. UJIKE,[a,b] A. NOMURA,[c] Y. TANAKA,[a] Y. MORITA,[a] K. OTANI,[a] M. KISHIMOTO,[a] M. HARANO,[b,d] T. INADA,[b,e] T. KOMIYAMA,[b,f] M. YAMADA,[b,g] Y. SEKINE,[b,h] N. IWATA,[b,i] M. IYO,[b,j] I. SORA,[b,k] N. OZAKI,[b,l] AND S. KURODA[a]

[a]*Department of Neuropsychiatry, Okayama University Graduate School of Medicine, Dentistry, and Pharmaceutical Sciences, Okayama 700-8558, Japan*

[b]*Japanese Genetics Initiative for Drug Abuse (JGIDA), Japan*

[c]*Kasaoka Hospital, Kasaoka, Japan*

[d]*Department of Neuropsychiatry, Kurume University School of Medicine, Kurume, Japan*

[e]*Department of Psychiatry, Teikyo University, School of Medicine, Ichihara Hospital, Ichihara, Japan*

[f]*Division of Psychiatry, National Center Hospital for Mental, Nervous, and Muscular Disorders, National Center of Neurology and Psychiatry, Tokyo, Japan*

[g]*Department of Psychogeriatrics, National Institute of Mental Health, National Center of Neurology and Psychiatry, Kodaira, Japan*

[h]*Department of Psychiatry and Neurology, Hamamatsu University School of Medicine, Hamamatsu, Japan*

[i]*Department of Psychiatry, Fujita Health University School of Medicine, Nagoya, Japan*

[j]*Department of Psychiatry, Graduate School of Medicine, Chiba University, Chiba, Japan*

[k]*Department of Psychobiology, Tohoku University Graduate School of Medicine, Sendai, Japan*

[l]*Department of Psychiatry, Nagoya University Graduate School of Medicine, Nagoya, Japan*

Address for correspondence: Hiroshi Ujike, M.D., Ph.D., Department of Neuropsychiatry, Okayama University Graduate School of Medicine, Dentistry, and Pharmaceutical Sciences, 2-5-1 Shikata-cho, Okayama 700-8558, Japan. Voice: +81-86-235-7242; fax: +81-86-235-7246.
e-mail: hujike@cc.okayama-u.ac.jp

Ann. N.Y. Acad. Sci. 1074: 411–417 (2006). © 2006 New York Academy of Sciences.
doi: 10.1196/annals.1369.041

ABSTRACT: Cocaine- and amphetamine-regulated transcript (CART) was originally discovered as a peptide that increased in the rat striatum after injection of a psychostimulant drug, such as cocaine or amphetamine, and is suggested to play potential roles in drug dependence. We tested the genetic association between the CART gene and methamphetamine (METH) dependence and/or psychosis. The subjects were 203 patients with METH dependence and 239 age- and gender-matched healthy controls. Two single nucleotide polymorphisms (SNPs) of the CART gene, −156A>G and IVS1 + 224G>A, were examined . There were no significant differences in genotype and allele distributions of the polymorphisms between patients with METH dependence and/or psychosis and controls. Neither were significant differences in subgroups of clinical phenotypes, for example, age at first consumption of METH, latency to onset of psychotic symptoms after the first consumption of METH, prognosis of psychosis after therapy, complication of spontaneous relapse to a psychotic state, or multisubstance abuse status, observed. The present findings suggest that the CART gene may not play a pivotal role in the development of METH dependence and psychosis, at least in a Japanese population.

KEYWORDS: cocaine- and amphetamine-regulated transcript; CART gene; methamphetamine dependence; polymorphism; association study

INTRODUCTION

Cocaine- and amphetamine-regulated transcript (CART) was identified as a peptide in the hypothalamus in 1981.[1] CART appears to play roles in reward, feeding, and stress, and it may mediate actions of psychostimulants in the brain or act as an endogenous psychostimulant.[2] As the peptide's name indicates, CART mRNA increased in the rat striatum after the injection of a psychostimulant drug, such as cocaine or amphetamine.[3,4] Cart mRNA and peptides are distributed throughout the brain except for the cerebellum, and are especially dense in the shell region of the accumbens and ventral tegmentum area (VTA),[5] which are key structures in substance dependence and substance-induced psychosis.[6] Intra-VTA injection of CART peptide 55–102 increased locomotor activity and conditioned place preference.[7] Intracerebroventricular injection of the peptide increased dopamine turnover in the accumbens and striatum.[8] These findings suggest that CART peptides may be involved in development of psychostimulant dependence.

The human CART gene, which was cloned in 1996, contains three exons, spans about 2.0 kb, and locates on 5q13.2.[9] Recently, a polymorphism of the human CART gene IVS1 + 224G>A was shown to be associated with alcoholism in a Korean population.[10] Therefore, we hypothesized that genetic variants of the human CART gene may affect individual vulnerability not only to alcohol dependence but also to psychostimulant dependence. In the present study, we examined a possible association between polymorphisms of the human CART gene and patients with methamphetamine (METH) dependence and/or psychosis in a Japanese population.

SUBJECTS AND METHOD

Subjects

The subjects consisted of 203 unrelated patients with METH dependence and/or psychotic disorder (166 males and 37 females, average age 36.9 $\pm$11.8 years) who met the ICD-10-DCR criteria (F15.2 and F15.5). They were out- or inpatients of psychiatric hospitals of the Japanese Genetics Initiative for Drug Abuse (JGIDA) . The healthy controls were 239 normal, unrelated, age-, gender-, and geographical origin-matched individuals (190 males and 49 females, average age 38.6 $\pm$ 12.6 years). Most were medical staff members who had no past history and no family history of drug dependence or psychotic disorder. All subjects were Japanese, born and living in restricted areas of Japan, including northern Kyushyu, Setouchi, Tokai, and Kanto. This study was initiated with the approval of the ethical committee of each attending member institution of the JGIDA. Written informed consent was obtained from all participating patients.

Clinical Phenotypes

The patients with METH dependence and/or psychosis were divided into five subgroups according to the following clinical phenotypes. Individual differences in certain phenotypes seem to be regulated, at least in part, genetically, and the rationale and methods of subgrouping were previously described.[11,12] Patients were divided by multisubstance-abuse status, age at first consumption of METH, latency to the onset of psychotic symptoms after the first consumption, prognosis of psychosis after therapy, and the complication of spontaneous relapse to a psychotic state.

Genotyping

Genomic DNA was extracted from the nuclei of leukocytes in peripheral blood. Genotyping of $-156A>G$ and IVS1 $+$ 224G$>$A was carried out according to the methods of Yamada *et al.*[13] and Jung *et al.*,[10] respectively, with minor modifications.

Statistical Analysis

Hardy–Weinberg equilibrium was tested using a chi-squared goodness-of-fit test. A χ^2 test was applied to obtain statistics of differences in genotype distributions and allele frequencies between controls and patients and between clinical subgroups of patients. The statistical significance level was chosen as 0.05. Linkage disequilibrium and haplotype analyses were performed using SNPAlyze software (Dynacom Co., Ltd., Kanagawa, Japan), and a global P value was adopted.

RESULTS

The genotype distributions of IVS1 + 224G>A and −156A>G of the CART gene were not significantly different from those expected according to Hardy–Weinberg equilibrium in any group or subgroup. There was no significant difference in the genotype and allele distribution of IVS1 + 224G>A and −156A>G of the CART gene between patients with METH dependence and/or psychosis and controls (TABLE 1. IVS1 + 224G>A, allele, $x^2 = 0.02$, df = 1, $P = 0.88$, genotype; $x^2 = 0.05$, df = 2, $P = 0.97$; −156A>G, allele, $x^2 = 0.43$, df = 1, $P = 0.51$, genotype; $x^2 = 0.50$, df = 2, $P = 0.78$). Neither was a significant difference in the relationship of either single nucleotide polymorphism (SNP) of the CART gene to any subgroup of clinical phenotypes of METH psychosis (TABLE 2) observed.

Multilocus analyses showed that two SNPs of the CART gene, IVS1 + 224G>A and −156A>G, were in strong linkage disequilibrium in controls and patients (controls, $D' = 0.96$, $r^2 = 0.16$, $P = 1.61 \times 10^{-15}$; patients, $D' = 0.91$, $r^2 = 0.15$, $P = 6.12 \times 10^{-17}$). Haplotype analysis showed there are four kinds of haplotype, and the estimated haplotype frequency showed that the AG haplotype at −156A>G and IVS1 + 224G>A loci was the major type, and that GG and AA haplotypes followed in frequency. The GA haplotype was rare. There was no significant difference of haplotype distribution between patients with METH dependence and/or psychosis and controls (TABLE 3. global P value = 0.82).

DISCUSSION

Yamada *et al.*[13] screened mutations in the coding regions of three exons of the CART gene in a Japanese population, but found no SNP. They found six SNPs in the 5′ flanking region and one SNP in the 3′ untranslated region of the gene. The CART upstream sequence displays strong promotor activity in GH3 cells by luciferase assay, and it contains several consensus sequences of transcription factor binding sites such as CRE/AP-1, SP1, AP-1, and AP-2.[14]

TABLE 1. Genotype and allele frequencies of –156A>G and IVS1 + 224G>A of the CART gene in patients with METH-use disorders and controls

SNP			Genotypes (%)				Alleles (%)		
−156A>G	Group	*n*	AA	AG	GG	*p*	A	G	*p*
	Patients	203	46.3	41.4	12.3		67.0	33.0	
	Controls	233	48.5	41.2	10.3	0.78	69.1	30.9	0.51
IVS1 + 224G>A			GG	GA	AA	*p*	G	A	*p*
	Patients	199	53.3	39.7	7.0		73.1	26.9	
	Controls	238	52.5	39.9	7.6	0.97	72.5	27.5	0.88

TABLE 2. Association analyses between subgroups of METH dependence and/or psychosis according to clinical phenotype

	−156A>G							
		Genotypes (%)				Alleles (%)		
Clinical phenotype	*n*	AA	AG	GG	*p*	A	G	*p*
Multisubstance abuse								
Yes	139	46.8	42.4	10.8		63.0	37.0	
No	57	45.6	36.9	17.5	0.41	64.0	36.0	0.48
Age at first consumption								
<20	100	50.0	38.0	12.0		69.0	31.0	
≥20	99	42.4	45.5	12.1	0.53	65.2	34.8	0.46
Latency to onset of psychosis								
<3 years	77	40.3	41.5	18.2		61.0	39.0	
≥3 years	97	47.4	44.3	8.3	0.14	69.6	30.4	0.26
Prognosis of psychosis								
Transient	105	44.8	43.8	11.4		66.7	33.3	
Prolonged	79	43.0	43.0	14.0	0.88	64.6	35.4	0.91
Spontaneous relapse of psychosis								
Yes	79	38.0	50.6	11.4		63.3	36.7	
No	108	50.9	38.0	11.1	0.18	70.0	30.0	0.18
	IVS1 + 224G>A							
		GG	GA	AA		G	A	
Multisubstance abuse								
Yes	135	49.6	43.0	7.4		71.1	28.9	
No	57	61.4	31.6	7.0	0.31	77.2	22.8	0.26
Age at first consumption								
<20	98	56.1	35.7	8.2		74.0	26.0	
≥20	96	49.0	45.8	5.2	0.31	71.9	28.1	0.65
Latency to onset of psychosis								
<3 years	76	48.7	44.7	6.6		71.1	28.9	
≥3 years	97	57.7	38.2	4.1	0.45	76.8	23.2	0.26
Prognosis of psychosis								
Transient	103	52.4	41.8	5.8		73.3	26.7	
Prolonged	79	55.7	38.0	6.3	0.88	74.7	25.3	0.81
Spontaneous relapse of psychosis								
Yes	78	62.8	32.1	5.1		78.8	21.2	
No	105	46.7	26.7	6.6	0.09	70.0	30.0	0.07

While the SNP −156A>G did not change these consensus sequences, it seems to be physiologically functional because it was significantly associated with obesity.[13] Therefore, −156A>G may be in linkage disequilibrium with other SNPs in the promotor region, such as −390T>C or −484T>G, that change the consensus sequence of the CRE/AP-1 site. IVS1 + 224G>A locates in intron 1, but it is relatively close to exon 1. Actually, the SNP was shown to be

TABLE 3. Haplotype analysis at –156A>G and IVS1 + 224G>A of the CART gene in METH dependence

−156A>G	IVS1 + 224G>A	Controls	Patients	Global *P* value
A	G	0.42	0.41	
G	G	0.31	0.32	
A	A	0.27	0.26	
G	A	0.004	0.008	0.82

associated with patients with alcoholism, which implies that IVS1 + 224G>A is potentially functional.

In the present study, using these polymorphisms of the human CART gene, we examined its association with METH dependence and/or psychosis. However, there was no association of the CART gene with METH-use disorders or with any clinical phenotype of the disorders, such as rapid onset of psychosis, severity of prognosis, or susceptibility to relapse. These findings suggest that the CART gene may not play pivotal roles in the development of METH dependence and METH-induced psychosis. Alternatively, it is possible that lack of association of METH-use disorders with the CART gene may be a type II error due to less power. Statistical power analysis showed that our sample size has powers of 0.84 and 0.44 to detect a small effect size ($w = 0.10$) in detecting a significant difference in allele and genotype distributions, respectively. In the case of subgroups of METH patients, the power was considerably reduced. Therefore, our findings must be qualified by studies with a larger number of subjects. Further, additional polymorphisms of the CART gene must be examined.

ACKNOWLEDGMENTS

We thank the METH dependence/psychosis patients and controls for participating in this study. We also acknowledge support from the Japanese Ministry of Health, Labor and Welfare, and the Zikei Institute of Psychiatry (Okayama, Japan).

REFERENCES

1. Spiess, J., J. Villarreal & W. Vale. 1981. Isolation and sequence analysis of a somatostatin-like polypeptide from ovine hypothalamus. Biochemistry **20:** 1982–1988.
2. Kuhar, M., J. Adams, S. Dominguez, *et al.* 2002. CART peptides. Neuropeptides **36:** 1–8.
3. Douglass, J., A. McKinzie & P. Couceyro. 1995. PCCR differential display identifies a rat brain mRNA that is transcriptionally regulated by cocaine and amphetamine. J. Neurosci. **15:** 2471–2481.

4. FAGERGREN, P. & Y.L. HURD. 1999. Mesolimbic gender differences in peptide CART mRNA expression: effects of cocaine. Neuroreport **10:** 3449–3452.
5. KOYLO, E.O., P.R. COUCEYRO, P.D. LAMBERT, *et al.* 1998. Cocaine- and amphetamine-regulated transcript peptide immunohistochemical localization in the rat brain. J. Comp. Neurol. **391:** 115–132.
6. UJIKE, H. 2002. Stimulant-induced psychosis and schizophrenia: the role of sensitization. Curr. Psychiatry Rep. **4:** 177–184.
7. KIMMEL, H.L., W. GONG, S.D. VECHIA, *et al.* 2000. Intra-ventral tegmental area injection of rat cocaine and amphetamine-regulated transcript peptide 55–102 induces locomotor activity and promotes conditioned place preference. J. Pharmacol. Exp. Ther. **294:** 784–792.
8. YANG, S.C., J.T. PAN & H. LI. 2004. CART peptide increases the mesolimbic dopaminergic neuronal activity: a microdialysis study. Eur. J. Pharmacol. **494:** 179–182.
9. DOUGLASS, J. & S. DAOUD. 1996. Characterization of the human cDNA and genomic DNA encoding CART: a cocaine- and amphetamine-regulated transcript. Gene **169:** 241–245.
10. JUNG, S.K., M.S. HONG, G.J. SUH, *et al.* 2004. Association between polymorphism in intron 1 of cocaine-and-amphetamine-regulated transcript gene with alcoholism, but not with bipolar disorder and schizophrenia in Korean population. Neurosci. Lett. **365:** 54–57.
11. UJIKE, H. & M. SATO. 2004. Clinical features of sensitization to methamphetamine observed in patients with methamphetamine dependence and psychosis. Ann. N. Y. Acad. Sci. **1025:** 279–287.
12. UJIKE, H., M. HARANO, T. INADA, *et al.* 2003. Nine- or fewer repeat alleles in VNTR polymorphism of the dopamine transporter gene is a strong risk factor for prolonged methamphetamine psychosis. Pharmacogenomics J. **3:** 242–247.
13. YAMADA, K., X. YUAN, S. OTABE, *et al.* 2002. Sequencing of the putative promoter region of the cocaine- and amphetamine-regulated transcript gene and identification of polymorphic sites associated with obesity. Int. J. Obes. Relat. Metab. Disord. **26:** 132–136.
14. DOMINGUEZ, G., A. LAKATOS & M.J. KUHAR 2002. Characterization of the cocaine- and amphetamine-regulated transcript (CART) peptide gene promoter and its activation by a cyclic AMP-dependent signaling pathway in GH3 cells. J. Neurochem. **80:** 885–893.

Differential Effects of Donepezil on Methamphetamine and Cocaine Dependencies

YUKIO TAKAMATSU,[a] YOSHIHARU YAMANISHI,[b] YOKO HAGINO,[a] HIDEKO YAMAMOTO,[a] AND KAZUTAKA IKEDA[a]

[a]*Division of Psychobiology, Tokyo Institute of Psychiatry, Tokyo 156-8585, Japan*

[b]*Tsukuba Research Laboratories, Eisai Co., Ltd, Tsukuba, Tsukuba 300-2635, Japan*

ABSTRACT: Donepezil, a choline esterase inhibitor, has been widely used as a medicine for Alzheimer's disease. Recently, a study showed that donepezil inhibited addictive behaviors induced by cocaine, including cocaine-conditioned place preference (CPP) and locomotor sensitization to cocaine. In the present study, we investigated the effects of donepezil on methamphetamine (METH)-induced behavioral changes in mice. In counterbalanced CPP tests, the intraperitoneal (i.p.) administration of 3 mg/kg donepezil prior to 2 mg/kg METH i.p. failed to inhibit METH CPP, whereas pretreatment with 3 mg/kg donepezil abolished the CPP for cocaine (10 mg/kg, i.p.). Similarly, in locomotor sensitization experiments, i.p. administration of 1 mg/kg donepezil prior to 2 mg/kg METH i.p. failed to inhibit locomotor sensitivity to METH, whereas pretreatment with 1 mg/kg donepezil significantly inhibited locomotor sensitivity to cocaine (10 mg/kg, i.p.). These results suggest that donepezil may be a useful tool for treating cocaine dependence but not for treating METH dependence. The differences in the donepezil effects on addictive behaviors induced by METH and cocaine might be due to differences in the involvement of acetylcholine in the mechanisms of METH and cocaine dependencies.

KEYWORDS: methamphetamine; cocaine; donepezil; conditioned place preference; sensitization; mice

INTRODUCTION

Methamphetamine (METH) and cocaine are widely abused in the world.[1] Since METH and repeated administration of cocaine frequently induce psychotic states with symptoms similar to those seen in schizophrenia of the

Address for correspondence: Kazutaka Ikeda, Division of Psychobiology, Tokyo Institute of Psychiatry, 2-1-8 Kamikitazawa, Setagaya-ku, Tokyo 156-8585, Japan. Voice: +81-3-3304-5701, ext. 508; fax: +81-3-3329-8035.
e-mail: ikedak@prit.go.jp

**Ann. N.Y. Acad. Sci. 1074: 418–426 (2006). © 2006 New York Academy of Sciences.
doi: 10.1196/annals.1369.042**

paranoid type,[2] such psychotic states are mainly treated in hospitals, thus resulting in large medical costs. Therefore, there is great need for the discovery of new medications for METH and cocaine abuse,[3] as the current treatments are primarily oriented toward the treatment of the psychosis with no treatments available to prevent relapse to METH and cocaine abuse.

Acetylcholine (ACh) is released from cholinergic interneurons within the nucleus accumbens (NAc),[4,5] a key brain region implicated in the reinforcement and addiction of abusive drugs, and acts concertedly, but in an opposite direction, to dopamine on the NAc neural circuit.[6–8] Mice lacking cholinergic neurons in their NAc as a result of immunotoxin-mediated cell targeting[9] show enhanced preference for and enhanced sensitization to cocaine,[10] suggesting that ACh in the NAc plays a pivotal role in preventing cocaine reinforcement and addiction. Recently, donepezil, an ACh esterase inhibitor with the trade name of Aricept, was reported to reduce preference for cocaine and morphine and sensitization to cocaine in mice.[11]

In the present study, we investigated whether donepezil reduces preference for and sensitization to METH as well as cocaine by conducting the conditioned place preference (CPP) test and locomotor sensitization test.

MATERIALS AND METHODS

Male C57BL/6J mice (9–13 weeks old) were purchased from CLEA Japan, Inc. (Tokyo, Japan) and were housed for 1–2 weeks before the experiments were begun in an animal facility maintained at 24 ± 1°C and 50% relative humidity under a 12/12 hour light:dark cycle with lights on at 8:00 AM and off at 8:00 PM. Food and water were available *ad libitum*. The experimental procedures and housing conditions were approved by the Institutional Animal Care and Use Committee of the Tokyo Institute of Psychiatry, and all animals were cared for and treated humanely in accordance with our institutional animal experimentation guidelines.

CPP Test

The CPP test was carried out according to the method of Hoffman and Beninger[12] with some modifications. For this test, we used a two-compartment Plexiglas chamber (Neuroscience Inc., Osaka, Japan), one compartment of which was black with a smooth floor and the other was of the same dimensions, but white with a textured floor. The compartmented chamber was placed in a sound- and light-attenuated box under conditions of dim illumination (about 40 Lx). There was no significant difference between time spent in the black compartment and that spent in the white compartment, indicating that there was no preference for either side under the present conditions before conditioning.

We selected a counterbalanced protocol in order to nullify each mouse's initial preference, as described previously.[13]

METH CPP

On day 1, the mice were allowed to freely explore the two compartments for 15 min. On day 2, again the mice were allowed to explore the compartments freely for 15 min, and the time spent in each compartment and the number of transitions between compartments were measured. Then, conditioning sessions were conducted once daily for four consecutive days (days 5–8). Mice were intraperitoneally (i.p.) injected with METH (2 mg/kg) and immediately confined to the black or white compartment for 50 min on day 5. On day 6, the mice were injected with saline and immediately confined to the opposite compartment for 50 min. On days 7 and 8, the same conditioning as on days 5 and 6 was repeated. Donepezil (1 mg/kg or 3 mg/kg, i.p.) or distilled water (DW) was injected 20 min before METH or saline treatment. On day 9, the mice were allowed to freely explore the two compartments for 15 min without drug injection, and the time spent in each compartment and the number of transitions between compartments were measured. The CPP score was designated as the time spent in the METH-paired compartment on day 9 minus the time spent in the same compartment in the preconditioning phase on day 2.

Cocaine CPP

On day 1, mice were allowed to freely explore the two compartments for 30 min, and the time spent in each compartment and the number of transitions between compartments were measured. Then, conditioning sessions were conducted twice daily for three consecutive days (days 2–4). On day 2, mice were injected with saline and immediately confined to the black or white compartment for 20 min. Four hours later, they were injected with cocaine (10 mg/kg, i.p.) and immediately confined to the opposite compartment for 20 min. Donepezil (1 mg/kg or 3 mg/kg, i.p.) or DW was injected 20 min before cocaine treatment. On days 3 and 4, the same conditioning as on day 2 was repeated. On day 5, the mice were allowed to freely explore the two compartments for 30 min without drug injection, and the time spent in each compartment and the number of transitions between compartments were measured. The CPP score was designated as the time spent in the cocaine-paired compartment on day 5 minus the time spent in the same compartment in the preconditioning phase on day 1.

Locomotor Activity

METH- or cocaine-induced locomotor activity sensitization was examined in mice injected with METH (2 mg/kg, i.p.) or cocaine (10 mg/kg, i.p.) once daily for five consecutive days. Donepezil (1 mg/kg) or DW was i.p. injected 10 min before the METH or cocaine treatment in a home cage. The animals were i.p. injected with METH or cocaine and placed at the center of the test chamber (250 mm in diameter and 270 mm in height; Muromachi Kikai Co., Tokyo, Japan). Then the treated mice were allowed to freely explore the chamber for 60 min and 10 min, respectively, while locomotor activity was being recorded by using an infrared activity monitor. On day 6, donepezil- and DW-pretreatment group mice were pretreated in an opposite manner with DW and donepezil, respectively, 10 min before METH or cocaine administration.

Drugs

Cocaine hydrochloride and methamphetamine hydrochloride were purchased from Takeda (Osaka, Japan) and Dainippon Pharmaceutical (Osaka, Japan), respectively. Donepezil hydrochloride was provided by Eisai (Tokyo, Japan). METH and cocaine were dissolved in saline, and donepezil was dissolved in DW. Drugs and vehicles were administered (i.p.) in a volume of 0.1 mL/10 g of body weight.

Statistical Analyses

In the CPP test, the time the mouse spent in the drug-paired compartment before and after conditioning was compared by within-group paired *t*-tests. The CPP scores of mice pretreated with DW or 1 or 3 mg/kg donepezil in the conditioning phase and treated with METH or cocaine were subjected to a one-way analysis of variance (ANOVA). Locomotor activity was subjected to repeated measures ANOVA followed by *post hoc* comparisons with the Scheffe test. The locomotor activity with opposite pretreatment on day 6 was compared with the locomotor activity on day 5 by the within-group paired *t*-test.

RESULTS

Effects of Donepezil on the METH and Cocaine CPP

Mice pretreated with DW, 1 mg/kg donepezil, or 3 mg/kg donepezil in the conditioning phase spent significantly longer time in the METH-paired compartment after the conditioning than before it ($df = 29$, $t = -7.510$, $P <$

0.0001; $df = 14$, $t = -3.173$, $P = 0.0068$; and $df = 14$, $t = -4.461$, $P = 0.0005$; respectively) (FIG. 1 A). Donepezil pretreatment during conditioning had no significant effects on the number of transitions between the compartments (data not shown).

Mice pretreated with DW and 1 mg/kg donepezil in the conditioning phase showed significant cocaine CPP ($df = 29$, $t = -7.009$, $P < 0.0001$; $df = 14$, $t = -4.585$, $P = 0.0004$; respectively; FIG. 1 B). By contrast, mice pretreated with 3 mg/kg donepezil in the conditioning phase did not show cocaine CPP ($df = 14$, $t = -1.624$, $P = 0.1268$). Furthermore, the one-way ANOVA showed that the effects of donepezil pretreatment tended to decrease the CPP score ($F_{2,57} = 2.780$, $P = 0.0705$). The Scheffe *post hoc* test showed that the CPP score of the mice pretreated with 3 mg/kg donepezil tended to be lower than that of the mice pretreated with DW ($P = 0.0905$). Donepezil pretreatment had no significant effect on the number of transitions between the compartments (data not shown).

Effects of Donepezil on METH-Induced Hyperlocomotion and Locomotor Sensitization

Locomotor activity in a novel environment was not inhibited by 1 mg/kg donepezil on day 0 (FIG. 2 A). Donepezil did not prevent METH-induced hyperlocomotion on day 1 ($F_{1,30} = 1.407$, $P = 0.2448$). The repeated measures ANOVA showed that the administration of METH led to sensitization to the locomotor-activating effects of METH as reflected by a main effect of Day ($F_{5,30} = 89.305$, $P < 0.0001$). Pretreatment with donepezil did not significantly affect the METH-induced increase in locomotor activity ($F_{5,30} = 1.355$, $P = 0.2447$).

To further investigate the effects of donepezil on METH-induced locomotor sensitization, on day 6 donepezil- and DW-pretreatment group mice were pretreated in an opposite manner with DW and donepezil, respectively, 10 min before METH administration. The opposite pretreatment with DW and donepezil did not significantly affect the locomotor activity when compared with that of the same group mice on day 5 ($df = 15$, $t = -2.107$, $P = 0.0523$; $df = 15$, $t = 1.465$, $P = 0.1635$; respectively).

Effects of Donepezil on Cocaine-Induced Hyperlocomotion and Locomotor Sensitization

Donepezil (1 mg/kg) prevented cocaine-induced hyperlocomotion on day 1 ($F_{1,29} = 4.581$, $P = 0.0409$). The repeated measures ANOVA showed that the administration of cocaine led to sensitization to the locomotor-activating effects of cocaine, as reflected by a main effect of Day ($F_{5,29} = 30.092$, $P <$

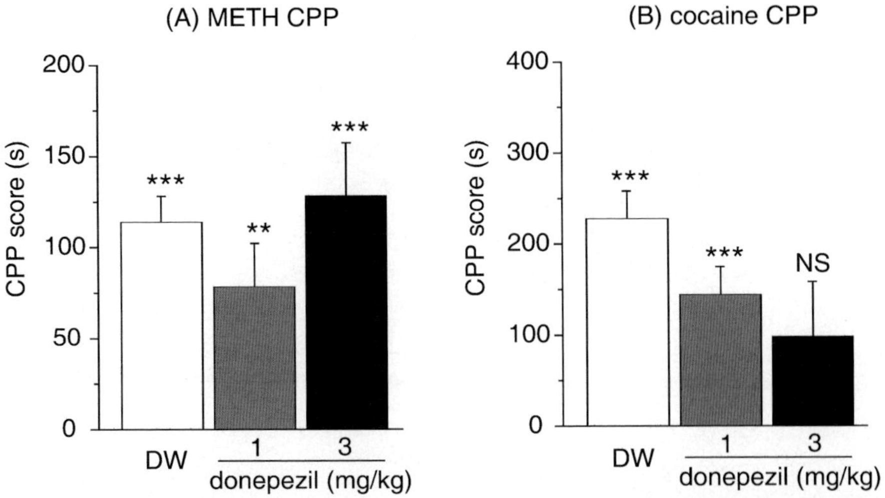

FIGURE 1. Effects of donepezil on CPP for METH (**A**) or cocaine (**B**). (**A**) Lack of a significant effect of donepezil on METH CPP. The CPP score was designated as the time spent in the drug-paired compartment minus the time spent in the same compartment in the preconditioning phase. METH CPP was significant regardless of the donepezil pretreatments ($n = 30$ for DW pretreatment, $n = 15$ for 1 mg/kg donepezil pretreatment, and $n = 15$ for 3 mg/kg donepezil pretreatment). (**B**) Abolishment of cocaine CPP by 3 mg/kg donepezil pretreatment. Cocaine CPP was not significant when 3 mg/kg donepezil was used for the pretreatment ($n = 15$), whereas it was significant when DW or 1 mg/kg donepezil was used ($n = 30$ for DW pretreatment and $n = 15$ for 1 mg/kg donepezil pretreatment). The CPP score of the mice pretreated with 3 mg/kg donepezil tended to be lower than that of the mice pretreated with DW. The CPP scores were expressed as means ± SEM. $^{**}P < 0.01$, $^{***}P < 0.001$, NS: not significant ($P > 0.05$).

0.0001). Pretreatment with donepezil significantly inhibited the cocaine-induced increase in locomotor activity ($F_{5,29} = 4.070$, $P = .0017$).

To further investigate the effects of donepezil on cocaine-induced locomotor sensitization, on day 6 donepezil- and DW-pretreatment group mice were pretreated in an opposite manner with DW and donepezil, respectively, 10 min before the cocaine administration. Locomotor activity of mice pretreated with DW on day 6 was significantly higher than that of the same group mice on day 5 ($df = 14$, $t = -3.984$, $P = 0.0014$). By contrast, the locomotor activity of the animals pretreated with donepezil on day 6 was significantly lower than that of the same group on day 5 ($df = 15$, $t = 5.377$, $P < 0.0001$).

DISCUSSION

Donepezil significantly abolished cocaine CPP and also reduced cocaine-induced hyperlocomotion and locomotor sensitization to cocaine in the present

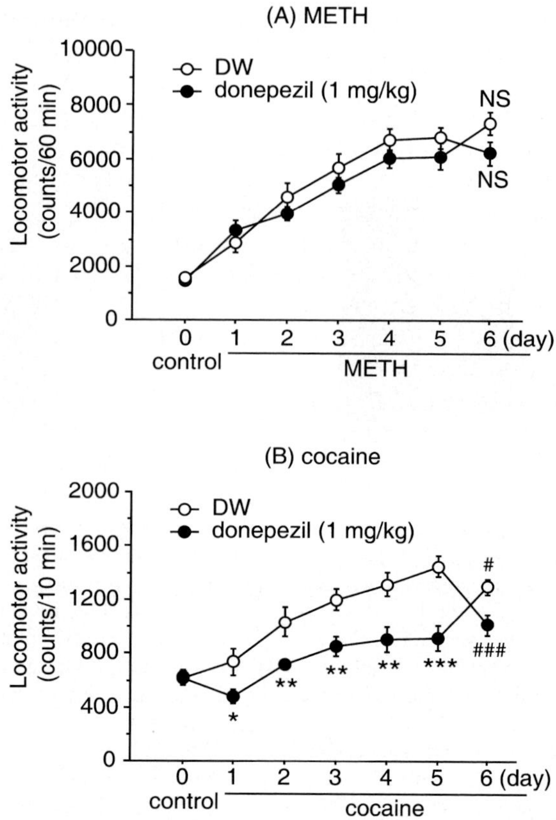

FIGURE 2. Effects of donepezil on METH- or cocaine-induced hyperlocomotion and locomotor sensitization. (**A**) Locomotor activity after 1 mg/kg METH injection with 1 mg/kg donepezil ($n = 15$) or DW ($n = 15$) pretreatment. Locomotor activity in a novel environment (day 0) and after METH treatment (days 1–5) was not affected by donepezil or DW pretreatment. The opposite pretreatment with DW or donepezil on day 6 did not affect the locomotor activity of mice when compared with that of the same mouse group on day 5. (**B**) Locomotor activity after 10 mg/kg cocaine injection with 1 mg/kg donepezil ($n = 15$) or DW ($n = 15$) pretreatment. Locomotor activity after cocaine injection on days 1–5 was decreased by donepezil pretreatment when compared with that in the case of DW pretreatment. The opposite pretreatment with donepezil on day 6 decreased the locomotor activity of mice when compared with that of the same mouse group on day 5, whereas pretreatment with DW on day 6 increased the locomotor activity of mice when compared with that of the same mouse group on day 5. The locomotor activity was expressed as mean ± SEM. $^{*}P < 0.05$, $^{**}P < 0.01$, $^{***}P < 0.001$, $\#P < 0.05$, $\#\#\#P < 0.001$, NS: not significant ($P > 0.05$).

study, findings that are consistent with those of a previous report.[11] By contrast, donepezil failed to abolish METH CPP or to reduce METH-induced hyperlocomotion and locomotor sensitization to METH. Cocaine inhibits monoamine transporters on the plasma membrane, such as those for dopamine, serotonin, and norepinephrine.[14] On the other hand, METH acts on these monoamine transporters to induce a reverse flow of monoamines through the transporters.[14] Furthermore, METH inhibits other molecules, such as vesicular monoamine transporter 2, which is localized on synaptic vesicle membranes and transports monoamines and monoamine oxidases that metabolize monoamines.[14] The differential effects of donepezil on METH- and cocaine-induced behaviors may be due to a difference in action between METH and cocaine on these target molecules. Further investigation of the molecular and neurobiological mechanisms underlying the difference in these donepezil effects will lead to a better understanding of the differences between METH and cocaine dependencies.

We found that mice pretreated with donepezil and treated with cocaine for 5 days showed significant hyperlocomotion after cocaine treatment with saline pretreatment on day 6 (FIG. 2 B), suggesting that donepezil can transiently inhibit cocaine-induced hyperlocomotion but not the development of locomotor sensitization to cocaine. Interestingly, similar results were obtained for mice treated with METH instead of cocaine, although the donepezil effects were not statistically significant (FIG. 2 A).

In conclusion, we found that donepezil, a widely used medication for Alzheimer's disease, inhibited preference and sensitization to cocaine, but not to METH, in mice. We propose that donepezil may be a useful tool for treating dependence on cocaine but not METH.

ACKNOWLEDGEMENTS

We are grateful to Dr. Keiko Matsuoka for animal care, and Yasukazu Ogai for the statistical analysis. This work was supported by a research grant (17025054) from MEXT of Japan and by grants (H17-pharmaco-001, H16-iyaku-029, H15-kou-3–03) from MHLW of Japan.

REFERENCES

1. UNITED NATIONS OFFICE FOR DRUG CONTROL AND CRIME PREVENTION ed. 2005. World Drug Report 2005. Oxford University Press, New York, NY.
2. UJIKE, H. 2002. Stimulant-induced psychosis and schizophrenia: the role of sensitization. Curr. Psychiatry Rep. **4:** 177–184.
3. NATIONAL INSTITUTE ON DRUG ABUSE (NIDA) ed. 2002. Research Report Series: Methamphetamine Abuse and Addiction. National Institutes of Health, Maryland, MD.
4. PENNARTZ, C.M. *et al.* 1994. The nucleus accumbens as a complex of functionally distinct neuronal ensembles: an integration of behavioral, electrophysiological and anatomical data. Prog. Neurobiol. **42:** 719–761.
5. KAWAGUCHI, Y. *et al.* 1995. Striatal interneurones: chemical, physiological and morphological characterization. Trends Neurosci. **18:** 527–535.

6. Di Chiara, G. *et al.* 1994. Modulatory functions of neurotransmitters in the striatum: ACh/dopamine/NMDA interactions. Trends Neurosci. **17:** 228–233.
7. Nisenbaum, L.K. *et al.* 1994. Dopaminergic and muscarinic regulation of striatal enkephalin and substance P messenger RNAs following striatal dopamine denervation: effects of systemic and central administration of quinpirole and scopolamine. Neuroscience **63:** 435–449.
8. Wang, J.Q. & J.F. McGinty. 1996. Muscarinic receptors regulate striatal neuropeptide gene expression in normal and amphetamine-treated rats. Neuroscience **75:** 43–56.
9. Kobayashi, K. *et al.* 1995. Immunotoxin-mediated conditional disruption of specific neurons in transgenic mice. Proc. Natl. Acad. Sci. USA. **92:** 1132–1136.
10. Hikida, T. *et al.* 2001. Increased sensitivity to cocaine by cholinergic cell ablation in nucleus accumbens. Proc. Natl. Acad. Sci. USA. **98:** 13351–13354.
11. Hikida, T. *et al.* 2003. Acetylcholine enhancement in the nucleus accumbens prevents addictive behaviors of cocaine and morphine. Proc. Natl. Acad. Sci. USA. **100:** 6169–6173.
12. Hoffman, D.C. & R.J. Beninger. 1989. Preferential stimulation of D1 or D2 receptors disrupts food-rewarded operant responding in rats. Pharmacol. Biochem. Behav. **34:** 923–925.
13. Ide, S. *et al.* 2004. Buprenorphine antinociception is abolished, but naloxone-sensitive reward is retained, in mu-opioid receptor knockout mice. Neuropsychopharmacology **29:** 1656–1663.
14. Meyer, J.S. & L.F. Quenzer. 2005. Psychopharmacology: Drugs, The Brain, and Behavior. J.S. Meyer and L.F. Quenzer Eds. 275–297. Sinauer Associates, Inc. Sunderland, MA.

Hippocampal Synaptic Plasticity and Water Maze Learning in Cocaine Self-Administered Rats

N. DEL OLMO,[a] A. HIGUERA-MATAS,[a] M. MIGUÉNS,[a]
C. GARCÍA-LECUMBERRI,[a] E. BORCEL,[a] J.M. SOLÍS,[b]
AND E. AMBROSIO[a]

[a]*Departamento de Psicobiología, UNED, 28040 Madrid, Spain*

[b]*Departamento de Investigación, Hospital Ramón y Cajal, 28034 Madrid, Spain*

ABSTRACT: Previously, we have shown that long-term potentiation (LTP) in hippocampus of Lewis rats was significantly modulated by cocaine self-administration. Using a single train of high-frequency stimulation of 100 Hz for 1s (HFS), we found an enhancement of LTP after cocaine self-administration that was maintained even during the extinction of this behavior. However, the effects of cocaine self-administration on a hippocampal-dependent spatial learning task were unknown. Therefore, in the present study our first objective was to analyze if cocaine self-administration might affect the performance in a hippocampus-dependent task, such as the Morris water maze test. Male adult Lewis (LEW) rats self-administered cocaine (1 mg/kg/injection) or saline (0.9% NaCl) for 3 weeks. Three hours after finishing the last self-administration session, animals were submitted to Morris water maze training for 3 consecutives days. A memory test was carried out 24 h after the last training session. No significant differences were found in escape latencies and time spent in the quadrant where the platform was located during training. Given that we did not find any cocaine effect on this spatial learning task, our second objective was to estimate indirectly if brain cocaine levels have failed to modulate LTP in animals that were performing the water maze trials. To this end, we tested if cocaine application to hippocampal slices of naïve subjects was able to evoke LTP. The results indicated that cocaine produced an enhanced LTP in these hippocampal slices. Taking together, the results of the present study suggest that hippocampal LTP-like processes generated after cocaine self-administration are not related to spatial learning hippocampal-dependent tasks, such as the water maze test.

KEYWORDS: cocaine self-administration; LTP; water maze; hippocampus; spatial learning

Address for correspondence: Emilio Ambrosio, Fac. Psicología, Dpto. Psicobiología, UNED, C/ Juan del Rosal n°10, 28040 Madrid, Spain. Voice: +34913987974; fax: +34913986287.
e-mail: eambrosio@psi.uned.es

Ann. N.Y. Acad. Sci. 1074: 427–437 (2006). © 2006 New York Academy of Sciences.
doi: 10.1196/annals.1369.043

INTRODUCTION

It is well accepted that repeated exposure to drugs of abuse influences neuronal plasticity and that neural adaptations leading to addiction involve similar cellular mechanisms that enable learning and memory.[1] In addition, drugs of abuse and learning processes have been found to activate common signal pathways and neural circuits.[2] To this respect, it has bccn proposed that hippocampus could play a critical role in rewarding response[2] and in drug-seeking behavior,[3] due to its key role in information encoding and retrieving in CNS. Although the hipoccampus is not considered an integral component of the addiction pathways, it has been described that the nucleus accumbens (NAcc) and the ventral tegmental area can be activated by the hippocampus.[4–7] In addition, it has been shown that hippocampal stimulation can reinitiate cocaine-seeking behavior,[3] and the inactivation of the subiculum, the major source of hippocampal innervation to NAcc,[8] reduces cocaine-seeking[9,10] and cocaine-taking behavior.[10]

Long-term potentiation (LTP) is the most studied form of synaptic plasticity in hippocampus that occurs at its synapses after high-frequency stimulation. LTP is considered one of the molecular substrates of learning and memory.[11] A great number of studies have demonstrated the involvement of LTP-like mechanisms in spatial learning,[12] specifically in Morris water maze test,[13,14] that is considered as a paradigm to assess spatial learning and memory associated with hippocampal function.[15,16] Thus, it has been demonstrated in transgenic mice that an enhancement of hippocampal LTP was closely related to a better performance in the water maze test.[17] Similarly, it has been found that hippocampal LTP blockade as well as LTP saturation impairs spatial learning in this behavioral test.[13,18]

Previous results obtained in our laboratory have shown that LTP in hippocampus of Lewis rats was significantly modulated by cocaine self-administration.[19] Using a single 100 Hz for 1 s (HFS) train, we found an enhancement of LTP after cocaine self-administration that was maintained even during the extinction of this behavior. However, we did not know the effects of cocaine self-administration on a hippocampal-dependent spatial learning task. Therefore, the first purpose of this study was to analyze whether cocaine self-administration might affect the performance in a hippocampus-dependent task, such as the Morris water maze test. Given that we did not find any cocaine effect on this spatial learning task, we decided to estimate indirectly if brain cocaine levels have failed to induce LTP in animals that were performing the water maze trials. In consequence, the second purpose of this work was to test if cocaine application to hippocampal slices of naïve subjects was able to evoke LTP. The results indicated that cocaine produced an enhanced LTP in these hippocampal slices, suggesting that hippocampal LTP-like processes generated after cocaine self-administration are not related to spatial learning hippocampal-dependent tasks, such as the water maze test.

METHODS

Cocaine Self-Administration Study

Animals used in this study were maintained in facilities according to European Union Laboratory Animal Care Rules (86/609/ECC directive). Male Lewis rats (n=17) were trained to self-administer i.v. cocaine (1 mg/kg/injection) or saline (0.9% NaCl) under a fixed ratio 1 schedule of reinforcement (FR1). Cocaine-reinforced behavior was run according to previously described procedure.[20] Before surgical implantation of the i.v. catheter, animals were trained to lever press for food under the same FR1 schedule of reinforcement. When operant behavior for food was established, a catheter of polyvinylchloride tubing (0.064 i.d.) was surgically implanted in the jugular vein approximately at the level of the atrium under anesthesia. Twelve operant chambers (Coulburn Instruments, Allentown, PA) were used for cocaine self-administration studies. Two levers designed to register a response when 3.0 g of force was applied were placed 14 cm apart on the front wall of the chamber. A microliter injection pump (Harvard 22) was used to deliver i.v saline or cocaine injections. Animals were allowed to self-administer cocaine or saline in daily 2-h sessions between 11:00 and 14:00 h 7 days a week for 3 weeks. No priming injections were given to the subjects at the beginning of the sessions, and no cues were associated with active lever presses. Only animals with stable self-administration behavior were taken into account for water maze testing. Drug delivery, operant data acquisition, and storage were accomplished on PC computers (Med Associates Inc., St. Albans, VT).

Morris Water Maze Test

Three hours after finishing the last self-administration session, animals were submitted to water maze testing. The Morris water maze was a black circular pool (2 m diameter, 45 cm high) filled with water (30 cm depth at 25°C) and divided into four quadrants. The pool was situated in a room with numerous extra maze cues. An invisible escape platform was placed in the middle of one of the quadrants and was kept in the same position during training. Individual behavior was monitored by a video camera and a computerized tracking system (Ethovision 1.90, Noldus Information Technology, The Netherlands). Animals were firstly submitted to water maze training for 3 days and three consecutive trials each day. Each trial lasted 120 s or until the animal found the platform. All animals were left in the platform during 30 s (including those who failed to locate it) and then taken away from the pool for 30-s rest period before the next trial. Animals kept on self-administering cocaine during the 3 days of the training to avoid that cocaine abstinence could affect the learning of the task. Twenty-four hours after the last training session, rats were submitted to memory test for 90 s. In the memory trial, the platform was removed from the pool and the time spent looking for the platform in each quadrant was measured two times, at 30 and 90 s.

In Vitro *Cocaine Effects on Electrophysiological Hippocampal Responses*

In order to estimate indirectly if brain circulating cocaine levels might be inducing electrophysiological responses in the hippocampus that could be affecting the performance in water maze training, we analyzed the effects of adding cocaine to hippocampal slices of Lewis naïve rats ($n = 4$ for control group; and $n = 4$ for cocaine group). After decapitation, animal brains were removed and immediately dropped into a bubbled (95% O_2 – 5% CO_2) and ice-cold Krebs–Ringer bicarbonate (KRB) solution in mM; 109 NaCl, 2.5 KCl, 1 KH_2PO_4, 1.3 $MgSO_4$, 2.5 $CaCl_2$, 26.2 $NaHCO_3$, and 11 glucose. As it has been previously described,[21,22] transverse slices (400 μm thick) were cut with a manual tissue chopper from the dorsal portion of each hippocampus and placed in a humidified interface chamber at room temperature (20–25°C). After 2-h incubation period, slices were submerged in a recording chamber and continuously perfused with a standard KRB solution at 2 mL/min. Evoked field excitatory postsynaptic potentials (fEPSPs) were monitored for 200 min in the CA1 stratum radiatum of the hippocampal slices preparations in response to electric stimulation of Schaffer collaterals. The electric stimulation was generated by a pulse generator (Master-8; AMPI, Israel) connected to an isolating stimulus unit (Cibertec, Spain) and tungsten electrodes (1 μm tip; 1 MΩ). Synaptic responses were firstly recorded for a 20-min period to establish baseline values. In cocaine group, once the baseline period elapsed, 1-μM cocaine was added to the KRB solution for 40 min. Twenty minutes after cocaine application, a single HFS train was applied to induce LTP, as previously described.[19] In control slices, LTP was studied 20 min after the baseline period. A single slice for each animal was considered as $n = 1$. Evoked fEPSPs were recorded and amplified by a CyberAmp 320 (Axon Instruments, Sunnyvale, CA) amplifier. Synaptic responses were visualized in a digital oscilloscope and stored in a PC computer using the pClamp 8.02 software (Axon Instruments). Data were normalized respect to the mean values of the responses obtained by each animal at the 20-min baseline period.

Data Analysis

In the self-administration study, a repeated measures analysis of variance (ANOVA) with the between subjects factor "group" and the within subjects factor "session" was used to test if there were significant differences in the number of injections self-administered by saline and cocaine rats. Student's *t*-test was used to reveal significant differences between both groups in each self-administration session. In Morris water maze test, a repeated measures ANOVA with the between subjects factors "group" and the within subjects factor "trial" was performed to analyze escape latencies to find the platform during training sessions. Student's *t*-test was runned to prove if there were significant differences between saline and cocaine self-administered rats in each trial of the training sessions as well as in the memory test. In the *in vitro* electrophysiological study, the averaged values of the initial rising slope of the fEPSP measured during 5 consecutive minutes were the dependent variable. The mean value of fEPSP 5 min after tetanization and the last 5 min of the recording assay were analyzed by Student's *t*-test. In all the cases, statistical differences were considered significant if the probability of error was $< 5\%$. All calculations were performed using SPSS statistical package 12.0 version.

RESULTS

FIGURE 1 shows the number of injections self-administered by saline and cocaine animals under an FR1 schedule of reinforcement for 3 weeks. Repeated measures ANOVA revealed a statistically significant effect of "group" ($F_{1,15} = 51.9, P < 0.001$), "session" ($F_{1,15} = 51.9, P < 0.05$), and "session" × "group" interaction ($F_{20,300} = 2.89, P < 0.001$). As it can be observed, cocaine animals self-administered a significant higher number of injections compared to saline group throughout all the sessions of the study, showing that LEW rats are responsive to reinforcing properties of cocaine.

In FIGURE 2 are represented the escape latencies to find the platform of saline and cocaine self-administered animals during the training sessions in Morris water maze test. FIGURE 3 shows the performance of the subjects in the memory test 24 h after the last training session. The figure represents the percentages of time spent by the animals in the quadrant where the platform was located during training, measured at 30 and 90 s from the beginning of the memory test. Repeated measures ANOVA only revealed a statistically significant effect of "trial" along the training sessions ($F_{8,8} = 14.03, P \leq 0.001$). There were not statistically significant differences between saline and cocaine self-administered animals in the escape latencies to find the platform during the training sessions. However, it can be noted that it seems to exist a tendency in the first session, especially in the second trial, in the escape latencies to be lesser in cocaine respect to saline self-administered animals ($P < 0.056$).

Significant differences were not found in memory test 24 h after the last training session either at 30 s or at 90 s. Cocaine self-administered animals spent similar percentages of time in the quadrant where the platform was located during training than saline animals when it was measured at 30 s

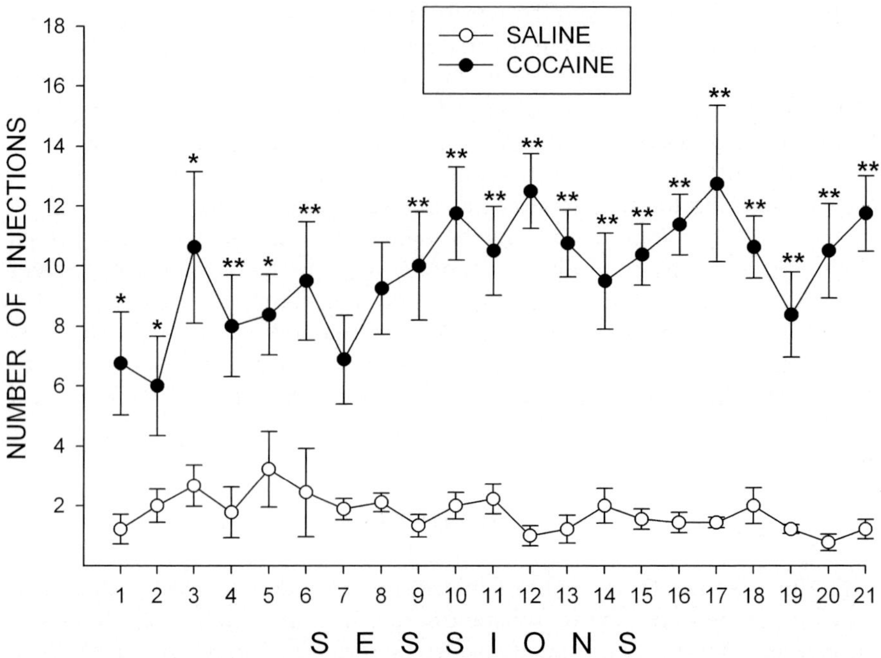

FIGURE 1. Cocaine self-administration behavior. Averaged number of injections self-administered by saline and cocaine animals per session under an FR1 schedule of reinforcement for 3 weeks. Data are expressed as the mean ± s.e.m. in cocaine ($n = 8$) and saline groups ($n = 9$). $^{*}P < 0.05$, $^{**}P < 0.01$, Student's t-test.

(saline: 37.4 ± 4.7%; cocaine: 36.8 ± 4.1%) and 90 s (saline: 33.7 ± 3.1%; cocaine: 32.3 ± 2.5%).

FIGURE 4 shows the synaptic transmission in absence or presence of cocaine (1 μM) in hippocampal slices of naïve rats. As it can be seen, basal synaptic transmission was not affected by cocaine when it was added to the KRB solution. However, the application of an HFS train in cocaine presence resulted in higher potentiation of the fEPSP compared to their respective controls 5 min after tetanization ($P < 0.05$; control: 158 ± 17%, cocaine: 231.6 ± 34.2%). This cocaine-induced LTP enhancement was maintained until the end of the recording assay ($P < 0.05$; at 5 min before final, control: 102 ± 21.17, cocaine: 172 ± 9.37).

DISCUSSION

We have found in this study that cocaine self-administration does not affect spatial learning and memory performance in a hippocampal-dependent task, such as the Morris water maze test. Both cocaine and saline self-administering

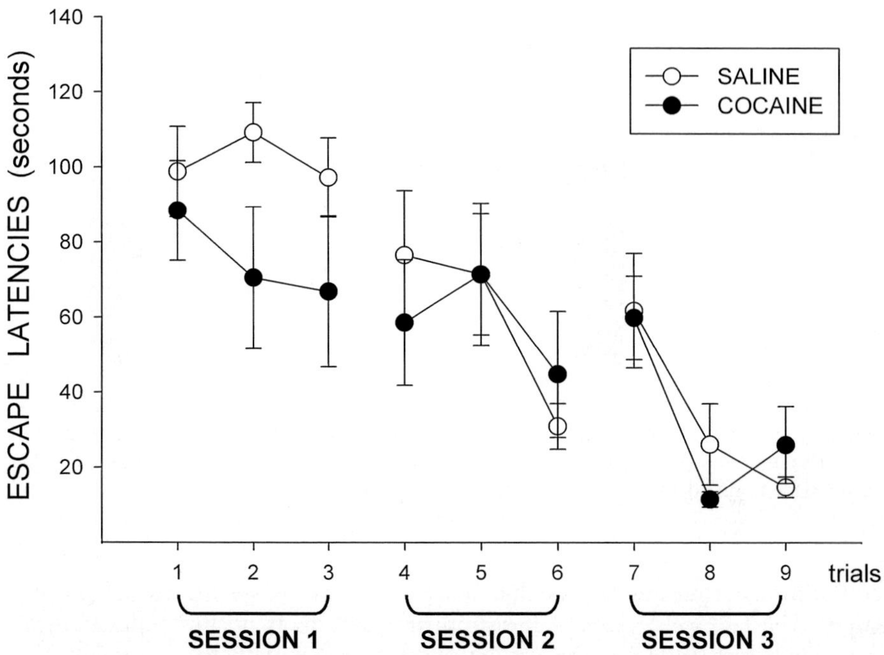

FIGURE 2. Morris water maze training. Escape latencies to find the platform in three trials during the three training sessions in saline and cocaine self-administered animals. Data are expressed as the mean ± s.e.m. in cocaine ($n = 8$) and saline groups ($n = 9$).

groups exhibited decreased escape latencies to find the platform in the water maze, suggesting that all the subjects learned adequately the task, but cocaine and saline animals did not differ in any of the parameters measured. The literature on this subject is scarce, but our data are in accordance with the results found by Kantak *et al.*,[23] who have shown that cocaine self-administration did not alter the speed or accuracy of learning in a hippocampus-related task. Other authors, however, using a cocaine experimenter-administered procedure, have found that subchronic cocaine administration prior to and during training impaired learning and memory in water maze test.[24] Similarly, Goto and Grace[25] have shown that repeated cocaine administration disrupted goal-directed behavior in a spatial maze task. Thus, it seems that passive versus self-administration is an important factor that may account for the described differences found among the cited studies. In this regard, we and others have demonstrated that differences in several neurobiological cocaine effects depend upon contingent or noncontingent drug administration.[20,26–29]

In a previous work,[19] we showed that cocaine self-administration induced an enhanced and perdurable LTP in hippocampal slices. Given that Morris water maze test has been considered a hippocampal-dependent spatial learning task,[15,16] we were interested in analyzing the performance of cocaine

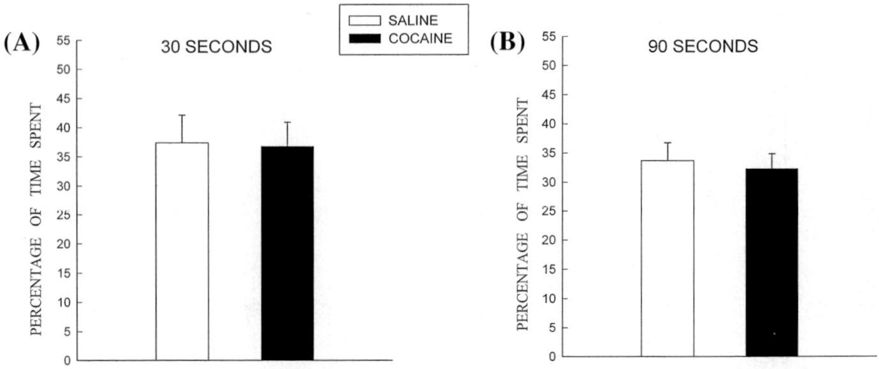

FIGURE 3. Morris water maze memory test. Percentage of time spent 24 h after the last training session in the quadrant where the platform was located during training, measured at 30 **(A)** and 90 s **(B)** from the beginning of the memory test. Data are expressed as the mean ± s.e.m. in cocaine ($n = 8$) and saline groups ($n = 9$).

self-administering animals in that behavioral test, as we did in the present study. The lack of cocaine self-administration effects on this hippocampal-dependent task found in the present work together with the increased hippocampal synaptic plasticity induced by cocaine self-administration shown in our previous study[19] suggests that cocaine-induced LTP enhancement in the hippocampus may participate in cocaine reinforcing effects, but not in spatial associative learning, at least as measured in the particular conditions of our study. It is also possible that hippocampal synaptic plasticity changes induced by cocaine were well established after 3 weeks of self-administration of this study, and that it could reflect a hippocampal modulation of synaptic connections with other brain regions rather than an unique activation of hippocampal synapses.

The animals of the present work were submitted to the water maze test 3 h after self-administration sessions ended, and it is reasonable to assume that enough circulating blood cocaine levels were still acting in the brain while they were performing the task. In contrast, in our already described previous study cocaine-induced LTP enhancement was obtained 24 h after finishing the last cocaine self-administration session and after 10 days of extinction of cocaine self-administration behavior,[19] suggesting that this cocaine-induced LTP increment was independent of brain circulating cocaine levels. Considering that water maze trials were carried out after cocaine self-administration session, it was speculated that brain circulating cocaine levels might have interfered with spatial learning processing. In a bid to estimate indirectly whether or not these cocaine levels might have affected water maze learning through an LTP modulation, we analyzed the induction of LTP in hippocampal slices of naïve animals when cocaine was added to the perfusion solution. The

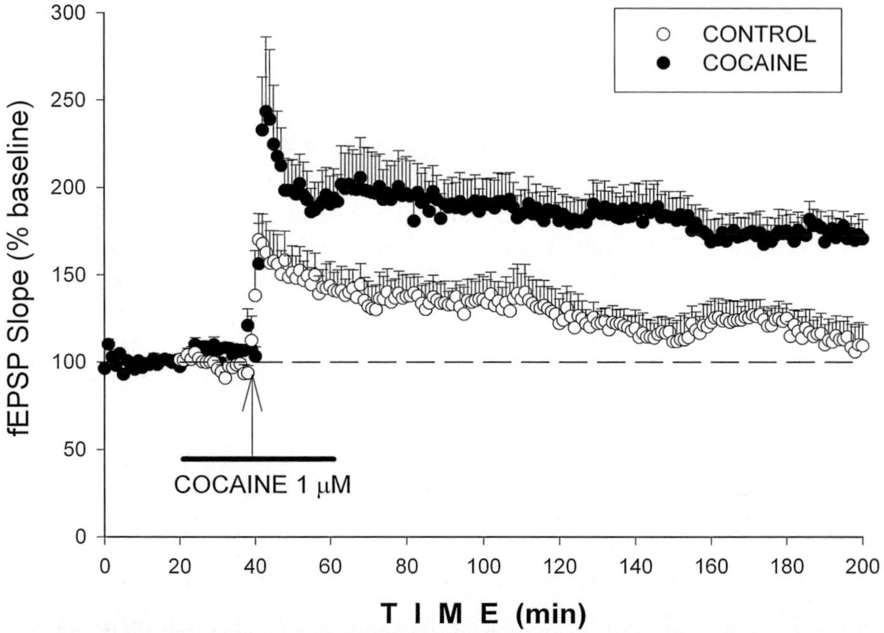

FIGURE 4. Hippocampal LTP induced by *in vitro* cocaine addition to hippocampal slices from naïve rats. Time course of changes in fEPSP slope expressed as the percentages of the baseline values in control and cocaine-exposed slices. In cocaine group, 20 min after the baseline period, cocaine (1 μM) was added to the perfusion solution for 40 min (indicated by a solid line). A single high-frequency train of 100 Hz/sec (indicated by arrow) was applied 20 min after cocaine addition. In control group, the HFS train was applied once the 20 min baseline period elapsed. Electrophysiological responses were recorded for 200 min in both groups. Data are expressed as the mean ± s.e.m. of cocaine-exposed (n = 4) and control slices (n = 4).

presence of cocaine induced a greater LTP, an effect that was not found in the absence of cocaine. This enhanced LTP was verified 5 min after tetanization and maintained until the end of the recording assay, beyond the 40 min of drug exposition period. Thus, cocaine addition facilitated the induction and maintenance of hippocampal LTP in naïve rats, without altering basal synaptic transmission as other authors have reported.[19,30,31] These results suggest that the probable cocaine-induced changes in hippocampal plasticity during cocaine self-administration were still present when the animals were being trained in the water maze. However, it appears that these synaptic changes are not related to spatial learning processing in this test.

In summary, cocaine self-administration does not affect performance in a hippocampal-related task, such as the Morris water maze test. Given that we have also shown that the mere presence of cocaine in the hippocampus produced an LTP facilitation, the results of this study suggest that hippocampal synaptic plasticity changes induced by cocaine self-administration are not related to spatial learning, at least in the water maze test.

ACKNOWLEDGMENTS

The authors are grateful to R. Ferrado and A. Marcos for technical assistance. This research has been supported by Plan Nacional sobre Drogas 2001–2003 and 2004–2006; FIS (01–005–01 and Red de Trastornos Adictivos-G03/05) and BSO2001–1099 grants. Cocaine hydrochloride was kindly provided by Dirección General de Estupefacientes (Spain).

REFERENCES

1. Wolf, M.E. 2002. Addiction: making the connection between behavioural changes and neuronal plasticity in specific pathways. Mol. Interv. **2:** 146–157.
2. Nestler, E.J. 2001. Neurobiology: total recall—the memory of addiction. Science **292:** 2266–2267.
3. Vorel, S.R. *et al.* 2001. Relapse to cocaine-seeking after hippocampal theta burst stimulation. Science **292:** 1175–1178.
4. Kelley, A.E. & V.B. Domesick. 1982. The distribution of the projection from the hippocampal formation to the nucleus accumbens in the rat: an anterograde- and retrograde-horseradish peroxidase study. Neuroscience **7:** 2321–2335.
5. Sesack, S.R. & V.M. Pickel. 1990. In the rat medial nucleus accumbens, hippocampal and catecholaminergic terminals converge on spiny neurons and are in apposition to each other. Brain Res. **527:** 266–279.
6. O'Donnell, P. & A.A. Grace. 1995. Synaptic interactions among excitatory afferents to nucleus accumbens neurons: hippocampal gating of prefrontal cortical input. J. Neurosci. **15:** 3622–3639.
7. Legault, M., P.P. Rompre & R.A. Wise. 2000. Chemical stimulation of the ventral hippocampus elevates nucleus accumbens dopamine by activating dopaminergic neurons of the ventral tegmental area. J. Neurosci. **20:** 1635–1642.
8. Yang, C.R. & G.J. Mogenson. 1984. Electrophysiological responses of neurones in the nucleus accumbens to hippocampal stimulation and the attenuation of the excitatory responses by the mesolimbic dopaminergic system. Brain Res. **324:** 69–84.
9. Sun, W. & G.V. Rebec. 2003. Lidocaine inactivation of ventral subiculum attenuates cocaine-seeking behaviour in rats. J. Neurosci. **23:** 10258–10264.
10. Black, Y.D. *et al.* 2004. Hippocampal memory system function and the regulation of cocaine self-administration behaviour in rats. Behav. Brain Res. **151:** 225–238.
11. Bliss, T.V. & G.L. Collingridge. 1993. A synaptic model of memory: long-term potentiation in the hippocampus. Nature **361:** 31–39.
12. Eichenbaum, H. & T. Otto. 1993. LTP and memory: can we enhance the connection? Trends Neurosci. **16:** 163–164.
13. Moser, E.I. *et al.* 1998. Impaired spatial learning after saturation of long-term potentiation. Science **281:** 2038–2042.

14. RICHTER-LEVIN, G. *et al.* 1998. Dissociation between genes activated in long-term potentiation and in spatial learning in the rat. Neurosci. Lett. **251:** 41–44.
15. MORRIS, R. *et al.* 1982. Place navigation impaired in rats with hippocampal lesions. Nature **24:** 681–683.
16. TSIEN, J., P.T. HUERTA, S. TONEGAWA. 1996. The essential role of hippocampal CA1 NMDA receptor dependent synaptic plasticity in spatial memory. Cell **87:** 1327–1338.
17. TANG, Y.P. *et al.* 1999. Genetic enhancement of learning and memory in mice. Nature **401:** 63–69.
18. MORRIS, R.G. *et al.* 1986. Selective impairment of learning and blockade of long-term potentiation by an N-methyl-D-aspartate receptor antagonist, AP5. Nature **319:** 774–776.
19. DEL OLMO, N. *et al.* 2006. Enhancement of hippocampal long-term potentiation induced by cocaine self-administration is maintained during the extinction of this behaviour. Brain Res. Submitted.
20. CRESPO, J.A. *et al.* 2001. Extinction of cocaine self-administration produces a differential time-related regulation of proenkephalin gene expression in rat brain. Neuropsychopharmacology **25:** 185–194.
21. DEL OLMO, N. *et al.* 2000. Taurine-induced synaptic potentiation: role of calcium and interaction with LTP. Neuropharmacology **39:** 40–54.
22. DEL OLMO, N. *et al.* 2003. Taurine-induced synaptic potentiation and the late phase of long-term potentiation are related mechanistically. Neuropharmacology **44:** 26–39.
23. KANTAK, K. *et al.* 2005. Influence of cocaine self-administration on learning related to prefrontal cortex or hippocampus functioning in rats. Psychopharmacology (Berl.) **181(2):** 227–236.
24. QUIRK, P.L., R.R.W. RICHARDS & D.D. AVERY. 2001. Subchronic cocaine produces training paradigm-dependent learning deficits in laboratory rats. Pharmacol. Biochem. Behav. **68:** 545–553.
25. GOTO, Y. & A.A. GRACE. 2005. Dopaminergic modulation of limbic and cortical drive of nucleus accumbens in goal-directed behaviour. Nat. Neurosci. **8:** 805–812.
26. WILSON, J.M. *et al.* 1994. Amygdala dopamine levels are markedly elevated after self- but not passive-administration of cocaine. Brain Res. **668:** 39–45.
27. DWORKIN, S.I. *et al.* 1995. Rat brain neurotransmitter turnover rates altered during withdrawal from chronic cocaine administration. Brain Res. **682:** 116–126.
28. HEMBY, S.E. *et al.* 1997. Differences in extracellular dopamine concentrations in the nucleus accumbens during response-dependent and response-independent cocaine administration in the rat. Psychopharmacology (Berl.) **133:** 7–16.
29. CRESPO, J.A. *et al.* 2003. Extinction of cocaine self-administration produces alterations in corticotropin releasing factor gene expression in the paraventricular nucleus of the hypothalamus. Brain Res. Mol. Brain Res. **117:** 160–167.
30. THOMPSON, A.M., B.A. GOSNELL & J.J. WAGNER. 2002. Enhancement of long-term potentiation in the rat hippocampus following cocaine exposure. Neuropharmacology **42:** 1039–1042.
31. THOMPSON, A.M. *et al.* 2004. Modulation of long-term potentiation in the rat hippocampus following cocaine self-administration. Neuroscience **127:** 177–185.

Comparison between Heroin and Heroin–Cocaine Polyabusers

A Psychopathological Study

ADOLFO BANDETTINI DI POGGIO,[a] FRANCESCO FORNAI,[a,b] ANTONIO PAPARELLI,[a] MATTEO PACINI,[c,d] GIULIO PERUGI[c,d] AND ICRO MAREMMANI[c,d]

[a]*Department of Human Morphology and Applied Biology, University of Pisa, 56126 Pisa, Italy*

[b]*Laboratory of Neurobiology of Movement Disorders I.R.C.C.S. I.N.M. Neuromed, 86077 Pozzilli, Isernia, Italy*

[c]*Institute of Behavioral Sciences 'G. De Lisio,' 54031 Carrara, Italy*

[d]*PISA-SIA (Study and Intervention on Addictions) Group 'Santa Chiara,' University Hospital, Department of Psychiatry, Neurobiology, Pharmacology and Biotechnologies, University of Pisa, I-56127 Pisa, Italy*

ABSTRACT: The concomitant use of cocaine by heroin-dependent subjects, or by patients on methadone maintenance treatment, is a relevant phenomenon that determines the negative consequences on health, social adjustment, and outcome of opioid addiction treatment. Little is known about the patterns of co-use of these two substances and the pathophysiological alterations following this condition. Only a few studies have evaluated the neurochemical effects in subjects carrying this specific pattern of abuse. Similarly, the impact of cocaine abuse on psychiatric and social function in subjects already affected by opioid addiction is still poorly understood and further studies are necessary to investigate this specific area that could profoundly affect methadone maintenance treatment. The aim of this article is to investigate the psychopathological symptoms of heroin–cocaine abuse in a group of heroin addicts applying for treatment. Results show a direct relationship between cocaine abuse and a higher rate of psychiatric disorders, but a negative correlation with the severity of self-rated psychopathology.

KEYWORDS: heroin; cocaine; polyabuse; methadone maintenance treatment; psychiatric comorbidity; double diagnosis

Address for correspondence: Adolfo Bandettini di Poggio, Department of Human Morphology and Applied Biology, Via Roma 55, 56126 Pisa, Italy. Voice: +39-0502218627; fax: +39-0502218606. e-mail: dipoggio@yahoo.it

Ann. N.Y. Acad. Sci. 1074: 438–445 (2006). © 2006 New York Academy of Sciences. doi: 10.1196/annals.1369.044

INTRODUCTION

Concurrent substance abuse during methadone maintenance treatment (MMT) occurs frequently, holds down retention rates, and interferes with the achievement of satisfactory clinical outcomes both in terms of relapsing behavior, general health status, and social adjustment.[1–11] As for cocaine, the prevalence among patients in MMT in the United States increased threefold in the 1980s with respect to previous estimates[2,12,13]; thus cocaine has become the most frequently abused substance in heroin addicts. The prevalence of cocaine use in untreated opioid addicts ranges from 30% to 80%, and this phenomenon persists for up to 6 years of methadone therapy. In the 1990s, it was proposed that cocaine abuse during MMT might result from inadequate methadone dosage,[14–17] although, even when daily doses of methadone are adequate to prevent opiate abuse they fail to prevent or reduce the concomitant cocaine abuse. This was alleged to occur when dosage was enough to control withdrawal symptoms and block opiate-induced euphoria, but was too low to affect drug craving. It has been hypothesized that patients initiate or increasingly resort to cocaine in order to achieve an alternative tool to modify their mood. While such a theory has not been clearly analyzed, data show that, when heroin abuse continues in MMT patients, cocaine use may be associated with it, over a wider range of methadone doses.[18–20] On the contrary, the counterbalancing effect of a tonic opiate may render individuals more tolerant to cocaine loads.

There is a large body of work suggesting that a preexistent psychiatric morbidity or even a personality disorder could influence the addiction process and determine different patterns of drug abuse.[21–27] Also, many authors described the coexistence of psychiatric disease and drug abuse and the reciprocal detrimental role of each condition.

The aims of this research study are (*a*) to evaluate the occurrence of cocaine abuse in heroin addicts and (*b*) the incidence of psychiatric comorbidity when cocaine adds on opioid abusers treated with methadone.

METHODS

Setting

In Italy, clinical facilities for drug addicts constantly provide opiate agonists at low doses, due to cultural reasons and despite existing guidelines.

Since 1993, the PISA-SIA group has been testing an experimental protocol that is characterized by a higher dosage pattern for opiate addiction ruled by the achievement of the absence of withdrawal symptoms. According to such a protocol, after a short period, the dose of methadone is gradually increased until drug abuse dwindles below one positive weekly urine drug screen per month. Abuse of a CNS depressant is considered equivalent to ongoing opiate use.

As long as this requirement is met, the patient is defined as "stabilized" and the dose at which this goal has been accomplished is referred to as the "stabilizing dose..." Thus, the dosage limit is not defined *a priori*. Nonetheless, patients who cannot be stabilized within 1 year are terminated and move back to their local treatment services.

Sample

The patients included in the study were consecutively selected among opiate abusers newly applying for opiate addiction treatment at the Unit for the Treatment of Drug Abuse, working within the Department of Psychiatry, University of Pisa (Italy) from March 2003 up to December 2004.

Inclusion criteria were:

1. A DSM-IV diagnosis for opioid dependence;
2. absence of severe physical illness.

All patients signed informed consent to protocol rules before being started on the increasing-dose phase. Those who denied consent were excluded and referred to the nearest addiction facilities units.

The sample consisted of 612 patients. Participants were classified into heroin-only users (HO, $n = 283$) or cocaine plus heroin users (HC, $n = 329$) according to the Drug Addiction History Rating Scale (DAH-RS) (see below).[28]

Mean age was 30 ± 6 years (range 18–53 years). The majority was male (474, 77.5%), never married (422, 69.0%), low education level (<13 years) (477, 77.9%), and unemployed (315, 51.5%). According to the DAH-RS, the average age at first heroin use was 20 ± 4 years (range 13–31 years); regular use had set on at 22 ± 6 years (range 13–40 years); and the average duration of addiction was 75 ± 64 months (range 1–240 months).

Instruments

Sociodemographic and clinical features were registered using a standardized form DAH-RS,[28] an instrument that is tailored for the collection of clinical information in cases of heroin abuse. The DAH-RS is a multiscale questionnaire assessing the following issues: somatic health, mental health, typology of abused substances, current and lifetime features of opiate use, treatment history, social adjustment, and environmental factors. Ten subscores are calculated: physical disorders, mental disorders, polysubstance abuse, previous treatments, current treatments, working status, family adjustment, sexual dysfunctions, socialization and leisure time, and legal problems. The specific variables addressed are: hepatic, vascular and lymphatic pathology, gastrointestinal disorders, sexual disorders, dental pathology, and HIV status; awareness of illness, memory disorders, anxiety disorders, mood disorders, aggression, thought disorders, and sensory disorders; employment, family, sex, socialization and leisure time, and legal problems; use of alcohol, opiates, CNS depressants, CNS stimulants, hallucinogens, phencyclidine, cannabis, inhalants, and poly-substance abuse; rate and pattern of drug use, and previous therapies; current therapy; and methadone dosage.

Psychopathological symptoms were investigated by the SCL-90.[29] SCL-90 is a self-administered rating scale including 90 items, each with scores ranging from 0 to 4, on the basis of subjective intensity. SCL-90 items can be grouped in nine factors corresponding to the following psychopathological dimensions: Somatic symptoms, Interpersonal sensitivity, Obsessive-Compulsive, Depression, Anxiety, Hostility, Phobic Anxiety, Paranoid Ideation, and Psychotic features. The rating scale also provides a global score index as the sum of all items divided by the number of items; a positive symptoms index as number of items rated positively (i.e., not zero in a 0–4 Likert scale); a positive symptoms' severity as sum of all items divided by the positive symptoms index. SCL-90-related information is meant to be referred to the previous week.

The presence of psychiatric symptoms as registered by the DAH-RS allows composing of different symptoms into profiles, which likely to correspond to diagnostic areas. Such a preliminary diagnostic procedure allows approaching the correct diagnosis approximately along symptoms typology, when it would be awkward and premature to define DSM-IV categories, due to concurrent substance intoxication or withdrawal. Attenuated syndromes, such as hypomania, may be underestimated, and a Bipolar II or Cyclothymic disorder may result in a preliminary depressive disorder diagnosis. However, such a trend does mirror the actual difficulty in the index assessment of minor bipolarity.

Preliminary diagnostic groups are Schizophrenia, Schizoaffective disorders, Bipolar Disorders, Depressive Disorders, Anxiety Disorders.

Urine drug screens for heroin and cocaine were performed at study entrance.

Statistical Analysis

Comparisons between the two groups were performed by a Student's *t*-test or by a chi-square test for continuous and categorical variables, respectively, with *post hoc* Scheffé when required. Differences on SCL-90 between groups were also explored by means of discriminant analysis. All the analyses were performed using SPSS Software ver 9. (SPSS Inc.).

RESULTS

No statistical differences between the two groups were found for demographic data or addiction chronology. HC were more likely than HO to report at least one somatic concern (56% versus 44% $P < 0.001$). The impact of

TABLE 1. Presence of psychiatric disorders registered by the DAH-RS

	HO	CH	Total
Psychiatric disorders*	43.6%	63.8%	
Schizophrenia*	0.4%	1.2%	0.8%
Schizoaffective*	8.8%	12.8%	10.9%
Depressive disorders*	22.6%	29.5%	26.3%
Bipolar disorder *	15.2%	17.9%	16.7%
Anxiety disorders	8.8%	6.7%	7.7%

*$P > 0.05$.

cocaine was substantial and significant for social aspects that were grouped in the generic item "problems at work" (59.4% versus 45.9%, $P < 0.005$). Unemployment was more likely among HC subjects (57.8% versus 47.0% in HO subjects, $P < 0.005$). Legal problems (recent incarceration, illegal activities and probation/parole status, as measured by the ASI legal subscale) were reported by 61.0% of HC patients versus 38.2% of HO peers ($P < 0.001$).

The SCL90 psychopathological scores were similar between groups. The discriminant profile showed HC to be rather displaying symptoms of Somatization Anxiety, Hostility, Phobic Anxiety, General Anxiety, Paranoid Ideation, and Psychosis, whereas Interpersonal sensitivity, Obsessive-Compulsive, and Depression were rather characteristic of non-polyabusers ($P = 0.03$).

With reference to the DAH-RS preliminary diagnostic grouping, Schizophrenia, Schizoaffective Disorders, Bipolar Disorders, Depressive disorders, Anxiety Disorders (that are countered all together), and no disorders, a higher rate was found among CH subjects for all diagnostic categories except for anxiety disorders, and for the presence of any disorder (43.6% in HO subjects versus 63.8% in the HC subjects, $P < 0.05$) (TABLE 1).

DISCUSSION

In agreement with previous data, our study confirms that polyabuse is a detrimental factor for social life and health in drug addicts. Moreover, a pattern of concurrent cocaine and heroin use is predictably related with a higher incidence of legal problems compared with what was observed in patients abusing only heroin.

The presence of higher rates of psychiatric disorders, beyond what was expected from literature data, may be justified by the peculiarity of this study setting. Higher rates of Axis I Disorders in patients that used both the two drugs are in line with what has been described in the literature.[30–33] Dual diagnosis may itself be a limit for some measures of the outcome, but recent evidence showed that it may not interfere with treatment retention and heroin use, as long as adequate dosages are employed.[34]

Curiously, current self-rated psychiatric discomfort does not seem to mirror higher level of impairment. HC abusers do not rate themselves as highly impaired on psychopathological grounds, despite their higher rate of psychiatric diagnosis and their poor social adjustment. Such a psychopathological paradox may be explained by the enhanced state of drug-induced euphoria (due to the add-on of cocaine), which amplifies the discrepancy between objective (DAH-RS) and subjective (SCL90) rating. Conversely to what was expected for nonaddicted users, the combination of heroin and cocaine in addicts does not results in mutual neutralization of toxic effects, but in the exacerbation of a state of behavioral excitement and the diminishing of insight.[22,32]

The discriminant psychopathological dimensions of HC subjects include two dimensions that are typical of heroin addicts, that is somatization, anxiety, and aggressiveness, whereas depression, also common, rather points at HO subjects. Despite the fact that self-rated severity of symptoms is not higher, subjects perceive themselves correctly for symptom typology.

CONCLUSIONS

Cocaine does not appear to counterbalance the toxic effects of heroin, but it is likely to grant further impairment of insight toward addiction. On psychopathological grounds, such a detrimental effect may be related to the enhancement of euphoria and the reduction of depression.

Comorbid psychiatric disorders may play a role in promoting such an enhancement in these types of polydrug abusers.

REFERENCES

1. ROWAN-SZAL, G.A. *et al.* 2000. Importance of identifying cocaine and alcohol dependent methadone clients. Am. J. Addict. **9:** 38–50.
2. MEANDZIJA, B. *et al.* 1994. HIV infection and cocaine use in methadone mantained and untreated intravenous drug users. Drug Alcohol Depend. **36:** 109–113.
3. MAGURA, S. *et al.* 1998. Changes in HIV risk behaviours among cocaine-using methadone patients. J. Addict. Dis. **17:** 71–90.
4. BUX, D.A. *et al.* 1995. Cocaine use and HIV risk behaviour in methadone maintenance patients. Drug Alcohol Depend. **37:** 29–35.
5. AVANTS, S.K. *et al.* 2000. A path analysis of cognitive, affective, and behavioral predictors of treatment response in a methadone maintenance program. J. Subst. Abuse **11:** 215–230.
6. BALL, J.C. *et al.* 1989. Cocaine and heroin use by methadone maintenance patients. NIDA Res. Monogr. **95:** 328.
7. FINNEGAN, L.P. 2000. Women, pregnancy and methadone. Heroin Addict. Related Clin. Prob. **2:** 1–8.
8. KANG, S.Y. & G. DE LEON. 1993. Criminal involvement of cocaine users in a methadone treatment program. Addiction **88:** 395–404.

9. GRELLA, C.E. *et al.* 1995. Cocaine and crack use and HIV risk behaviours among high-risk methadone maintenance clients. Drug Alcohol Depend. **37:** 15–21.
10. KOSTEN, T.R. *et al.* 1988. Antecedents and consequences of cocaine abuse among opioid addicts: a 2.5 year follow-up. J. Nerv. Ment. Dis. **176:** 176–181.
11. GUADAGNINO, G. *et al.* 1995. Relevance of intravenous cocaine use in relation to prevalence of HIV, hepatitis B and C virus markers among intravenous drug abuser in Southern Italy. J. Clin. Lab. Immunol. **47:** 1–9.
12. KOLAR, A.F. *et al.* 1991. A treatment crisis: cocaine use by clients in methadone maintenance programs. J. Subst. Abuse Treat. **7:** 101–107.
13. DES JARLAIS, D.C. *et al.* 1992. Crack cocaine use in a cohort of methadone maintenance patients. J. Subst. Abuse Treat. **9:** 319–325.
14. STINE, S.M. *et al.* 1992. Effects of methadone dose on cocaine abuse in a methadone program. Am. J. Addict. **1:** 294–303.
15. GRABOWSKI, J. *et al.* 1993. Methadone dosage, cocaine and opiate abuse. Am. J. Psychiatry **150:** 675.
16. HARTEL, D.M. *et al.* 1995. Heroin use during methadone maintenance treatment: the importance of methadone dose and cocaine use. Am. J. Public Health **85:** 83–88.
17. TENNANT, F. & J. SHANNON. 1995. Cocaine abuse in methadone maintenance patients is associated with low serum methadone concentration. J. Addict. Dis. **14:** 67–74.
18. FOLTIN, R.W. & M.W. FISCHMAN. 1996. Effects of methadone or buprenorphine maintenance on the subjective and reinforcing effects of intravenous cocaine in humans. J. Pharmacol. Exp. Ther. **278:** 1153–1164.
19. MAREMMANI, I. *et al.* 2003. Substance (ab)use during methadone and naltrexone treatment. Interest of adequate methadone dosage. J. Maint. Addict. **2:** 19–36.
20. PELES, E. *et al.* 2005. Correlation between high methadone dose and methadone blood level in methadone maintenance treatment patients. Heroin Addict. Related Clin. Prob. **7:** 27–32.
21. RUTHERFORD, M.J. *et al.* 1999. Antisocial personality disorder and psychopathy in cocaine-dependent women. Am. J. Psychiatry **156:** 849–856.
22. LEMERE, F. & J.W. SMITH. 1990. Hypomanic personality trait in cocaine addiction. Br. J. Addict. **85:** 575–576.
23. YATES, W.R. *et al.* 1989. Personality risk factors for cocaine abusers. Am. J. Public Health **79:** 891–892.
24. MAREMMANI, I. *et al.* 2002. Psico(pato)logia dell'addiction. Un'ipotesi interpretativa. Ann. Ist Super. Sanita **38:** 241–257.
25. VUKOV, M. *et al.* 1995. Personality dimensions of opiate addicts. Acta Psychiatr. Scand. **91:** 103–107.
26. MAREMMANI, I. *et al.* 2004. Addiction and bipolar spectrum: dual diagnosis with a common substrate? Addict. Dis. Treat. **3:** 156–164.
27. MAREMMANI, I. *et al.* 2005. Addictive disorders, bipolar spectrum and the impulsive link: the psychopathology of a self-regenerating pathway. Heroin Addict. Rel. Clin. Prob. **7:** 33–46.
28. MAREMMANI, I. & P. CASTROGIOVANNI. 1989. DAH-RS: Drug Addiction History Rating Scale. University Press, Pisa.
29. DEROGATIS, L.R. *et al.* 1974. The Hopkins Symptom Checklist (HSCL)—A self report symptom inventory. Behav. Sci. **19:** 1–16.
30. WEISS, R.D. *et al.* 1988. Psychopatology in cocaine abusers: changing trends. J. Nerv. Ment. Dis. **176:** 719–725.

31. NUNES, E.V. *et al.* 1989. Psychiatric diagnosis in cocaine abuse. Psychiatry Res. **28:** 105–114.
32. KLEINMAN, P.H. *et al.* 1990. Psychopatology among cocaine abusers entering in treatment. J. Nerv. Ment. Dis. **178:** 442–447.
33. CANNON, D.S. *et al.* 1992. Affective correlates of alcohol and cocaine use. Addict. Behav. **17:** 517–524.
34. PANI, P.P. *et al.* 2003. Psychiatric severity and treatment response in methadone maintenance treatment programmes: new evidence. Heroin Addict. Rel. Clin. Prob. **5:** 22–36.

Persistent and Reversible Morphine Withdrawal-Induced Morphological Changes in the Nucleus Accumbens

MARCO DIANA,[a] SATURNINO SPIGA,[b] AND ELIO ACQUAS[c]

[a] *"G. Minardi" Cognitive Neuroscience Laboratory http://lns.uniss.it, Department of Drug Sciences University of Sassari, 07100 Sassari, Italy*

[b] *Department of Animal Biology and Ecology, University of Cagliari, 09124 Cagliari, Italy*

[c] *Department of Toxicology and Centre of Excellence on Neurobiology of Addiction, University of Cagliari, 09123 Cagliari, Italy*

ABSTRACT: Morphine withdrawal produces a hypofunction of mesencephalic dopamine (DA) neurons which impinge upon medium spiny neurons (MSN) of the forebrain. After chronic treatment rats were either spontaneously or pharmacologically withdrawn from chronic morphine: under these two distinct conditions we studied the effects of withdrawal on spine density of MSN of the core and shell of the nucleus accumbens (NAcc) at various times (1–3–7–14 days). MSN were stained with the Golgi–Cox procedure and analyzed by a confocal laser-scanning microscope. Our analysis shows that both spontaneous and naloxone-induced withdrawal produces a long-lasting but reversible reduction in spines' density in shell MSN, as compared with core MSN. This effect is selectively localized at the level of second-order dendritic trunks and persists up to 14 days when spine density was found within control (pretreatment) values. By contrast, spine density counts of NAcc MSN from rats chronically treated with morphine, did not reveal any change over time. Collectively, the results of the present article suggest that spontaneous and pharmacologically precipitated withdrawal, but not chronic morphine, persistently but reversibly reduce spines' density under a condition of reduced mesolimbic DA transmission, and the reduction of spines' density in second-order dendritic trunks is selectively segregated in the MSN of the shell of the NAcc. Morphine withdrawal dramatically, lastingly, and reversibly reduces spine density, selectively in second-order dendritic trunks of NAcc shell MSN, thereby further impoverishing the already abated DA transmission. These results may be relevant in the most harmful consequences of drug addiction such as craving and loss of control over intake and are in line with recent views suggesting the hypodopaminergic state as a cardinal feature of drug dependence.

Address for correspondence: Marco Diana, M.D., Department of Drug Sciences University of Sassari, Via Muroni n. 23, 07100 Sassari, Italy. Voice: +39-079-228711; fax: +39-079-228712. e-mail: dsfdiana@uniss.it

Ann. N.Y. Acad. Sci. 1074: 446–457 (2006).
doi: 10.1196/annals.1369.045

KEYWORDS: neuronal plasticity; morphine withdrawal; dendritic spines; medium spiny neurons; nucleus accumbens; drug addiction

INTRODUCTION

A general consensus has emerged on drug dependence as a drug-induced, aberrant form of neural pasticity.[1–8]

Among others, the mesolimbic dopamine (DA) system,[9] which originates in the ventral tegmental area (VTA) and projects to forebrain areas, such as the nucleus accumbens (NAcc), seems to play a crucial role in conveying reward of pleasant stimuli of various addicting drugs.[10–14] Accordingly, DAergic transmission is activated by drugs of abuse when administered acutely[14] and activity is reduced upon withdrawal[6,8] of diverse addicting chemicals, such as cannabinoids,[15] ethanol,[16] and morphine.[17] In particular, previous work has shown that spontaneous neuronal activity of antidromically identified, NAcc-projecting DA neurons is abated by morphine withdrawal in rats.[17] The reduction in spontaneous activity may be the result of an increased GABA release from local interneurons[18] and/or a reduction in excitatory postsynapticcurrents from glutamatergic terminals impinging upon DA neurons.[19] These electrophysiological changes may, in turn, contribute to the reduction in DA release, as measured by the microdialysis method.[20–22] Further, a reduction in DA cells' size has been documented[23] suggesting a structural abnormality induced by morphine withdrawal, although not induced by chronic morphine,[24] which accompanies the physiological changes described above. These modifications appear to be long-lasting in nature[25–27] and are likely to significantly contribute to the most harmful consequences of chronic drug intake and subsequent withdrawal.[6–9,27]

On the other hand, DA-receiving areas, such as the NAcc,[28–30] are populated mainly by medium spiny neurons (MSN)[31,32] which represent the principal dopaminoceptive cell type[33] in the basal ganglia.[31,32] At present, little information is available concerning the effects produced by morphine withdrawal, although recent studies have reported a reduction in dendritic branching, in the number of NAcc dendritic spines after long-term (24–25 days) intermittent morphine withdrawal,[26] and region-specific differences related to the mode of morphine administration.[34] In addition, we recently found a reduction in spine density highly localized at the level of secondary dendrites of MSN selectively in the shell.[35] However, since these morphological alterations correlated with somatic signs of withdrawal, we decided to investigate on the persistence and reversibility of these changes over time, in order to gain some further insight on the functional effects of these structural abnormalities.[35] Thus, in the present article we sought to determine if morphine withdrawal-induced spines' alteration of MSN in the subdivisions of the NAcc would persist over time and would eventually be reversible. This information would permit speculations on the functional significance of these structural abnormalities.

MATERIALS AND METHODS

Subjects and Morphine Treatment

Male Sprague–Dawley albino rats ($n = 16$; 4/group) (Charles River, Como, Italy) weighing 200–225 g at the beginning of treatment, were used. Rats were kept on a 12-h light/12-h dark cycle with food and water available *ad libitum*. Experimental protocols were approved by the Ethical Committee at the University of Sassari and performed in strict accordance with the E.C. regulations for the use of experimental animals [CEE no. 86 (609)] and recommended guidelines for the care and use of experimental animals approved by the Society for Neuroscience. Morphine hydrochloride was dissolved in sterile saline and administered twice daily (at 08.00 and 20.00 h) for 14 days, as already described in Reference [17]. As has been reported in Reference 36, that repeated intake of opioids is associated with dose escalation and self-regulated dosing of morphine is also associated with rapid escalation of daily consumption, the initial dose administered was 20 mg/kg and it was increased by 20 mg/kg every other day until the 14th day of treatment. Control rats received an equal volume of saline. Rats were chronically treated for 14 days and then assigned to one of the following groups: (*a*) controls (CTRL): chronically treated with saline. (*b*) Chronically treated with morphine (CH-M): last morphine administration 1 h before sacrifice. (*c*) Spontaneous morphine withdrawal (S-W_1): last morphine administration 1 day (24 h) before sacrifice. (*d*) Spontaneous morphine withdrawal (S-W_3): last morphine administration 3 days (72 h) before sacrifice. (*e*) Spontaneous morphine withdrawal (S-W_7): last morphine administration 7 days (168 h) before sacrifice. (*f*) Spontaneous morphine withdrawal (S-W_{14}): last morphine administration 14 days (336 h) before sacrifice. (*g*) Naloxone-induced morphine withdrawal (NLX-W): last morphine administration 1 h before sacrifice and NLX 30 min. later. Before sacrifice, rats were tested for signs of opiate withdrawal, such as wet dog shakes, weight loss, diarrhea, teeth chattering, and ptosis by an experimentor blind to treatment. Withdrawal severity was assessed according to a point-scoring technique.[37]

Golgi–Cox Procedure and Confocal Microscopy

Animals were deeply anesthetized with urethane (1.3 g/kg, i.p.) and transcardially perfused with 0.9% saline. Brains were rapidly removed and placed in a Golgi–Cox solution. The solution was changed after 2 days and the brains left in Golgi–Cox for additional 14 days. Brains were cryoprotected in a 30% sucrose solution for 2–3 days. Ninety micrometer thick coronal slices, beginning at 1.60 and ending at 0.50 from bregma, according to Paxinos *et al.*,[38] were obtained with a cryostat (Microm Cryo-Star HM 560, Walldorf, Germany). Slices were developed using a procedure described by Kolb and McCliman.[39] Slices were dehydrated through 55%, 75%, and 95% ethanol solutions for 1 min each and two changes of 100% ethanol, and 3 min each; 2 changes of xylene, and 3 min each, coverslipped as usual for frozen tissue.

Quantitative analysis was performed 24–36 h later using a Leica 4D confocal laser-scanning microscope (CLSM) with an argon–krypton laser (Leica, Heidelberg, Germany). Confocal images were generated using 40 × oil (n.a. = 1.00–0.5) and 100 × oil (n.a. = 1.3) in reflection mode (488 excitation wavelength). Each frame (512 lines and 512 columns) was acquired eight times and then averaged to obtain noise-free images. Confocal images were obtained from the maximum number of scans allowed by the cell thickness. Optical sections, usually at consecutive intervals of 0.5–1 μm, were imaged through the depth of the labeled neurons and saved as image stacks. All confocal images were white-labeled on a black background, in a grayscale ranging from 0 (black) to 255 (white) and processed in a grayscale value with Scanware 4.2a Leica.

Counts

Spine counts are performed by two independent observers blind to pharmacological treatments. For each treatment group, about 50 (at least 20 μm long) dendritic segments for primary and secondary dendrites, respectively, are analyzed by CLSM three-dimensional reconstructions. Spine density was calculated by tracing a 10–15 μm long "sp-line" curve, along the dendritic trunk and the number of spines was recorded. The procedure was repeated along the entire detectable dendritic length. Spines were counted in primary dendrites, from the soma to the first ramification and in secondary dendrites from bifurcation to the first branch of tertiary dendrites.

Statistics

Preliminary evaluations among means have been performed with Bartlett's test for multiple comparisons and Fisher's test for comparisons between two samples. The *t*-test and ANOVA were applied for comparisons between two samples and multiple comparisons, respectively.

RESULTS

FIGURE 1 shows the effect of chronic treatment with morphine and of naloxone-precipitated (1 mg/kg) and spontaneous withdrawal (at different time

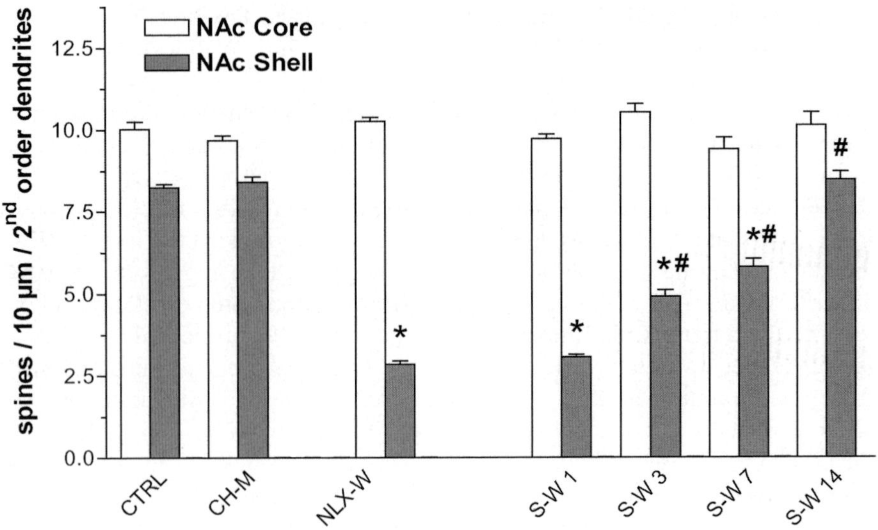

FIGURE 1. Spine densities counts of second-order dendrites of MSN of NAcc core (white histograms) and shell (gray histograms) of CTRL, CH-M, S-W_1, S-W_3, S-W_7, S-W_{14}, and NLX-W groups. Averages ± SEM are from at least 25 counts/group of treatment. * indicates $P < 0.05$ with respect to CTRL group at aTukey's post hoc test; # indicates $P < 0.05$ with respect to S-W_1 and NLX-W groups at Tukey's post hoc test.

intervals: 1, 3, 7, and 14 days) on spines' density of second-order dendrites of MSN of the NAcc core and shell. Two-way ANOVA of the results of chronic morphine and spontaneous and naloxone-precipitated withdrawal revealed a main effect of treatment [$F(6,343) = 69.23$, $P < 0.001$], area [$F(1,343) = 1117.36$, $P < 0.001$], and a significant treatment by area interaction [$F(6,343) = 67.9$, $P < 0.001$]. Tukey's post hoc analysis ($P < 0.05$) applied to treatment as main effect showed that spines' densities of MSN of S-W_1, S-W_3, S-W_7, and NLX-W groups were significantly different from densities of S-W_{14}, CTRL, and CH-M groups. Tukey's post hoc analysis ($P < 0.05$) applied to the treatment by area interaction showed that specifically NAcc shell density counts for S-W_1, S-W_3, and S-W_7 groups were significantly different from S-W_{14}, CTRL, and CH-M groups. Tukey's post hoc analysis, furthermore, failed to reveal any significant difference between NAcc shell density counts of NLX-W and S-W_1 groups and between NAcc core density counts of all groups.

FIGURE 2 provides representative images of MSN from the shell of the NAcc of rats belonging to various experimental groups. Counts revealed that the spines' loss peaked at 63.1% for S-W_1 group with respect to spines' density counts in the NAcc shell of the CTRL group and at 65.7% for the NLX-W group, while it was at 40.5% for S-W_3, at 70.1% for S-W_7, and recovered to 102.6% for S-W_{14} group.

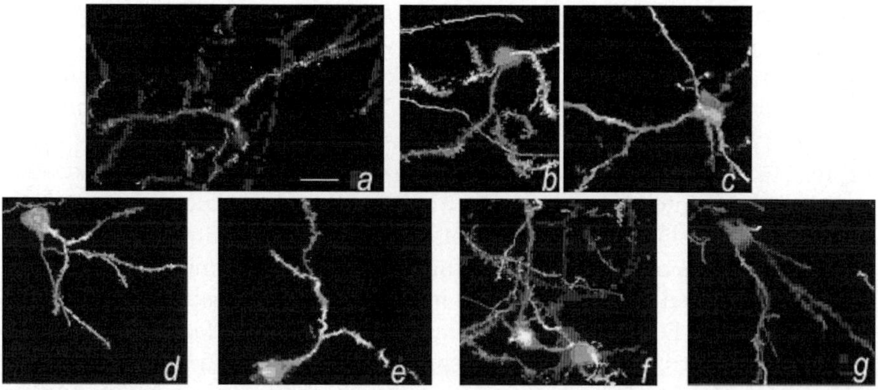

FIGURE 2. Confocal images of Golgi–Cox stained, representative MSN in the shell of the NAcc. Each is a reconstruction, frame by frame, of two adjacents scans. **a:** CTRL; **b:** CH-M; **c:** S-W_1; **d:** S-W_3; **e:** S-W_7; **f:** S-W_{14}, and **g:** NLX-W. The scale bar equals 20 μm. Note relative smoothness in second-order dendrites in panels **c**, **d**, and **e**.

DISCUSSION

The reduction in spine density under withdrawal conditions, but not chronic morphine *per se*, was selectively localized at the level of second-order dendrites of MSN only in the shell of the NAcc and was found to last up to 14 days after last morphine administration when spine density was observed to be within control values. In contrast, somatic indices of withdrawal were not present longer than 33 h[40] and were undetectable at 3 days after morphine suspension. This dichotomy (between somatic indices and spine density) suggests a lack of correlation thereby excluding the possibility that spine loss may be relevant in somatic aspects of opiate withdrawal/dependence. In contrast, the longer-lasting spine loss observed here may bear relevance in the enduring changes typical of psychological symptoms of dependence, such as craving, relapse, loss of control, etc. Incidentally, the time-course of the spine loss coincides with the abatement of DA presynaptic terminal observed electrophysiologically[27] and biochemically with the microdialysis method.[20]

Role of DAergic Tone

Considering that spines are the preferential postsynaptic target of DAergic terminals in the NAcc, the spine loss suggests a selective reduction of DA transmission specifically in the shell, in line with a primary role of this structure in the motivational properties generally ascribed to drugs of abuse,[41,42] and particularly to opiate withdrawal.[42–45] Indeed, the reduced electrophysiological activity of NAcc-projecting DA cells in the VTA[17] and the consequent decreased DA release in the NAcc, as estimated by microdialysis studies,[20–22,46] may contribute to the negative motivational state typical of opiate withdrawal,[47] as well as that of other drug withdrawal states.[6,8] Thus, the enduringly reduced spine density observed here would ultimately contribute to further *impoverish* the already abated DA transmission by depriving presynaptic DA terminals from their physiological postsynaptic target. Likewise, striatal DA receptors mRNA levels were found to be reduced during abstinence from morphine in dependent rats, and a downregulation of both D1 and D2 receptors was observed.[48] In addition, 6-hydroxydopamine (6-OHDA) lesioned rats showed similar reductions in spine density,[30] raising the possibility that the reduced DA tone may play a causal role in this effect. However, it is currently unclear if the reduction in spine density is caused by a reduced DA transmission, or is a direct effect of morphine withdrawal on MSN. Further experiments are needed to clarify this issue, although the selectivity observed (shell versus core) would seem to favor the latter possibility. Additional support for a DA-independence of these effects stems from recent studies in rats chronically treated with the DA-receptor blocker, haloperidol, which show persistent increases in dendritic spines in the NAcc shell.[49]

Functional Considerations

Irrespective of the role played by DA in this effect, which is the object of current experiments, the reduction in spine density occurring only at the level of second-order dendrites of MSN of the shell of the NAcc is likely to alter the physiological properties of these neurons. Indeed, the previous work suggests that synaptic inputs differentially affect neuronal activity depending on synaptic location on the dendritic tree.[50–52] In the present context, the disappearance of dendritic spines would reduce distal synaptic contact, thereby favoring proximal synaptic activity, with, presumably, profound alterations in action potential output capacity. It has been shown in different neuronal types, such as neocortical pyramidal neurons, that as inputs became more distal, somatic excitatory postsynaptic potential (EPSP) amplitude decreased, whereas use-dependent depression increased.[53] In CA1 pyramidal neurons, somatic EPSP seems to be location-independent,[54] although it was found that dendritic EPSP amplitude increases with the distance from the soma, counterbalancing the filtering effects of the dendrites and reducing the location dependence of somatic EPSP amplitude.[54]

A similar analysis applies to glutamate terminals: NAcc receives extensive glutamatergic projections directly from the prefrontal cortex and limbic structures,[29,55] which mainly terminate on the MSN spine head with asymmetric contacts.[56] Thus, the reduced number of dendritic spines would also reduce cortical glutamatergic inputs on MSN, thereby depriving them from an important excitatory drive, and further altering their physiological status.

Accordingly, though the release of glutamate has been reported to increase during morphine withdrawal,[57] as measured by the microdialysis method, functional electrophysiological experiments have reported a blockade of long-term depression in slices of the NAcc obtained from morphine withdrawn mice.[58] Further support for this possibility comes from studies on the neostriatum of 6-OHDA-lesioned rats[59] in which the loss of the spines was accompanied by a (quantitatively) similar loss of asymmetric glutamatergic synapses, rather than by the movement of synapses from spines to other postsynaptic targets.[59]

CONCLUSIONS

Collectively, the present structural findings suggest that a persistent, but reversible, reduction in spine density, selectively in second-order dendrites of NAcc shell MSN, affects MSN, thereby altering, in principle, their physiological activity, synaptic inputs, and, DAergic and glutamatergic transmissions as a result—both major targets of withdrawal from morphine[60] and other drugs of abuse.[6,8,61]

The present observations provide visual evidence of a structural plasticity affecting MSN, the principal DAceptive[33] neuronal type in the NAcc, during morphine withdrawal, crucial phase of the entire opiate dependence cycle. These results are in line with and support recent suggestions indicating a hypodopaminergic state as a cardinal feature of animal models[8] and human studies[62] of drug addiction.

ACKNOWLEDGMENTS

This work was supported, in part, by a grant from MIUR (2004052392_001) to M.D. and (2004052392_003) to E.A. The authors wish to thank Bernadette Valdes, Maria Antonietta Fradelloni, and Elena Sias for their expert technical assistance and Miriam Melis for valuable discussions. We thank William Dunn III for proofreading the manuscript.

REFERENCES

1. Nestler, E.J. 1993. Cellular responses to chronic treatment with drugs of abuse. Crit. Rev. Neurobiol. **7:** 23–39.
2. Nestler, E.J. 2001. Molecular basis of long-term plasticity underlying addiction. Nat. Rev. Neurosci. **2:** 119–128.
3. Nestler, E.J. & G.K. Aghajanian. 1997. Molecular and cellular basis of addiction. Science **278:** 58–63.
4. Diana, M. 1996. Dopaminergic neurotransmission and drug withdrawal: relevance to drug craving. *In* The Basal Ganglia V. Advances in Behavioral Biology, Vol.

47. V.C. Ohye, M. Kimura & J. McKenzie, Eds.: 123–130. Plenum Press. New York.
5. DIANA, M. 1998. Drugs of abuse and dopamine cell activity. *In* Catecholamines, Bridging Basic Science with Clinical Medicine. Advances in Pharmacology, Vol. 42. D.S. Goldstein, G. Ad Eisenhofer & R. McCarthy, Eds.: 998–1001. Academic Press. San Diego.
6. PULVIRENTI, L. & M. DIANA. 2001. Drug dependence as a disorder of neural plasticity: focus on dopamine and glutamate. Rev. Neurosci. **12:** 41–59.
7. HYMAN, S.E. & R.C. MALENKA. 2001. Addiction and the brain: the neurobiology of compulsion and its persistence. Nat. Rev. Neurosci. 695–703.
8. MELIS, M., S. SPIGA & M. DIANA. 2005. The dopamine hypothesis of drug addiction: hypodopaminergic state. Int. Rev. Neurobiol. **63:** 101–152.
9. DIANA, M. & J.M. TEPPER. 2002. Electrophysiological pharmacology of mesencephalic dopaminergic neurons. *In* Handbook of Experimental Pharmacology, Vol. 154, Part II. G. Di Chiara, Ed.: 1–62. Springer-Verlag. Berlin.
10. YOKEL, R.A. & R.A. WISE. 1975. Increased lever pressing for amphetamine after pimozide in rats: implications for a dopamine theory of reward. Science **187:** 547–549.
11. YOKEL, R.A. & R.A. WISE. 1976. Attenuation of intravenous amphetamine reinforcement by central dopamine blockade in rats. Psychopharmacology **48:** 311–318.
12. BOZARTH, M.A. & R.A. WISE. 1981. Intracranial self-administration of morphine into the ventral tegmental area in rats. Life Sci. **28:** 551–555.
13. DE WIT, H. & R.A. WISE. 1977. Blockade of cocaine reinforcement in rats with the dopamine receptor blocker pimozide, but not with the noradrenergic blockers phentolamine or phenoxybenzamine. Can. J. Psychol. **31:** 195–203.
14. DI CHIARA, G. & A. IMPERATO. 1988. Drugs abused by humans preferentially increase synaptic dopamine concentrations in the mesolimbic system of freely moving rats. Proc. Natl. Acad. Sci. USA **85** 5274–5278.
15. DIANA, M., M. MELIS, A.L. MUNTONI & G.L. GESSA. 1998. Mesolimbic dopaminergic decline after cannabinoid withdrawal. Proc. Natl. Acad. Sci. USA **95:** 10269–10273.
16. DIANA, M., M. PISTIS, S. CARBONI, *et al.* 1993. Profound decrement of mesolimbic dopaminergic neuronal activity during ethanol withdrawal syndrome in rats: electrophysiological and biochemical evidence. Proc. Natl. Acad. Sci. USA **90:** 7966–7969.
17. DIANA, M., M. PISTIS, A. MUNTONI & G. GESSA. 1995. Profound decrease of mesolimbic dopaminergic neuronal activity in morphine withdrawn rats. J. Pharmacol. Exp. Ther. **272:** 781–785.
18. BONCI, A. & J.T. WILLIAMS. 1997. Increased probability of GABA release during withdrawal from morphine. J. Neurosci. **17:** 796–803.
19. MANZONI, O.J. & J.T. WILLIAMS. 1999. Presynaptic regulation of glutamate release in the ventral tegmental area during morphine withdrawal. J. Neurosci. **19:** 6629–6636.
20. ACQUAS, E. & G. DI CHIARA. 1992. Depression of mesolimbic dopamine transmission and sensitization to morphine during opiate abstinence. J. Neurochem. **58:** 1620–1625.
21. POTHOS, E., P. RADA, G.P. MARK & B.G. HOEBEL. 1991. Dopamine microdialysis in the nucleus accumbens during acute and chronic morphine,

naloxone-precipitated withdrawal and clonidine treatment. Brain Res. **566:** 348–350.
22. ROSSETTI, Z.L., Y. HMAIDAN & G.L. GESSA. 1992. Marked inhibition of mesolimbic dopamine release: a common feature of ethanol, morphine, cocaine and amphetamine abstinence in rats. Eur. J. Pharmacol. **221:** 227–234.
23. SPIGA, S., G.P. SERRA, M.C. PUDDU, *et al.* 2003. Morphine withdrawal-induced abnormalities in the VTA: confocal laser scanning microscopy. Eur. J. Neurosci. **17:** 605–612.
24. SKLAIR-TAVRON, L., W.X. SHI, S.B. LANE, *et al.* 1996. Chronic morphine induces visible changes in the morphology of mesolimbic dopamine neurons. Proc. Natl. Acad. Sci. USA **93:** 11202–11207.
25. ROBINSON, T.E. & B. KOLB. 1997. Persistent structural modifications in nucleus accumbens and prefrontal cortex neurons produced by previous experience with amphetamine. J. Neurosci. **17:** 8491–8497.
26. ROBINSON, T.E. & B. KOLB. 1999. Morphine alters the structure of neurons in the nucleus accumbens and neocortex of rats. Synapse **33:** 160–162.
27. DIANA, M., A.L. MUNTONI, M. PISTIS, *et al.* 1999. Lasting reduction in mesolimbic dopamine neuronal activity after morphine withdrawal. Eur. J. Neurosci. **11:** 1037–1041.
28. DEUTCH, A.Y. & D.S. CAMERON. 1992. Pharmacological characterization of dopamine systems in the nucleus accumbens core and shell. Neuroscience **46:** 49–56.
29. MEREDITH, G.E., C.M. PENNARTZ & H.J. GROENEWAGEN. 1993. The cellular framework for chemical signalling in the nucleus accumbens. Prog. Brain Res. **99:** 3–24.
30. MEREDITH, G.E., P. YPMA & D.S. ZAHM. 1995. Effects of dopamine depletion on the morphology of medium spiny neurons in the shell and core of the rat nucleus accumbens. J. Neurosci. **15:** 3808–3820.
31. SMITH, A.D. & J.P. BOLAM. 1990. The neural network of the basal ganglia as revealed by the study of sinaptic connections of identified neurones. Trends Neurosci. **13:** 259–265.
32. WILSON, C.J. 2004. Basal ganglia. *In* The Synaptic Organization of the Brain, 5th ed. G.M. Shepherd, Ed.: 361–414. Oxford University Press. Oxford.
33. FREUND, T.F., J.F. POWELL & A.D. SMITH. 1984. Tyrosine hydroxylase-immunoreactive boutons in synaptic contact with identified striatonigral neurons, with particular reference to dendritic spines. Neuroscience **13:** 1189–1215.
34. ROBINSON, T.E., G. GORNY, V.R. SAVAGE & B. KOLB. 2002. Widespread but regionally specific effects of experimenter—versus self-administered morphine on dendritic spines in the nucleus accumbens, hippocampus, and neocortex of adult rats. Synapse **46:** 271–279.
35. SPIGA, S., M.C. PUDDU, M. PISANO, *et al.* 2005. Morphine withdrawal-induced morphological changes in the nucleus accumbens. Eur. J. Neurosci. **22(9):** 2332–2340.
36. KRUZICH, P.J., A.C. CHEN, E.M. UNTERWALD & M.J. KREEK. 2003. Subject-regulated dosing alters morphine self-administration behavior and morphine-stimulated [35S]GTPgammaS binding. Synapse **47:** 243–249.
37. FREDERICKSON, R.C. & S.E. SMITS. 1973. Time course of dependence and tolerance development in rats treated with "slow release" morphine suspensions. Res. Commun. Chem. Pathol. Pharmacol. **5:** 867–870.

38. PAXINOS, G. & C. WATSON. 1997. The Rat Brain in Stereotaxic Coordinates, 3rd ed. Academic Press. Sydney.
39. KOLB, B. & J. MCCLIMANS. 1986. Cryostat sectioning of Golgi-Cox tissue. Stain Technol. **61:** 379–380.
40. MUNTONI, A.L., M. DIANA, G.L. GESSA. 1996. Repeated naltrexone administration accelerates resolution of morphine somatic withdrawal signs in morphine-dependent rats. Eur. J. Pharmacol. **301:** R9–R10.
41. DI CHIARA, G., V. BASSAREO, S. FENU, *et al.* 2004. Dopamine and drug addiction: the nucleus accumbens shell connection. Neuropharmacology **47:** 227–241.
42. GERRITS, M.A., P. PETROMILLI, H.G. WESTENBERG, *et al.* 2002. Decrease in basal dopamine levels in the nucleus accumbens shell during daily drug-seeking behaviour in rats. Brain Res. **924:** 141–150.
43. AHMED, S.H., J.R. WALKER & G.F. KOOB. 2000. Persistent increase in the motivation to take heroin in rats with a history of drug escalation. Neuropsychopharmacology **22:** 413–421
44. SHAW-LUTCHMAN, T.Z., M. BARROT, T. WALLACE, *et al.* 2002. Regional and cellular mapping of cAMP response element-mediated transcription during naltrexone-precipitated morphine withdrawal. J. Neurosci. **22:** 3663–3672.
45. FRENOIS, F., L. STINUS, F. DI BLASI, *et al.* 2005. A specific limbic circuit underlies opiate withdrawal memories. J. Neurosci. **25:** 1366–1374.
46. CRIPPENS, D. & T.E. ROBINSON. 1994. Withdrawal from morphine or amphetamine: different effects on dopamine in the ventral-medial striatum studied with microdialysis. Brain Res. **650:** 56–62.
47. FRENOIS, F., M. CADOR, S. CAILLE, *et al.* 2002. Neural correlates of the motivational and somatic components of naloxone-precipitated morphine withdrawal. Eur J Neurosci. **16:** 1377–1389.
48. GEORGES, F., L. STINUS, B. BLOCH & C. LE MOINE. 1999. Chronic morphine exposure and spontaneous withdrawal are associated with modifications of dopamine receptor and neuropeptide gene expression in the rat striatum. Eur. J. Neurosci. **11:** 481–490.
49. MEREDITH, G.E., I.E. DE SOUZA, T.M. HYDE, *et al.* 2000. Persistent alterations in dendrites, spines, and dynorphinergic synapses in the nucleus accumbens shell of rats with neuroleptic-induced dyskinesias. J. Neurosci. **20:** 7798–7806.
50. MAGEE, J.C. 2000. Dendritic integration of excitatory synaptic input. Nat. Rev. Neurosci. **1:** 181–190.
51. WILLIAMS, S.R. & G.J. STUART. 2003. Role of dendritic synapse location in the control of action potential output. Trends Neurosci. **26:** 147–154.
52. SEGAL, M. 2001. Rapid plasticity of dendritic spine: hints to possible functions? Prog. Neurobiol. **63:** 61–70.
53. WILLIAMS, S.R. & G.J. STUART. 2002. Dependence of EPSP efficacy on synapse location in neocortical pyramidal neurons. Science **295:** 1907–1910.
54. MAGEE, J.C. & E.P. COOK. 2000. Somatic EPSP amplitude is independent of synapse location in hippocampal pyramidal neurons. Nat. Neurosci. **3:** 895–903.
55. CHRISTIE, M.J., R.J. SUMMERS, J.A. STEPHENSON, *et al.* 1987. Excitatory amino acid projections to the nucleus accumbens septi in the rat: a retrograde transport study utilizing D[3H]aspartate and [3H]GABA. Neuroscience **22:** 425–439.
56. SHEPHERD, G.M. 1996. The dendritic spine: A multifunctional integrative unit. J. Neurophysiol. **75:** 2197–2210.
57. SEPULVEDA, M.J., L. HERNANDEZ, P. RADA, *et al.* 1998. Effect of precipitated withdrawal on extracellular glutamate and aspartate in the nucleus accumbens of

chronically morphine-treated rats: an in vivo microdialysis study. Pharmacol. Biochem. Behav. **60:** 255–262.
58. Robbe, D., J. Bockaert & O.J. Manzoni. 2002. Metabotropic glutamate receptor 2/3-dependent long-term depression in the nucleus accumbens is blocked in morphine withdrawn mice. Eur. J. Neurosci. **16:** 2231–2235.
59. Ingham, C.A., S.H. Hood, P. Taggart & G.W. Arbuthnott. 1998. Plasticity of synapses in the rat neostriatum after unilateral lesion of the nigrostriatal dopaminergic pathway. J. Neurosci. **18:** 4732–4743.
60. Williams, J.T., M.J. Christie & O.J. Manzoni. 2001. Cellular and synaptic adaptations mediating opioid dependence. Physiol. Rev. **81:** 299–343.
61. Kalivas, P.W. & N.D. Volkow. 2005. The neural basis of addiction: a pathology of motivation and choice. Am. J. Psychiatry **162:** 1403–1413.
62. Volkow, N.D., J.S. Fowler, G.J. Wang & J.M. Swanson. 2004. Dopamine in drug abuse and addiction: results from imaging studies and treatment implications. Mol. Psychiatry **9:** 557–569.

Expression of NR1/NR2B *N*-Methyl-D-Aspartate Receptors Enhances Heroin Toxicity in HEK293 Cells

ANTÓNIO DOMINGUES,[a,*] TERESA CUNHA OLIVEIRA,[a,*] MÁRIO L. N. LAÇO,[a] TICE R.A. MACEDO,[b] CATARINA R. OLIVEIRA,[a] AND A. CRISTINA REGO[a]

[a]*Institute of Biochemistry, Faculty of Medicine and Center for Neuroscience and Cell Biology of Coimbra, University of Coimbra, 3004-504 Coimbra, Portugal*

[b]*Institute of Pharmacology and Experimental Therapeutics, Faculty of Medicine, University of Coimbra, 3004-504 Coimbra, Portugal*

[*]*A.D. and T.C.O. contributed equally to this work.*

ABSTRACT: Repeated use of drugs of abuse, namely opiates, has been shown to affect glutamate-releasing neurons. Moreover, blockade of *N*-methyl-D-aspartate (NMDA) receptors (NMDAR) prevents cell death by apoptosis induced by morphine, a heroin metabolite. Thus, in this article we investigated the involvement of different NMDAR subunits in heroin cytotoxicity. Human embryonic kidney (HEK293) cells, which do not express native NMDAR, were transfected with NR1/NR2A or NR1/NR2B subunits. As a control, cells were transfected with NR1 alone, which does not form functional channels. Incubation with heroin for 24 h induced a dose-dependent decrease in cell viability both in NR1-transfected and nontransfected cells. The loss of membrane integrity induced by heroin was more evident in cells transfected with NR1/NR2B than in cells transfected with NR1 alone or NR1/NR2A. This decrease in cell viability was blocked by MK-801, a selective and noncompetitive antagonist of NMDAR. Nevertheless, no significant changes in intracellular adenosine 5′-triphosphate (ATP) were observed in cells treated with heroin. These data implicate NR2B-composed NMDAR as important mediators of heroin neurotoxicity.

KEYWORDS: cytotoxicity; drugs of abuse; HEK203 cells; heroin; NMDA receptors

Address for correspondence: A. Cristina Rego, Institute of Biochemistry, Faculty of Medicine and Center for Neuroscience and Cell Biology of Coimbra, University of Coimbra, 3004-504 Coimbra, Portugal. Voice: 351-239-820190; fax: 351-239-822776.
e-mail: acrego@cnc.cj.uc.pt

Ann. N.Y. Acad. Sci. 1074: 458–465 (2006).
doi: 10.1196/annals.1369.046

INTRODUCTION

The abuse of opioids and other drugs of abuse is associated with severe physical and mental health problems. These drugs interact with the central nervous system, inducing changes in the release of neurotransmitters, namely in the dopaminergic system. Many evidences also suggest the involvement of glutamatergic neurotransmission in the mechanisms of drug dependence involving the dopaminergic reward circuit in the brain.[1] On the other hand, some drugs of abuse, such as methamphetamine, are responsible for neurodegenerative mechanisms that lead to the irreversible loss of neurons, with the involvement of dopaminergic and/or glutamatergic systems.[2] Under this perspective, heroin is able to induce cell death in PC12 cells[3,4] and morphine, a heroin metabolite, induces cell death by apoptosis in the spinal cord [5] and in human cerebrocortical neurons.[6]

Among the processes leading to cell death, the excitotoxic mechanism, which involves the hyperactivation of ionotropic glutamate receptors, has been largely studied due to its involvement in ischemia and several neurodegenerative diseases.[7] *N*-methyl-D-aspartate (NMDA) receptors (NMDAR) have an outstanding role in excitotoxic processes, due to their high permeability to calcium, which is responsible for the activation of several intracellular enzymes, leading to mitochondrial dysfunction and cell death. NMDAR are composed by NR1 subunits which can interact with NR2 (A–D) subunits, and less frequently with NR3 (A, B). NR1 subunits contain the glycine-binding site, whereas the NR2 subunits contain the glutamate-binding site, conferring heterogeneity to these receptors. Previous studies demonstrated that NR2B subunits, which are mainly localized in extrasynaptic sites, are associated to increased toxicity in comparison with NR2A synaptic subunits.[8]

It was previously suggested that glutamatergic neurotransmission involving the NMDAR contributes to opioid dependence in humans.[9] Moreover, the NMDAR antagonist MK-801 was shown to specifically block morphine tolerance and neuronal apoptosis in the spinal cord.[5] In this context, in this work we analyzed the involvement of NR1/NR2A and NR1/NR2B subunits in heroin cytotoxicity.

MATERIAL AND METHODS

Cell Culture and Transfection

Human embryonic kidney (HEK293) cells were obtained from the American Type Culture Collection (Manassas, VA) and were grown in Dulbecco's modified Eagle's medium (DMEM; Sigma Chemical Co., St. Louis, MO) supplemented with 10% fetal bovine serum (Biochrom AG, Berlin, Germany), penicillin (100 U/mL), and streptomycin (100 μg/mL). Cells were grown to

50–75% confluence in poly-L-lysine-coated multiwells and transfected using the superfect transfection reagent (Qiagen, Hilden, Germany) according to the manufacturer's instructions. In cotransfections the NR1:NR2 plasmid ratio was 1:4. Cells were transfected with the DNA-superfect mixture for 4 h and further incubated for 24 h with heroin (provided by the *Instituto da Droga e da Toxicodependência*, Lisbon, Portugal) and/or 10 μM dizocilpine maleate (MK-801), in fresh culture media. The rat NR1 (NR1a), NR2A, and NR2B cDNA clones inserted respectively in pEGFP-N3, pcDNAI, or pDP3 were a generous gift from Dr. John Woodward (Medical University of South Carolina, Charleston, SC). NR1 is expressed as a fusion protein with enhanced green fluorescent protein (EGFP), which is referred throughout the manuscript as NR1-GFP.

Cell Reducing Capacity Assay

Cell reducing capacity was assessed by the 3-(4,5-dimethylthiazol-2-yl)-2,5-diphenyltetrazolium bromide (MTT) colorimetric assay for cell survival. MTT (0.5 mg/mL) in Na^+ medium (in mM: 132 NaCl, 1.2 NaH_2PO4, 1.4 $MgCl_2$, 4 KCl, 10 HEPES, 6 glucose, and 1 $CaCl_2$, pH 7.4) was added to the cultures and incubated for 2 h at 37°C in the dark. When taken up by living cells, MTT is converted to a water-insoluble blue product (formazan). The precipitated dye was dissolved in 0.04 M HCl in isopropanol and was colorimetrically quantified at 570 nm. Data were expressed as the percentage of optical density of untransfected HEK293 cells or NR1-GFP-expressing cells, in the absence of heroin.

Lactate Dehydrogenase Leakage Assay

The integrity of the plasma membrane was determined by monitoring the activity of the cytoplasmic enzyme lactate dehydrogenase (LDH) in the extracellular incubation medium. Intracellular LDH activity was assessed after cell lysis with 10 mM HEPES (pH 7.4) supplemented with 0.01% Triton X-100 (Sigma Chemical Co.), and further freezing at −80°C. Cell debris in both aliquots (intracellular and extracellular) were removed by centrifugation at 20,800 *g*, for 10 min (0–4°C). LDH activity was determined spectrophotometrically, by following the rate of conversion of reduced nicotinamide adenine dinucleotide (NADH) to oxidized NAD^+ at 340 nm. LDH released into the extracellular medium was expressed as a percentage of total LDH activity in the cells (percentage of LDH released = extracellular LDH/[extracellular LDH + intracellular LDH]).

Determination of Adenosine Triphosphate Intracellular Levels

The intracellular content of the adenine nucleotide adenosine 5′-triphosphate (ATP) was determined after cell extraction with 0.3 M perchloric acid (0–4°C). The cells were centrifuged at 20,800 *g* for 5 min, and the pellet was solubilized with 1 M NaOH for total protein analysis using *Bio-Rad Protein Assay Dye* (Bio-Rad Laboratories, Hercules, CA). The supernatants were neutralized with 5 M KOH in 2.5 M Tris and centrifuged at 15,800 *g* for 10 min (0–4°C). The resulting supernatants, stored at −80°C, were assayed for ATP determination, by separation in a reverse phase high-performance liquid chromatography (HPLC) and absorbance was monitored at 254 nm. Peak identity was determined by the comparison with the retention time of an ATP standard.

Statistical Analysis

Data are the mean ± SEM from at least three experiments, performed in duplicate or triplicate. Statistical analysis was performed by one-way ANOVA followed by Tukey post-test (a $P < 0.05$ was considered significant).

RESULTS AND DISCUSSION

Previously, we showed that heroin induces a dose-dependent decrease in cell viability in PC12 cells[3] and in primary cortical neurons (unpublished results). In the present study we observed a dose-dependent decrease in cell reducing capacity after 24 h exposure to heroin in both untransfected and NR1-GFP-transfected HEK293 cells (FIG. 1). The decrease in cell reducing capacity was statistically significant for both populations at a high heroin concentration (1 mM). A decrease in cell viability was also observed in untransfected ($P < 0.05$) and NR1-GFP transfected (nonstatistically significant) HEK293 cells exposed to 100 μM heroin. This concentration of heroin was used in the following experiments, because a moderate decrease in cell viability was observed under these conditions. These results demonstrated that heroin is toxic to HEK293 cells. Furthermore, expression of nonfunctional NR1 did not affect heroin toxicity.

Next we evaluated the effect of functional NMDAR, composed of NR1/NR2A or NR1/NR2B, on heroin-induced toxicity. NMDAR expression in the non-neuronal cell line *per se* led to a nonstatistical increase (approximately 5–10%) in LDH release, indicative of some loss of membrane integrity (FIG. 2). Exposure to heroin (100 μM, for 24 h) did not significantly change membrane integrity of NR1-GFP- or NR1/NR2A-expressing cells (FIG. 2). However, NR1/NR2B-transfected cells showed a significant increase in membrane permeability in the presence of the drug ($P < 0.05$), and this effect was completely prevented by the NMDAR antagonist MK-801 (FIG. 2). The

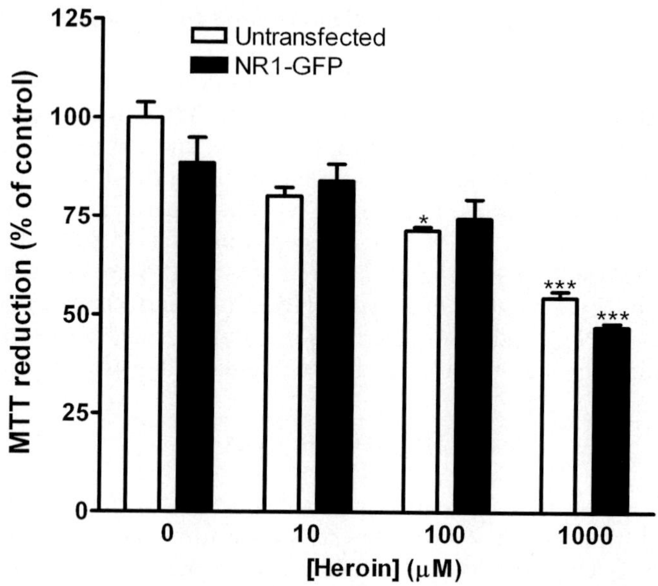

FIGURE 1. Analysis of cell viability in HEK293 cells exposed to street heroin. The viability of untransfected HEK293 cells and cells transfected with NR1-GFP was evaluated upon exposure to increasing concentrations of street heroin (10–1000 μM) for 24 h, by using the MTT reduction assay. Data were presented as mean ± SEM of at least three experiments, performed in triplicate, and were normalized in percentage of nontreated untransfected cells (control). Statistical analysis: $^{*}P < 0.05$ and $^{***}P < 0.001$ compared to the respective untreated cells.

protective effect of MK-801 suggests that activation of NR1/NR2B receptor is necessary for heroin-induced increase in membrane permeability, because MK-801 is an open-channel blocker of NMDAR. Interestingly, NR1/NR2B subtype was previously linked to cellular demise that occurs both in an excitotoxic paradigm[8] and in Huntington´s disease.[10]

Cellular energy deficits are often associated with NMDAR mediated excitotoxicity. Overactivation of NMDAR leads to an excessive increase in intracellular calcium concentration, which is exacerbated by a dysfunction of calcium extrusion mechanisms. This has been suggested to occur as a consequence of mitochondrial dysfunction and resulting decrement in ATP production.[7] Nevertheless, neither the presence of heroin nor the expression of functional NMDAR subtypes, NR1/NR2A or NR1/NR2B, affected ATP intracellular levels significantly (FIG. 3). Because intact cellular energy levels are needed for the prosecution of apoptotic cell death,[11] we hypothesize that NR1/NR2B-mediated increase in heroin cytotoxicity is initially mediated through apoptosis, rather than necrosis. Later stages of apoptosis also involve increase of membrane permeability,[12] explaining the loss of membrane integrity observed in FIGURE 2.

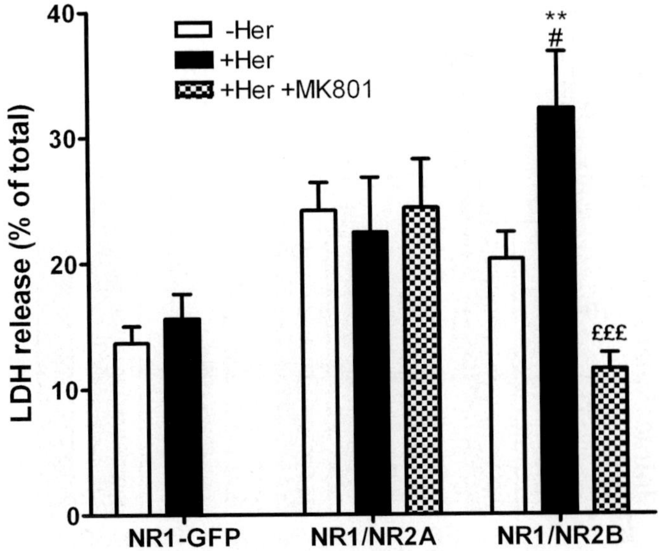

FIGURE 2. Analysis of plasma membrane integrity in HEK293 cells transfected with different subunits of the NMDAR upon acute exposure to street heroin. The cells were transfected with NR1/NR2A or NR1/NR2B subunits of the NMDAR or with NR1-GFP (transfection control) and exposed to 100 μM street heroin and/or 10 μM MK-801 for 24 h. The integrity of the plasma membrane was evaluated by the LDH leakage assay. Data were expressed as a percentage of total LDH and presented as mean ± SEM of at least three experiments, performed in triplicate. Statistical significance: $^{**}P < 0.01$ as compared to NR1-GFP, $\#P < 0.05$ compared to the respective untreated cells, and £££$P < 0.001$ compared to heroin-treated cells expressing NR1/NR2B.

Taken together our results indicate that the NR1/NR2B subtype of NMDAR is a mediator of heroin-induced cytotoxicity. Previously, chronic exposure to morphine, a heroin metabolite that can co-exist in heroin solutions,[13] was reported to alter NMDAR subunit composition in rat nucleus accumbens neurons. Neuroadaptation to chronic morphine exposure was shown to increase NR2A activity and decrease NR2B activity.[14] In the present work we hypothesize that overactivation of NR2B-composed receptors is responsible for the deleterious cellular effects induced by heroin. It is possible that the decrease in the activity of NR2B-composed NMDAR observed by Martin *et al.*[14] is due to selective cell death of neurons exhibiting higher expression levels of this NMDAR subunit. In this case, these neurons may be more susceptible to toxic insults, similarly to what was reported in Huntington´s disease.[10]

ACKNOWLEDGMENTS

The authors would like to thank Dr. Sancha Santos (Center for Neuroscience and Cell Biology, University of Coimbra) for helping with the analysis of

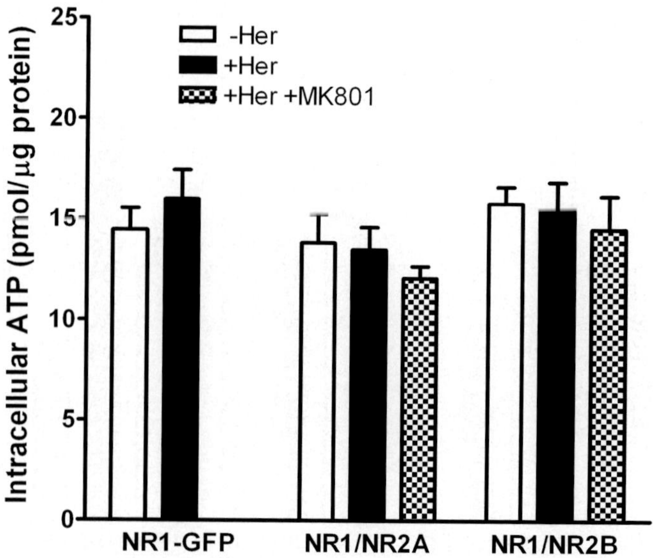

FIGURE 3. Measurement of intracellular ATP levels in HEK293 cells transfected with different subunits of the NMDAR upon acute exposure to street heroin. Cells transfected with NR1-GFP (transfection control) or with the different subunits of the NMDAR (NR1/NR2A or NR1/NR2B) were treated as described in FIGURE 2. Intracellular ATP levels were analyzed by HPLC with UV detection. Data were expressed as pmol/μg protein and presented as mean ± SEM of at least three experiments, performed in triplicate.

ATP by HPLC. This work was supported by Project GAI 09/04, Faculty of Medicine, University of Coimbra, Portugal; and by *Fundação para a Ciência e a Tecnologia* (FCT), Portugal (PhD fellowships SFRH/BD/10910/2002 and SFRH/BD/17275/2004 and project POCTI/SAU-FCF/58330/2004).

REFERENCES

1. TZSCHENTKE, T.M. & W.J. SCHMIDT. 2003. Glutamatergic mechanisms in addiction. Mol. Psychiatry **8**: 373–382.
2. OHMORI, T., T. ABEKAWA & T. KOYAMA. 1996. The role of glutamate in behavioral and neurotoxic effects of methamphetamine. Neurochem. Int. **29**: 301–307.
3. OLIVEIRA, M.T., A.C. REGO, M.T. MORGADINHO, *et al.* 2002. Toxic effects of opioid and stimulant drugs on undifferentiated PC12 cells. Ann. N. Y. Acad. Sci. **965**: 487–496.
4. OLIVEIRA, M.T., A.C. REGO, T.R. MACEDO & C.R. OLIVEIRA. 2003. Drugs of abuse induce apoptotic features in PC12 cells. Ann. N. Y. Acad. Sci. **1010**: 667–670.
5. MAO, J., B. SUNG, R.R. JI & G. LIM. 2002. Neuronal apoptosis associated with morphine tolerance: evidence for an opioid-induced neurotoxic mechanism. J. Neurosci. **22**: 7650–7661.

6. Hu, S., W.S. Sheng, J.R. Lokensgard & P.K. Peterson. 2002. Morphine induces apoptosis of human microglia and neurons. Neuropharmacology **42**: 829–836.
7. Rego, A.C. & C.R. Oliveira. 2003. Mitochondrial dysfunction and reactive oxygen species in excitotoxicity and apoptosis: implications for the pathogenesis of neurodegenerative diseases. Neurochem. Res. **28**: 1563–1574.
8. Hardingham, G.E., Y. Fukunaga & H. Bading. 2002. Extrasynaptic NMDARs oppose synaptic NMDARs by triggering CREB shut-off and cell death pathways. Nat. Neurosci. **5**: 405–414.
9. Bisaga, A., S.D. Comer, A.S. Ward, *et al.* 2001. The NMDA antagonist memantine attenuates the expression of opioid physical dependence in humans. Psychopharmacology (Berl.) **157**: 1–10.
10. Zeron, M.M., O. Hansson, N. Chen, *et al.* 2002. Increased sensitivity to N-methyl-D-aspartate receptor-mediated excitotoxicity in a mouse model of Huntington's disease. Neuron **33**: 849–860.
11. Nicotera, P. & G. Melino. 2004. Regulation of the apoptosis-necrosis switch. Oncogene **23**: 2757–2765.
12. Schwab, B.L., D. Guerini, C. Didszun, et al. 2002. Cleavage of plasma membrane calcium pumps by caspases: a link between apoptosis and necrosis. Cell Death Differ. **9**: 818–831.
13. Hutchinson, M.R. & A.A. Somogyi. 2002. Diacetylmorphine degradation to 6-monoacetylmorphine and morphine in cell culture: implications for in vitro studies Eur. J. Pharmacol. **453**: 27–32.
14. Martin, G., A. Guadano-Ferraz, B. Morte, *et al.* 2004. Chronic morphine treatment alters N-methyl-D-aspartate receptors in freshly isolated neurons from nucleus accumbens. J Pharmacol. Exp. Ther. **311**: 265–273.

Brain Blood Flow SPET Imaging in Heroin Abusers

MARIA FILOMENA BOTELHO,[a] JOÃO S. RELVAS,[b]
MARGARIDA ABRANTES,[a] MARIA JOÃO CUNHA,[c]
TIAGO R. MARQUES,[b] EUGÉNIA ROVIRA,[c]
CARLOS A. FONTES RIBEIRO,[d] AND TICE MACEDO[d]

[a]*Department of Biophysics and Biomathematics, IBILI, Faculty of Medicine, University of Coimbra, Coimbra, 3000-548 Coimbra, Portugal*

[b]*Psychiatry Department, HUC/Faculty of Medicine, University of Coimbra*

[c]*Nuclear Medicine, HUC, Coimbra, 3000-548 Coimbra, Portugal*

[d]*Pharmacology Institute, IBILI, Faculty of Medicine, University of Coimbra, Azinhaga de Santa Comba, Celas, 3000-548, Coimbra, Portugal*

ABSTRACT: To assess whether chronic heroin abuse may generate vascular central nervous deficits, we studied the profile of vascular alterations in 17 heroin addicts (14 males mean age 31 years, range 23–39 years and 3 females mean age 33 years, range 30–35 years) before and, in one of them, 10 weeks after an ultra-rapid heroin detoxification. Using the functional technique of single-photon emission tomography (SPET) with 740 MBq of ^{99m}Tc-hexametazine (HMPAO) and computational brain-mapping techniques by means of a Talairach analysis, we determined the pattern of vascular brain alterations associated with chronic heroin abuse. Compared with controls, subjects who had used heroin chronically showed a decrease of global brain perfusion that was more significant in the frontal cortex—mainly in orbito-frontal regions, as well as in the occipital and temporal lobes. All patients showed marked asymmetric perfusion of the basal ganglia and the majority of them showed also an asymmetric perfusion of cerebellum. In addition, there were small activated areas dispersed in the occipital lobe (3 of 17) and apex region (4 of 17). In conclusion, decreased perfusion in heroin addicts was found in regions involved in the control of attention, motor speed, memory and visual–spatial processing. The prefrontal cortex is involved in decision making and inhibitory control, processes disturbed in heroin addicts who have stopped heroin consumption. A reduction in regional perfusion may reflect ongoing subtle neurocognitive deficits, which are consistent with the maintenance of asymmetry of the basal nuclei.

KEYWORDS: heroin abuse; cerebral blood flow; SPET

Address for correspondence: Tice Macedo, Pharmacology Institute, IBILI, Faculty of Medicine of Coimbra, Azinhaga de Santa Comba, Celas, 3000–548 Coimbra, Portugal. Voice: +351-239-480207; fax: +351-239-480258.
e-mail: tice@ci.uc.pt

**Ann. N.Y. Acad. Sci. 1074: 466–477 (2006). © 2006 New York Academy of Sciences.
doi: 10.1196/annals.1369.047**

INTRODUCTION

Heroin abuse is epidemic in Portugal as in many other countries and the use of the intranasal route of administration is growing in popularity among heroin abusers. Just as the pharmacokinetic profile of intranasal-administered heroin mimics that of injected heroin, the adverse neurological and systemic effects may be very similar and as potentially dangerous. Vascular cerebral complications are not usually thought to be associated with heroin abuse. However, toxic disorders related to heroin may cause neuropathological changes including hypoxic and ischemic changes with cerebral edema, ischemic neuronal damage, and neuronal loss which are assumed to occur under conditions of prolonged heroin respiratory depression, stroke due to, for example, thromboembolism, vasculitis, septic emboli, hypotension, and positional vascular compression.[1–5]

The exact etiology of different neuropathological alterations associated with heroin abuse is still unclear, but may also be related to additional substances used as adulterants as well as with the occasional consumption of others drugs. All these neuropathological entities could have consequent brain vascular lesions.

This article aims to characterize possible persistent abnormalities in 17 heroin addicts, immunodeficiency virus negative, with a history of episodic use of cocaine and cannabis and regular use of tobacco and alcohol.

METHODS

A total of 17 subjects participated in this study, which was approved by the Institutional Ethics Committee of Coimbra University Hospital (Coimbra, Portugal). Informed consent was obtained.

The heroin-dependent subjects (14 males and 3 females; mean; age 31.11 years) were recruited from a program of ultra-rapid heroin detoxification from the Psychiatric Department of Coimbra University Hospital. All the subjects underwent an extensive medical and neurological examination, a routine blood work-up, and HIV antibody testing to rule out existing medical or neurological illness. All the patients were free of psychotropic medication, except three who were receiving buprenorphine (mean dosage of 7.4 mg/day) for several weeks. Exclusion criteria consisted of any significant past or current medical or neurological condition including epilepsy, migraine, unexplained loss of consciousness, or severe head trauma. All results of medical, psychiatric, and clinical laboratory evaluations were unremarkable.

Detailed clinical histories of drug and alcohol consumption were obtained for each patient. Diagnosis of opioid dependence was performed in all cases according to the criteria of the Diagnostic and Statistical Manual, Version 4 (DSM-IV) (304.00). None met DSM-IV criteria for any other Axis I diagnosis, with the exception of nicotine dependence (305.10).

TABLE 1. Clinical and demographic characteristics of the group of subjects

Patients studied	17 patients (14 males; 3 females)
Mean age	31.11 years; range (22–39 years)
Mean age of initiation	21.18 years; range (16–31 years)
Mean years of consumption	9.81 years; range (3–18 years)
Mean daily heroin	0.66 g; (smoked: 9 patients; i.v.: 5 patients)
Mean daily buprenorphine (3 patients)	7.4 mg
Sporadic use	Cocaine 7 patients; cannabis 4 patients
Mean period of time between last consumption of substances with opioid action and performance of SPET	11.93 h

All patients reported sporadic use of other illicit drugs (mainly cocaine and cannabis) but none met the criteria for abuse or dependence.

TABLE 1 summarizes the clinical and demographic characteristics of the group of subjects.

Imaging Protocol

Patients were studied using the functional technique of single-photon emission tomography (SPET) and computational brain-mapping techniques through a Talairach analysis to determine the patterns of vascular brain alterations associated with chronic heroin abuse.

In a quiet, dark room, each patient received 740 MBq of ^{99m}Tc-hexametazine (HMPAO) (Ceretec®, Amersham, United Kingdom) via an intravenous line, to avoid noxious stimuli and cerebral activation. To prevent frontal lobe activation as a result of total sensory deprivation, the patients were allowed to leave the ears unplugged. Oppositely, the patients close their eyes to avoid the activation of visual areas.

These environmental conditions were maintained during the ^{99m}Tc-HMPAO uptake period (~30 min). After the uptake period, patients were transported in bed to the gantry room to reduce voluntary movements. One of the male patients repeated the protocol 10 weeks after suppression due to an ultra-rapid heroin detoxification with naloxone.

Imaging of the brain, via a gamma camera with three detectors (Neurocam, GE, Milwaukee, WI) connected to a computer, began 30 min after tracer injection in all 17 patients.

Tomography was performed in a 128 $\times$ 128 matrix using 128 stops at 30 s per view in a 360° circular rotation. The energy setting was 140 keV with a 20% window. The time required for SPET data acquisition was 25 min. Images were reconstructed by filtered back-projection with a Butherworths filter of 0.5 Nyquist cutoff frequency associated with a ramp filter without attenuation correction. Image pixel size was 4 mm in a 128 $\times$ 128 array.

Neurogam software was used to evaluate the cerebral blood flow (CBF) using statistical parametric mapping. This program contains a database of CBF normal results with which we can compare our findings.

RESULTS

In general terms, the most evident change was a marked decrease of perfusion in some preferential lobes, with minus 3 or 4 standard deviation when compared with the normal controls included in the software database. Compared with those controls, subjects who had used heroin chronically showed a decrease of global brain perfusion that was more significant in the frontal cortex (12 of 17), mainly in orbito-frontal (FIG. 1) and temporal regions (12 of 17). The occipital (7 of 17) and parietal lobes (5 of 17) have also hypoperfused areas (FIG. 2). All the studied patients showed marked asymmetric perfusion of the basal ganglia (FIG. 3). Cerebellum showed also decreased perfusion in 16 patients, 7 with symmetric (FIG. 4) and 9 with asymmetric (FIG. 1) alterations. Simultaneously, there were small activated areas dispersed in the frontal lobes (10 of 17), temporal lobes (4 of 17), occipital lobes (3 of 17), and apex region (4 of 17) (FIG. 4). The patient who had repeated brain perfusion study 10 weeks later did not show any improvement on the second scan.

DISCUSSION AND CONCLUSIONS

Functional neuroimaging techniques, such as positron emission tomography (PET), single photon emission computerized tomography (SPECT), and magnetic resonance imaging (MRI) have revealed altered regional cerebral activity by all drugs of abuse.[6]

Several groups have found that opioids, such as morphine or heroin, decrease global or regional CBF after acute administration in normal laboratory animals.[1,7–13]

The effect of chronic administration of heroin in animals and in patients is less clear. Morphine has usually a vasodilator effect on cerebral arterial circulation but this effect could be related with hypercapnia as a consequence of alveolar hypoventilation induced by the drug.[14–16] The cerebral circulation is not modified by therapeutic doses of morphine. However, the respiratory depression and CO_2 retention induced by opioids could originate cerebral vasodilation and rise LCR pression.[17]

The symmetrical involvement of functional brain systems strongly indicates a toxic or metabolic etiology.[18,19] Chemical agents may damage functional brain systems selectively. Certain brain regions and systems have a greater sensitivity to specific types of toxins. These regions of identical vulnerability frequently involve a whole functional chain of neurons and tracks and

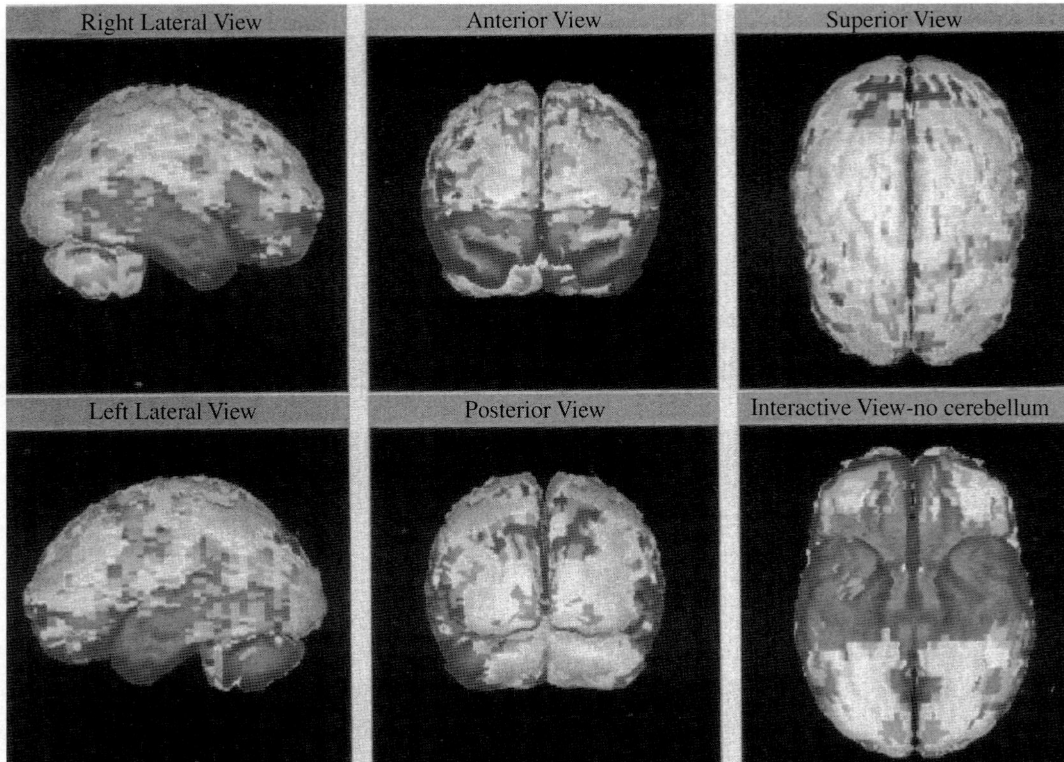

FIGURE 1. Example of a patient studied before ultra-rapid heroin detoxification with naloxone. The images show decreased brain perfusion in the frontal cortex mainly in orbito-frontal regions and temporal lobes. Notice that the cerebellum also shows decreased perfusion in an asymmetric way.

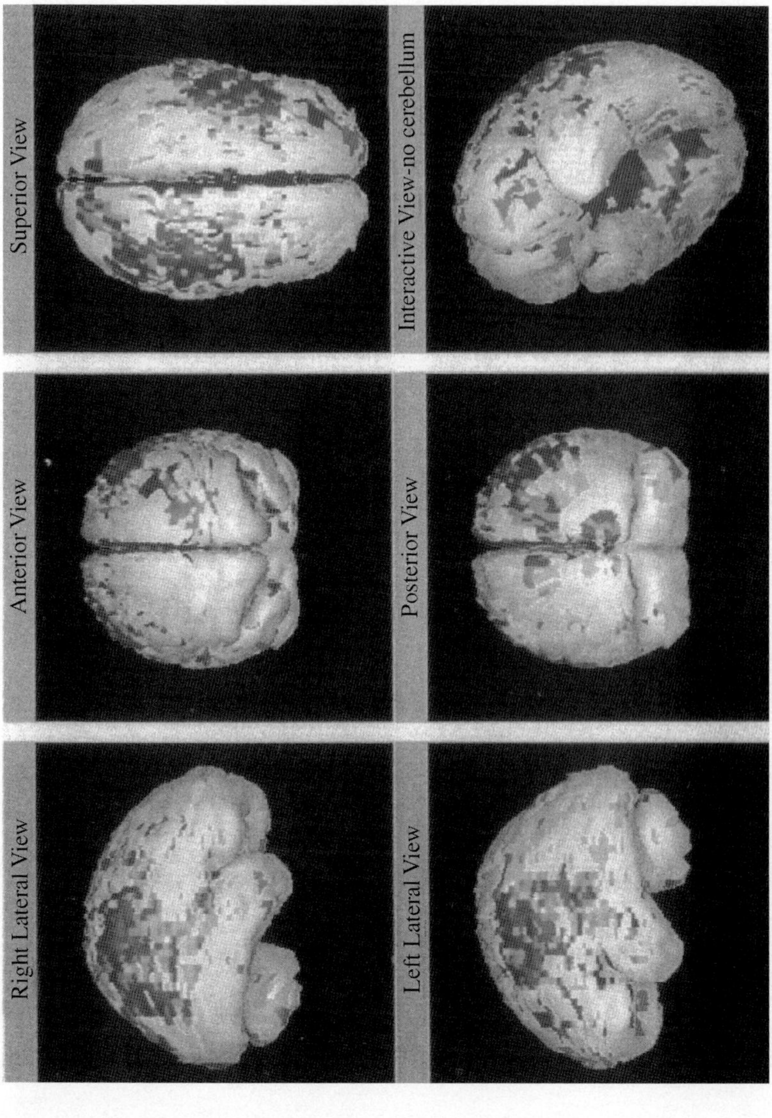

FIGURE 2. Example of a patient studied before ultra-rapid heroin detoxification with naloxone. The images show decreased brain perfusion in the parietal and occipital lobes.

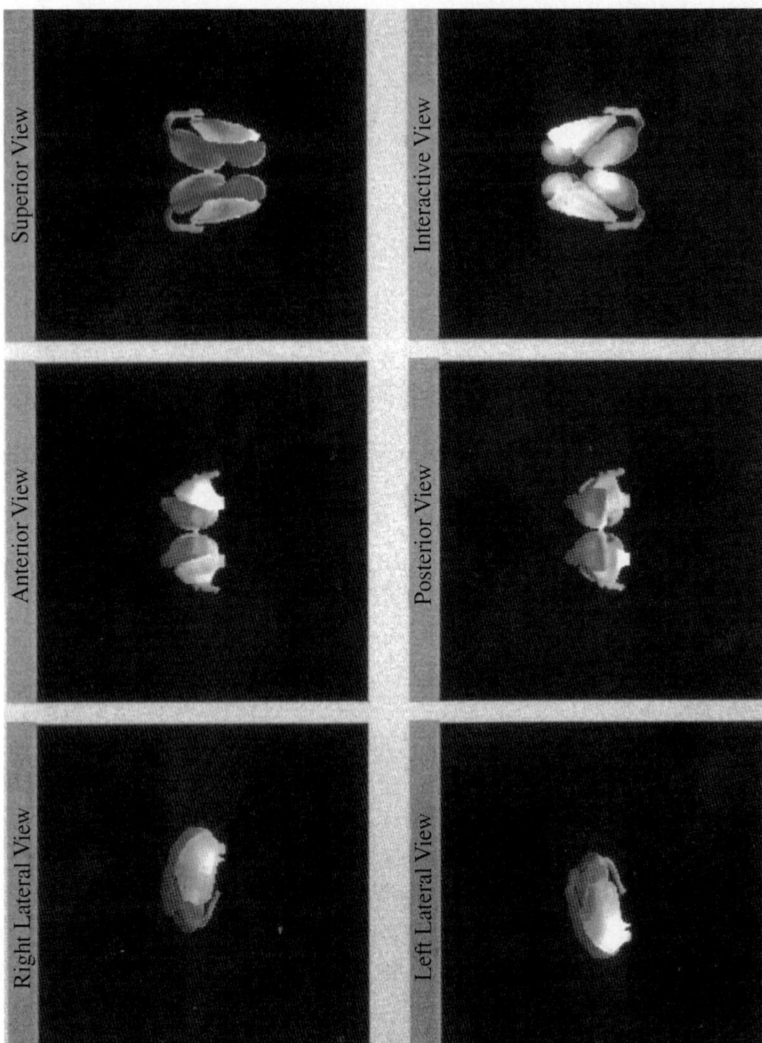

FIGURE 3. In this patient, a marked asymmetric perfusion of the basal ganglia is apparent. This event was seen in all the studied patients.

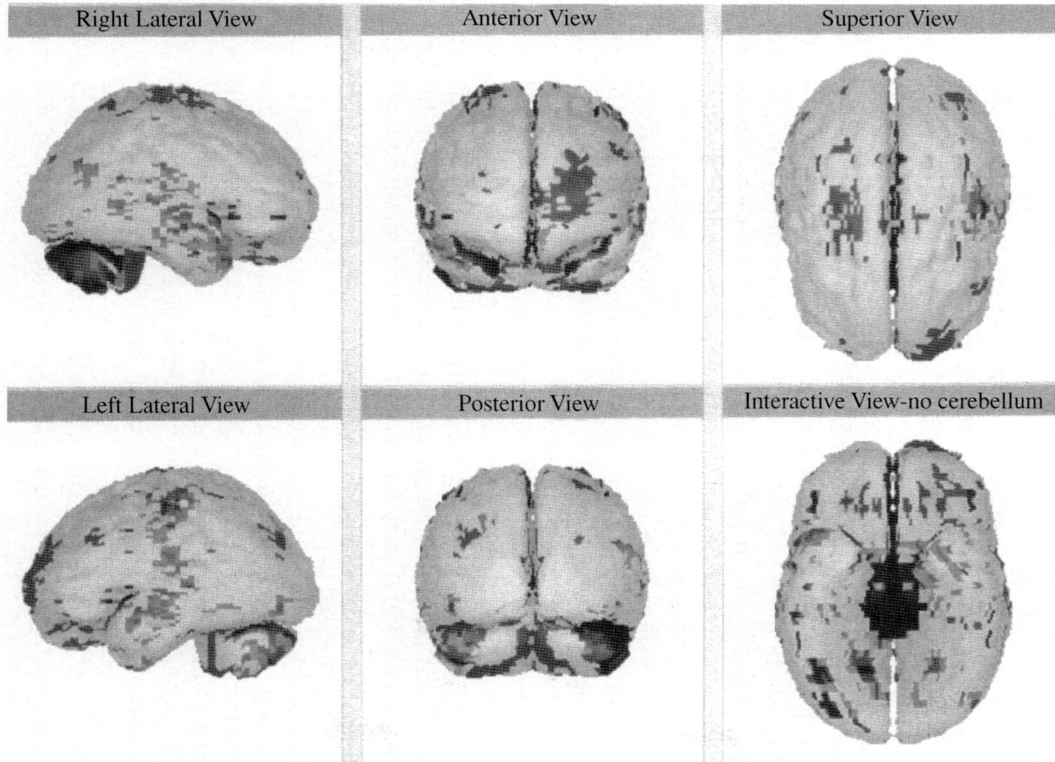

FIGURE 4. Images obtained in a male patient studied before ultra-rapid heroin detoxification with naloxone, showing dispersed small activated areas in frontal and occipital cortex and apex region. In this example, we can appreciate a symmetric cerebellar decreased perfusion.

not a single structure. Brain areas that form functional systems show a synchronous development, including myelination, during phylo- and ontogenesis. Demyelination due to degeneration or toxic damage may also be synchronous. Selective vulnerability may also be related to similarity and particular characteristics (e.g., oxygen requirements, chemical composition, and neurotransmitters). The selective vulnerability of myelin to lipophilic agents results from a specific chemical composition. Myelin[20] is characterized by a higher specific lipid content and a slow turnover.[20] Once in the blood, heroin is rapidly hydrolyzed to monoacetylmorphine (MAM) which is then hydrolyzed to morphine. Heroin and MAM are more lipid soluble than morphine and enter the brain more readily. Morphine and MAM are believed to be responsible for the pharmacologic action of heroin. Cone *et al.*[21] found that the intranasal administration of heroin resulted in a rapid appearance of heroin, MAM, and morphine in blood. Morphine was present for a longer time (2–4 h) than heroin or MAM because of its lower clearance rate. Morphine time course coincided with the observed–induced effects of intranasal heroin.

The imaging findings after heroin consumption are highly specific. The neurological deficit is, as a rule, irreversible. There is no effective therapy. The image findings are almost always unchangeable at follow-up examinations.

Our results differ, however, from those obtained in a group on 16 heroin-dependent patients where the CBF was measured using SPET with ^{99m}Tc-HMPAO showing that the temporal lobes were the most affected area; hypoperfusions of the right and left temporal lobe were observed in five and five patients, respectively. Three of the patients had a hypoperfusion of the right frontal lobe, two patients showed perfusion defects in the left frontal lobe, right parietal lobe, and left parietal lobe.[22] In another study, the heroin addicts showed a nonsignificant reduction of whole brain perfusion values. Significant hypoperfusion in the right frontal and left temporal lobes was found in addicts with comorbid depression, and a significant decrease in CBF in the right frontal lobe was observed in those with antisocial tendencies.[23]

In our group, the symmetrical findings in cortical CBF may mainly be attributed to substance abuse per se than to mood and behavioral traits, where the asymmetrical findings are more common.[23]

The patients in this study were nicotine dependent, many for several years, and it was uncertain how cerebral perfusion would be affected by heroin plus nicotine.

Using ^{99m}Tc-HMPAO and Talairach analysis, heroin abuse associated with cigarette smoke was found to have an effect on CBF, similar to that obtained by cigarette smoke alone.[24] The results indicate that heroin and smoking induce a significant reduction in CBF related to normals of the same gender and age, included in the database.

In fact, a chronic smoking habit is known to be significantly associated with a reduction in CBF, and smoking is known to accelerate cerebral arteriosclerosis.[5] The influence of cigarette smoking on CBF seems likely to be a net effect of not only nicotine but also the other constituents of main stream cigarette smoke (e.g., tar, phenol, acetic acid, CO, CO_2, NO, and NO_2) and some vasoconstrictors—thromboxane A2, plasma endothelin, and cerebral cortex serotonin, that have been found to be elevated after smoking.[25] So, smoking in heroin users also reduced central blood flow as assessed by SPET. Since cerebral perfusion decreased, will ultimately result in a high incidence of cerebral vascular disease in smokers, our study seems to appoint to a sum effect of the two drugs.

Young drug abusers also have very high alcohol consumption parallel to narcotic drug abuse.[26] A magnetic resonance study[27] in 23 drug abusers always combined with heavy alcohol consumption demonstrated that chronic drug abusers may develop structural brain changes early in life consisting of cerebral atrophy, both manifesting itself as cortical atrophy, a mild enlargement of the lateral ventricles, and atrophy of the cerebellum. In our group of patients, the decrease of cerebellar perfusion could be consistent with the changes referred above.

Cerebral perfusion, studied with ^{99m}Tc-HMPAO SPET, in cocaine dependent-women, 40 of whom were also heroin dependent, was abnormal. The concurrent abuse of heroin and cocaine was associated with more perfusion abnormalities in both sexes, located in anterior brain structures, such as the frontal and temporal cortex and the basal ganglia.[28–30]

Basal ganglia dysfunction has been associated with disturbances of movement and in addition to motor dysfunction cognitive abnormalities were described.[31] In our study, decrease perfusion in the occipital cortex was not associated with a strong cognitive decline and we were unable to find consistent relationships between motor scores and topographic network in the brain for heroin abuse, suggesting that various levels of regional activity may exist and pointing to the complexity of studying the underlying pathophysiology with a direct topographic analytic approach directed at functional localization.[31]

In this study, only relative CBF values were used, which are susceptible to general arousal, years of consumption of heroin, and other drug effects; in view of the differences found, this still indicates that additional differential diagnostic information can be obtained using clinically available relative perfusion measurements.

Our images show some regions of hyperperfusion in another wise normal cortex and this increase did not vary significantly by location; it is likely that these changes could reflect the different emotional status of opioid-dependent patients.[32]

In conclusion, this ^{99m}Tc-HMPAO SPET and Talairach analysis suggest that the chronic use of opiates results in a decrease of global brain perfusion abnormalities more significant in frontal cortex, mainly in orbito-frontal regions, as well as in temporal and occipital lobes. All the studied patients showed marked asymmetric perfusion of basal ganglia. Simultaneously dispersed small activated areas in the occipital lobes and apex region were observed. The decreased perfusion is found in regions mediating attention, motor speed, memory, and visual and spatial processing. The prefrontal cortex is involved in decision making and inhibitory control, processes that are disturbed in heroin addicts. The decrease of regional perfusion may reflect continuing subtitle neurocognitive deficits that are sustained with the maintenance of basal nuclei asymmetry.

REFERENCES

1. Büttner, A., G. Mall, R. Penning & S. Weiss 2000. The neuropathology of heroin abuse. Foresinc Sci. Int. **113**: 435–422.
2. Kaye, B. & M. Fainstat. 1987. Cerebral vasculitis associated with cocaine abuse. JAMA **258**: 2104–2106.
3. Niehaus, L. & B.U. Meyer 1998. Bilateral borderzone brain infarctions in association with heroin abuse. J. Neurol. Sci. **160**: 180–182.
4. Wang, Q. & B.X. Lu. 2002. Single photon emission computerized tomography of spongiform leukoencephalopathy heroin addicts: analysis of 10 cases. Di Y Jun Yi Da Xue Bao **22**: 659–660.
5. Yamashita, K., S. Kobayashi, S. Yamaguchi, *et al.* 1988. Effect of smoking on regional blood flow in the normal aged volunteers. Gerontology **34**: 1999–2004.
6. Volkow, N.D., J.S. Fowler & G.J. Wang. 2003. The addicted human brain: insights from imaging studies. J. Clin. Invest. **111**: 1444–1451.
7. Anderson, S.N. & K. Skullerud. 1999. Hypoxic/ischemic brain damage, especially pallidal lesions, in heroin addicts. Forensic Sci. Int. **102**: 51–59.
8. Buchweitz, E., L. Grandison & H.R. Weiss. 1984. Effect of morphine on regional cerebral oxygen consumption and supply. Brain Res. **291**: 301–308.
9. Dohi, S., N. Matsumiya & T. Abe. 1983. Mechanism of morphine-induced suppression of central nervous system blood flow. No to Shinkei **35**: 1083–1088.
10. Hœhner, P.J., J.T. Whitson, J.R. Kirsch & R.J. Traystman. 1993. Effect of intracarotid and intraventricular morphine on regional cerebral blood flow and metabolism in pentobarbital-anesthetized dogs. Anesth. Analg. **76**: 266–273.
11. Matsumiya, N. & S. Dohi 1983. Effects of intravenous subarachnoid morphine on cerebral and spinal cord hemodynamics and antagonism with naloxone in dogs. Anesthesiology **59**: 175–181.
12. Rose, J.S., M. Branchey, L. Buydens-Branchey, *et al.* 1996. Cerebral perfusion in early and late opiate withdrawal: a technetium-99m-HMPAO SPECT study. Psychiatry Res. **67**: 39–47.
13. Sandor, P., J. Cox-van Put, W. de Jong & D. de Wied 1986. Continuous measurement of cerebral blood volume in rats with the photoelectric technique: effect of morphine and naloxone. Life Sci. **39**: 1657–1665.
14. Daglish, M.R., A. Weinstein, A.L. Malizia, *et al.* 2001. Changes in regional cerebral blood flow elicited by craving memories in abstinent opiate-dependent subjects. Am. J. Psychiatry **158**: 1680–1686.
15. Eckenhoff, J.E. & R. Deh. 1960. The effects of narcotics and antagonists upon respiration and circulation in man. Clin. Pharmacol. Ther. **1**: 483–494.
16. Hattori, N., Y. Yonekure, F. Tanaka, *et al.* 1996. One day protocol for cerebral perfusion reserve with acetazolamide. J. Nucl. Med. **37**: 2057–2061.
17. Goldstein, R.Z. & N.D. Volkow. 2002. Drug addiction and its underlying neurobiological basis: neuroimaging evidence for the involvement of the frontal cortex. Am. J. Psychiatry **159**: 1642–1652.

18. VALK, J. & M.S. VAN DER KNAAP. 1989. Magnetic Resonance of Myelin, Myelination and Disorders, p. 268–272, Springer. Berlin, Heidelberg, New York.
19. VALK, J. & M.S. VAN DER KNAAP. 1992. Toxic encephalopathy. AJNR **13**: 747–760.
20. WEBER, W., H. HENKES, P. MÖLLER, *et al.* 1998. Toxic spongiform leucoencephalopathy after inhaling heroin vapor. Eur. Radiol. 8: 749–755.
21. CONE, E., B. HOLICKY, T. GRANT, *et al.* 1993. Pharmacokinetics and pharmacodynamics of intranasal "snorted" heroin. J. Anal. Toxicol. **17**: 327–337.
22. DANOS, P., S. KASPER, F. GRUNWALD, *et al.* 1998. Pathological regional cerebral blood flow in opiate-dependent patients during withdrawal: a HMPAO-SPECT study. Neuropsychobiology **37**: 194–199.
23. GERRA, G., B. CALBIANI, A. ZAIMOVIC, *et al.* 1998. Regional cerebral blood flow and comorbid diagnosis in abstinent opioid addicts. Psychiatry Res. **83**: 117–126.
24. YAMAMOTO, Y., Y. NISHIYANA, T. MONDEN, *et al.* 2003. A study of the acute effect of smoking on cerebral blood flow using ^{99m}Tc-ECD SPET. Eur. J. Nucl. Med. Mol. Imaging **30**: 612–614.
25. IIDA, M., H. IIDA, S. DOHI, M. TAKENAKA & H. FUJIWARA. 1998. Mechanisms underlying cerebrovascular effects of cigarette smoking in rats *in vivo*. Stroke **29**: 1656–1665.
26. SELL, L.A., J.S. MORRIS, L. BEARN, *et al.* 2000. Neural responses associated with cue evoked emotional states and heroin in opiate addicts. Drug. Alcohol Depend. **60**: 207–216.
27. AASLY, J., O. STORSAETER, G. NIELSEN, *et al.* 1993. Minor structural brain changes in young drug abusers. Acta Neurol. Scand. **87**: 210–214.
28. LEVIN, J.M., B.L. HOLMAN, J.H. MENDELSON, *et al.* 1994. Gender differences in cerebral perfusion in cocaine abuse: technetium-99m-HMPAO SPECT study of drug-abusing women. J. Nucl. Med. **35**: 1902–1909.
29. LEVIN, J.M., J.H. MENDELSON, B.L. HOLMAN, *et al.* 1995. Improved regional cerebral blood flow in chronic cocaine polydrug users treated with buprenorphine. J. Nucl. Med. **36**: 1211–1215.
30. VOLKOW, N.D., J.S. FOWLER & G.J. WANG. 2003. Positron emission tomography and single-photon emission computed tomography in substance abuse research. Semin Nucl. Med. **33**: 114–128.
31. VAN LAERE, K., P. SANTENS, T. BOSMAN, *et al.* 2004. Statistical parametric mapping of ^{99mTc}-ECD SPECT in idiopatic Parkinson's disease and multiple system atrophy with predominant parkinsonian features: correlation with clinical parameters. J. Nucl. Med. **45**: 933–944.
32. PEZAWAS, L., G. FISCHER, J. PODREKA, *et al.* 2002. Opioid addiction changes cerebral blood flow symmetry. Neuropsychibiology **45**: 67–73.

The Comet Assay as a Method of Assessment of Neurotoxicity

Usefulness for Drugs of Abuse

GIADA FRENZILLI,[a] VITTORIA SCARCELLI,[a] FRANCESCO FORNAI,[a,b] ANTONIO PAPARELLI,[a] AND MARCO NIGRO[a]

[a]*Department of Human Morphology and Applied Biology, University of Pisa, I-56126 Pisa, Italy*

[b]*Laboratory of Neurobiology of Movement Disorders I.R.C.C.S. I.N.M. Neuromed, 86077 Pozzilli, Isernia, Italy*

ABSTRACT: Comet assay is a quick and versatile method for assessing DNA damage in individual cells. It allows the detection of single and double DNA strand breaks, as well as the presence of alkali labile sites. DNA breaks may represent the direct effect of some damaging agent, or they may be intermediates in cellular repair. DNA strand breaks may also come from the action of free radicals generated by oxidative stress processes. The present article summarizes some data from our and other groups underlining the suitability of the Comet assay in assessing neurotoxicity and its potential in evaluating drugs of abuse-related genotoxicity.

KEYWORDS: DNA damage; neurotoxicity; Comet assay; drugs of abuse; brain cells

INTRODUCTION

Preservation of genomic stability is an essential biological function. Cells recruit very efficiently mechanisms involving DNA surveillance/repair proteins that work to maintain the inherited nucleotide sequence of genomic DNA over time. It is well known that the mutation of genes related to DNA damage repair is associated with specific cancer-prone syndromes. Interestingly, as recently pointed out by Rolig and McKinnon,[1] many human pathological conditions with genetic defects in DNA damage responses are also characterized by neurological deficits.

Over the past decade the Comet assay has become one of the standard methods for assessing DNA damage with applications spreading in different

Address for correspondence: Giada Frenzilli, Ph.D., Dipartimento di Morfologia Umana, E Biologia Applicata, Università di Pisa, Via Volta, 4, I-56126 Pisa, Italy. Voice: +39-050-2219111; fax: +39-050-2219101.
e-mail: giada@biomed.unipi.it

**Ann. N.Y. Acad. Sci. 1074: 478–481 (2006). © 2006 New York Academy of Sciences.
doi: 10.1196/annals.1369.048**

fields of research. This electrophoretic technique allows the detection of single and double DNA strand breaks, as well as the presence of alkali labile sites in individual cells, carrying out the assay at pH12.1, pH8, and pH $>$ 13, respectively, and potentially any kind of cell can be used.

COMET ASSAY: PRINCIPLES AND APPLICATIONS

Cells embedded in agarose on a microscope slide are lysed with detergent and high salt to form nucleoids containing supercoiled loops of DNA linked to the nuclear matrix. Electrophoresis at high pH results in structures resembling comets, observed by fluorescence microscopy; the intensity of the comet tail relative to the head reflects the number of DNA breaks. The rationale for this is that the loops containing in a break lose their supercoil and become free to extend toward the anode. DNA breaks may represent the direct effect of some damaging agent, or they may be intermediates in cellular repair. DNA strand breaks may also come from the action of free radicals indirectly generated by oxidative stress processes.[2] A modified version of the technique includes the use of enzymes that are able to cut oxidized bases in order to detect the loss of DNA integrity, specifically due to oxidative stress.[3]

The Comet assay has applications in testing novel chemicals for genotoxicity, monitoring environmental contamination with genotoxins, human biomonitoring, molecular epidemiology, and fundamental research in DNA damage and repair.

When the amount of DNA damage overwhelms DNA repair capabilities, the process of programmed cell death or apoptosis can occur. It is characterized by fragmentation of DNA to the size of nucleosome oligomers and such small pieces of DNA would disappear during lysis or electrophoresis. A modified version of Comet assay, described by Singh,[4] named Diffusion assay, is a visualization method for apoptotic cells in which cells are embedded in agarose, lysed, and then the DNA is precipitated with ethanol, instead of undergoing electrophoresis. Cells treated with an agent known to induce apoptosis appeared with a halo of granular DNA and a hazy outer boundary, related to the presence of diffusing small fragments.

Due to the versatility of the technique, the Comet assay has been successfully applied to the study of neurotoxicity during the last years. A group of studies evaluated the *in vitro* effects induced by chemical compounds like ethanol, acethaldeide, cycloheximide[5–7] or physical compounds like gamma rays or magnetic radiation[8,9] in cell cultures, neurons, and blood leukocytes. Cardile *et al.*[10] focused their attention on the possible genotoxicity of the antiepileptic drug, tiagabine, in cultured rat astrocytes, looking for the proper range of doses useful for the treatment but unable to induce DNA fragmentation. Another group of studies showed data obtained after *in vivo* treatments of rats or mice with chemicals like acrilamide, apomorphine, food color additives, aromatic amines, carcinogens and physical agents,[11–16] looking at the possible effects on several organs, including brain. As oxidative stress is known to play a key role in a number of neurodegenerative disorders like Alzheimer's disease (AD), Parkinson's disease (PD), and amyotrophic lateral sclerosis (ALS), recent studies applied Comet assay to evaluate the possible loss of DNA integrity in such patients.

The presence of spontaneous chromosome and oxidative DNA damage was found by Migliore *et al.*[17] in peripheral blood leukocytes of patients with untreated PD. Moreover, higher levels of primary DNA damage in leukocytes of AD and also of mild cognitive impairment patients compared to control individuals were detected by the same group, indicating that oxidative stress, at least at the DNA level, is an earlier event in the pathogenesis of AD.[18]

Increasing attention has been paid to the genotoxic potential of the drugs of abuse in target areas. Significant increases in single strand breaks in rat brain cells were found after ethanol administration.[19] Also, Shafer *et al.*[20] demonstrated by Comet assay that while brief ethyl methansulphonate exposure can be repaired by human cell cultures, if morphine exposures persists through one or more cell cycles, direct or indirect mutagenesis is initiated. Indeed, they had previously showed chromosomal aberrations in heroin addicts.[21]

The alkaline version of the Comet assay has been used to evaluate the possible genotoxicity of 3,4-methylenedioxymethamphetamine (MDMA) in mouse brain cells.[22] Data obtained in our lab indicated that MDMA was able to induce DNA fragmentation and oxidized bases to monoaminergic as well as non-monoaminergic neurons in the nigrostriatal pathway, indicating a final common pathway involving the generation of free radicals and oxidative stress.

Such findings lead to the underlying neurotoxic consequence of MDMA intake and might help to explain the occurrence of movement disorders in chronic MDMA abusers. Overall, this report confirms the suitability of the Comet assay in assessing neurotoxicity and its potential in evaluating drugs of abuse-related genotoxicity.

REFERENCES

1. ROLIG, R.L. & P.J. MCKINNON. 2000. Linking DNA damage and neurodegeneration. Trends Neurosci. **23:** 417–424.
2. TICE, R.R. *et al.* 2000. Single cell gel/Comet Assay: guidelines for in vitro and in vivo genetic toxicology testing. Environ. Mol. Mutagen. **31:** 113–124.
3. COLLINS, A.R. 2004. The Comet Assay for DNA damage and repair. Principles, applications, and limitations. Molec. Biotechnol. **26:** 249–261.
4. SINGH, N.P. 2000. A simple method for accurate estimation of apoptotic cells. Exp. Cell. Res. **256:** 328–337.
5. SIGNORINI-ALLIBE, N. *et al.* 2005. Chronic consumption of ethanol leads to substantial cell damage in cultured rat astrocytes in conditions promoting acetaldehyde accumulation. Alcohol Alcohol. **40:** 163–171.

6. LAMARCHE, F. *et al.* 2003. Acute exposure of cultured neurones to ethanol results in reversible DNA single-strand breaks; whereas chronic exposure causes loss of cell viability. Alcohol Alcohol. **38:** 550–558.
7. CHAO, K.S. *et al.* 1999. Differential effect of cycloheximide on neuronal and glioma cells treated with chemotherapy and radiation. J. Neurooncol. **45:** 19–26.
8. MORRIS, E.J. *et al.* 1999. Optimization of single-cell gel electrophoresis (SCGE) for quantitative analysis of neuronal DNA damage. Biotechniques **26:** 282–283, 286-289.
9. MALYAPA, R.S. *et al.* 1997. Measurement of DNA damage after exposure to 2450 MHz electromagnetic radiation. Radiat. Res. **148:** 608–617.
10. CARDILE, V. *et al.* 2001. Tiagabine treatment and DNA damage in rat astrocytes: an *in vitro* study by comet assay. Neurosci. Lett. **306:** 17–20.
11. MANIERE, I. *et al.* 2005. DNA damage and DNA adduct formation in rat tissues following oral administration of acrylamide. Mutat. Res. **580:** 119–129.
12. PICADA, J.N. *et al.* 2003. DNA damage in brain cells of mice treated with an oxidized form of apomorphine. Brain Res. Mol. Brain Res. **114:** 80–85.
13. MUT, M. *et al.* 2004. Effects of ionizing radiation on brain tissue surrounding arteriovenous malformations: an experimental study in a rat caroticojugular fistula model. Neurosurg. Rev. **27:** 121–127.
14. SASAKI, Y.F. *et al.* 2002. The comet assay with 8 mouse organs: results with 39 currently used food additives. Mutat. Res. **519:** 103–119.
15. MCNAMEE, J.P. *et al.* 2002. DNA damage and apoptosis in the immature mouse cerebellum after acute exposure to a 1 mT, 60 Hz magnetic field. Mutat. Res. **513:** 121–133.
16. SASAKI, Y.F. *et al.* 1998. Detection of *in vivo* genotoxicity of haloalkanes and haloalkenes carcinogenic to rodents by the alkaline single cell gel electrophoresis (comet) assay in multiple mouse organs. Mutat. Res. **419:** 13–20.
17. MIGLIORE, L. *et al.* 2002. Oxidative damage and cytogenetic analysis in leukocytes of Parkinson's disease patients. Neurology **58:** 1809–1815.
18. MIGLIORE, L. *et al.* 2005. Oxidative DNA damage in peripheral leukocytes of mild cognitive impairment and AD patients. Neurobiol. Aging **26:** 567–573.
19. SINGH, N.P. *et al.* 1995. Ethanol-induced single-strand DNA breaks in rat brain cells. Mutat. Res. **345:** 191–196.
20. SHAFER, D.A. *et al.* 1994. Detection of opiate-enhanced increases in DNA damage, HPRT mutants, and the mutation frequency in human HUT-78 cells. Environ. Mol. Mutagen. **23:** 37–44.
21. SHAFER, D.A. *et al.* 1990. Enhanced assays detect increased chromosome damage and sister-chromatid exchanges in heroin addicts. Mutat. Res. **234:** 327–336.
22. FORNAI, F. *et al.* 2004. DNA damage and neuronal inclusions in the substantia nigra and striatum associated with nigrostriatal dopamine denervation following MDMA (ecstasy). Psychopharmacology **173:** 353–363.

A Potent Serotonin-Modulating Compound AP-267 Attenuates Morphine Withdrawal-Induced Blood–Brain Barrier Dysfunction in Rats

HARI S. SHARMA,[a,b] TORBJÖRN LUNDSTEDT,[c,d] ARNE BOMAN,[c] PER LEK,[c] ELISABETH SEIFERT,[c] LARS WIKLUND,[b] AND SYED F. ALI[a]

[a]*Laboratory of Neurochemistry, Division of Neurotoxicology, National Center for Toxicology Research, Food and Drug Administration Laboratories, Jefferson 72079, Arkansas*

[b]*Laboratory of Cerebrovascular Research, Department of Surgical Sciences, Anaesthesiology and Intensive Care Medicine, University Hospital, Uppsala University, SE-75185 Uppsala, Sweden*

[c]*Acure Pharma AB, Ulleråkersv. 38, SE-756 43 Uppsala, Sweden*

[d]*Department of Organic and Pharmaceutical Chemistry, Uppsala University, SE-741 23 Uppsala, Sweden*

ABSTRACT: The possibility that a serotonin 5-HT2c receptor-modulating compound, AP-267, will influence spontaneous morphine withdrawal symptoms and the alterations in the brain fluid microenvironment was examined in a rat model. Daily administration of morphine (10 mg/kg, i.p.) for 10 days resulted in dependence of rats as seen by loss of analgesic response. On the 11th day, no morphine administration was given. This resulted in profound withdrawal symptoms 24 h after morphine withdrawal. The magnitude and severity of these symptoms were increased further 48 h after withdrawal. Measurement of the blood-brain barrier (BBB) permeability, a measure of perturbed brain fluid microenvironment showed leakage of Evans blue and radioiodine tracers in several parts of the brain in rats showing withdrawal symptoms. Whereas, rats treated with AP-267 either on the 1st day or 2nd day morphine withdrawal showed much less symptoms and leakage of the BBB. Taken together, these observations suggest that (*a*) stress associated with the withdrawal symptoms are sufficient enough to induce breakdown of the BBB function, and (*b*) modulation of serotonin 5-HT2c receptors may have some protective influence on the stress symptoms and the BBB disruption.

Address for correspondence: Hari Shanker Sharma, Dr Med Sci, Laboratory of Cerebrovascular Research, Department of Surgical Sciences, Anaesthesiology and Intensive Care Medicine, University Hospital, Uppsala University, SE-75185 Uppsala, Sweden. Voice and fax: +46-18-243899.
e-mail: Sharma@surgsci.uu.se

Ann. N.Y. Acad. Sci. 1074: 482–496 (2006).
doi: 10.1196/annals.1369.049

KEYWORDS: morphine; withdrawal symptoms; dependence; spontaneous withdrawal; AP-267; serotonin; 5-HT2c receptor; blood-brain barrier; Evans blue; radioiodine

INTRODUCTION

Blood-brain barrier (BBB) maintains the fluid microenvironment of the brain and spinal cord strictly within a narrow limit.[1] Thus, breakdown of the BBB permeability alters the brain fluid microenvironment resulting in abnormal brain function.[2] Abnormal cell and tissue reaction occurs following BBB disruption leading to long-term consequences and brain damage depending on the magnitude, severity, and duration of the barrier breakdown. Studies carried out in our laboratory show that morphine dependence and withdrawal is a severe stressful situation in which breakdown of the BBB to large molecules, such as proteins occur (see Refs. 3 and 4 in this volume). Morphological examinations suggest abnormal nerve cell and glial cell reaction in specific parts of the brain involving amygdala, cerebellum, hippocampus, thalamus, brain stem, and the cerebral cortex.[3] Since 5-HT2c receptors are known to influence BBB function[5] and are localized in high concentration in most of the above brain regions (see Ref. 5), it appears that compounds having modulating effects on this receptor may have some influence on morphine dependence and withdrawal responses.

Interaction of serotonergic and opioid mechanisms play important roles in morphine-induced tolerance and dependence (see TABLE 1). One possibility is that serotonin containing neurons and nerve terminals can modify the mesolimbic dopamine pathways[6] via 5-HT3 receptors.[7–9] Furthermore, the areas involved in morphine analgesia and dependence, e.g., the basal ganglia, particularly globus pallidus and substantia nigra in the rat, and olfactory nucleus, cingulate cortex, hippocampus, lateral habenula, and subthalamic nucleus in humans are very rich in 5-HT2c receptors.[10] Activation of 5-HT2c receptors induces hypolocomotion and hypophagia.[11] In addition, the serotonergic nerve terminals are also present on the walls of the cerebral ventricles (see TABLE 1). The epithelial cells of the choroid plexus contain 5-HT2c receptors in abundance[12] and may be involved in the regulation of the cerebrospinal fluid (CSF) volume and its composition.[13] Taken together, it appears that serotonin through specific 5-HT receptors could play important roles in drugs of abuse induced alteration in brain fluid microenvironment. However, the role of serotonin and its receptors on brain function in morphine-induced dependence and withdrawal is still not known in all details.

It is interesting to note that although, large numbers of investigations were done on drugs of abuse induced alterations in physiological function, the changes in brain microfluid environment during morphine dependence or withdrawal are still not examined in details (see Ref. 4 in this volume). Thus, our

TABLE 1. Distribution of 5-HT2 receptors in brain areas sensitive to morphine due to presence of multiple opioid receptors

5-HT2 receptor type	Regions of the brain	Density of 5-HT receptors	Probable function	Opioid receptors density
5-HT2a	Vascular smooth muscles	++	↑Head-twitch, wet-dog shake, neuronal depolarization	±?
	Peripheral tissues	++	Depolarization	+
	Neocortex (layer I and IV, rat)	+++	Release of glutamate, β-endorphin,	+++
	Neocortex (layer III and V, human)	++++	corticosterone, leutinizing hormone, prolactin	+++
	Claustrum, parts of limbic	+++	↑Phosphatidylinositol turnover, phospholipase C,	++
	system and basal ganglia	++	inositol phospholipid hydrolysis, Ca^{2+} mobilization	+++
5-HT2c	basal ganglia, globus pallidus,	+++	Emotion, stress, behavior	++++
	substantia nigra,	+++	↑Inositol phosphatase,	++++
	olfactory nucleus,	++	phospholipase C, chloride channels	
	cingulate cortex,	++++		++
	hippocampus, lateral habenula,	+++		++++
	subthalamic nucleus	+++		+++
	Epithelial cells of choroid plexus	++	CSF production?	±?

Low (+) to high (++++) intensity; ±? = presence not confirmed yet; ↑ = stimulation induced effects; CSF = cerebrospinal fluid; # = largely rich in μ− and δ− receptors, some regions also contain κ− receptors. Compiled from various sources, see Sharma (Refs. 3 and 5).

knowledge regarding brain-barrier system in such an important psychosocial problem in our society is largely unexplored.[4] It is quite likely that investigations in this novel area will certainly help to explore therapeutic strategies to treat this menace of our society.

Keeping these views in consideration, we have initiated a series of experiments in our laboratory to find out whether the brain-barrier system is compromised following morphine dependence or withdrawal. Secondly, whether this alteration in the brain-barrier system is mediated via neurochemicals and the second messenger systems. Finally, whether morphine dependence or withdrawal is associated with structural changes in the brain. This investigation was undertaken to find out whether a potent serotonin receptor-modulating compound, AP-267, may have some influence on morphine-induced spontaneous withdrawal symptoms and the BBB function in our rat model.

MATERIALS AND METHODS

Animals

Experiments were carried out on male Sprague Dawley rats (220–250 g) housed at controlled room temperature (21 ± 1°C) with 12 h light and 12 h dark schedule. Food and tap water were supplied *ad libitum*.

The Model

We used rat model[14] to study changes in the microvascular permeability disturbances in the CNS following morphine tolerance and dependence. The morphine abstinence was used to develop spontaneous withdrawal symptoms. All experiments were carried out according to the NIH Guidelines for Care and Maintenance of Laboratory Animals.

Development of Morphine Tolerance

Morphine tolerance was developed in rats by injecting morphine hydrochloride (10 mg/kg, i.p., calculated as free base) dissolved in sterilized water under aseptic conditions once at 8:00 AM daily for 12 days. On each day, the tail flick latency to thermal stimulus was examined 30 min after the administration of morphine.[4,14] Rats were made morphine dependent by administration of morphine (10 mg/kg, i.p.) daily for 12 days.[3,14]

Morphine Withdrawal Symptoms

To induce spontaneous morphine withdrawal symptoms, the morphine administration was withdrawn on the day 12 and the symptoms were noted daily for 72 h. Each rat was observed for 30 min and the gross abnormal behavior, e.g., wet-shakes, piloerection, writhing, teeth chattering, diarrhea, aggressive behavior, and loss of body weight as described earlier.[3,4,15,16]

Measurement of BBB Permeability

The BBB permeability was measured using Evans blue and $^{[131]}$Iodine as described earlier.[17] In brief, the tracers were administered into the right femoral vein at the end of experiments under anesthesia as described earlier and allowed to circulate for 10 min. The intravascular tracer was washed out with sterile 0.9% saline perfused through heart (at 90 torr). After perfusion, the brains were removed, examined for Evans blue leakage and the radioactivity determined in selected brain regions.[18] The dye entered into the brain was also measured colorometrically.[19]

Treatment with AP-267

The compound AP-267 (Acure Pharma, Sweden) was dissolved in sterile saline and administered (1 mg/kg, s.c.) in the morning hours (8:00 to 8:30 AM) beginning on the 1st day (0 h), after morphine withdrawal. A repeat administration was done 24 h after the morphine withdrawal. In another group, AP-267 was administered on the 2nd day (24 h after morphine withdrawal). The same dose was repeated on the 3rd day (48 h after withdrawal). The animals were treated with AP-267 compound (1 mg/kg, s.c.) on the 1st and the 2nd day of morphine withdrawal. The BBB permeability was examined on the 2nd and 3rd day of morphine withdrawal using Evans blue albumin and radioactive iodine (see Ref. 4). The withdrawal symptoms were observed every day and the BBB function was determined 24 and 48 h after morphine withdrawal (see TABLE 2).

Statistical Evaluation of the Data

The semiquantitative data were evaluated using nonparametric χ^2 test. The quantitative data obtained were analyzed for statistical significance using analysis of variance (ANOVA) followed by Dunnet test for multiple group comparison from one control group.

RESULTS

Morphine Dependence and Withdrawal Symptoms

The animals developed tolerance and dependence when one daily dose of morphine (10 mg/kg, i.p.) was used.[4] The onset of development of tolerance was found on the 4th day onwards and the full tolerance was developed on the day 12th day.[3] Thus, these animals did not exhibit any morphine analgesia tested using thermal pain stimulus according to standard protocol.[14]

When the morphine administration was stopped in these rats on the 13th day, appearance of spontaneous withdrawal symptoms were seen within 12 h (TABLE 2). The withdrawal symptoms include loss of body weight, "wet-shake" phenomena, piloerection, writhing, teeth chattering, diarrhea, aggressive behavior, and jumping (TABLE 2) that were progressive in nature. Thus, the symptoms were aggravated at 24 and 48 h after the discontinuation of morphine administration that was continued with more or less similar intensity until 72 h after the cessation of morphine injection (TABLE 1).

Stress Symptoms

The stress symptoms, e.g., hyperactivity and hyperlocomotion, were most severe following 24 and 48 h after the cessation of morphine administration.

TABLE 2. Effect of AP-267 on morphine dependence and withdrawal on stress symptoms and physiological variables

Parameters Stress symptoms	Control $n = 6$	MD12 $n = 6$	MWD1 $n = 8$	MWD2 $n = 8$	AP-267 +MWD1 $n = 6$	AP-267 +MWD2 $n = 6$
Wet-shakes	Nil	Nil	4 ± 2	8 ± 3a	2 ± 2	2 ± 3
Piloerection	Nil	Nil	+++	+++++	++	++
Writhing	Nil	Nil	+++	+++++	++	++
Teeth chattering	Nil	Nil	+++	+++++	++	++
Diarrhea	Nil	Nil	+++	+++++	+	Nil
Aggressive behavior	Nil	?	+++	+++++	±?	±?
Microhemorrhages in stomach	Nil	$48 \pm 12^{**}$	$68 \pm 18^{a**\#}$	$85 \pm 14^{a**\#}$	$23 \pm 8^{a,b**\#}$	$28 \pm 6^{a,b**\#}$

Values are mean ± SD.

$^{\#}$Many microhemorrhages; ^{a}Significantly different ($P < 0.05$) from morphine withdrawal 12 h; (+ to +++++) + = mild; ++ = moderate; +++ = high; +++++ = severe; ? = unclear; Nil = absent; MD12=morphine dependent day 12; MWD1=morphine withdrawal day 1; MWD2=morphine withdrawal day 2.

$^{**}P < 0.01$, chi-square test from control; ^{a}Significantly different from MD12; ^{b}Significantly different from MWD1.

The occurrence of diarrhea was most prominent on the 2nd day of morphine withdrawal. At postmortem, many microhemorrhages were noted in the mucosal wall of the stomach indicating formation of stress ulcers (TABLE 2).

BBB Permeability

Animals subjected to morphine withdrawal showed profound extravasation of Evans blue albumin and radioiodine tracers in several parts of the brain 24 h after morphine withdrawal. At this time, the spontaneous withdrawal symptoms are much more prominent (see TABLE 3). The magnitude and intensity of the BBB leakage further increased during 48 h and 72 h withdrawal in a progressive manner. Although, no significant differences in the BBB permeability to these tracers can be seen between 48 and 72 h after withdrawal (results not shown). A close parallelism was observed between the magnitude of withdrawal symptoms with the intensity of BBB leakage in various brain regions (see Ref. 4 in this volume).

Effect of AP-267 Treatment

Withdrawal Symptoms

Pretreatment with AP-267 administered on the 1st day (0 h) of cessation of morphine administration slightly attenuated the spontaneous withdrawal symptoms, e.g., jumping and circular motion (see TABLE 1). Whereas, rats that received 2 consecutive days of AP-267 treatment (first; and second day after morphine 1 mg/kg, s.c.), the withdrawal symptoms were significantly reduced 48 h after discontinuation of morphine administration.

Stress Symptoms

The animals that received AP-267 treatment significantly attenuated hyperthermia following morphine withdrawal (TABLE 2) that was most pronounced in animals that received the compound for 2 consecutive days following cessation of morphine administration. At postmortem, the number of gastric ulceration seen on the mucosal lining of the stomach in rats subjected to morphine withdrawal was also markedly reduced by AP-267 (see TABLE 2).

BBB Permeability

Pretreatment with AP-267 significantly attenuated the leakage of Evans blue albumin and radioiodine tracers into the brain of rats subjected to spontaneous

TABLE 3. Effect of AP-267 on morphine withdrawal-induced changes in the BBB permeability

	Control $n = 6$		MWD1 $n = 8$		MWD2 $n = 8$		AP-267+MWD1 $n = 6$		AP-267+MWD2 $n = 6$	
CNS regions	EBA mg%	$^{[131]}$I%	EBA mg%	$^{[131]}$I%	EBA mg%	$^{[131]}$I%	EBA mg%	$^{[131]}$I%	EBA mg%	$^{[131]}$I%
Cingulate cortex	0.24 ± 0.06	0.38 ± 0.04	0.54 ± 0.04**	0.68 ± 0.08**	0.89 ± 0.10**	0.98 ± 0.13**	0.44 ± 0.08*b	0.52 ± 0.08**b	0.62 ± 0.10**c	0.72 ± 0.06**c
Cerebellum	0.08 ± 0.02a	0.09 ± 0.04a	0.34 ± 0.12*	0.44 ± 0.12**	0.54 ± 0.18**	0.62 ± 0.16**	0.22 ± 0.10**b	0.26 ± 0.12**b	0.34 ± 0.12**c	0.46 ± 0.13**
Hippocampus	0.26 ± 0.06	0.36 ± 0.04	0.58 ± 0.11*	0.67 ± 0.14*	0.87 ± 0.12**	0.94 ± 0.08**	0.46 ± 0.12*	0.54 ± 0.08**b	0.65 ± 0.11*c	0.71 ± 0.14**c
Thalamus	0.45 ± 0.08a	0.56 ± 0.06a	0.48 ± 0.08	0.64 ± 0.06	0.78 ± 0.10*	0.89 ± 0.12*	0.48 ± 0.09	0.53 ± 0.08b	0.62 ± 0.08*c	0.68 ± 0.06**c
Hypothalamus	0.52 ± 0.08a	0.67 ± 0.05a	0.76 ± 0.11*	0.87 ± 0.15*	0.89 ± 0.21*	0.96 ± 0.19*	0.63 ± 0.07*b	0.73 ± 0.06**b	0.78 ± 0.10*c	0.82 ± 0.10**c
Brain stem	0.23 ± 0.06	0.28 ± 0.05	0.34 ± 0.05*	0.42 ± 0.06*	0.44 ± 0.08**	0.56 ± 0.06**	0.32 ± 0.10	0.35 ± 0.14	0.40 ± 0.12	0.48 ± 0.16
Spinal cord C-5	0.20 ± 0.04	0.28 ± 0.06	0.48 ± 0.08*	0.59 ± 0.08*	0.76 ± 0.10**	0.88 ± 0.09**	0.36 ± 0.08*b	0.44 ± 0.12*b	0.56 ± 0.14*c	0.64 ± 0.12*c

Data from 6–8 animals in each group; values are mean ± SD; EBA=Evans blue albumin; MWD1 = morphine withdrawal day 1; MWD2 = morphine withdrawal day 2, for details see text.
a = significantly different ($P < 0.05$) from cingulate cortex; $^*P < 0.05$, $^{**}P < 0.01$ significantly different from control group; b = significantly different from MWD1; c = significantly different from MWD2; ANOVA followed by Dunnet test from multiple group comparison.

withdrawal of morphine. This effect was most pronounced in rats that received 2 consecutive days of AP-267 treatment (TABLE 3). The compound itself did not influence BBB function to Evans blue or radioiodine when administered in normal rats (results not shown).

DISCUSSION

Our results are the first to show that pretreatment with a potent serotonin 5-HT2c receptor-modulating compound AP-267 significantly thwarted the morphine withdrawal symptoms and the BBB breakdown. This effect was most pronounced when the compound was administered for 2 consecutive days indicating that repeated administration of the compound is necessary to attenuate morphine withdrawal symptoms and its consequences on the brain dysfunction. These observations suggest that the new serotonin 5-HT2c receptor-modulating compound AP-267 has some therapeutic value in drugs of abuse that require additional investigations.

This investigation further confirms our finding that the magnitude of withdrawal symptoms is closely associated with the intensity of the BBB disruption.[3,4] This indicates that stress associated with withdrawal symptoms play important roles in the breakdown of the BBB permeability.

Previous observations from our laboratory suggest that stress associated with immobilization, forced swimming, or hyperthermia is associated with specific and selective breakdown of the BBB to Evans blue and radioiodine in the rat brain.[17–23] Interestingly, this increase in the BBB permeability closely corresponds to the increased plasma and brain's serotonin levels following stress (see Refs.18–22). Elevation of circulating serotonin in doses comparable to that seen during the stress situation in the anesthetized rats resulted in breakdown of the BBB function[23–26] is in line with this hypothesis. Although, morphine dependence and withdrawal is known to influence serotonergic mechanisms in the brain, to our knowledge, measurement of plasma and brain serotonin in morphine dependence and/or withdrawal has not been reported so far. Thus, it would be interesting to see whether increased circulating serotonin or its release in brain is somehow contributing to the BBB disruption during morphine withdrawal, a feature currently being examined in our laboratory.

Increased permeability of the BBB in stress, trauma or ischemia is known to be mediated through serotonin 5-HT2 receptors.[27–32] Thus, blockade of 5-HT2 receptors with classical compounds, such as ketanserin, ritanserin, cyproheptadine, methysergide, and mianserin are known to attenuate BBB dysfunction and brain edema formation in CNS injuries (for review see Ref. 5). Our present results further suggest that the compound AP-267 is also able to attenuate BBB dysfunction in morphine withdrawal indicating an important role of 5-HT2c receptors in BBB dysfunction in drugs of abuse, not reported earlier.

Previously, the potent 5-HT2 receptor antagonist, ketanserin, attenuated 3,4-methylenedioxy-methamphetamine (MDMA, ecstasy) induced neurotoxicity.[33] The MDMA is well known to release serotonin and has the affinity for 5-HT2 receptors.[34,35] Thus, coadministration of another 5-HT2 receptor antagonist, ritanserin, was able to reduce the MDMA-induced serotonergic deficits in the cortex, striatum, and hippocampus (see Ref. 36). The action of 5-HT2 receptor is linked to increased intracellular Ca^{2+} through a second messenger phosphatidylinositol (PI) hydrolyses[35] that induce apoptosis.[37] Since, serotonin is a well-known stimulator of PI-hydrolysis through 5-HT2 receptors, modulation of 5-HT2 receptors appears to be neuroprotective in several animal models as well as in cell culture studies.[33–36] It would be interesting to see whether AP-267 is also able to attenuate nerve cell, glial cell, or myelin dysfunction seen during morphine withdrawal in this model (see Ref. 4 in this volume).

Serotonin is involved in behavioral functions in drugs of abuse, e.g., morphine through specific receptors. Activation of 5-HT3 receptors leads to psychosis, anxiety, reward, and withdrawal effect from drugs of abuse.[37] Stimulation of 5-HT3 receptors causes vasodilatation and respiratory disturbances.[3,4,38,39] The 5-HT3 receptor antagonists attenuate place-preference due to effects of morphine.[40,41] Few reports in the past used 5-HT3 receptor antagonists, ondansetron, to influence morphine-induced withdrawal symptoms in rodents.[42,43] Chronic treatment with ondansetron (0.1 mg/kg, i.p.) suppressed the development of naloxone-precipitated withdrawal symptoms in mice.[42,43] The 5-HT3 receptor antagonist also attenuated the development of tolerance to the analgesic effects of morphine. It would be interesting to examine whether 5-HT3 receptors have any role in spontaneous morphine withdrawal-induced BBB dysfunction.

The probable mechanisms underlying morphine withdrawal-induced BBB disruption is not clear from this study. However, our results with AP-267 suggest that serotonin is somehow involved in the BBB disruption during morphine withdrawal. Serotonin is a known mediator of the BBB permeability and brain edema formation (see Ref. 44). It appears that serotonin either directly or indirectly stimulates of cyclic adenosine monophosphate (cAMP) synthesis resulting in BBB disruption.[24,25,45–48] The amine, after binding to its receptors on the cerebral microvessels, will induce signal transduction mechanisms either directly or through other neurotransmitters, e.g., prostaglandins (PG) or nitric oxide (NO) to induce microvascular leakage.[49–51] Stimulation of PG and NO in cerebral vessels increases the synthesis of cAMP or cyclic guanosine monophosphate (cGMP).[52–54] An increased level of cAMP or cGMP is associated with breakdown of the BBB probably by enhancing the cell membrane permeability and/or vesicular transport within the cerebral capillaries.[55–61] Alternatively, PGs can influence NO production that can induce BBB disruption via cGMP production (for details see Refs. 4, 62, 63). To further confirm this hypothesis, expression of enzymes responsible for NO and PG synthesis (nNOS or COX-2) in AP-267 treated animals are needed that require additional investigation.

CONCLUSION

In summary, our observations suggest that the compound AP-267, a potent 5-HT2c receptor-modulating agent, is able to thwart morphine withdrawal-induced symptoms and the BBB dysfunction. This indicates that serotonin 5-HT2c receptors are involved in physiological mechanisms of morphine withdrawal symptoms and consequently the BBB disruption, not reported earlier. However, further studies are needed to understand the molecular mechanisms of AP-267-induced beneficial effects on morphine withdrawal to explore the potential therapeutic value of the compound in drugs of abuse, a feature currently being investigated in our laboratory.

ACKNOWLEDGMENTS

This study is supported by Swedish Medical Research Council (2710, HSS); Astra-Zeneca, Mölndal (HSS), Sweden; Acure Pharma, Uppsala (HSS), Sweden; The University Grants Commission (HSS), New Delhi, India; and Indian Council of Medical Research (HSS), New Delhi, India. Technical assistance of Mrs. Becky Divine and Mrs. Bonnie Robinson is gratefully acknowledged. The secretarial assistance of Mrs. Aruna Sharma is highly appreciated.

REFERENCES

1. SHARMA, H.S. & J. WESTMAN. 2004. The Blood-Spinal Cord and Brain Barriers in Health and Disease. Academic Press. San Diego, CA.
2. SHARMA, H.S. 2004. Blood-brain and spinal cord barriers in stress. *In* The Blood-Spinal Cord and Brain Barriers in Health and Disease. H.S. Sharma & J. Westman, Eds.: 231–298. Elsevier Academic Press. San Diego, CA.
3. SHARMA, H.S., R. PATNAIK, A.K. RAY & P.K. DEY. 2004. Blood-central nervous system barriers in morphine dependence and withdrawal. *In* The Blood-Spinal Cord and Brain Barriers in Health and Disease. H.S. Sharma & J. Westman, Eds.: 299–328. Elsevier Academic Press. San Diego, CA.
4. SHARMA, H.S. & S.F. ALI. 2006. Alterations in blood-brain barrier function by morphine and methamphetamine. Ann. N. Y. Acad. Sci. (in this volume).
5. SHARMA, H.S. 2004. Influence of serotonin on the blood-brain and blood-spinal cord barriers. *In* The Blood-Spinal Cord and Brain Barriers in Health and Disease. H.S. Sharma & J. Westman, Eds.: 117–158. Elsevier Academic Press, San Diego, CA.
6. GUAN, X.M. & W.J. MCBRIDE. 1989. Serotonin microinfusion into the ventral tegmental area increases accumbens dopamine release. Brain Res. Bull. **23:** 541–547.

7. KILPATRICK, G.J., B.J. JONES & M.B. TYERS. 1987. Identification and distribution of 5-HT3 receptors in rat brain using radioligand binding. Nature **330:** 746–748.
8. BARNES, J.M., N.M. BARNES, S. CHAMPANERIA, *et al.* 1990. Characterisation and autoradiographic localisation of 5-HT3 receptor recognition sites identified with [3H]-(S)-zacopride in the forebrain of the rat. Neuropharmacology **29:** 1037–1045.
9. PERRY, D.C. 1990. Autoradiography of [3H]quipazine in rodent brain. Eur. J. Pharmacol. **187:** 75–85.
10. MENGOD, G., M. POMPEIANO, M.I. MARTINEZ-MIR & J.M. PALACIOS. 1990. Localisation of the mRNA for the 5-HT2 receptor by in situ hybridisation histochemistry. Correlation with the distribution of receptor sites. Brain Res. **524:** 139–143.
11. CURZON, G. & G.A. KENNETT. 1990. m-CPP: a tool for studying behavioural responses associated with 5-HT(1C) receptors. Trends Pharmacol. Sci. **11:** 181–182.
12. YAGALOFF, K.A. & P.R. HARTIG. 1985. 125I-lysergic acid diethylamide binds to a novel serotonergic site on rat choroid plexus epithelial cells. J. Neurosci. **5:** 3178–3183.
13. PAZOS, A., D. HOYER & J.M. PALACIOS. 1984. The binding of serotonergic ligands to the porcine choroid plexus: characterisation of a new type of serotonin recognition site. Eur. J. Pharmacol. **196:** 539–546.
14. RAY, A.K. & P.K. DEY. 1980. Morphine analgesia following its infusion into different liquor spaces in rat brain. Arch. Int. Pharmacodyn. Ther. **246:** 108–117.
15. GIANUTSOS, G., M.D. HYNES, R.B. DRAWBAUGH & H. LAL. 1975a. Paradoxical absence of aggression during naloxone-precipitated morphine withdrawal. Psychopharmacologia **43:** 43–46.
16. GIANUTSOS, G., M.D. HYNES, R.B. DRAWBAUGH & H. LAL. 1975b. The narcotic withdrawal syndrome in rats. *In* Methods in Narcotic Research. S. Ehrenpreis & A. Neidle, Eds.: 293–309. Marcel Dekker Inc. New York, NY.
17. SHARMA, H.S. 1987. Effect of captopril (a converting enzyme inhibitor) on blood-brain barrier permeability and cerebral blood flow in normotensive rats. Neuropharmacology **26:** 85–92.
18. SHARMA, H.S. & J. CERVÓS-NAVARRO. 1990. Nimodipine improves cerebral blood flow and reduces brain edema, cellular damage and blood-brain barrier permeability following heat stress in young rats. *In* Pharmacology of Cerebral Ischemia 1990. J. Krieglstein & H. Oberpichler, Eds.: 303–310. CRC Press. Boca Raton, FL.
19. SHARMA, H.S. & P.K. DEY. 1986. Influence of long-term immobilization stress on regional blood-brain barrier permeability, cerebral blood flow and 5-HT level in conscious normotensive young rats. J. Neurol. Sci. **72:** 61–76.
20. SHARMA, H.S. & P.K. DEY. 1987. Influence of long-term acute heat exposure on regional blood-brain barrier permeability, cerebral blood flow and 5-HT level in conscious normotensive young rats. Brain Res. **424:** 153–162.
21. SHARMA, H.S., J. CERVÓS-NAVARRO & P.K. DEY. 1991. Increased blood-brain barrier permeability following acute short-term forced-swimming exercise in conscious normotensive young rats. Neurosci. Res. **10:** 211–221.
22. SHARMA, H.S., J. WESTMAN, J. CERVÓS-NAVARRO, *et al.* 1995. Probable involvement of serotonin in the increased permeability of the blood-brain barrier by

forced swimming. An experimental study using Evans blue and 131I-sodium tracers in the rat. Behav. Brain Res. **72:** 189–196.
23. SHARMA, H.S. 2005. Selective neuronal vulnerability and heat shock protein expression in stress Invited Review. *In* Recent Modalities of Brain Research with Special Reference to Depression and Dementia. S. N. Sarbadhikari, Ed.: 97–152. Nova Science Publishers, Inc. NY.
24. SHARMA, H.S. 1999. Pathophysiology of blood-brain barrier, brain edema and cell injury following hyperthermia: new role of heat shock protein, nitric oxide and carbon monoxide. An experimental study in the rat using light and electron microscopy. Acta Universitatis Upsaliensis **830:** 1–94.
25. SHARMA, H.S., P.K. DEY & Y. OLSSON. 1989. Brain edema, blood-brain barrier permeability and cerebral blood flow changes following intracarotid infusion of serotonin: modification with cyproheptadine and indomethacin. *In* Pharmacology of Cerebral Ischemia 1988. J. Krieglstein Ed.: 317–323. CRC Press. Boca Raton, FL.
26. SHARMA, H.S., Y. OLSSON & P.K. DEY. 1990. Blood-brain barrier permeability and cerebral blood flow following elevation of circulating serotonin level in the anaesthetized rats. Brain Res. **517:** 215–223.
27. SHARMA, H.S. 2004. Pathophysiology of the blood-spinal cord barrier in traumatic injury. *In* The Blood-Spinal Cord and Brain Barriers in Health and Disease. H.S. Sharma & J. Westman Eds.: 437–518. Elsevier Academic Press, San Diego, CA.
28. SHARMA, H.S. 2003. Neurotrophic factors attenuate microvascular permeability disturbances and axonal injury following trauma to the rat spinal cord. Acta Neurochir. Suppl. **86**: 383–388.
29. SHARMA, H.S. 2005. Neuroprotective effects of neurotrophins and melanocortins in spinal cord injury: an experimental study in the rat using pharmacological and morphological approaches. Ann. N. Y. Acad. Sci. **1053:** 407–421.
30. SHARMA, H.S. 2005. Pathophysiology of blood-spinal cord barrier in traumatic injury and repair. Curr. Pharm. Des. **11:** 1353–1389.
31. SHARMA, H.S., Y. OLSSON & P.K. DEY. 1990. Early accumulation of serotonin in rat spinal cord subjected to traumatic injury. Relation to edema and blood flow changes. Neuroscience **36:** 725–730.
32. SHARMA, H.S., P.J. HOOPES. 2003. Hyperthermia induced pathophysiology of the central nervous system. Int. J. Hypertherm. **19:** 325–354.
33. AZMITIA, E.C., R.B. MURPHY & P.M. WHITAKER-AZMITIA. 1990. NDMA (ecstasy) effects on cultured serotonergic neurons: evidence for Ca2(+)-dependent toxicity linked to release. Brain Res. **510:** 97–103.
34. ANANTH, U.S., U. LETTI. 1987. Stimulation of phosphoinositide hydrolysis by serotonin in C6 glioma cells. J. Neurochem. **48:** 253–261.
35. LUCAITES, V.L., D.L. NELSON, D.B. WAINSCOTT & M. BAEZ. 1996. Receptor subtype and density determine the coupling repertoire of the 5-HT2 receptor subfamily. Life Sci. **59:** 1081–1095.
36. AZMITIA, E.C. 2001. Modern views on ancient chemical: serotonin effects on cell proliferation, maturation, and apoptosis. Brain Res. Bull. **56:** 413–424.
37. BARNES, N.M., C.H. CHENG, B. COSTALL, *et al.* 1992. Differential modulation of extracellular levels of 5-hydroxytryptamine in the rat frontal cortex by (R)- and (S)-zacopride. Br. J. Pharmacol. **107:** 233–239.
38. BLAUW, G.J., P. VAN BRUMMELEN & P.A. VAN ZWIETEN. 1988. Serotonin induced vasodilatation in the human forearm is antagonized by the selective 5-HT3 receptor antagonist ICS 205–930. Life Sci. **43:** 1441–1449.

39. HOYER, D., D.E. CLARKE, J.R. FOZARD, *et al.* 1994. International union of pharmacology classification of receptors for 5-hydroxytryptamine (serotonin). Pharmacol. Rev. **46:** 157–203.
40. CARBONI, E., E. ACQUAS, P. LEONE, *et al.* 1988. 5-HT3 receptor antagonists block morphine- and nicotine-induced place-preference conditioning. Eur. J. Pharmacol. **151:** 159–160.
41. HIGGINS, G.A., N. JOHARCHI, P. NGUYEN & E.M. SELLERS. 1992. Effect of the 5-HT3 receptor antagonists, MDL72222 and ondansetron on morphine place conditioning. Psychopharmacology (Berl.) **106:** 315–320.
42. ROYCHOUDHURY, M. & S.K. KULKARNI. 1986. Prevention of morphine discontinuation phenomenon in mice by ondansetron, a selective 5-HT3 antagonist. Methods Find Exp. Clin. Pharmacol. **18:** 677–683.
43. HUI, S.C., E.L. SEVILLA & C.W. OGLE. 1993. 5-HT3 antagonists reduce morphine self-administration in rats. Br. J. Pharmacol. **110:** 1341–1346.
44. WAHL, M., A. UNTERBERG, A. BAETHMANN & L. SCHILLING. 1988. Mediators of blood-brain barrier dysfunction and formation of vasogenic brain edema. J. Cereb. Blood Flow Metab. **8:** 621–634.
45. WESTERGAARD, E. 1975a. Enhanced vesicular transport of exogenous peroxidase across cerebral vessels, induced by serotonin. Acta Neuropathol. (Berl.) **32:** 27–42.
46. WESTERGAARD, E. 1977. The blood-brain barrier to horseradish peroxidase under normal and experimental conditions. Acta Neuropathol. **39:** 181–188.
47. WESTERGAARD, E. 1980. Ultrastructural properties of cerebral microvasculature under normal and experimental conditions after application of tracers. Adv. Neurol. **28:** 55–74.
48. WINKLER, T., H.S. SHARMA, E. STÅLBERG, *et al.* 1995. Impairment of blood-brain barrier function by serotonin induces desynchronisation of spontaneous cerebral cortical activity. Experimental observations in the anaesthetised rat. Neuroscience **68:** 1097–1104.
49. AUER, L.M., K. LEBER & I. SAYAMA. 1985. Effect of serotonin and its antagonist ketanserin on pial vessels. J. Cereb. Blood Flow Metab. **5:** 517–525.
50. EDVINSSON, L. & E.T. MACKENZIE. 1977. Amine mechanisms in the cerebral circulation. Pharmacol. Rev. **28:** 275–348.
51. SHARMA, H.S., J. WESTMAN & F. NYBERG. 1998. Pathophysiology of brain edema and cell changes following hyperthermic brain injury. *In* Brain Functions in Hot Environment, Vol. 115. H.S. Sharma & J. Westman Eds.: 351–412. Progress in Brain Research. Elsevier, North Holland, B. V. Amsterdam.
52. GERZER, R., A.R. BRASH & J.G. HARDMAN. 1986. Activation of soluble guanylate cyclase by arachidonic acid and 15-lipoxygenase products. Biochim. Biophys. Acta. 29;**886:** 383–389.
53. HAUBRICH, D.R., J. PEREZ-CRUET & W.D. REID. 1973. Prostaglandin E1 causes sedation and increases 5-HT turnover in rat brain. Br. J. Pharmacol. **48:** 80–87.
54. DAWSON, V.L., V.M. KIZUSHI, P.L. HUANG, *et al.* 1996. Resistance to neurotoxicity in cortical cultures from neuronal nitric oxide synthase-deficient mice. J. Neurosci. **16:** 2479–2487.
55. BACA, G.M. & G.C. PALMER. 1978. Presence of hormonally-sensitive adenylate cyclase receptors in capillary-enriched fractions from rat cerebral cortex. Blood Vessels **15:** 286–296.

56. Gullis, R.J., C.E. Rowe. 1975. The stimulation by transmitter substances and putative transmitter substances of the net activity of phospholipase A2 of synaptic membrane of cortex of guinea-pig brain. Biochem. J. **148:** 197–198.
57. Huang, M. & O.P. Rostad. 1983. Effects of vasoactive intestinal polypeptide, monoamines, prostaglandins and 2-chloroadenosine on adenylate cyclase in rat cerebral microvessels. J. Neurochem. **40:** 719–726.
58. Joó, F. 1985. The blood-brain barrier in vitro: ten years of research on microvessels isolated from the brain. Neurochem. Int. **7:** 1–25.
59. Joó, F., P. Temesvári & E. Dux. 1983. Regulation of the macromolecular transport in the brain microvessels: the role of cyclic GMP. Brain Res. **278:** 165–174.
60. Karnushina, I., I. Toth, E. Dux & F. Joó. 1980. Presence of the guanylate cyclase in brain capillaries: histochemical and biochemical evidences. Brain Res. **189:** 588–592.
61. Palmer, G.C. 1983. Biochemical mechanisms of the microvasculature. Physiol. Pharmacol. Microcirc. **1:** 1–37.
62. Manyhan, W.G. 1999. VEGF increases permeability of the blood-brain barrier via a nitric oxide synthase/cGMP-dependent pathway. Am. J. Physiol. **276:** C1148–C1153.
63. Sharma, H.S., P. Alm & Westman. 1998. Nitric oxide and carbon monoxide in the pathophysiology of brain functions in heat stress. *In* Brain Functions in Hot Environment, Vol. 115. H.S. Sharma & J. Westman Eds.: 297–333. Progress in Brain Research. Elsevier, North Holland, P. V. Amsterdam.

Peri-Response Pharmacokinetics of Remifentanil during a Self-Administration Session Indicates That Neither Blood nor Brain Levels Are Titrated

JOSE A. CRESPO,[a] LEIGH V. PANLILIO,[b] CHARLES W. SCHINDLER,[b] KATJA STURM,[a] ALOIS SARIA,[a] AND GERALD ZERNIG[a]

[a]*Division of Neurochemistry, Department of Psychiatry, Medical University Innsbruck, A-6020 Innsbruck, Austria*

[b]*Preclinical Pharmacology Section, Behavioral Neuroscience Branch, Intramural Research Program, National Institute on Drug Abuse, NIH, DHHS, Baltimore, Maryland, 21224 USA*

ABSTRACT: An individual's drug abuse pattern is determined by a multitude of factors. Among these, simple pharmacological determinants of within-binge drug consumption are sorely underinvestigated. We therefore determined if within-session operant responding to the ultra-short-acting mu opioid agonist remifentanil (RMF) was determined by blood or brain RMF levels or changes thereof. Our peri-response analysis did not detect any "threshold" RMF level, either in blood or in the nucleus accumbens (NAc) core as a deep brain region that might determine a rat's "decision" to re-emit a response during a multiple-injection drug self-administration session. The peri-response analysis also failed to find any peak RMF level, either in blood or in the NAc core, which could serve as a "ceiling" level. Thus, our findings strongly suggest that titration of blood or brain RMF levels does not determine a rat's intra-session operant response.

KEYWORDS: remifentanil; pharmacokinetics; accumbens; core; dopamine; titration; threshold; satiation; reinforcement; self-administration; mu; opioid; brain; blood; plasma; contingent; noncontingent

Address for correspondence: Dr. Gerald Zernig, Division of Neurochemistry, Department of Psychiatry, Medical University Innsbruck, Anichstrasse 35, A-6020 Innsbruck, Austria. Voice: +43-512-504-23711; fax: +43-512-504-25866.

e-mail: gerald.zernig@uibk.ac.at

Ann. N.Y. Acad. Sci. 1074: 497–504 (2006). © 2006 New York Academy of Sciences.
doi: 10.1196/annals.1369.050

INTRODUCTION

Among the multitude of factors that influences an individual's drug abuse pattern, one might assume that simple pharmacological determinants would be among the most thoroughly studied. This, however, is not the case, even for the controlled conditions of the animal behavioral laboratory. In addition, the scarce literature is confusing with respect to how drug levels in specific pharmacokinetic compartments—blood, brain, or certain brain regions—influence an animal's "decision" to re-emit a response during a multiple-injection lever press-based drug self-administration session, the experimental paradigm that is most often used to assess a drug's abuse liability. To add to the confusion, many of these studies have used cocaine as the prototypical drug of abuse, employing the pharmacokinetic data of a single seminal study by Pan and coworkers[1] without clear identification of the respective pharmacokinetic compartment and, for most purposes, using a monoexponential cocaine elimination half-life [$t(1/2)$] of around 7–9 min and an association rate $t(1/2)$ of around 2 min. Close inspection of the data presented by Pan and coworkers,[1] however, reveals a monoexponential elimination of cocaine from the nucleus accumbens (NAc), as determined by *in vivo* microdialysis, with a $t(1/2)$ of 8.5 min (upon acute cocaine administration) or 9 min (after chronic cocaine administration), and a *bi*exponential elimination of cocaine from blood, with 80% of the cocaine being eliminated with a $t(1/2)$ of 1.6 min and 20% with a $t(1/2)$ of 11 min upon acute cocaine administration and 87% versus 13% of cocaine being eliminated with a $t(1/2)$ of 1.6 min versus 11 min after chronic cocaine administration. The $t(1/2)$ for cocaine elimination from the NAc determined by Pan *et al.*[1] is in good agreement with a $t(1/2)$ of around 10 min (regardless of contingent or noncontingent i.v. administration) extrapolated from an *in vivo* microdialysis study by Hemby *et al.*,[2] and is very similar to the NAc $t(1/2)$ of 10 min for remifentanil (RMF), an ultra-short-acting mu opioid agonist,[3] also determined by *in vivo* microdialysis and also unaffected by contingent versus noncontingent administration. In that study, noncontingent RMF was eliminated from blood with a $t(1/2)$ of 0.3 min or less. To summarize, cocaine and RMF share a very fast elimination from blood [$t(1/2)$s, 0.3–1.1 min] and a very slow elimination from the NAc as a deep brain structure [$t(1/2)$ around 10 min].

Therefore, in order to answer the question of whether an individual's decision to re-emit an operant response during an experimental session is based on titration of either blood or brain levels of a drug of abuse, we used RMF as a prototypical drug of abuse, and calculated the changes in NAc RMF and blood RMF levels during an actual self-administration session.[4,5] In an extension of a previous pharmacokinetic study that analyzed RMF changes over the whole experimental session at a more descriptive level[3] and in accordance with the more refined peri-event analysis commonly used by electrophysiologists,[6–9] we performed a peri-response analysis of changes in RMF levels in blood and the NAc during self-administration of RMF. The RMF unit doses for which the peri-response analysis was performed were (*a*) 0.00025 mg/kg, i.e., the lowest dose that maintained RMF response which, furthermore, occurred at more irregular intervals than for higher RMF doses; (*b*) 0.001 mg/kg RMF, i.e., the unit dose that maintained the highest rate of response; and (*c*) 0.0032 mg/kg RMF, the highest tested RMF dose, which engendered highly regular but low-rate response.[4,5]

MATERIALS AND METHODS

Raw data of an individual rat responding to various doses of RMF (see Fig. 1B of Ref. 5) were used to calculate intra-session RMF levels in blood and in the NAc core with the software AutoKinetic® version 3.4 (toennes@em.uni-frankfurt.de). The following pharmacokinetic parameters were employed: Cmax, 10 s; Vd in the NAc (core), 2.68 L/kg; $t(1/2)$ from the NAc (core), 10 min; $t(1/2)$ from blood, 1.1 min; rat weight, 308 g[3]; and a Vd of 1 L/kg for blood.[10] RMF levels before and after eight consecutive responses that occurred immediately after the first 30 min had elapsed (i.e., after steady-state response was firmly established, see Fig. 1B of Ref. 5) were entered into a peri-response analysis. Concentrations of RMF in blood or NAc at response emission (i.e., at time point zero) were further analyzed by one-factor ANOVA (factor = RMF unit dose self-administered) followed by the Newman–Keuls *post hoc* test using Prism® (www.graphpad.com). All other statistical tests and curve fitting were also performed with Prism®. Unless indicated otherwise, values are given as means ± SEM of N determinations.

RESULTS

FIGURE 1 shows pre- and post-response levels of RMF concentrations in blood and in the NAc core for eight consecutive responses that were emitted under a fixed ratio 1 timeout 5 s (FR1 TO5s) schedule of reinforcement after a stable response was established, i.e., after the first 30 min of the session had passed (see Fig. 1B of Ref. 5).

The only feature consistently observed (and clearly based on the pharmacological principle) was that RMF levels fell before the response and rose after the response. Pre-response RMF levels did not converge to the same (threshold) level (FIG. 1). At the low RMF unit dose, pre-response RMF levels seemed to be more variable than at the intermediate RMF unit dose. At the highest RMF unit dose, most pre-response RMF levels in blood were zero, suggesting that zero blood RMF might be a "zero threshold" level at this RMF unit dose, but the pre-response time span for which RMF was at zero before the response

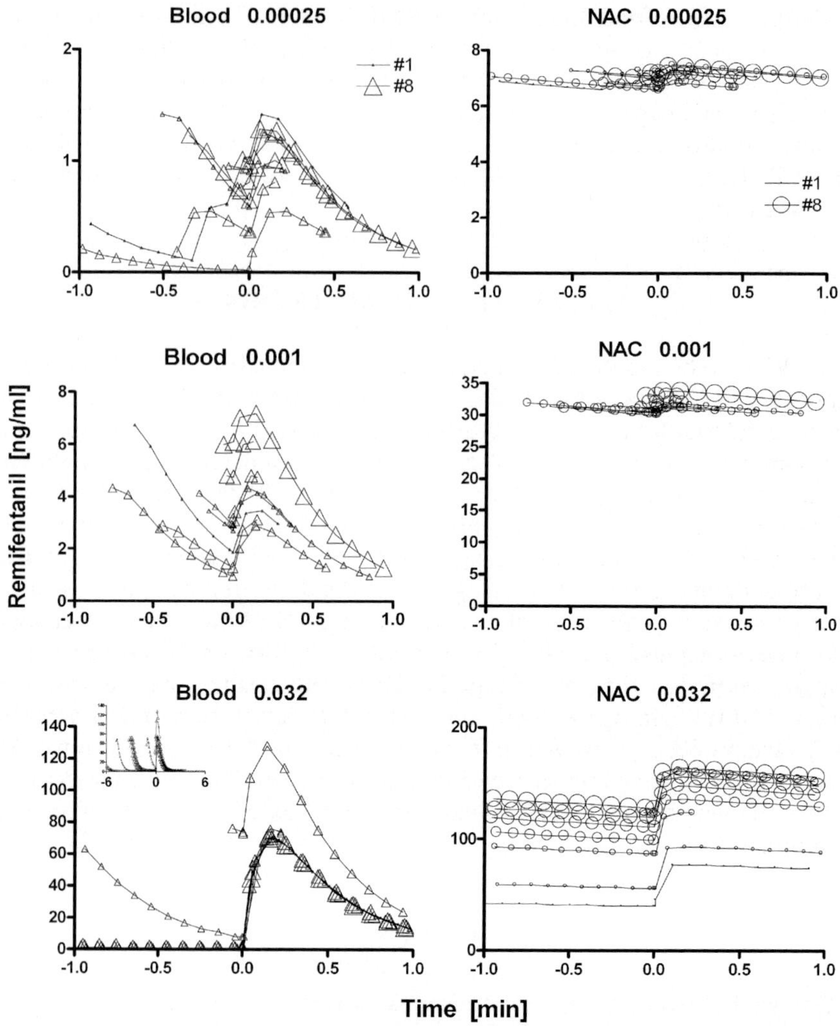

FIGURE 1. Peri-response analysis of blood and RMF levels at different unit doses. Calculated concentrations (ng/mL) of RMF in blood (left side, triangles) and in the NAc core (right side, circles) before and after the first eight responses that occurred after 30 min into the experimental session (i.e., after steady-state responding was firmly established for all investigated doses) at unit doses of 0.00025 mg/kg i.v. RMF (top row), 0.001 mg/kg RMF (middle row), and 0.032 mg/kg RMF (bottom row) are shown. Symbol size represents response order, with the smallest symbol indicating response 1 and the largest symbol indicating response 8. Time zero designates the emission of the operant response, i.e., a lever press, under a fixed ratio 1 timeout 5 s (FR1 TO5s) schedule of reinforcement. The inset in the bottom left panel shows the peri-response blood RMF levels at a unit dose of 0.032 covering –6 to + 6 min, i.e., a time window that is sixfold larger than that depicted in the larger panel (*y*-axis range for both, 0–140 ng/mL). For pharmacokinetic parameters used to calculate RMF levels, see Materials and Methods.

was emitted varied considerably, rendering the notion of a "zero threshold" unlikely (see inset in bottom left panel of FIG. 1). RMF concentrations (ng/mL) at response emission (i.e., at timepoint zero) and at RMF unit doses of 0.00025, 0.001, and 0.032 mg/kg i.v. were 0.67 $\pm$ 0.12, 3.0 $\pm$ 1.7, and 10 $\pm$ 9 ng/mL in blood (ANOVA, $P = 0.43$) and 7.0 $\pm$ 0.1, 31 + 0.4, and 95 $\pm$ 11 ng/mL (ANOVA, $P < 0.0001$) in the NAc core region. These mean values also show that pre-response RMF levels did not converge to a single threshold level but that pre-response RMF levels in blood and NAc depended on RMF unit dose in a hyperbolic function ($r^2 = 0.994$ for blood and $r^2 = 0.991$ for NAc RMF levels) instead. This hyperbolic function predicts that the maximum attainable pre-RMF levels would be 11 $\pm$ 3 ng/mL in blood and 109 $\pm$ 32 ng/mL in the NAC ($N = 3$ each), with half-maximum RMF levels being obtained at a RMF unit dose that is almost identical for blood and brain, i.e., 0.0032 $\pm$ 0.0012 mg/kg for blood RMF and 0.0029 $\pm$ 0.0012 mg/kg for NAC core RMF.

Post-response RMF levels in blood also showed no consistent pattern except for the highest RMF dose (0.032 mg/kg) at which six out of eight responses led to the same blood RMF post-response fluctuations (FIG. 1, bottom left panel), reflecting the fact that at this high RMF unit dose, response occurred at such a low frequency that blood RMF had long returned to zero before re-emission of a response, effectively rendering each RMF injection as a unique event with respect to blood RMF levels. At this RMF unit dose, both pre- and post-response intra-accumbens RMF levels continuously rose over the eight consecutive responses (FIG. 1, bottom right panel), indicating that RMF accumulation occurred in the brain at this unit dose. At the two lower RMF unit doses, pre-response RMF levels in the NAc differed very little from their respective post-response NAc RMF levels. The lack of any appreciable NAc RMF change before the response emission also strongly indicated that there was no pre-response RMF threshold level in this brain region.

DISCUSSION

Peri-response analysis of pre- and post-response RMF levels in the blood and the NAc core of a rat during a RMF self-administration session did not yield any indication that pre-response RMF levels converged to a certain fixed level, refuting the concept that the fall in the drug level below a certain blood or brain "threshold" level drives response for the next drug injection during a self-administration session.[11,12] Quite on the contrary, pre-response RMF levels both in blood and the NAc depended simply on the RMF unit dose (i.e., the dose available to the rat for self-administration). In the NAc core, the lack of any threshold RMF level was even more obvious as pre-response RMF levels (which were also dependent on the self-administered RMF unit dose) did not change appreciably in the last minute before the emission of the response.

The lack of RMF level titration in the blood or the NAc, a deep brain structure, suggests that other, *non*pharmacological, factors determine within-session operant response. These factors are the focus of a very active research field[8,13–23] the coverage of which is beyond the scope of the present study.

There are two methodological shortcomings of our study. First, the half-life (i.e., 10 min) of RMF's elimination from the NAc core, determined by *in vivo* microdialysis,[3] although essentially identical to that of cocaine,[1,2] was found to be much longer than RMF's elimination $t(1/2)$ from the whole brain (i.e., 1.1 min), as determined from brain tissue extracts.[3] Adsorption to and diffusion across the microdialysis membrane might lead to RMF dialysate changes that are slower than the actual intra-accumbens RMF changes, possibly explaining the ninefold difference in $t(1/2)$ as detailed above. However, this possibility would not explain the fact that after either contingent or noncontingent i.v. administration, measured NAc levels of RMF (movement across the microdialysis possibly being slowed down) peaked 10 min *before* DA (movement across the microdialysis membrane did not slow down).[3]

Second, in order to minimize brain trauma, we determined the intra-cerebral RMF pharmacokinetics in the NAc[3] instead of the ventral tegmental area (VTA), i.e., the brain area thought to be the main site of mu opioid agonist reinforcement (see, e.g., Ref. 24). However, when directly compared, striatal levels of the mu opioid agonist morphine did not differ significantly from its midbrain levels.[25] It is therefore plausible that the observed NAc RMF changes can be generalized to RMF kinetics in most deep brain structures, including the VTA.

One could argue that i.v. RMF injections cause large but very transient distribution-based fluctuations in the NAc RMF that our *in vivo* microdialysis approach could not detect due to its relatively large sampling interval (i.e., 10 min) and that these short-lived large fluctuations might have determined the animal's decision to press the lever for the next RMF injection. On pharmacokinetic principle,[26,27] however, it would not be expected that such quick and large RMF fluctuations would be overlaid on an elimination occurring with a half-life of 10 min, or furthermore that such fluctuations would occur 7–11 min after the onset of RMF elimination, which was the time range at which the next response for 0.032 mg/kg RMF was emitted.[5]

In conclusion, the present peri-event analysis did not detect any "threshold" RMF level, either in blood or in the NAc core as a deep brain region, which might determine a rat's decision to re-emit a response during a multiple-injection drug self-administration session. The present analysis also failed to find any peak RMF level, either in blood or in the NAc core, which could serve as a "ceiling" level. Thus, with the caveats described above, our findings strongly suggest that titration of blood or brain RMF levels does not determine a rat's intra-session operant responding.

ACKNOWLEDGMENTS

This work was supported by the Austrian Science Fund Grant P16394-B05 and by the Verein für Experimentelle Psychiatrie, Psychotherapie und Pharmakologie (VEPPP) and in part by the Intramural Research Program of the NIH, National Institute on Drug Abuse.

REFERENCES

1. PAN, H.T., S. MENACHERRY & J. JUSTICE JR. 1991. Differences in the pharmacokinetics of cocaine in naive and cocaine-experienced rats. J. Neurochem. **56:** 1299–1306.
2. HEMBY, S.E., C. CO, T.R. KOVES, *et al.* 1997. Differences in extracellular dopamine concentrations in the nucleus accumbens during response-dependent and response-independent cocaine administration in the rat. Psychopharmacology (Berl.) **133:** 7–16.
3. CRESPO, J.A., K. STURM, A. SARIA & G. ZERNIG. 2005. Simultaneous intra-accumbens remifentanil and dopamine kinetics suggest that neither determines within-session operant responding. Psychopharmacology (Berl.) **183:** 201–209. http://dx.doi.org/10.1007/s00213-005–0180-7
4. PANLILIO, L.V. & C.W. SCHINDLER. 2000. Self-administration of remifentanil, an ultra-short-acting opioid, under continuous and progressive-ratio schedules of reinforcement in rats. Psychopharmacology (Berl.) **150:** 61–66.
5. PANLILIO, L.V., J.L. KATZ, R.W. PICKENS & C.W. SCHINDLER. 2003. Variability of drug self-administration in rats. Psychopharmacology (Berl.) **167:** 9–19.
6. NICOLA, S.M. & S.A. DEADWYLER. 2000. Firing rate of nucleus accumbens neurons is dopamine-dependent and reflects the timing of cocaine-seeking behavior in rats on a progressive ratio schedule of reinforcement. J. Neurosci. **20:** 5526–5537.
7. HAMPSON, R.E. & S.A. DEADWYLER. 2003. Temporal firing characteristics and the strategic role of subicular neurons in short-term memory. Hippocamipus **13:** 529–541.
8. ROBINSON, D.L., B.J. VENTON, M.L. HEIEN & R.M. WIGHTMAN. 2003. Detecting subsecond dopamine release with fast-scan cyclic voltammetry *in vivo*. Clin. Chem. **49:** 1763–1773.
9. CARELLI, R.M. & R.M. WIGHTMAN. 2004. Functional microcircuitry in the accumbens underlying drug addiction: insights from real-time signaling during behavior. Curr. Opin. Neurobiol. **14:** 763–768.
10. COX, E.H., M.W. LANGEMEIJER, J.M. GUBBENS-STIBBE, *et al.* 1999. The comparative pharmacodynamics of remifentanil and its metabolite, GR90291, in a rat electroencephalographic model. Anesthesiology **90:** 535–544.
11. TSIBULSKY, V.L. & A.B. NORMAN. 1999. Satiety threshold: a quantitative model of maintained cocaine self-administration. Brain Res. **839:** 85–93.
12. SIZEMORE, G.M. & T.J. MARTIN. 2000. Toward a mathematical description of dose-effect functions for self-administered drugs in laboratory animal models. Psychopharmacology (Berl.) **153:** 57–66.
13. STUBER, G.D., M.F. ROITMAN, P.E. PHILLIPS, *et al.* 2005. Rapid dopamine signaling in the nucleus accumbens during contingent and noncontingent cocaine administration. Neuropsychopharmacology **30:** 853–863.

14. PHILLIPS, P.E., G.D. STUBER, M.L.A.V. HEIEN, *et al.* 2003. Subsecond dopamine release promotes cocaine seeking. Nature **422:** 614–618.
15. MATEO, Y., E.A. BUDYGIN, D. MORGAN, *et al.* 2004. Fast onset of dopamine uptake inhibition by intravenous cocaine. Eur. J Neurosci. **20:** 2838–2842.
16. SCHULTZ, W., L. TREMBLAY & J.R. HOLLERMAN. 2003. Changes in behavior-related neuronal activity in the striatum during learning. Trends Neurosci. **26:** 321–328.
17. DEADWYLER, S.A. & R.E. HAMPSON. 1997. The significance of neural ensemble codes during behavior and cognition. Annu. Rev. Neurosci. **20:** 217–244.
18. KOOB, G.F., S.H. AHMED, B. BOUTREL, *et al.* 2004. Neurobiological mechanisms in the transition from drug use to drug dependence. Neurosci. Biobehav. Rev. **27:** 739–749.
19. KALIVAS, P.W. 2004. Recent understanding in the mechanisms of addiction. Curr. Psychiatry Rep. **6:** 347–351.
20. EVERITT, B.J., R.N. CARDINAL, J.A. PARKINSON & T.W. ROBBINS. 2003. Appetitive behavior: impact of amygdala-dependent mechanisms of emotional learning. Ann. N. Y. Acad. Sci. **985:** 233–250.
21. DICHIARA, G., V. BASSAREO, S. FENU, *et al.* 2004. Dopamine and drug addiction: the nucleus accumbens shell connection. Neuropharmacology **47:** 227–241.
22. REED, B., N. CHEN & J.B. JUSTICE JR. 2003. Dual-electrode voltammetry of catecholamine transport: simultaneous monitoring of uptake and efflux. J. Neurosci. Methods **126:** 127–135.
23. PHILLIPS, A.G., S. AHN & J.G. HOWLAND. 2003. Amygdalar control of the mesocorticolimbic dopamine system: parallel pathways to motivated behavior. Neurosci. Biobehav. Rev. **27:** 543–554.
24. DEVRIES, T.J. & T.S. SHIPPENBERG. 2002. Neural systems underlying opiate addiction. J. Neurosci. **22:** 3321–3325.
25. BHARGAVA, H.N., A.K. LARSEN, N.H. RAHMANI & V.M. VILLAR. 1993. Naltrexone-induced alterations of the distribution of morphine in brain regions and spinal cord of the rat. Brain Res. **607:** 1-8.
26. WAGNER, J.G. 1993. Pharmacokinetics for the Pharmaceutical Scientist. Technomic Publishing AG. Missionsstrasse 44, CH-4055 Basel.
27. HARDMAN, J.G., L.E. LIMBIRD, P.B. MOLINOFF, *et al.* 1996. Goodman & Gilman's The Pharmacological Basis of Therapeutics. McGraw-Hill. New York.

Nicotine Alters Nicotinic Receptor Subunit Levels Differently in Developing Mammalian Sympathetic Neurons

MALATHI SRIVATSAN,[a] JONATHAN TREECE,[a] AND EZEKIEL E. SHOTTS[b]

[a]*Department of Biological Sciences, Arkansas State University, Jonesboro, Arkansas 72401, USA*

[b]*University of Arkansas for Medical Sciences, Little Rock, Arkansas 72205, USA*

ABSTRACT: The subunit specific expression of nicotinic acetylcholine receptors (nAChRs) undergo changes in the superior cervical sympathetic ganglion (SCG) of rat pups during neonatal growth. Since nAChRs play a significant role in sympathetic transmission, and the effect of nicotine on the expression of nAChR subunits in neurons of neonatal SCG is not known, we determined the effects of nicotine on receptor profiles using primary cultures of SCG neurons of 1-day-old rat pups. Neurons in culture were exposed to 1 and 10 μM of nicotine in the presence and absence of nerve growth factor (NGF). After 24 h, protein from the control and experimental neuron cultures was analyzed for the presence of nAChR containing α7 and α3 subunits using subunit specific antibodies. Exposure to 1 μM of nicotine marginally increased α7 subunits only in the absence of NGF. However it increased the level of α3 subunits significantly by 18% and 33.6% in the presence and absence of NGF, respectively. Exposure to 10 μM of nicotine did not alter the levels of either of the subunits. Interestingly, when the neurons were pre-exposed to α-bungarotoxin (antagonist of α7 nAChR), exposure to 10 μM of nicotine resulted in significant increases not only in α7 nAChR (25.5%) but also in α3 nAChR (32.2%). These results show that exposure to nicotine alters the nAChR levels differently in the neonatal sympathetic neurons in a subunit specific manner and suggest that the level of α7 as well as α3 nAChR is linked to the functional status of α7 nAChR in these neurons.

KEYWORDS: nicotinic receptor; rat sympathetic neuron; neonatal development; survival and growth

Address for correspondence: Malathi Srivatsan, Ph.D., Department of Biological Sciences, Arkansas State University, PO Box 599, State University, AR 72467. Voice: 870-972-3167; fax: 870-972-2638. e-mail: msrivatsan@astate.edu

Ann. N.Y. Acad. Sci. 1074: 505–513 (2006). © 2006 New York Academy of Sciences.
doi: 10.1196/annals.1369.051

INTRODUCTION

Nicotine in tobacco contributes to addiction to cigarette smoking.[1,2] Although the adverse health consequences of smoking are well known, many pregnant women are unable to quit smoking due to addiction. Smoking among women of childbearing age is of special concern because of its deleterious effect on the fetal and neonatal development of the infant. Unfortunately the fastest growing segment of smokers in the United States is women younger than 23 years of age and approximately 30% of the women who smoke are between 18–44 years of age.[3] Children of smokers exhibit hyperactivity, attention deficit disorder, and retarded educational achievement when compared to unexposed children.[4,5] In addition, the children exposed to cigarette smoke may exhibit disrupted noradrenergic functioning and enhancement of cholinergic receptors that inhibit cardiac functioning.[6] Perinatal exposure to environmental tobacco smoke (ETS) has adverse effects on respiratory function associated with changes in autonomic responses.[7] Thus the developing nervous system, especially its sympathetic autonomic component, is adversely affected by exposure to nicotine. Nicotine binds to nicotinic acetylcholine receptors (nAChRs) which belong to a family of ligand-gated cation channels and are formed by the assembly of subunits derived from several genes encoding the different α (α2–α9) and β (β2–β4) subunits of nAChR in neurons. Superior cervical sympathetic ganglion (SCG) neurons of rat express predominantly α7, α3, and β4 subunits.[8,9] Interestingly, the effect of nicotine on nAChR runs counter to the principle observed in other systems in which receptors are downregulated after repeated exposure to agonists. Chronic exposure to nicotine induces cell-specific upregulation of neuronal nAChR in most neurons of the brain.[10–13] However in the SCG of adult rat, it does not induce upregulation of nAChR.[14,15] Unlike the adult sympathetic neurons, in the developing or neonatal SCG neurons, nicotinic influence on nAChR might be different because a rapid change in the subunit expression of nAChR occurs during neonatal growth.[16] In the SCG of neonatal rat, expression of α3 and α7 subunits increases in the first 2 weeks of postnatal life while mRNA levels for only α3 and β4 subunits predominate in adult SCG indicating that α7 subunits are replaced during subsequent growth.[17] Further, the presence of nerve growth factor (NGF) which is essential for the survival of neonatal SCG neurons is shown to stabilize the levels of α3 subunits in these neurons.[18] Since nAChRs play a significant role in sympathetic transmission in the SCG, and information on the direct effects of nicotine exposure on the expression of nAChR subunits in neonatal neurons of SCG is lacking, we determined the levels of α3 and α7 subunits of nAChR in neonatal SCG neurons with and without NGF. We chose the primary culture of neurons from SCG of neonatal rat pups for nicotine exposure since the *in vitro* condition enables the investigation of the direct effect of nicotine on the developing neurons by avoiding the confounding effects of acute hypoxia and ischemia resulting from systemic administration of nicotine.

MATERIALS AND METHODS

Timed pregnant *Sprague-Dawley* rats were purchased from Harlan Co. (Indianapolis, IN). Culture supplies such as DMEM, Leibowitz 15 medium, neurobasal medium, B27 supplement, calcium- and magnesium-free Hank's balanced salt solution, collagenase, trypsin, and NGF were purchased from GIBCO (Carlsbad, CA). Antibiotics (Penicillin–Streptomycin 100×), Bradford protein assay reagent, nicotine hydrogen tartrate, poly-D-lysine, 5-fluoro-5′-deoxyuridine, uridine were purchased from Sigma-Aldrich (St. Louis, MO). α-Bungarotoxin (α-Bgt) was purchased from Molecular Probes (Eugene, OR). Monoclonal anti-α7 nAChR (clone M-220) and polyclonal anti-α3 nAChR (N2565) were purchased from Sigma and US Biologicals (Swampscott, MA), respectively. Alkaline phosphatase conjugated secondary antibodies were purchased from CHEMICON (Temecula, CA). Mammalian protein extraction buffer and Halt protease inhibitor cocktail were purchased from Pierce Biotechnology (Rockford, IL).

Cell Culture

Primary cultures of SCG neurons were established from 1-day-old rat pups delivered by Sprague-Dawley timed pregnant rats. The pups were decapitated after anesthesia over ice. The right and left SCG were dissected out under sterile conditions. The dissected ganglia were enzymatically dissociated by first treating with collagenase (1 mg/mL) in Leibowitz 15 (L-15) medium for 20 min at 37°C followed by treating with trypsin (0.25%) in calcium and magnesium-free Hank's balanced salt solution for 20 min at 37°C. Ganglia were then washed in L-15 + 1 mg/mL of bovine serum albumin (BSA) followed by trituration with a sterile pipette tip. Cells were pre-plated on uncoated sterile dishes and incubated for 30 min to isolate neurons in suspension from supporting cells that were attached to the uncoated dishes. Neurons in suspension were carefully removed and cell density was determined using a hemocytometer. Neurons were plated on poly-D-lysine (60 μM)-coated 100-mm dishes (100,000 cells/dish). Serum-free neurobasal culture medium with B-27 supplement containing uridine mix (5-fluoro- 5′-deoxyuridine and uridine, 10 μM) to eliminate non-neuronal cells (control medium) and β-NGF, 25 ng/mL was added and the dishes were incubated at 37°C in 5% CO_2. After 24 h, the appropriate pharmacological agents were added to the control medium with and without NGF, and pH of the medium was checked and adjusted before feeding the experimental cultures.

Nicotine Treatment

SCG neurons in culture were exposed to nicotine hydrogen tartrate to give a final concentration of 1.0 and 10 μM of nicotine for 24 h with and without

NGF. Some dishes were pretreated with α-Bgt (1 μM) as an antagonist for blocking α7 subtype nAChR for 20 min before being exposed to nicotine, since α-Bgt has been used by investigators routinely as an α7 antagonist and is not known to exert any non-nAChR-mediated effects.

Determination of Receptor Protein Levels

At the end of 24 h of treatment with nicotine in the presence or absence of NGF, and in the presence or absence of α-Bgt, the culture medium was removed, and the neurons were rinsed with buffer (phosphate buffered saline, pH 7.4, at 37°C). Cells were lysed and protein was isolated by treating the cells with mammalian protein extraction buffer containing protease inhibitor cocktail and detergent Triton X-100 (Sigma-Aldrich (0.5%). The extracts were centrifuged for 15 min at 10,000 *g* at 4°C to pellet the membranes. The supernatant containing the extracted proteins was quickly frozen and stored at –80°C till ready for analysis. Protein concentration of these samples was determined by Bradford protein microplate assay procedure. Protein samples from the different groups from equal number of cells (based on plating density) and equal total protein concentration were used for ELISA to determine the levels of α7 and α3 nicotinic receptor proteins expressed in these cells using subunit specific antibodies.

Data Collection and Analysis

Measurement of receptor levels from eight cultures was performed in each condition, two per experiment, four independent replicates of each experiment. Differences between the means of controls and each treatment groups were analyzed by a two-tailed Student's *t*-test. For comparison of multiple treatment groups, data were analyzed using analysis of variance (ANOVA) followed by *post hoc* analysis as required. Means were considered to be significantly different when $P < 0.05$.

RESULTS AND DISCUSSION

We have begun to study the time and dose-dependent effects of nicotine exposure on nAChR expression profiles in neonatal sympathetic neurons and are reporting here our results on 24-h exposure to 1 and 10 μM of nicotine. Twenty-four hours after plating and incubating neurons in the presence of NGF (25 ng/mL), the culture medium was changed. To one-half of the cultures, medium containing NGF and nicotine (1 μM and 10 μM) was added and to the other half, medium containing only nicotine was added as described in Methods. After exposing the SCG neurons for 24 h to nicotine, protein was extracted and the levels of α7 and α3 nAChR subunits were determined

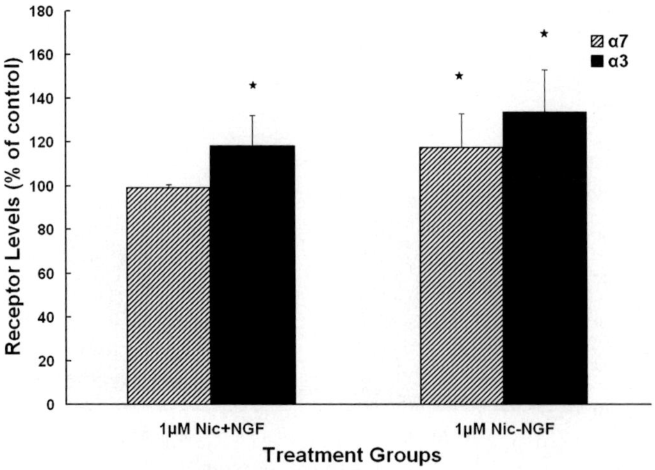

FIGURE 1. The protein levels of α7 and α3 subunits of nAChRs present in sympathetic neurons of SCG of postnatal day 1 rat pups exposed for 24 h to 1 μM of nicotine in the presence and absence of NGF.

by ELISA. Exposure to 1 μM of nicotine did not change α7 subunits in the presence of NGF and lead to a marginal increase in α7 subunits (17%, $P <$ 0.09) only in the absence of NGF (FIG. 1). However it increased the level of α3 subunits significantly by 18.4% ($P < 0.04$) in the presence of NGF and 33.6% ($P < 0.02$) in the absence of NGF (FIG.1). Thus the absence of NGF almost doubled the increase in α3 subunits when SCG neurons were exposed to 1 μM of nicotine whereas it had a marginal effect on the α7 subunits under the same conditions.

Unlike 1 μM of nicotine, 24 h of exposure to 10 μM of nicotine did not alter the levels of both α3 and α7 subunits in the presence or absence of NGF. However the levels of α3 subunits were slightly reduced when compared to that of α7 subunits (FIG. 2). To isolate and understand the role of nAChR consisting of α7 subunits in nicotine-mediated changes in receptor protein levels, we pretreated some cultures for 20 min with 1 μM of α-Bgt (antagonist of α7 nAChR) before adding nicotine. α-Bgt by itself did not affect the levels of nAChRs (FIG. 3). Interestingly, when the neurons were pre-exposed to α-Bgt, exposure to 10 μM of nicotine resulted in a significant increase not only in α7 nAChR but also in α3 nAChR (FIG. 3). When nAChRs consisting of the α7 subunits were prevented from binding to nicotine, nicotine binding to the other subunits of nAChRs appears to significantly increase α7 subunits by 25.5% ($P < 0.04$) and α3 subunits by 32.2% ($P < 0.001$). Overall, exposure to nicotine altered the levels of nAChRs consisting of α3 subunits more significantly as shown by ANOVA, $F(4, 19) = 4.519, P < 0.03$ while it did not have a significant effect on the α7 protein levels, $F(4, 19) = 1.581, P < 0.3$.

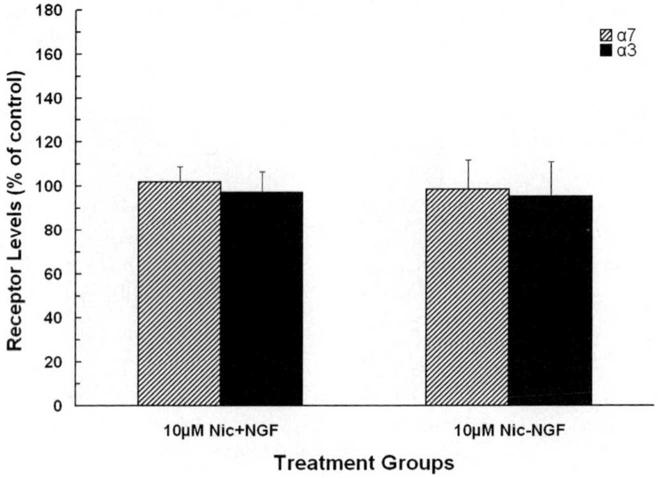

FIGURE 2. The protein levels of α7 and α3 subunits of nAChRs present in sympathetic neurons of SCG of postnatal day 1 rat pups exposed for 24 h to 10 μM of nicotine in the presence and absence of NGF.

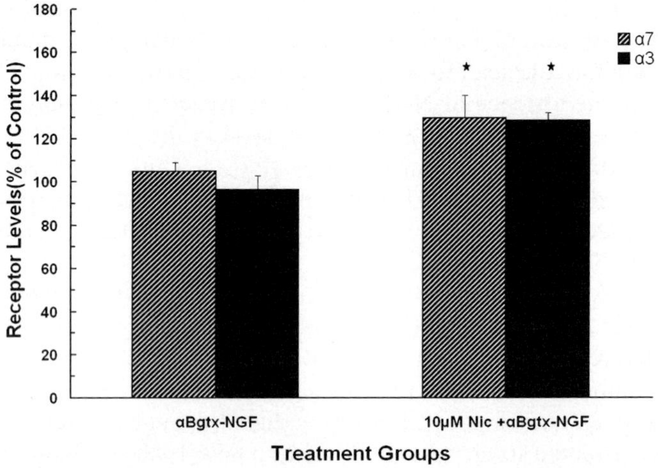

FIGURE 3. The protein levels of α7 and α3 subunits of nAChRs present in sympathetic neurons of SCG of postnatal day 1 rat pups pre-incubated with 1 μM of α-Bgt and then exposed to 10 μM of nicotine in the presence and absence of NGF.

We observed that on postnatal day 1, the ratio of α7 to α3 subunits present in nAChRs was 4:5 in SCG neurons of rat pups. Although α7 subunits were present in significant numbers, the protein levels of α7 subunits did not undergo any significant change to either concentration of nicotine exposure. It appears that nicotine exposure regulates the presence of α7 nAChR differently in the cortical and in the sympathetic neurons. Thus nicotine treatment for 2 weeks resulted in the upregulation of α-Bgt binding α7 subunits in rat hippocampal neurons in culture,[19] yet chronic administration of nicotine for 2 weeks did not change the nAChR levels in the SCG of adult rat.[15] While our results showing no change in α7 nAChR in response to nicotine exposure agrees with the above, it is possible that extended duration of nicotine exposure might alter α7 nAChR levels in neonatal sympathetic neurons. In contrast, our results show that the levels of α3 nAChR increased significantly when neonatal SCG neurons were exposed to low concentration of nicotine. This is different from the finding in adult rat sympathetic neurons. It was reported that chronic administration of nicotine did not change the level of any of the nAChRs in SCG of adult rat.[15] It is possible that the regulation of the levels of α3 nAChR in neonatal SCG neurons in response to nicotine exposure is different from that of the adult neurons. Our results agree with the study on PC12 cells that resemble sympathetic neurons in the expression and function of nAChR. PC12 cells when exposed to nicotine showed a significant increase in the levels of α3 subunits of nAChR.[20] Nicotine was found to be neuroprotective in a dose-dependent manner to neonatal SCG neurons during NGF withdrawal[21] and the increase in α3 subunits in response to 1 μM of nicotine in the cultures in which NGF was withdrawn suggests that in the rat neonatal SCG neurons nicotine may interfere with apoptosis via α3 nAChR. This is supported by findings in neonatal cortical neurons in which nicotine provided neuroprotection through α4β2 nAChR.[22] In contrast, activation of α7 nAChR, which is protective in adult animals, was deleterious to neonatal neurons.[22] Thus our results strengthen the notion that neuroprotective strategies must consider these opposite properties of distinct nAChR isoforms in neonates versus adults. High concentration of nicotine (10 μM) resulted in no change in either type of subunits. However when the neurons were pre-exposed to α-Bgt, exposure to the same high concentration of nicotine resulted in significant increases not only in α7 nAChR but also in α3 nAChR. Since α-Bgt is an antagonist of α7 nAChR, an increase in the level of α7 nAChR was expected. Interestingly it resulted in an increase in α3 subunits as well suggesting that the expression level of α7 as well as α3 nAChR is linked to the functional status of α7 nAChR in these neurons. Thus it appears that powerful compensatory mechanisms to retain nicotinic receptor function are activated during loss of function of one type of nAChR. Hence antagonist binding to α7 subunits might have activated mechanisms which upregulate both α7 and α3 protein levels.

ACKNOWLEDGMENTS

This study was supported by research funding to M. Srivatsan from Arkansas Bioscience Institute and also by funding from Arkansas IDeA Network of Biomedical Research Excellence (Arkansas INBRE) by a grant from the NCRR/NIH. We thank Ms Swati Mishra for her technical help.

REFERENCES

1. ROBINSON, J.H. & W.S. PRITCHARD. 1992. The role of nicotine in tobacco use. Psychopharmacology (Berl.) **108**: 397–407.
2. Center for disease control—The health consequences of smoking 1988. Nicotine Addiction: A Report of the Surgeon General. Washington, D.C.: Government Printing Office, DHHS publication no. (CDC) 88–8406.
3. Centers for Disease Control and Prevention, National Center for Health Statistics, healthy women: State trends in health and mortality. http://www.4woman.gov/pub/steps/HTMLMapsChart/TobaccoUsebyState.htm (last accessed on 11-9-2005).
4. BUTLER, N.R. & H. GOLDSTEIN. 1973. Smoking in pregnancy and subsequent child development. Br. Med. J. **4**: 573–574.
5. MAKIN, J., P.A. FRIED & B.A. WATKINSON. 1991. A comparison of active and passive smoking during pregnancy: long-term effects. Neurotoxicol. Teratol. **13**: 5–12.
6. RAINE, A. 2002. Annotation: the role of prefrontal deficits, low autonomic arousal, and early health factors in the development of antisocial and aggressive behavior in children. J. Child Psychol. Psychiatry **43**: 417–434.
7. SLOTKIN, T.A., K.E. PINKERTON & F.J. SEIDLER FJ. 2000. Perinatal exposure to environmental tobacco smoke alters cell signaling in a primate model: autonomic receptors and the control of adenylyl cyclase activity in heart and lung. Brain Res. Dev. Brain Res. **124**: 53–58.
8. SI, M.L. & T.J.F. LEE. 2003. Pb2+ inhibition of sympathetic α7-nicotinic acetylcholine receptor-mediated nitrergic neuronic dilation in porcine basilar arteries. J. Pharmacol. Exp. Ther. **305**: 1124–1131.
9. SIGNORE, A.D., C. GOTTI, A. RIZZO, *et al.* 2004. Nicotinic acetylcholine receptor subtypes in the rat sympathetic ganglion: pharmacological characterization, subcellular distribution, and effect of pre- and postganglionic nerve crush. J. Neuropathol. Exp. Neurol. **63**: 138–150.
10. BENWELL, M.E.M., D.J.K. BALFOUR & J.M. 1988. Evidence that tobacco smoking increases the density of (-)-[^{3}H]nicotine binding sites in human brain. J. Neurochem. **50**: 1243–1247.
11. MARKS, M.J., J.R. PAULY, S.D. GROSS, *et al.* 1992. Nicotine binding and nicotinic receptor subunit RNA after chronic nicotine treatment. J. Neurosci. **12**: 2765–2784.
12. MARKS, M.J., S.R. GRADY & A.C. COLLINS. 1993. Down-regulation of nicotinic receptor function after chronic nicotine infusion. J. Pharmacol. Exp. Ther. **266**: 1268–1276.
13. NARAHASHI, T., C.P. FENSTER, M.W. QUICK, *et al.* 2000. Mechanism of action of nicotine on neuronal acetylcholine receptors, from molecule to behavior. Toxicol. Sci. **57**: 193–202.
14. FLORES, C.M., M.I. DÁVILA-GARCÍA, Y.M. ULRICH, *et al.* 1997. Differential regulation of neuronal nicotinic receptor binding sites following chronic nicotine administration. J. Neurochem. **69**: 2216–2219.
15. DAVILA-GARCIA, M.I., J.L. MUSACHIO & K.J. KELLER. 2003. Chronic nicotine administration does not increase nicotinic receptors labeled by [i125] epibatidine in adrenal gland, superior cervical ganglia, pineal or retina. J. Neurochem. **85**: 1237–1246.

16. Mandelzys, A., B. Pié, E.S. Deneris, *et al.* 1994. The developmental increase in Ach current densities on rat sympathetic neurons correlates with changes in nicotinic ACh receptor α-subunit gene expression and occurs independent of innervation. J. Neurosci. **14**: 2357–2364.
17. Rust, G., J.M. Burgender, T.E. Lauterburg, *et al.* 1994. Expression of neuronal nicotinic acetylcholine receptor subunit genes in the rat autonomic nervous system. Eur. J. Neurosci. **6**: 478–485.
18. Yeh, J., M. Ferrira, S. Ebert, *et al.* 2001. Axotomy and nerve growth factor regulate levels of neuronal nicotinic acetylcholine receptor α3 subunit protein in the rat superior cervical ganglion. J. Neurochem. **79**: 258–265.
19. Rogers, A. & S. Wonnacott. 1995. Nicotine-induced up-regulation of α-bungarotoxin (α-Bgt) binding sites in rat hippocampal neurons. Biochem. Soc. Trans. **23**: 48S.
20. Avila, A.M., M.I. Davila-Garcia, V.S. Ascarrunz, *et al.* 2003. Differential regulation of nicotinic acetylcholine receptors in PC12 Cells by nicotine and nerve growth factor. Mol. Pharmacol. **64**: 974–986.
21. Srivatsan, M., B.M. Prabhu, C. Cavenaugh, *et al.* 2004. Nicotine influences survival and neurite growth differently in neonatal sympathetic neurons. Soc. Neurosci. Abstr. **34**: E43.
22. Laudenbach, V., F. Medja, M. Zoli, *et al.* 2002. Selective activation of central subtypes of the nicotinic acetylcholine receptor has opposite effects on neonatal excitotoxic brain injuries. FASEB J. **16**: 423–425.

Discovery of the Presence and Functional Expression of Cannabinoid CB2 Receptors in Brain

EMMANUEL S. ONAIVI,[a,b] HIROKI ISHIGURO,[c] JIAN-PING GONG,[b] SEJAL PATEL,[a] ALEX PERCHUK,[a] PAUL A. MEOZZI,[a] LESTER MYERS,[a] ZOILA MORA,[a] PATRICIA TAGLIAFERRO,[d] EILEEN GARDNER,[a] ALICIA BRUSCO,[d] BABATUNDE E. AKINSHOLA,[e] QING-RONG LIU,[b] BRUCE HOPE,[f] SHINYA IWASAKI,[c] TADAO ARINAMI,[c] LINDSEY TEASENFITZ,[a] AND GEORGE R. UHL[b]

[a]*William Paterson University, Wayne, New Jersey 07470, USA*

[b]*MNB, NIDA, Baltimore, Maryland 21224, USA*

[c]*Institute of Basic Medical Sciences, University of Tsukuba, Tsukuba Japan*

[d]*Universidad de Buenos Aires, Buenos Aires, Argentina*

[e]*Howard University, Washington, DC 20059, USA*

[f]*Behavioral Neuroscience Branch, NIDA, Baltimore, Maryland 21224, USA*

ABSTRACT: Two well-characterized cannabinoid receptors (CBrs), CB1 and CB2, mediate the effects of cannabinoids and marijuana use, with functional evidence for other CBrs. CB1 receptors are expressed primarily in brain and peripheral tissues. For over a decade several laboratories were unable to detect CB2 receptors in brain and were known to be intensely expressed in peripheral and immune tissues and have traditionally been referred to as peripheral CB2 CBrs. We have reported the discovery and functional presence of CB2 cannabinoid receptors in mammalian brain that may be involved in depression and drug abuse and this was supported by reports of identification of neuronal CB2 receptors that are involved in emesis. We used RT-PCR, immunoblotting, hippocampal cultures, immunohistochemistry, transmission electron microscopy, and stereotaxic techniques with behavioral assays to determine the functional expression of CB2 CBrs in rat brain and mice brain exposed to chronic mild stress (CMS) or those treated with abused drugs. RT-PCR analyses supported the expression of brain CB2 receptor transcripts at levels much lower than those of CB1 receptors. *In situ* hybridization revealed CB2 mRNA in cerebellar neurons of wild-type but not of CB2 knockout mice. Abundant CB2 receptor immunoreactivity (iCB2) in neuronal and

Address for correspondence: Dr. Emmanuel S. Onaivi, Department of Biology, William Paterson University, Wayne, NJ 07470. Voice: 973-720-3453; fax: 973-720-2338.
e-mail: Onaivie@wpunj.edu

Ann. N.Y. Acad. Sci. 1074: 514–536 (2006).
doi: 10.1196/annals.1369.052

glial processes was detected in brain and CB2 expression was detected in neuron-specific enolase (NSE) positive hippocampal cell cultures. The effect of direct CB2 antisense oligonucleotide injection into the brain and treatment with JWH015 in motor function and plus-maze tests also demonstrated the functional presence of CB2 cannabinoid receptors in the central nervous system (CNS). Thus, contrary to the prevailing view that CB2 CBrs are restricted to peripheral tissues and predominantly in immune cells, we demonstrated that CB2 CBrs and their gene transcripts are widely distributed in the brain. This multifocal expression of CB2 immunoreactivity in brain suggests that CB2 receptors may play broader roles in the brain than previously anticipated and may be exploited as new targets in the treatment of depression and substance abuse.

KEYWORDS: CB2 cannabinoid receptor; brain; immunohistochemistry; CB2 polyclonal antibody; CB2 blocking peptide; hippocampal cultures; RT-PCR; *in situ* hybridization; mRNA; CB2 knockout mice; CB2 electron micrograph

INTRODUCTION

Research on the molecular and neurobiological basis of the physiological and neurobehavioral effects of marijuana and cannabinoids lagged behind those of other natural addictive products like opium and tobacco, because of the lack of specific molecular tools and technology. Now significant and rapid progress has transformed marijuana–cannabinoid research into mainstream science with the cloning of genes encoding cannabinoid receptors (CNRS) and the generation of cannabinoid receptor knockout mice. There are two currently well-characterized cannabinoid receptors, CB1 and CB2, with functional evidence for the existence of other subtypes, whose identities have been elusive. But these unknown subtypes may turn out to be splice variants of CB1 or CB2 receptor subtypes. The effects of cannabinoids and marijuana use are mediated by the activation of cannabinoid receptors. CB1 receptors were serendipitously discovered[1] while characterizing an orphan receptor that turned out to be CB1 cannabinoid receptor, which has turned out to be one of the most abundant binding site in the brain.[2] The CB1 receptors are expressed primarily in the brain and some peripheral tissues, while the CB2 receptors are thought to be expressed primarily by immune cells[3] in peripheral tissues. After more than a decade, definitive identification and functional characterization of neuronal CB2 cannabinoid receptors was also serendipitous. During the summer of 2004, we were interested in evaluating the involvement of cannabinoid receptors in depression, in line with the self-medication hypothesis of drug abuse. Because it was believed that only CB1 receptors are expressed in the brain, we wanted to measure CB1 protein expression in the brains of stressed mice in comparison with controls. As CB1 receptor antibodies were back ordered, we ordered the available CB2 receptor antibodies, since we had postulated several years back that CB2 receptors are expressed in the brain but are not well characterized. We identified and reported the functional presence and expression of peripheral cannabinoid CB2 receptors in brain[4–11] at several scientific conferences in abstract form and as a book chapter.

While abundant CB1 receptors are likely to represent the principal brain sites for the action of endogenous and exogenous cannabinoids, a number of lines of evidence support possible brain roles for CB2 and other as yet unidentified cannabinoid receptors. CB2 cannabinoid receptors are particularly enriched in immune tissues,[12–14] leading to the expectation that they are present in microglia. A number of laboratories were not been able to detect the presence of CB2 in healthy brains.[13,15–19] Other groups have demonstrated CB2 expression in rat microglial cells,[20] in cerebellar granule cells,[21] in mast cells,[22,23] in retina,[24] in human astrocytes,[25] in limited populations of microglial including plaque-associated glia in Alzheimer's disease brains,[26–28] and in human brain capillary and microvessel preparations.[29] CB2 receptors' expression is induced in the macaque brains by simian immunodeficiency virus infection[26] and induced in rat spinal cord in neuropathic but not inflammatory chronic pain models.[27,28,30,31] Despite this evidence that CB2 receptors might be present in the central nervous system (CNS), the expression of neuronal CB2 cannabinoid receptors in the CNS has been much less well established and characterized in comparison with the expression of abundant brain CB1 receptors. The availability of anti-CB2 affinity-purified polyclonal antibodies directed against amino acids 1–33 and 20–33 of the CB2 N terminus and a C-terminal CB2 receptor antibody provided an opportunity to study the brain expression of CB2 immunoreactivity (iCB2) using light and electron microscopy that can be documented in glial and neuronal patterns. In previous studies and even now the specificity of the available antibodies against both CB1 and CB2 cannabinoid receptors has been questionable and perhaps why many investigators who may have observed the presence of CB2 receptors in brain concluded that it was probably an artifact. Nevertheless, we reported the discovery and functional characterization of brain cannabinoid CB2 receptors using real-time polymerase chain reaction (RT-PCR), immunoblotting, hippocampal cultures, immunohistochemistry, and stereotaxic techniques with behavioral assays. This allowed us to determine the functional expression of CB2 CBrs in rat brain and in mice brain exposed to chronic mild stress (CMS) or those treated with abused drugs. Immunohistochemical observations of CB2 immunostaining (iCB2) in apparent neuronal and glial processes in a number of brain areas can be blocked by preadsorbing the sera and is absent from CB2 knockout mice. These observations receive support from *in situ* hybridization, Western blot, RT-PCR data, and transmission electron microscopy, which are consistent with significant multifocal neuronal iCB2 expression in brain, albeit at more restricted patterns and much lower levels than those previously reported for CB1 receptors.

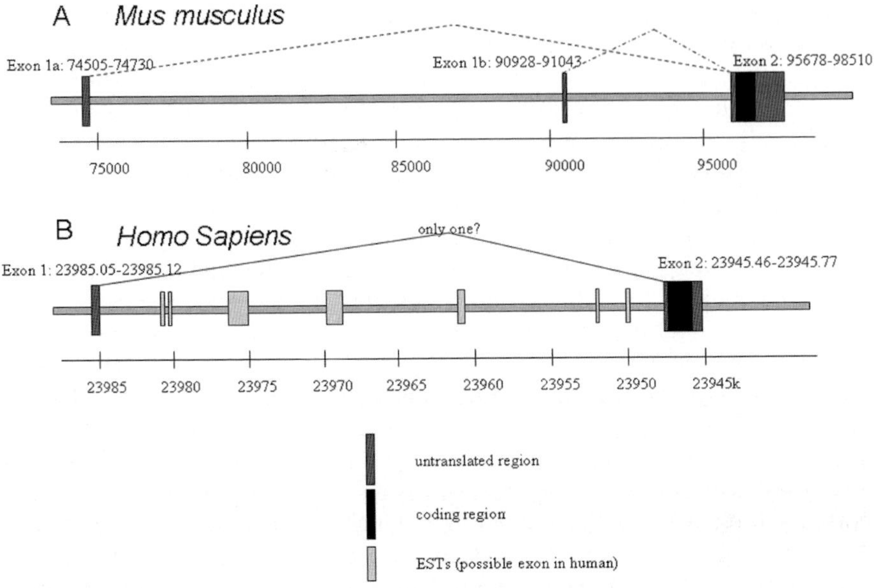

FIGURE 1. The human *CB2* gene and its mouse ortholog are located on chromosomes 1p36 and 4QD3, respectively. In humans (**B**), the *CB2* gene consists of a single translated exon flanked by 5′ and 3′ untranslated regions, and single untranslated exon and similar *CB2* gene structure is shown in mice but encodes two transcripts using different first exons (**A**). Most regions of the *CB2* gene are highly conserved, but the human has glutamine and mice and rats have arginine at position 63.

CANNABINOID RECEPTOR *CB2* GENE STRUCTURE

The *CB2* cannabinoid gene structure has been poorly defined thus far, but we have extensively analyzed and characterized the human cannabinoid receptor 1, CB1 and its 5′ exons, candidate regulatory regions, polymorphisms, haplotypes, and association with polysubstance abuse. The human CB1 receptor was found to have a number of splice variants, which may in part account for some of the myriad behavioral effects of marijuana and cannabinoid ligands, along with novel exons and candidate promotor region sequences that confer reporter gene expression. Interestingly, common polymorphisms reveal patterns of linkage disequilibrium and haplotype analysis that display significant allelic frequency differences between substance abusers and controls in European American, African American, and Japanese samples. The presence of CB2 cannabinoid receptor has been poorly characterized and is less well studied for the CNS function. However, many features of the cannabinoid *CB2* gene structure, regulation, and variation are beginning to emerge with the discovery and functional identification of CB2 receptors in the mammalian CNS. This prior poor definition could be related to the previously held view that *CB2* cannabinoid receptor gene was not expressed in the brain but that it was mainly expressed in immune cells and was less investigated for the roles in the CNS except for the association with brain cells of macrophage lineage. The human *CB2* gene and its mouse ortholog are located on chromosomes 1p36 and 4QD3 respectively. In humans the *CB2* gene is reported to consist of a single translated exon flanked by 5′ and 3′ untranslated regions,[32] and single untranslated exon and similar *CB2* gene structure is in mice but encodes two transcripts using different first exons (FIG. 1 A, B). Most regions of the *CB2* gene are highly conserved, but humans have glutamine and mice and rats have arginine at position 63.[32,33] Mice with the deletion of *CB2* gene have a decreased bone mass reminiscent of human osteoporosis[34] and in humans a number of polymorphisms in the *CB2* gene including (Q63R)[32,34] and (H316Y) have been linked to osteoporosis and autoimmune disorders. There is little or no information about the role of CB2 cannabinoid receptors in neuropsychiatric disorders as they were thought to be absent in the brain. But in neurological disorders associated with inflammation the expression of CB2 receptors has been reported in limited populations of microglial including plaque-associated glia in Alzheimer's disease brains.[27,28] Indeed, our studies provide the first evidence for a role of CB2 cannabinoid receptors in depression and substance abuse as described below.[35]

BEHAVIORAL EVIDENCE FOR THE FUNCTIONAL PRESENCE OF CB2 CANNABINOID RECEPTORS IN BRAIN

There are two currently well-characterized cannabinoid receptors and there is functional evidence of the existence of other subtypes of cannabinoid receptors.[2] Increasingly, functional evidence suggests that some cannabinoids mediate their effects independently of known CB1 and CB2 cannabinoid receptors. Initial characterization, functional distribution, and cloning of an orphan G protein coupled-cannabinoid receptor, GPR55, may be present in several CNS cell types and whose activation increases intracellular calcium.[36] This putative human GPR55 CBR is encoded by 319 amino acids and was mapped to chromosome 2q37. Human GPR transcripts have been isolated from brain and spleen, and specific mRNA is expressed in the caudate nucleus and putamen, but not in the hippocampus, thalamus, pons, cerebellum, frontal cortex of the brain or in the liver.[37] Curiously, in rats, mRNA transcripts of the GPR55 ortholog have been detected in spleen and intestine, and *in situ* hybridization has indicated some expression in the hippocampus, thalamic nuclei, and midbrain regions.[37] So far GPR55 orthologs have been identified in rat, mouse, dog, cow, chimpanzee, and human genomes. The mouse ortholog is located on chromosome 1 and encodes a 327 amino acid protein. These currently known cannabinoid receptors including CB1, CB2, GPR55, and CBn cannabinoid receptors are activated following the administration of cannabinoids or the use of marijuana known to induce a number of behavioral effects in animals and humans.

We have identified the presence and functional expression of the "peripheral" cannabinoid CB2 receptors in mammalian brain in animal models of chronic mild stress and substance abuse. In the behavioral studies we used mice subjected to CMS and another group of mice that had been exposed to capsaicin, the pungent ingredient in hot "chili" peppers. We measured anhedonia, a major feature in depression and determined the involvement and expression of CB2 cannabinoid receptors in the brains of CMS and control mice using Western blotting and RT-PCR. Anhedonia was established with a significant decrease in weekly sucrose and modification of alcohol consumption by animals subjected to CMS. CB2 cannabinoid receptors were found to be expressed in the brains of control mice and enhanced in the brains of CMS animals. The CB2 immunoreactivities detected in naïve untreated controls and the CMS animals were undetectable when the CB2 antibody was preadsorbed with the CB2 immunizing peptide. This was an indication of the involvement of CB2 receptors in the CMS model of depression. We also found that alcohol consumption was modified in the CMS animals compared to controls and curiously that alcohol consumption in stressed mice was significantly enhanced by chronic treatment with mixed CB1/CB2 agonist WIN55212-2 and JWH015, a putative CB2 cannabinoid receptor agonist, but not in control mice that were not subjected to CMS. Indeed, chronic unpredictable stress was shown to downregulate endocannabinoid signaling with reduced CB1 receptor expression and significantly reduced the content of the endocannabinoid, 2-arachidonylglycerol, within the hippocampus in the rat.[38] The deficient endocannabinoid signaling in this stress model was associated with cognitive impairments that were reversed by exogenous cannabinoid administration. In another study, the differential responses to acute and repeated stress in cannabinoid CB1 receptor knockout in newborn and adult mice provided additional evidence that the endocannabinoid physiological control system (EPCS) plays a vital role in the animal's ability to cope with stress during early development as well as in adulthood.[39] Furthermore, similarities between some symptoms of melancholic depression and those seen in animals with endocannabinoid deficiency as in CB1 mutant mice or those with pharmacological blockade of the CB1 receptors have also been reported.[40] Our data extends this deficiency in endocannabinoid signaling in the CMS model to the alteration of brain CB2 cannabinoid receptors, which is a component of the EPCS. Taken together with previous data, demonstrating that CB1 knockout mice exhibit enhanced susceptibility to anhedonic effects of chronic variable stress[40] suggests a functional interaction between the EPCS, with a contribution from both CB1 and CB2 cannabinoid receptors in the CMS model of depression.

In our current studies, the chronic treatment of mice with the mixed CB1 and CB2 agonist WIN55212-2 blocked anhedonia induced by CMS. Similar results were obtained with the putative CB2 agonist, JWH015, also known to have

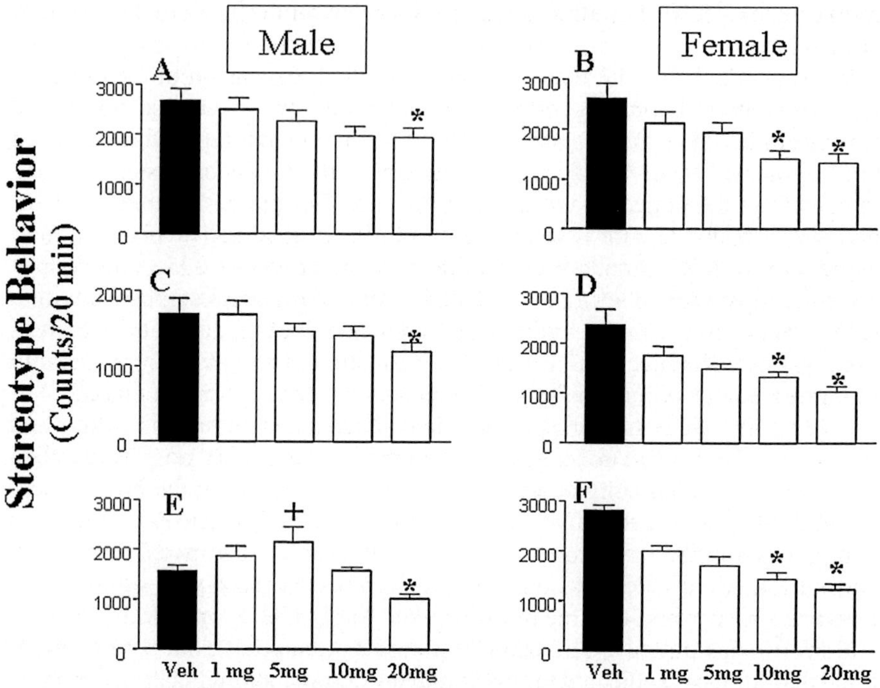

FIGURE 2. Modification of mouse stereotype behavior by the putative CB2 cannabinoid receptor agonist, JWH015, as assessed in activity monitors. Groups of male and female mice were acutely treated with JWH015 (1–20 mg/kg) for 10 min prior to placement in activity monitors and stereotypy evaluated for 20 min and compared to vehicle-treated animals. Data represent the mean ± SEM for 6–10 mice per group. Significant changes in stereotype behavior is indicated as $^{+}P < 0.05$ or $^{*}P < 0.05$ (one-way ANOVA followed by Dunnett's test for multiple comparison with controls).

effects on CB2 receptors (Onaivi *et al.*, unpublished data). We have also evaluated the effects of the putative CB2 agonist, JWH015, the mixed CB1/CB2 agonist WIN55212-2, and the antagonist SR144528 on mouse general activity, including, distance traveled, ambulatory activity, and stereotype behavior. The performance of mice in the two-compartment black and white box was also assessed following acute treatment with the agonist JWH015 and the antagonist SR144528. Acute treatment with CB2 agonist (JWH015) alters mouse spontaneous locomotor activities in a strain- and gender-dependent fashion. Increasing doses of JWH015 reduced activity in general. However, there was an increase in activity by the males and a reduction in activity by the females of the DBA/2 strain. The enhanced locomotor activity recorded in the DBA/2 males occurred at the lower doses of the agonist; however, a general pattern of depression in locomotor activity was induced by JWH 015 in both males and females in the three mouse strains tested as the dose was increased up to 20 mg/kg dose (FIG. 2). The effects of acute administration of JWH015 on stereotype behavior was similar to those described for locomotor activity with the females of the three C57BL/6, BALBc, and DBA/2 strains more susceptible to the locomotor depressant effects. Similar observations have been reported for the effects of a CB2 agonist, GW405833.[41] Curiously, the observation that CB2 agonists induce sedation and catalepsy only at higher doses has been interpreted by this group and others,[42,43] in rodent models of pain, to have a potential to treat pain without eliciting the centrally mediated side effects associated with nonselective cannabinoid agonists. While this view may be speculative, the recent reports of the functional presence of CB2 cannabinoid receptors in the CNS may indicate that CB2 and CB1 cannabinoid receptors work independently and/or cooperatively in different neuronal populations to regulate a number of physiological activities influenced by cannabinoids.

The performance of mice in the two-compartment black and white box was also evaluated. The CB2 agonist reduced mouse general activity, with increasing doses, demonstrating that JWH015 may inhibit mouse spontaneous locomotor activity probably through activation of CB2 CBrs. In the two-compartment black and white box the acute effects of the putative CB2 agonist, JWH015, at low doses (1–20 mg/kg) did not induce robust anxiolytic response; rather, this peripheral administration of JWH015 induced an anxiogenic profile of response in the black–white test box and the females of the C57BL/6 strain were more sensitive to the aversions in the white chamber. In contrast chronic treatment of control mice with JWH015 induced an anxiolytic profile of response in comparison with the CMS animals. The locomotor activities following acute treatment with JWH015 by the female C57BL/6 mice in the white chamber were significantly reduced compared to the males without significant modification in the black chamber by both male and female C57BL/6 mice in comparison with the vehicle-treated controls. However, the total zone entries into both chambers were significantly reduced with increasing dose with the female mice being more susceptible to the locomotor depressant effects of JWH015. Using the DBA/2 strain the spontaneous locomotor activity and stereotype behavior was enhanced by acute administration of low doses of SR144528, with the males more susceptible to enhanced locomotor behavior than the female mice except at the 20 mg/kg dose when the male mice were also more sensitive to the locomotor depressant effects of CB2 cannabinoid receptor antagonism. SR144528 did not induce stereotype behavior in female mice at the doses used. In the two-compartment black and white box test box treatment with SR144528 had little or no effect on the time spent in both chambers by male or female DBA/2 mice except a reduced time spent in the white chamber by the male mice at the highest dose used of 20 mg/kg. The spontaneous locomotor activities in both chambers by both DBA/2 male and female treated with SR144528 were also not significantly different from vehicle-treated control mice at 20 mg/kg when the locomotor activity was significantly reduced in the white chamber in comparison with control animals.

The transition between the chambers measured as total zone entries were also not significantly different from control mice, except at the lowest dose of 1 mg/kg of SR144528 when the transition between the chambers was significantly enhanced in the male mice. We then determined the performance of the stressed animals in behavioral measures of these motor function and emotionality tests with and without challenge with the mixed CB1 and CB2 agonist WIN55212-2 or JWH015 putative CB2 cannabinoid receptor agonist. Stress whether by CMS or prenatal exposure to capsaicin induced gender-specific aversions in the elevated plus-maze test and modulation of spontaneous locomotor activity in mice. While the modulation of locomotor activity induced in mice by stress was enhanced, the aversions of mice to the open arms of the plus-maze were reduced by treatment with WIN55212-2. In contrast the reduced spontaneous locomotor activities of mice subjected to CMS for 4 weeks was enhanced by acute or chronic daily treatment with the putative CB2 cannabinoid agonist, JWH015, in comparison with control mice that were not stressed but treated acutely or chronically with JWH015. On the other hand, stress and chronic treatment with JWH015 appeared to reduce the stereotypical response in control and stressed mice, while acute treatment significantly reduced stereotype behavior in stressed but not in control animals (FIG. 3). These effects of CB2 cannabinoid receptor ligands in *in vivo* behavioral tests are provided as functional evidence of CB2 cannabinoid receptors in the brain that plays a role in motor function and emotionality tests.

CB2 CANNABINOID RECEPTOR GENE TARGETING BY CB2 ANTISENSE OLIGONUCLEOTIDE MODIFIES BEHAVIOR

We speculated that if CB2 cannabinoid receptors are present in the brain, then antisense oligonucleotides complementary to CB2 mRNA transcript will block translation of or stimulate degradation of CB2 mRNA. It is therefore of importance to determine whether inhibition of CB2 gene expression in the brain will alter behavior as observed with the exogenous administration of CB2 ligands discussed above. Although antisense technologies have limitations, with appropriate controls and modifications, an antisense drug for human use is available in the clinic.[42] We therefore used the validated plus-maze test of anxiety to ascertain whether CB2 cannabinoid transcripts are functionally expressed in the brain to influence behavior. An underlying hypothesis for this test is the self-medication hypothesis that an affective syndrome, including stress associated with every day living, depression, and anxiety states may be associated with uncontrollable drug and alcohol dependency. Thus the plus-maze test that has been validated for use as a model for the assessment of emotionality was utilized in the determination of a functional role (if any) of CB2 cannabinoid receptors in the brain. The plus-maze consists of two enclosed arms and two open arms and the test is based on rodent's aversion to

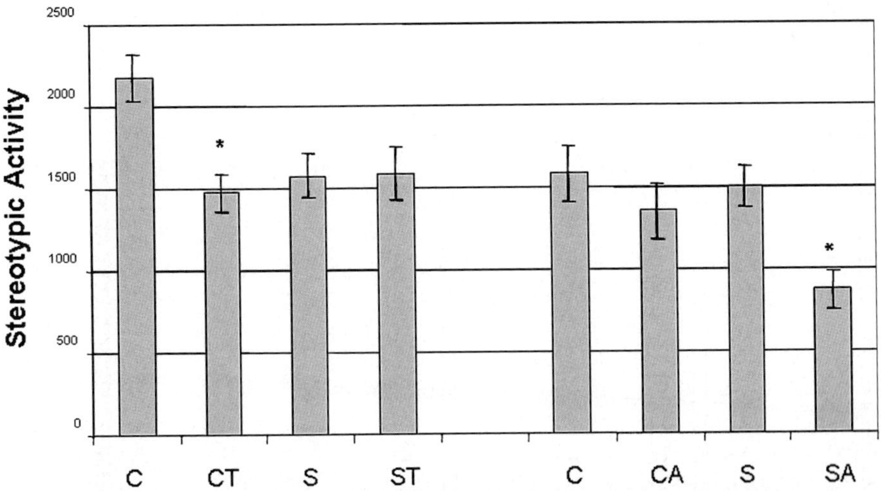

FIGURE 3. Modification of mouse stereotype behavior by the putative CB2 cannabinoid receptor agonist, JWH015, 20 mg/kg, as assessed in the activity monitors in stressed and nonstressed mice. Groups of stressed and nonstressed controls were chronically treated and other nontreated stressed and nonstressed groups were acutely challenged with 20 mg/kg JWH015. C is controls and CT is controls chronically treated while S is stressed group and ST is stressed animals chronically treated with JWH015. CA and SA are control or stressed animals acutely treated with 20 mg/kg JWH015. Stereotype behavior was evaluated for 20 min and compared to vehicle-treated animals. Data represent the mean ± SEM for 6–10 mice per group. Significant changes in stereotype behavior is indicated as $^{+}P < 0.05$ or $^{*}P < 0.05$ (one-way ANOVA followed by Dunnett's test for multiple comparison with controls).

open spaces. Standard anxiolytic drugs such as diazepam reduces the aversion to open arms by increasing the time spent and number of entries into the open arms. Direct intracerebroventricular cannabinoid CB2 oligonucleotide microinjection into the mouse brain reduced mouse aversion to open arms, further indicating the functional presence of CB2 cannabinoid receptors in the brain that influence behavior.

FUNCTIONAL PRESENCE AND CB2 CANNABINOID GENE TRANSCRIPT VARIATION IN BRAINS OF STRESSED AND ANIMALS TREATED WITH ABUSED SUBSTANCES

To determine whether *CB2* gene transcripts are present in the brain, we first compared the expression of *CB2* gene transcripts between the spleen and the brain as CB2 receptor mRNA was thought to be expressed primarily in immune cells but not in brain and that the message was most abundant in B cells.[17–19,33,44,45] Since CB2 receptors are intensely expressed in peripheral

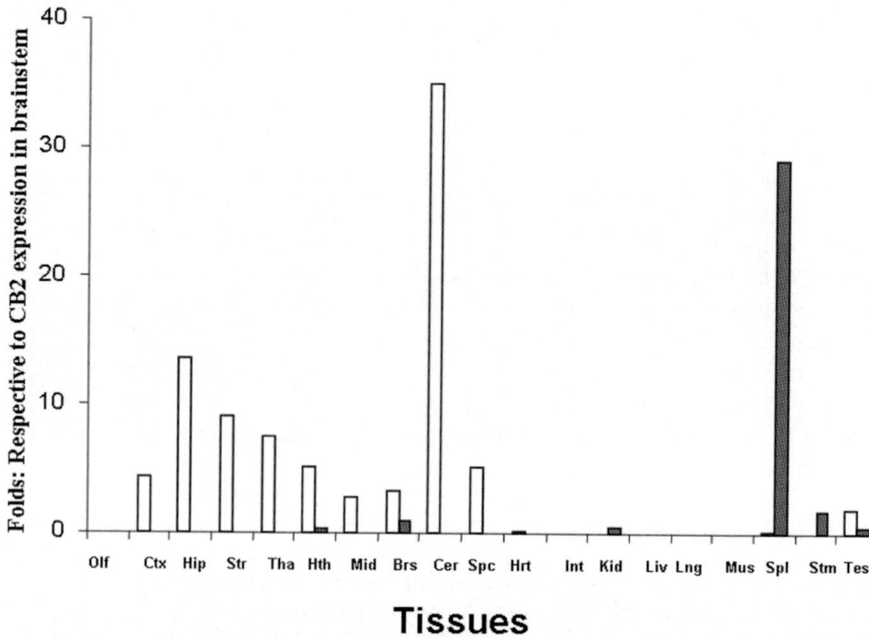

FIGURE 4. Relative quantification of *CB1* and *CB2* mRNA expression in mouse brain regions and peripheral tissues. CB1 mRNA expression levels (open bars) are represented in the scale of 100 × of CB2 mRNA expression levels (filled bars). Olf, Olfactory; Ctx, Cortex; Hip, Hippocampus; Str, Striatum; THa, Thalamus; Hth, Hypothalamus; Mid, Midbrain; Brs, Brain stem; Cer, Cerebellum; Spc, Spinal cord; Hrt, Heart; Int, Intestine; Kid, Kidney; Liv, Liver; Lng, Lung; Mus, Muscle; Spl, Spleen; Stm, Stomach; and Tes, Testis.

and immune tissues, expression in brain microglial has been anticipated. We found that the expression of *CB2* gene transcripts was about 100 times higher in the spleen than in the brain of rats using RT-PCR. Therefore, brain cells neuron plus glial cells express mRNA for *CB2* gene transcripts but at lower levels than peripheral tissues and immune tissues. Differences in the distribution of mouse, rat, and human[3,33] CB2 cannabinoid receptors have been reported, but in all cases these investigators could not detect CB2 receptors or their gene transcripts in the brain. We have previously demonstrated the differential expression of *CB1* gene transcripts in different mouse strains. Using CB2-specific probes and primers we compared the expression of *CB2* gene transcripts in three mouse strains BALBc, DBA/2, and C57BL/6 in which we previously reported the differential strain-specific brain distribution of *CB1* gene transcripts.[2] The expression of the *CB2* gene transcripts was present but varied insignificantly in the whole brains of these mouse strains and was enhanced by CMS. Furthermore, the expression of the *CB1* and *CB2* cannabinoid receptor gene transcripts was compared in different regions of the mouse brain.

The data obtained confirmed previously known distribution patterns of *CB1* gene transcripts enriched in the cerebellum, hippocampus, striatum, thalamus, cortex, hypothalamus, brain stem, midbrain, testis etc. The expression levels of the *CB1* gene as shown in a representative RT-PCR was 100 times of the *CB2* gene expression levels with reference to the brain stem. As reported here and by the others, the spleen has the most abundant *CB2* gene transcripts. Substantial detection of *CB2* gene transcripts was recorded in the stomach, brain stem, testis, lungs, kidney, heart, and hypothalamus (FIG. 4). To further understand the physiological relevance of the expression of CB2 cannabinoid receptors and their gene transcripts, we examined the expression of *CB2* gene transcripts in rodents treated with opioids, morphine or heroine, cocaine, and alcohol in comparison with saline-treated controls. Animals treated with cocaine or heroin showed increased expression of *CB2* gene transcripts in comparison with saline-treated controls. The modification of expression of *CB2* gene transcripts is notable, indicating the presence of *CB2* gene transcripts in the brain that is influenced by abused substances and stress.

CB2 CANNABINOID RECEPTOR GENE VARIATION IN DEPRESSION AND SUBSTANCE ABUSE: FROM MICE TO HUMANS

Reports by our group,[4–11,35] and others,[46,47] have identified the functional presence of cannabinoid CB2 receptors in neuronal and glial processes contrary to the view for more than a decade that the CB2 cannabinoid receptors were restricted to peripheral tissues and predominantly in immune tissues. We also found differential modification of *CB2* gene expression in various brain regions of animals treated with abused substances like cocaine, morphine, and alcohol and in those subjected to stressors, including chronic mild stress and prenatal capsaicin exposure. These findings are of importance as they open new areas in basic neuroscience research and approaches in our fundamental understanding of depression and addictive disorders for which pharmacological treatment has been disappointing. In view of our identification of functional expression and regulation of cannabinoid *CB2* receptor genes in mammalian brain, we tested the hypothesis that genetic variants of the *CB2* gene might have significant effects and association with depression and alcoholism. This hypothesis is supported by the identification of a missense polymorphism at *CB2* cDNA position 188–189, which results in a dinucleotide conversion of AA to GG and predicts a nonconservative amino acid substitution of glutamine by arginine at position 63 (Q63R). This tandem polymorphism is important as it has the potential to change function in the mature expressed cannabinoid CB2 receptor as demonstrated in the immune system by an *in vitro* assay.[32] In humans (Q63R) polymorphism has been associated with osteoporosis and autoimmune disorders.[32,34] The association of the *CB2* gene variation was probed in Japanese subjects to examine the nonsynonymous polymorphism, (Q63R), in the *CB2* gene for association with depression or alcoholism in the Japanese population. There was a significant difference in allelic frequency between cases and controls at (Q63R) polymorphism in the *CB2* gene in alcoholism and depressed subjects. Thus a high incidence of this polymorphism was found in Japanese alcoholics and depressed subjects. As many genetic variants play various roles in depression and/or substance abuse, variation in the *CB2* gene, (Q63R) polymorphism may be a previously unknown risk factor in depression and/or alcoholism at least in the Japanese population. If this can be generalized to other ethnicities, then the results support the possibility of targeting the cannabinoid system using CB2 ligands in depression and drug abuse and perhaps in their comorbidity. FIGURE 5 shows the computed structural changes with (Q63R) polymorphism in the *CB2* gene using three analysis of the computer program GENETYX. Chou-Fasman (FIG. A) and Robson (FIG. B) analysis indicated 5–6 amino acids' structural change between alpha-helix, beta-sheet, coiled-coil, or turn. (FIG. C) Hydrophilic or hydrophobic structure in codon 51–101 region of the *CB2* gene, indicating subtle but striking differences between the alleles. In the mouse model, the CB2 receptor and transcripts were regulated by chronic mild stressors. Chronic treatment with the mixed CB2 agonist, WIN55212-2 1.0 mg/day, or the putative CB2 agonist, JWH015 20 mg/kg, enhanced alcohol consumption in stressed but not in control mice. In animals that developed alcohol preference, *CB2* gene expression was downregulated in the midbrain and striatum. It is therefore tempting to speculate that the reported effects of alcohol may be associated with changes in the cannabinoid system, with CB2 cannabinoid receptors playing a regulatory role.

CB2 RECEPTOR IMMUNOHISTOCHEMICAL LOCALIZATION IN RAT BRAIN AND SPLEEN

Contrary to prior reports that CB2 cannabinoid receptors were not expressed in the brain, we report wide distribution of CB2 receptors in brain regions suggesting a reevaluation of the role of CB2 cannabinoid receptors in the CNS. Other reports have appeared indicating the functional presence in brain stem[46] and localization in rat cerebellum[47] in agreement with our reports.[4–11,35,48] Immunoblots from mouse brain and spleen lysates revealed a major band of approximately 53 kDa, with other visible bands around 37 kDa and 75 kDa, similar to those observed recently.[46] The use of three anti-CB2 affinity-purified polyclonal antibodies with peptide conjugates corresponding to different amino acid terminals and yielding similar patterns of staining indicated further specificity of CB2 receptor localization. The different antibodies showed very similar staining patterns in both the rat spleen and cerebellum sections supporting their specificity to CB2 receptor. Cannabinoid CB2 immunostaining (iCB2) was observed in many parts of the rat and mouse CNS.

Estimated CNR2 structural change by (Q63R) polymorphism in the *CNR2*.

A. Chou-Fasman

58. Ile(I)	h 1.08 0.96 *+	H 1.60 1.10 *+	0.47 0.98 0.0000142	b
59. Leu(L)	H 1.21 0.94 *+	h 1.30 0.92 *+	0.59 1.10 0.0000572	b
60. Ser(S)	i 0.77 0.91 *+	b 0.75 0.87 *+	1.43 1.20 0.0001520 *	b
61. Ser(S)	i 0.77 1.02 *+	b 0.75 1.01	1.43 0.99 0.0000146 *	a
62. His(H) +	I 1.00 1.08 *+	i 0.87 1.05	0.95 0.87 0.0000420 *	a
63. Gln(Q)	h 1.11 1.07 +	h 1.10 1.07	0.98 0.87 0.0000158 *	a
64. Leu(L)	H 1.21 1.08 +	h 1.30 0.98	0.59 0.88 0.0000608	a
65. Arg(R) +	i 0.98 0.92 +	i 0.93 0.79	0.95 1.11 0.0000363	a
66. Arg(R) +	i 0.98 0.87 +	i 0.93 0.74	0.95 1.23 0.0000290	a
67. Lys(K) +	h 1.16 0.80 +	b 0.74 0.88	1.01 1.27 0.0002587 *	t
68. Pro(P)	B 0.57 0.81	B 0.55 1.02	1.52 1.17 0.0001131 *	t

58. Ile(I)	h 1.08 0.96 *+	H 1.60 1.10 *+	0.47 0.98 0.0000142	b
59. Leu(L)	H 1.21 0.94 *+	h 1.30 0.92 *+	0.59 1.10 0.0000572	b
60. Ser(S)	i 0.77 0.88 *+	b 0.75 0.83 *+	1.43 1.19 0.0001319 *	b
61. Ser(S)	i 0.77 0.99 *+	b 0.75 0.96	1.43 0.98 0.0000391 *	c
62. His(H) +	I 1.00 1.04 *	i 0.87 1.01	0.95 0.86 0.0000454 *	c
63. Arg(R) +	i 0.98 1.04	i 0.93 1.02	0.95 0.86 0.0000147 *	c
64. Leu(L)	H 1.21 1.08	h 1.30 0.98	0.59 0.88 0.0000608	c
65. Arg(R) +	i 0.98 0.92	i 0.93 0.79	0.95 1.11 0.0000363	c
66. Arg(R) +	i 0.98 0.87	i 0.93 0.74	0.95 1.23 0.0000290	c
67. Lys(K) +	h 1.16 0.80	b 0.74 0.88	1.01 1.27 0.0002587 *	t
68. Pro(P)	B 0.57 0.81	B 0.55 1.02	1.52 1.17 0.0001131 *	t

B. Robson

58. Ile(I)	-14	167	-21	-18	b
59. Leu(L)	-65	108	-16	-5	b
60. Ser(S)	-114	63	11	40	b
61. Ser(S)	-116	33	36	70	c
62. His(H)	-60	45	42	61	c
63. Gln(Q)	-15	67	39	20	b
64. Leu(L)	17	18	14	-5	b
65. Arg(R)	11	-11	36	-22	t
66. Arg(R)	-6	-66	56	-12	t
67. Lys(K)	-52	-88	160	77	t
68. Pro(P)	-92	-98	136	120	t

58. Ile(I)	-59	117	-71	-68	b
59. Leu(L)	-95	58	-46	-35	b
60. Ser(S)	-124	23	1	30	c
61. Ser(S)	-116	3	46	60	c
62. His(H)	-65	25	52	41	t
63. Arg(R)	-34	59	56	13	b
64. Leu(L)	-3	18	19	-5	t
65. Arg(R)	-9	-1	26	-32	t
66. Arg(R)	-16	-61	41	-27	t
67. Lys(K)	-57	-88	140	57	t
68. Pro(P)	-92	-98	111	95	t

C. hydrophilic/ hydrophobic structure

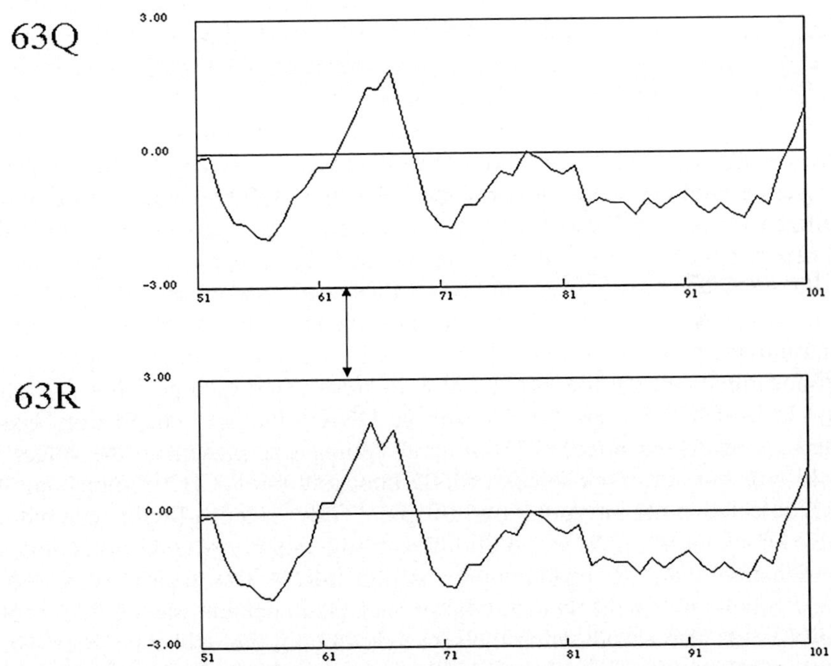

FIGURE 5. Shows the computed structural changes with (Q63R) polymorphism in the *CB2* gene using three analyses of the computer program GENETYX. Chou-Fasman (**A**) and Robson (**B**) analysis indicated 5–6 amino acids structural change between alpha-helix, beta-sheet, coiled-coil, or turn. (**C**) Hydrophilic or hydrophobic structure in codon 51–101 region of the *CB2* gene, indicating subtle but striking differences between the alleles.

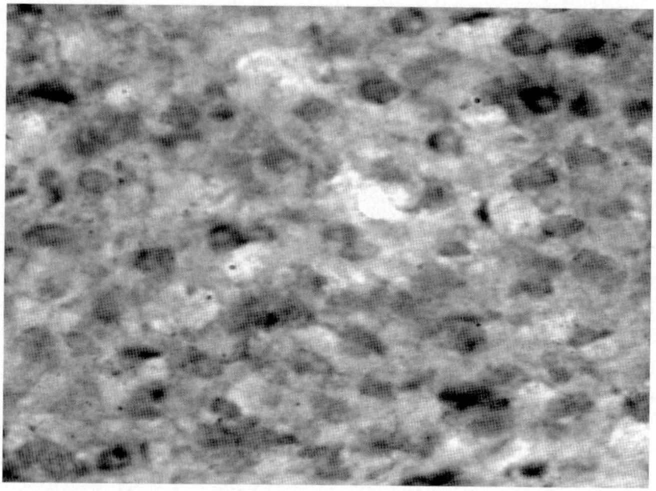

FIGURE 6. CB2-immunopositive staining was observed in the regions of cerebral cortex that we analyzed. Apical dendrites of pyramidal neurons were moderately to heavily stained. Other less heavily stained neurons and many blood cells do not show immunostaining.

Most iCB2 was found in patterns consistent with nerve cell bodies, neuronal processes, and glial cells and processes. The third CB2 receptor antibody was utilized for the CB2 knockout mice and their wild-type controls. This third antibody appeared more specific for mouse CB2 receptors and has an origin different from the first two antibodies that were initially utilized in the preliminary studies. The preadsorption and coincubation of the antibody with the immunizing peptide resulted in blocking CB2 staining in the rat hippocampus, hippocampal cell culture, HEK 293 cells transfected with pc DNA 3.1 CB2, and lack of iCB2 in HEK cells with pc DNA 3.1 mock transfection. Using the CB2 knockout mice, CB2 immunostaining was present in the spleen of wild-type but not in the spleen of CB2 knockout mice. CB2 immunostaining was detected in the interpolar part of spinal fifth nucleus of wild-type but not CB2 knockout mice. As an additional control, using *in situ* hybridization, we demonstrate that *CB2* cannabinoid receptor mRNA was clearly expressed in the cerebellum of wild-type and not in the CB2 knockout mice. *CB2* receptor mRNA was also absent using the sense controls in the wild-type mice. Antisense cRNA probe did not detect signals around the Purkinje and molecular layer in the CB2 knockout mice. However, strong signals were detected around the Purkinje cells and molecular layers with little or no expression in the granular layer of the cerebellum in the wild-type mice. Specifically, these studies and our initial RT-PCR analyses of brain *CB2* mRNAs of naïve and drug-treated

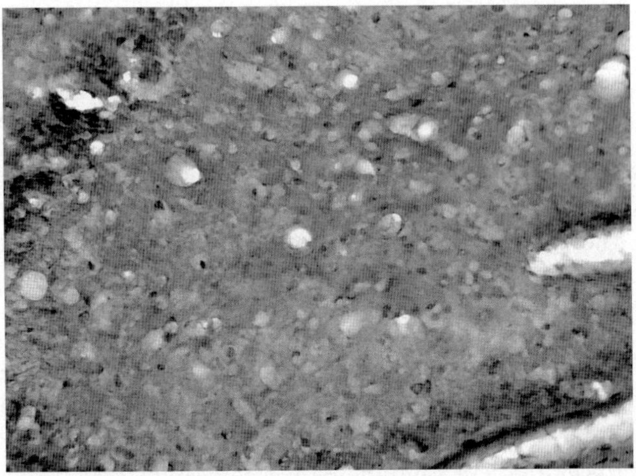

FIGURE 7. A moderate-to-dense CB2 immunostaining was observed in pyramidal neurons of hippocampal allocortex and some interneurons in the stratum oriens and stratum radiatum. Some glial cells also appeared to be immunostained for CB2 in the hippocampus.

mice[35] revealed brain *CB2* receptor gene transcript expression at levels much lower than those of the spleen, further indicating the presence CB2 receptors in the brain. The spleen *CB2* gene expression using RT-PCR was about 140 times higher than that in the brain. *CB2* receptor gene expression was also detected in mouse striatum, midbrain, and hippocampus at about the same expression levels. Using double labeling sequentially, tissues were first labeled with the CB2 receptor antibody, followed by a neuron marker, neuron-specific enolase (NSE). Confocal immunofluorescence image of iCB2, NSE on neurons, and overlay of CB2 receptor on neurons illustrate the presence of CB2 receptors on hippocampal neurons in the culture. CB2 immunoreactivity was also observed in the olfactory tubercle, islands of Calleja, cerebral cortex, striatum, thalamic nuclei, hippocampus, amygdala, substantia nigra, periaqueductal gray, paratrochlear nucleus, paralemniscal nucleus, red nucleus, pontine nuclei, inferior colliculus, and the parvicellular portion of the medial vestibular nucleus. CB2-immunopositive staining was observed in the regions of cerebral cortex in FIGURE 6, that we analyzed. Apical dendrites of pyramidal neurons were moderately to heavily stained. Other less heavily stained neurons and many blood cells do not show immunostaining. A moderate-to-dense CB2 immunostaining was observed in pyramidal neurons of hippocampal allocortex and some interneurons in the stratum oriens and stratum radiatum (FIG. 7). Some glial cells also appeared to be immunostained for CB2 in the hippocampus (FIG. 7). Therefore, CB2 are widely distributed in the brain areas examined.

ULTRASTRUCTURAL AND SUBCELLULAR LOCALIZATION OF CB2 RECEPTORS IN MOUSE CORTICAL NEURONS

As definitive electron microscopic evidence is needed to precisely determine the subcellular localization of CB2 receptors, our preliminary transmission electron micrograph data using immunoelectron microscopy approach shows a high-resolution definition of cortical CB2 cannabinoid receptor localization at the ultrastructural level. Electron micrographs from different cortical areas show dendrites with immunostaining for CB2 receptors with diffuse black deposits and mitochondria clearly visible. In some areas axon terminals were not immunoreactive for CB2 receptors and small rounded synaptic vesicles were seen. Two axon terminals making contact with a dendrite but without immunostaining for CB2 are apparent in FIGURE 8. The pattern of staining in most cortical areas appears to be mainly a post synaptic localization of CB2 cannabinoid receptors. For example, at the area of the two synaptic contacts seen in FIGURE 8, the synapses appear to be excitatory and possibly glutamatergic. While these data are preliminary and we cannot exclude that some of the CB2 receptors may be presynaptic, CB1 receptors are not exclusively presynaptic in the brain. CB1 receptors are known to be mainly presynaptic in the CNS where cannabinoids act at presynaptic CB1 receptors and endocannabinoids have emerged as one of the classes of retrograde messengers involved in the regulation of synaptic transmission. The functional implication of pre- and/or postsynaptic localization of CB2 cannabinoid receptors awaits further electrophysiological investigation and image analysis of this interesting component of the endocannabinoid physiological control system.

TECHNICAL CODA

The clinical and functional implication of the presence of CB2 cannabinoid receptors in the brain will gradually become clear as more research will certainly unravel additional role(s) as we have noted in this effort. As accumulating evidence from our studies and those of others indicate that CB2 cannabinoid receptors are present in the brain but have not been systematically characterized, our main goal was to localize CB2 cannabinoid receptors and their distribution patterns in the rat brain and to assess their functional implication. An initial publication[35] of data from this work has appeared and in abstract form.[4–11] Numerous previous studies for more than a decade since the cloning of CB2 cannabinoid receptors have failed to detect the presence of CB2 cannabinoid receptors in the brain,[3,13,15–19,43] and little was known about its neuronal function. With the availability of specific probes and primers we detected the presence of CB1[49] and CB2 mRNAs in the brains of rats and mice using RT-PCR.[4–11,35] We show that CB2 receptors are present in various regions of the adult rat and mouse brains. There were similar patterns of immunostaining in the spleen

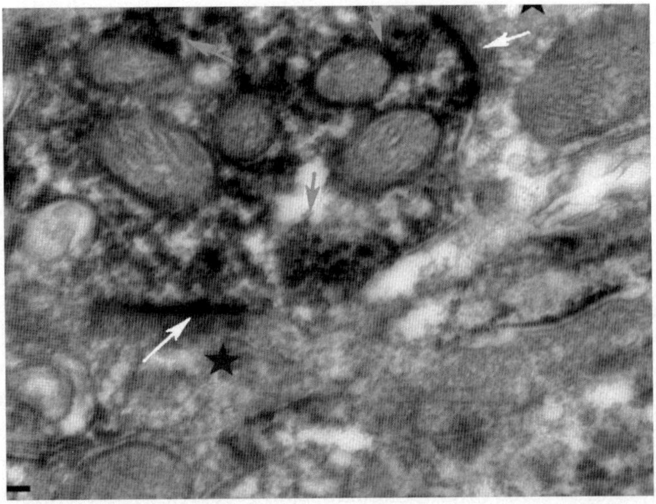

FIGURE 8. Ultrastructural and subcellular localization of CB2 receptors in mouse cortical neurons. Transmission electron micrograph shows a high-resolution definition of cortical CB2 cannabinoid receptor localization at the ultrastructural level. A representative micrograph of cortical areas showing axons and dendrites with CB2 receptors with diffuse black deposits and mitochondria is clearly visible. In some areas axon terminals were not immunoreactive for CB2 receptors and small rounded synaptic vesicles are present. Two axon terminals making contact with a dendrite but without immunostaining for CB2 are also apparent. Immunostaining for CB2 receptors on axon terminals establish asymmetrical synapses. The primary magnification is 10,000 X. White arrows show asymmetrical synaptic contacts; gray arrows show the diffuse dark DAB deposits indicating

and cerebellum using three different antibodies. Furthermore, in primary hippocampus cultures, CB2-positive expression was detected in NSE- positive cells. Immunohistochemical analyses revealed abundant CB2 immunostaining in apparent neuronal and glial cells in a number of brain areas. Previous studies have shown intense CB1 receptor immunoreactivity in hippocampal formation, basal ganglia, and the molecular and granular layers of the cerebellum with moderate staining in the olfactory bulb, piriform cortex, cerebral cortex, and many thalamic nuclei.[50,51] Our data indicate that CB1 and CB2 immunoreactivities may share localization in same brain structures with possible differences in the distribution patterns in neuronal elements where they are localized. For example, these previous studies,[50,51] and our data show that both CB1 and CB2 receptors are localized in the cerebellum, where CB1 was seen in the molecular layer and granular layers whereas CB2 receptors were observed in Purkinje cells and the molecular layer. In spite of the accumulating evidence using *in situ* hybridization, mRNA probes, specific CB2 antibodies, and data from our studies and those of others indicating the expression of CB2 receptors in the brain, much less is known about the specific cell types in which CB2 receptors are found and its subcellular localization in these cells in the brain remains to be determined. Such future studies will allow direct electrophysiological analysis for the specific definition of the specific roles of CB2 receptors in the brain.

The new knowledge from our data and those of other recent studies,[4–11,35,46–48] that CB2 receptors are present in the brain raises many questions about the possible roles that CB2 receptors may play in the nervous system. These results therefore extend the previous evidence that CB2 receptors are playing an important role in the immune function to other putative neuronal function by their apparent presence in neuronal processes. Our studies implicate neuronal and glial CB2 receptors in the CMS model of depression, substance abuse, and the brain stem CB1 and CB2 receptors that were demonstrated to be functionally coupled to inhibition of emesis in the ferret.[46] The immunohistochemical localization of CB2 receptors when compared to that of known CB1 receptor distribution in the brain may be an indication of other putative functional roles of CB2 cannabinoid receptors in the brain and spinal cord. Therefore, both CB1 and CB2 receptors seem likely to work both independently and/or cooperatively in differing neuronal populations to regulate important physiological activities in the CNS. From the CB2 electron micrograph data presented here and from the immunohistochemical distribution patterns in the cerebellum, it can be postulated that the presence of CB2 immunoreactivity in the Purkinje cell bodies and dendrites may be indicative of the mainly postsynaptic localization. This is because the dendritic trees arising from the Purkinje cells are positive for CB2 immunoreactivity. However, these dendrites have been shown not to be immunostained for CB1 receptors confirming the presynaptic localization of CB1 receptors while as demonstrated in our study, the cell bodies of the Purkinje cells are immunoreactive for CB2 but negative for CB1 receptors as noted by others,[50,51] again confirming the established presynaptic localization of CB1 receptors in the brain. Another possibility is that CB2 cannabinoid receptors may be synthesized in the cell body of the Purkinje cells to be transported to another location. It has been documented that CB1 receptors are present in the axons coming from the basket cells located in the molecular layer that forms the basket cells around the basal area of the Purkinje.[50,52] The report[46] on the identification and functional characterization of brain stem cannabinoid CB2 receptors is consistent, in part, with our findings and with other reports of brain CB2 receptor expression.[4–11,28,35,47] However, a focus on brain stem localizations and antiemetic functions of brain cannabinoid CB2 receptors[46] may understate the importance of CB2 receptors in the other brain areas in which we and others have identified CB2 mRNA and protein. Thus, the previous interpretation that because CB2 was not detected in the brain but enriched in the peripheral tissues, particularly in immune cells and therefore targeting CB2 receptors by specific CB2 ligands may result in therapeutic activity without psychoactivity and may be valid for the wrong reasons. It appears that cannabinoids may have a more significant role in controlling neuroinflammation than previously thought.[47] Nevertheless, the distribution of CB2 immunoreactivity in the brain may provide novel targets for the effects of cannabinoids in the nervous system beyond neuroimmunocannabinoid activity.

ACKNOWLEDGMENTS

This work was supported financially by NIDA/IRP, NIH, DHSS and ESO acknowledges financial support from William Paterson University center for research. The CB2 knockout and their wild-type control mice used in this study were developed by Buckley *et al.* (2000)[53], and obtained from the National Institutes of Health.

REFERENCES

1. Matsuda, L.A., S.J. Lolait, *et al.* 1990. Structure of a cannabinoid receptor and functional expression of the cloned cDNA. Nature **346:** 561–564.
2. Onaivi, E.S. 2002. Biology of Marijuana: from Gene to Behavior. Taylor and Francis, CRC Press. Boca Raton.
3. Munro, S., K.L. Thomas, *et al.* 1993. Molecular characterization of a peripheral receptor for cannabinoids. Nature **365:** 61–65.
4. Meozzi, P.A., S. Patel, *et al.* 2004. Decreased alcohol consumption and enhanced cannabinoid CB2 receptor expression in mouse chronic mild stress model of depression. 7th Annual Undergraduate Research Symposium in the Chemical and Biological Sciences, UMBC. Baltimore, MD.
5. Onaivi, E.S., H. Ishiguro, *et al.* 2005. Presence and functional expression of peripheral cannabinoid CB2 receptors in the brain. College on Problems of drug dependency. Orlando, FL.
6. Onaivi, E.S., H. Ishiguro, *et al.* 2005. Peripheral cannabinoid CB2 receptors are expressed in the brain and involved in depression and substance abuse. 66. ICRS Symposium on Cannabinoids. Vermont USA.
7. Onaivi, E.S., H. Ishiguro, *et al.* 2005. Presence and functional expression of CB2 cannabinoid receptors in brain that is involved in depression and substance abuse. International Society for Neurochemistry/European Society for Neurochemistry Satellite meeting. Isola di San Servolo. Venice, Italy.
8. Gong, J-P., E.S. Onaivi, *et al.* 2005. Cannabinoid CB2 receptors: Immunohistochemical localization in rat brain. 91. ICRS symposium on cannabinoids. Vermont USA.
9. Onaivi, E.S., H. Ishiguro, *et al.* 2005. Presence and functional expression of CB2 cannabinoid receptors in the brain that is involved in depression and substance abuse. International Narcotic Research Society Meeting. Annapolis, MD.
10. Gong, J-P., E.S. Onaivi, *et al.* 2005. Peripheral cannabinoid CB2 receptors: expression in neuronal patterns and localization in rat brain. International Narcotic Research Society Meeting. Annapolis, MD.
11. Onaivi, E.S., H. Ishiguro, *et al.* 2005. Discovery of the presence and functional expression of CB2 cannabinoid receptors in brain that is involved in

depression and substance abuse. Society for Neuroscience Abstracts. Washington, DC.

12. BERDYSHEV, E.V. 2000. Cannabinoid receptors and the regulation of immune response. Chem. Phys. Lipids **108:** 169–190.
13. SUIGIURA, T. & K. WAKU. 2000. 2-Arachidonoylglycerol and cannabinoid receptors. Chem. Phys. Lipids **108:** 89–106.
14. WILSON, R.I. & R. NICOLL. 2001. Endogenous cannabinoids mediate retrograde signaling at hippocampal synapses. Nature **410:** 588–592.
15. CARLISLE, S.J., F. MARCIANO-CABRAL, *et al.* 2002. Differential expression of the CB2 cannabinoid receptor by rodent macrophages and marcophage-like cells in relation to cell activation. Int. J. Immunopharmacol. **2:** 69–82.
16. DEROCQ, J.M., M.J. SEGUI, *et al.* 1995. Cannabinoids enhance human B-cell growth at low nanomolar concentrations. FEBS Lett. **369:** 177–182.
17. GALIEGUE, S., S. MARY, *et al.* 1995. Expression of central and peripheral cannabinoid receptors in human immune tissues and leukocyte subpopulations. Eur. J. Biochem. **232:** 54–61.
18. GRIFFIN, G., E.J. WRAY, *et al.* 1999. Evaluation of the cannabinoid CB2 receptor-selective antagonist, SR144528: further evidence for CB2 receptor absence in the rat central nervous system. Eur. J. Pharmacol. **377:** 117–125.
19. SHATZ, A.R., M. LEE, *et al.* 1997. Cannabinoid receptors CB1 and CB2: a characterization of expression and adenylate cyclase modulation within the immune system. Toxicol. Appl. Pharmacol. **142:** 278–287.
20. KEARN, C.S. & C.J. HILLIARD. 1997. Rat microglial cell express the peripheral-type cannabinoid receptor (CB2) which is negatively coupled to adenyl cyclase. 61. ICRS Symposium on Cannabinoids. Vermont USA.
21. SKAPER, S.D., A. BURIANI, *et al.* 1996. The ALIAmide palmitoylethanolamide and cannabinoids, but not anandamide, are protective in a delayed postglutamate paradigm of excitotoxic death in cerebral granule neurons. Proc. Natl. Acad. Sci. USA. **93:** 3984–3989.
22. FACCI, L., R. DAL TOSO, *et al.* 1995. Mast cells express a peripheral cannabinoid receptor with differential sensitivity to anandamide and palmitoylethanolamide. Proc. Natl. Acad. Sci. USA. **92:** 3376–3380.
23. SAMSON, M-T., A. SMALL-HOWARD, *et al.* 2003. Differential roles of CB1 and CB2 cannabinoid receptors in mast cells. J. Immunol. **170:** 4953–4962.
24. LU, Q., A. STRAIKER, *et al.* 2000. Expression of CB2 cannabinoid receptor mRNA in adult rat retina. Vis. Neurosci. **17:** 91–95.
25. SHENG, W.S., S. HU, *et al.* 2005. Synthetic cannabinoid WIN55212-2 inhibits generation of inflammatory mediators by IL-IB-stimulated human astrocytes. Glia **49:** 211–219.
26. BENITO, C., W.K. KIM, *et al.* 2005. A glial endogenous cannabinoid system is upregulated in the brains of macaques with simian immunodeficiency virus-induced encephalitis. J. Neurosci. **25:** 2530–2536.
27. NUNEZ, E., C. BENITO, *et al.* 2004. Cannabinoid CB2 receptors are expressed by perivascular microglia cells in the human brain: an immunohistochemical study. Synapse **53:** 208–213.
28. PAZOS, M.R., E. NUNEZ, *et al.* 2004. Role of the endocannabinoid system in Alzheimer's disease: new perspectives. Life Sci. **75:** 1907–1915.
29. GOLECH, S.A., R.M. MCCARRON, *et al.* 2004. Human brain endothelium: coexpression and function of vanilloid and endocannabinoid receptors. Molec. Brain Res. **132:** 87–92.

30. BEN-SHABAT, S., E. FRIDE, *et al.* 1998. An entourage effect: inactive endogenous fatty acid glycerol esters enhance 2-arachidonyl-glycerol cannabinoid activity. Eur. J. Pharmacol. **353:** 23–31.
31. BENITO, C., E. NUNEZ, *et al.* 2003. Cannabinoid CB2 receptors and fatty acid amide hydrolase are selectively overexpressed in neuritic plaque-associated glia in Alzheimer's disease brains. J. Neurosci. **23:** 11136–11141.
32. SIPE, J.C., N. ARBOUR, *et al.* 2005. Reduced endocannabinoid immune modulation by a common cannabinoid 2 (CB2) receptor gene polymorphism: possible risk for autoimmune disorders. J. Leukoc. Biol. **78:** 231–238.
33. BROWN, S.M., J. WAGNER-MILLER, *et al.* 2002. Cloning and molecular characterization of the rat CB2 cannabinoid receptor. Biochim. Biophys. Acta **1576:** 255–264.
34. KARSAK, M., M. COHEN-SOLAL, *et al.* 2005. Cannabinoid receptor type 2 gene is associated with human osteoporosis. Human Molec. Gen. **14:** 3389–3396.
35. ONAIVI, E.S., H. ISHIGURO, *et al.* 2006. Methods to study the behavioral effects and expression of CB2 cannabinoid receptors and its gene transcripts in chronic mild stress model of depression. *In* Marijuana and Cannabinoid Research: Methods and Protocols. E.S. Onaivi. Ed.: 291–298. Humana Press Inc. Totowa, NJ.
36. LAUCKNER, J.E., F. REYES, *et al.* 2005. Distribution and functional characterization of a novel cannabinoid receptor. Society for Neuroscience Abstracts. Washington, DC.
37. SAWZDARGO, M., T. NGUYEN, *et al.* 1999. Identification and cloning of three novel human G protein-coupled receptor genes GPR52, uGPR53 and GPR55: GPR55 is extensively expressed in human brain. Mol. Brain Res. **64:** 193–198.
38. HILL, M.N., E.J. PATEL, *et al.* 2004. Downregulation of endocannabinoid signaling in the hippocampus following chronic unpredictable stress. Neuropyschopharmacology **30:** 508–511.
39. FRIDE, E., R. SURIS, *et al.* 2005. Differential response to acute and repeated stress in cannabinoid CB1 receptor knockout newborn and adult mice. Behav. Pharmacol. **16:** 431–471.
40. HILL, M.N. & B.B. GORZALKA. 2005. Is there a role for the endocannabinoid system in the etiology and treatment of melancholic depression. Behav. Pharmacol. **16:** 333–352.
41. VALENZANO, K.J., L. TAFASSE, *et al.* 2005. Pharmacological and pharmacokinetic characterization of the cannabinoid receptor 2 agonist, GW405833, utilizing rodent models of acute and chronic pain, anxiety, ataxia and catalepsy. Neuropharmacology **48:** 658–672.
42. KURRECK, J. 2003. Antisense technologies. Improvement through novel chemical modifications. Eur. J. Biochem. **270:** 1628–1644.
43. IBRAHIM, M.M., H. DENG, *et al.* 2003. Activation of CB2 cannabinoid receptors by AM1241 inhibits experimental neuropathic pain: pain inhibition by receptors not present in the brain. Proc. Natl. Acad. Sci. USA **100:** 10529–10533.
44. KLEIN, T.W., C. NEWTON, *et al.* 2003. The cannabinoid system and immune modulation. J. Leukocyte Biol. **74:** 486–496.
45. LEE, S.F., C. NEWTON, *et al.* 2001. Differential expression of cannabinoid CB2 receptor mRNA in mouse immune cell subpopulation and following B cell stimulation. J. Pharmacol. **423:** 235–241.
46. VAN SICKLE M.D., M. DUNCAN, *et al.* 2005. Identification and functional characterization of brainstem cannabinoid CB2 receptors. Science **310:** 329–332.

47. ASHTON, J.C., D. FRIBERG, *et al.* 2005. Expression of the cannabinoid CB2 receptor in the rat cerebellum: an immunohistochemical study. Neurosci Lett. **396:** 113–116.
48. GONG, J.P., E.S. ONAIVI, *et al.* 2006. Cannabinoid CB2 receptors: immunohistochemical localization in rat brain. Brain Res. **1071:** 10–23.
49. ZHANG, P-W., H. ISHIGURO, *et al.* 2004. Human cannabinoid receptor1: 5″ exons, candidate regulatory regions, polymorphisms, haplotypes and association with polysubstance abuse. Molec. Psychiatry **9:** 916–931.
50. PETTIT, D.A., M.P. HARRISON, *et al.* 1998. Immunohistochemical localization of the neural cannabinoid receptor in rat brain. Neurosci. Res. **51:** 391–342.
51. TSOU, K., S. BROWN, *et al.* 1998. immunohistochemical distribution of cannabinoid CB1 receptors in the rat central nervous system. Neuroscience **83:** 393–411.
52. ONAIVI, E.S., C.M. LEONARD, H. ISHIGURO, *et al.* 2002. Endocannabinoids and cannabinoid receptor genetics. Prog. Neurobiol. **66:** 307–344.
53. BUCKLEY, N.E. & K.L. MCCOY. 2000. Immunomodulation by cannabinoids is absent in mice deficient for the cannabinoid CB2 receptor. Eur. J. Pharmacol. **396:** 141–149.

γ-Hydroxybutyrate (GHB), γ-Butyrolactone (GBL), and 1,4-Butanediol (1,4-BD) Reduce the Volume of Cerebral Infarction in Rodent Transient Middle Cerebral Artery Occlusion

SHANKAR SADASIVAN,[a] TIMOTHY J. MAHER,[a] AND LAWRENCE S. QUANG[b]

[a]*Department of Pharamaceutical Sciences, Massachusetts College of Pharmacy and Health Sciences, Boston, Massachusetts, 02115 USA*

[b]*Division of Pediatric Emergency Medicine, Children's Hospital Boston, Harvard Medical School, Boston, Massachusetts, 02115 USA*

ABSTRACT: γ-Hydroxybutyric acid (GHB), an endogenous organic acid catabolite of γ-aminobutyric acid (GABA), has been shown to have tissue-protective effects in various organs, including the brain. We examined the potential neuroprotective effect of GHB and its chemical precursors, γ-butyrolactone (GBL) and 1,4-butanediol (1,4-BD), in the rodent ischemic stroke model by intraluminal filament middle cerebral artery occlusion (MCAO). Adult male Sprague-Dawley rats underwent transient left-sided MCAO and received intraperitoneal treatment with 300 mg/kg of GHB, GBL, 1,4-BD, or control vehicle given at 30 min before, as well as 180 and 360 min after the onset of ischemia. Infarct volumes were determined 24 h after MCAO. In transient MCAO, the mean volume of infarction for control rats was 464.4 $\pm$ 17.9 cu.mm versus 273.6 $\pm$ 53.1, 233.3 $\pm$ 44.7, and 275.4 $\pm$ 39.9 cu.mm for rats treated with 1,4-BD ($P <$ 0.05), GBL ($P <$ 0.05), and GHB ($P <$ 0.05), respectively. We conclude that GHB, GBL, and 1,4-BD protect against rat focal cerebral ischemia from transient MCAO.

KEYWORDS: γ-hydroxybutyric acid (GHB); γ-butyrolactone (GBL); 1,4-butanediol (1,4-BD); stroke; transient focal cerebral ischemia; middle cerebral artery occlusion (MCAO)

Address for correspondence: Lawrence S. Quang, M.D., Division of Pediatric Emergency Medicine, Rainbow Babies & Children's Hospital/Case Western Reserve University School of Medicine, 11100 Euclid Avenue, Cleveland, OH 44106. Voice: 216-844-3310; fax: 216-844-5122.
e-mail: lawrence.quang@case.edu

Ann. N.Y. Acad. Sci. 1074: 537–544 (2006). © 2006 New York Academy of Sciences.
doi: 10.1196/annals.1369.054

INTRODUCTION

γ-Hydroxybutyric acid (GHB) and its chemical precursors, γ-butyrolactone (GBL) and 1,4-butanediol (1,4-BD), have become popular recreational drugs during the past 15 years as reports of its "natural" euphoric and hallucinogenic properties popularized its illicit abuse.[1] Despite their recent emergence as popular recreational "club drugs," GHB continues to be the subject of medical research seeking licit therapeutic uses. As a result, GHB was recently approved by the U.S. Food and Drug Administration (FDA) as a pharmacotherapy for narcolepsy-associated cataplexy.[2] In Europe, GHB continues to be used and investigated medically as an anesthetic agent[3–6] and as treatment for alcohol dependence and withdrawal.[7–11] Experimentally, GHB has been proposed to be a potential neuroprotective agent for cerebral ischemia, and interesting and compelling preclinical data have recently been generated to demonstrate the efficacy of GHB as a neuroprotective agent in traumatic brain injury,[12,13] spinal cord injury,[14] and stroke.[15–17]

Several laboratories have studied the neuroprotective effects of GHB and GBL in rodent models of permanent and transient global cerebral ischemia. However, no studies have evaluated GHB or GBL as a potential neuroprotectant in a rodent model of transient focal cerebral ischemia, or reperfusion injury. Furthermore, no studies have evaluated 1,4-BD as a potential neuroprotectant in either permanent or transient focal cerebral ischemia. In this study, we evaluated the potential neuroprotective effects of GHB, GBL, and 1,4-BD in the rodent model of focal reperfusion injury by transient intraluminal filament occlusion of the middle cerebral artery.

MATERIALS AND METHODS

Animal Preparation

Our Institutional Animal Care and Use Committee approved all experimental procedures. Adult male Sprague-Dawley rats (250–325 g, Charles River Laboratories, Wilmington, MA) were housed in our climate-controlled facility with 12-h alternating light and dark cycles and had *ad libitum* access to food (Purina 5001) and tap water. The animals were acclimated to our facility for at least 3 days and were fasted on the evening before surgery. On the day of the experiment, rats underwent induction and maintenance anesthesia with 1–3% isoflurane in a 60/40% air/oxygen mixture delivered by nosecone. The core body temperature of the study animals was monitored by a rectal thermistor probe and maintained at 37°C throughout the surgical procedure using a heating pad.

Protocol for Transient Middle Cerebral Artery Occlusion (MCAO)

We induced transient focal MCAO by using a modification of the method of Aspey *et al.*[18] Under a stereoscopic operating microscope (Zeiss Model OMP1; Thornwood, NY), the left common carotid artery (CCA), external carotid artery (ECA), and internal carotid artery (ICA) were exposed via a ventral midline cervical incision. To prevent cerebral collateral blood flow, the occipital artery branches of the ECA and the pterygopalatine artery branch of the ICA were dissected free, isolated, and coagulated. A 3/0 monofilament nylon suture (Ethicon, Johnson & Johnson, Somerville, NJ), with its tip flanged by flame heating to avoid endothelial damage to the vessels, was advanced from the proximal CCA into the lumen of the ICA until it entered the circle of Willis to block the origin of the MCA, a distance of approximately 20 mm from the carotid bifurcation according to the weight of the animal. After the intraluminal monofilament nylon occluder was positioned to produce MCAO, it was trimmed so as to leave a small tag portion out of the lumen and secured in place by a silk suture ligature at the CCA. Animals were allowed to awaken from anesthesia in a small animal recovery chamber. At 60 min after MCAO, animals were tested on a standardized neurobehavioral battery to confirm the occurrence of a high-grade neurological motor deficit. Rats that demonstrated contralateral upper forelimb paresis and spontaneous contralateral circling were considered to have suffered a high-grade neurological motor deficit from MCAO and were re-anesthetized for the removal of the intraluminal suture after 90 min of MCAO. Animals not exhibiting these deficits were excluded from further study.

Experimental Groups

Experimental animals were randomly assigned to receive treatment with GHB, GBL, 1,4-BD, or control vehicle ($n = 8$ each group). All drugs were of the highest available purity (Sigma-Aldrich, St. Louis, MO, USA), dissolved in a vehicle of normal saline at a concentration of 10 mg/mL, and administered at a dose of 300 mg/kg by intraperitoneal injection at 30 min before MCAO as well as 180 and 360 min after MCAO. Control animals were administered normal saline at these treatment times.

Histopathological Determination of Infarct Volume

Computer-assisted volumetry was used to quantify stroke volume at 24 h after MCAO, whereupon brains were harvested, placed into a stainless steel 1.0-mm rodent coronal brain matrix for sectioning, and the sections stained with a 2% solution of 2,3,5-triphenyltetrazolium chloride (TTC, Sigma-Aldrich) at 37°C for 30 min and fixed in neutralized buffered 10% formalin at pH 7.4.

Grossly, the presence of a TTC-negative stained area indicated a stroke-positive area. Histological sections were digitalized with a 5.0 megapixel digital camera (Sony MVC-CD500, New York), and the digitalized photographs of gross views of the brain sections were exported into a Windows-based workstation employing the computer-assisted image analysis system and software, SigmaScan Pro® 5.0 (SPSS Inc., Chicago, IL). For each TTC-reacted brain section, the perimeter of each stroke lesion was outlined, and the lesion area was analyzed and calculated by the software. The volumes of infarction for each brain were then integrated and calculated from the respective calibrated area measurements made on the digitalized images of the TTC-reacted coronal slices of a given animal's brain. To minimize the potential error introduced by edema, an indirect method for calculating infarct volume was used whereby the infarct volume is presented as a percentage of the volume of the entire brain.

Data Analysis

Data in the present study are presented as the mean ± standard error of the mean (SEM). Statistical significance between infarct volumes was determined by ANOVA and supplemented by the Newman Keuls multiple range test for comparison of more than two groups or by the Student's *t*-test for comparison between two groups. A probability level of $P < 0.05$ was considered statistically significant.

RESULTS

All animals exhibited neurobehavioral signs of a high-grade neurological motor deficit from transient MCAO. The mean volume of infarction for control rats was 464.4 ± 17.9 cu.mm versus 273.6 ± 53.1, 233.3 ± 44.7, and 275.4 ± 39.9 cu.mm for rats treated with 1,4-BD ($P < 0.05$), GBL ($P < 0.05$), and GHB ($P < 0.05$), respectively (TABLE 1). Cortical infarct volumes were reduced by

TABLE 1. Volumes of infarction and percentages of total brain infarcted in Sprague-Dawley rats undergoing transient intraluminal filament occlusion of the MCAO and treatment with GHB, GBL, 1,4-BD, or control vehicle at 30 min before and 180 and 360 min after MCAO

	Transient MCAO		
	Volume of infarction (cu.mm.)	Percentage of brain infarcted (%)	*P* value
Control	464.4 ± 17.9	37.9 ± 2.0	–
GHB	275.5 ± 39.9	22.9 ± 3.3	<0.05
GBL	233.3 ± 44.7	18.9 ± 3.6	<0.05
1,4-BD	273.6 ± 53.1	22.6 ± 4.4	<0.05

GHB, GBL, and 1,4-BD by a mean of 41%, 50%, and 41%, respectively. The mean percentage volume of total brain infarcted for control animals was 37.9 ± 2.0% versus 22.6 ± 4.4%, 18.9 ± 3.6%, and 22.9 ± 3.3% for rats treated with 1,4-BD ($P < 0.05$), GBL ($P < 0.05$), and GHB ($P < 0.05$), respectively (TABLE 1).

DISCUSSION

The main findings of the present study are: (*a*) a single pretreatment dose of GHB, GBL, and 1,4-BD did not prevent or reduce the occurrence of a high-grade neurological motor deficit observed immediately after the onset of the ischemic insult; (data not shown) (*b*) two additional postinfarction doses of GHB, GBL, and 1,4-BD significantly reduced infarct volumes in transient MCAO; and (*c*) there was an apparent equal efficacy among GHB, GBL, and 1,4-BD in reducing stroke volumes in transient MCAO.

These findings are consistent with the small body of published literature reporting GHB neuroprotective effects, as GHB has been shown to exert tissue protective effects in both *in vitro* and *in vivo* model systems. Specifically, GHB and GBL have been shown to be protective in gastrointestinal,[19] hepatic,[20] myocardial,[21,22] and cerebral[15–17,23–32] models of ischemia. With respect to the latter, past studies have reported that GHB and GBL produce cerebral neuroprotection by decreasing cerebral energy metabolism and oxygen consumption in the hypoxic-ischemic rodent, canine, and human brain.[23–32] While previous *in vivo* animal data support the role for GHB and GBL as neuroprotectants in acute ischemic stroke, none of these studies employed a focal cerebral ischemia model that more closely mimics the clinical situation of human stroke, where stroke lesions are generally focal and the middle cerebral artery is the most frequently embolized artery. Furthermore, no prior studies have evaluated GHB, GBL, or 1,4-BD neuroprotection in cerebral models of focal transient ischemia, or stroke reperfusion injury. Last, no prior studies have evaluated 1,4-BD as a potential neuroprotectant in any model of cerebral ischemia.

To our knowledge, the present study is the first to evaluate the neuroprotective effects of GHB and GBL in the rodent model of *focal transient* cerebral ischemia by MCAO. Delayed, secondary neuronal tissue injury following primary recovery after recanalization, or reperfusion injury, is a common pathophysiologic feature that has been well described in experimental stroke models. Several mechanisms are associated with reperfusion injury, including free radical formation, protein synthesis inhibition, apoptosis, glutamate-related excitotoxicity, and blood–brain barrier disruption.[33] While the present study does not provide a mechanistic explanation, it demonstrates GHB, GBL, and 1,4-BD to exert significant neuroprotective effects in rats with experimentally induced reperfusion injury by transient MCAO. Furthermore, this is the first study to demonstrate a neuroprotective effect of 1,4-BD in any model of cerebral ischemia. Future studies will need to assess the efficacy of GHB, GBL, and 1,4-BD as a neuroprotectant solely in the post-infarct epoch as well as their efficacy in preserving or minimizing stroke neurocognitive and sensorimotor deficits.

ACKNOWLEDGMENTS

This research was supported by National Institutes of Health (NIH)/National Institute of Child Health and Human Development (NICHHD) grant 1T32 HD40128-02 (Dr. Quang) and NIH/National Institute on Drug Abuse (NIDA) grant 1RO3 DA14951-02 (Dr. Quang).

REFERENCES

1. SHANNON, M. & L. QUANG. 2000. Gamma-hydroxybutyrate, gamma-butyrolactone, and 1,4-butanediol: a case report and review of the literature. Ped. Emerg. Care **16:** 435–440.
2. FULLER, D.E., C.S. HORNFELDT, J.S. KELLOWAY, *et al.* 2004. The Xyrem risk management program. Drug Saf. **27:** 293–306.
3. KLEINSCHMIDT, S., U. GRUNDMANN, U. JANNECK, *et al.* 1997. Total intravenous anesthesia using propofol, gamma-hydroxybutyrate or midazolam in combination with sufentanil for patients undergoing coronary artery bypass surgery. Eur. J. Anaesthesiol. **14:** 590–599.
4. KLEINSCHMIDT, S., U. GRUNDMANN, T. KNOCKE, *et al.* 1998. Total intravenous anaesthesia with gamma-hydroxybutyrate (GHB) and sufentanil in patients undergoing coronary artery bypass graft surgery: a comparison in patients with unimpaired and impaired left ventricular function. Eur. J. Anaesthesiol. **15:** 559–564.
5. KLEINSCHMIDT, S., C. SCHELLHASE & F. MERTZUFFT. 1999. Continuous sedation during spinal anaesthesia: gamma-hydroxybutyrate vs propofol. Eur. J. Anaesthesiol. **16:** 23–30.
6. EUROPEAN MONITORING CENTRE FOR DRUGS AND DRUG ADDICTION. Report on the risk assessment of GHB in the framework of the joint action on new synthetic drugs (electronic source). http://www.emcdda.eu.int/?nnodeid=2821 (accessed April 2005).
7. GALLIMBERTI, L., M.R. SPELLA, C.A. SONCINI, *et al.* 2000. Gamma-hydroxybutric acid in the treatment of alcohol and heroine dependence. Alcohol **20:** 257–262.
8. GALLIMBERTI, L., G. CANTON, N. GENTILE, *et al.* 1989. Gamma-hydroxybutyric acid for treatment of alcohol withdrawal syndrome. Lancet **2:** 787–789.
9. GALLIMBERI, L., M. FERRI, S.D. FERRARA, *et al.* 1992. Gamma-hydroxybutyric acid in the treatment of alcohol dependence: a double blind study. Alcohol Clin. Exp. Res. **16:** 673–676.
10. ADDOLORATO, G., M. CIBIN, E. CAPRISTA, *et al.* 1999. Maintaining abstinence from alcohol with gamma-hydroxybutyric acid. Lancet **351:** 38.

11. Addolorato, G., E. Castelli, G.F. Stefanini, *et al.* 1996. An open multicentric study evaluating 4-hydroxybuytric acid sodium salt in the medium-term treatment of 179 alcohol dependent subjects. Alcohol Alcohol. **31:** 341–345.
12. Yosunkaya, A., H. Bariskaner, M.E. Ustun, *et al.* 2004. Effect of gamma-hydroxybutyric acid on lipid peroxidation and tissue lactate level in experimental head trauma. J. Trauma **56:** 585–590.
13. Yosunkaya, A., M.E. Ustun, H. Bariskaner, *et al.* 2004. Effect of gamma-hydroxybutyric acid on tissue Na+,K- ATPase levels after experimental head trauma. Acta Anaesthesiol. Scand. **48:** 631–636.
14. Guney, O., J. Bengi Celik, M. Arazi, *et al.* 2004. Effects of gamma-hydroxybutyrate on cerebrospinal fluid lactate and glucose levels after spinal cord trauma. J. Clin. Neurosci. **11:** 517–520.
15. Vergoni, A.V., A. Ottani, A.R. Botticelli, *et al.* 2000. Neuroprotective effect of γ-hydroxybutyrate in transient global cerebral ischemia in the rat. Eur. J. Pharmacol. **397:** 75–84.
16. Ottani, A., S. Saltini, M. Bartiromo, *et al.* 2003. Effect of gamma-hydroxybutyrate in two rat models of focal cerebral damage. Brain Res. **986:** 181–190.
17. Ottani, A., A.V. Vergoni, S. Saltini, *et al.* Effect of late treatment with gamma-hydroxybutyrate on the histological and behavioral consequences of transient brain ischemia in the rat. Eur. J. Pharmacol. **485:** 183–191.
18. Aspey, B.S., F.L. Taylor, M. Terruli, *et al.* 2000. Temporary middle cerebral artery occlusion in the rat: consistent protocol for a model of stroke and reperfusion. Neuropathol. Appl. Neurobiol. **26:** 232–242.
19. Boyd, A.J., I.A. Sherman, F.G. Saibil, *et al.* 1990. The protective effect of gamma-hydroxybutyrate in regional intestinal ischemia in the hamster. Gastroenterology **99:** 860–862.
20. Sherman, I.A., F.G. Saibil & T.I. Janossy. 1994. Gamma-hydroxybutyrate mediated protection of liver function after long-term hypothermic storage. Transplantation **57:** 8–11.
21. Boyd, A.J., I.A. Sherman & F.G. Saibil. 1992. The cardiovascular effects of gamma-hydroxybutyrate following hemorrhage. Circ. Shock **38:** 115–121.
22. Dosmugambetova, R.S. 1983. Prevention of stress-related disorders in the contractile function of non-ischemic areas of the heart during myocardial infarction using gamma-hydroxybutyric acid. Bull. Exp. Biol. Med. **96:** 28–30.
23. Wolfson, L.I., O. Sakurada & L. Sokolorff. 1977. Effects of gamma-butyrolactone on local cerebral glucose utilization in the rat. J. Neurochem. **29:** 777–783.
24. Escuret, E., B. Roquefeuil, P. Frerebean, *et al.* 1977. Effect of hyperventilation associated with administration of central nervous depressants in brain injuries. Acta. Neurol. Scand. **56:** 154–155.
25. Escuret, E., C. Chapron, C. Geniez-Bouscarel, *et al.* 1982. Cerebral metabolic depression induced by sodium gamma-hydroxybutyrate in the treatment of severe traumatic comas. Agressologie **23:** 51–56.
26. Escuret, E., B. Roquefeuil, P. Frerebeau, *et al.* 1981. Cerebral metabolic effect of gamma-hydroxybutyrate in neurosurgical patients on artificial respiration. Agressologie **22:** 163–167.
27. MacMillan, V. 1978. The effects of gamma-hydroxybutyrate and gamma-butyrolactone upon the energy metabolism of the normoxic and hypoxic rat brain. Brain Res. **146:** 177–187.

28. MacMillan, V. 1979. A comparison of γ-hydroxybutyrate and γ-butyrolactone on cerebral carbohydrate metabolism. Can. J. Physiol. Pharmacol. **57:** 787–797.
29. Bralet, J., P. Beley, A.M. Bralet, *et al.* 1979. Influence of various agents on the development of brain edema in the rat following microembolism: protective effect of gamma-butyrolactone. Stroke **10:** 653–656.
30. Artru, A.A., P.A. Steen & J.D. Michenfelder. 1980. γ-Hydroxybutyrate: cerebral metabolic, vascular, and protective effects. J. Neurochem. **35:** 1114–1119.
31. Lavyne, M.H., R.J. Hariri, T. Tankosic, *et al.* 1983. Effect of low dose γ-butyrolactone therapy on forebrain neuronal ischemia in the unrestrained, awake rat. Neurosurgery **12:** 430–434.
32. MacMillan, V. 1980. Effects of gamma-hydroxybutyrate and gamma-butyrolactone on cerebral energy metabolism during exposure and recovery from hypoxemia-oligemia. Stroke **11:** 271–277.
33. Lo, E.H., T. Dalkara & M.A. Moskowitz. 2003. Mechanisms, challenges and opportunities in stroke. Natl. Rev. Neurosci. **4:** 399–415.

Evaluation for the Withdrawal Syndrome from γ-Hydroxybutyric Acid (GHB), γ-Butyrolactone (GBL), and 1,4-Butanediol (1,4-BD) in Different Rat Lines

LAWRENCE S. QUANG,[a] GIANCARLO COLOMBO,[b] CARLA LOBINA,[b] PAOLA MACCIONI,[b,c] ALESSANDRO ORRU`,[b,c] GIAN LUIGI GESSA,[b] TIMOTHY J. MAHER,[d] AND MAURO A.M. CARAI[b]

[a]*Divisions of Pediatric Pharmacology & Critical Care and Pediatric Emergency Medicine, Rainbow Babies and Children's Hospital/Case Western Reserve University School of Medicine, Cleveland, Ohio 44106, USA*

[b]*CNR Institute of Neuroscience, I-09126 Cagliari, Italy*

[c]*Department of Neuroscience, University of Cagliari, I-09126 Cagliari, Italy*

[d]*Massachusetts College of Pharmacy and Health Sciences, Boston, Massachusetts, 02115 USA*

ABSTRACT: A severe and life-threatening γ-hydroxybutyric acid (GHB) withdrawal syndrome, clinically similar to the alcohol withdrawal syndrome, is increasingly being reported in GHB addicts. We investigated for the occurrence of withdrawal in Wistar and Sprague-Dawley rats, and in the selectively bred lines of GHB-sensitive (GHB-S) and Sardinian alcohol-preferring (sP) rats, following chronic administration of GHB, γ-butyrolactone (GBL), and/or 1,4-butanediol (1,4-BD). Using validated rodent alcohol withdrawal scoring scales, little to no spontaneous or pharmacologically precipitated withdrawal effects were observed in Wistar, Sprague-Dawley, or GHB-S rats. Conversely, sP rats displayed both spontaneous and precipitated audiogenic seizures following abrupt cessation of chronic GHB or 1,4-BD administration and following pharmacological challenge with the $GABA_B$ receptor-selective antagonist, SCH 50911, respectively.

KEYWORDS: γ-hydroxybutyric acid (GHB); γ-butyrolactone (GBL); 1,4-butanediol (1,4-BD); withdrawal syndrome; $GABA_B$ receptor-selective antagonist SCH 50911; Sardinian alcohol-preferring (sP) rats; GHB-sensitive (GHB-S) rats

Address for correspondence: Lawrence S. Quang, M.D., Division of Pediatric Pharmacology & Critical Care, Rainbow Babies & Children's Hospital, 11100 Euclid Avenue, Cleveland, OH 44106. Voice: 216-844-3310; fax: 216-844-5122.
e-mail: lawrence.quang@case.edu

Ann. N.Y. Acad. Sci. 1074: 545–558 (2006).
doi: 10.1196/annals.1369.055

INTRODUCTION

Recently, there has been a dramatic surge in the clinical reporting of a severe withdrawal syndrome following the abrupt cessation of chronic, high-dose abuse with the recreational drug γ-hydroxybutyric acid (GHB) and its precursors, 1,4-butanediol (1,4-BD), and γ-butyrolactone (GBL). The rapid and recent emergence of the GHB withdrawal syndrome represents a significant shift in the clinical paradigm of GHB-related toxicity. Prior to 2000, reports of clinical toxicity from abuse of GHB, GBL, and 1,4-BD, were overwhelmingly related to poisonings in the setting of acute overdose and rarely from complications of addiction, such as withdrawal. As of this writing, there are 101 published case reports of GHB withdrawal in the clinical literature.[1–30] Only eight of these GHB withdrawal case reports can be traced to the clinical literature between 1994 and 1999[1–6]; the remaining 93 GHB withdrawal case reports have been published in the clinical literature since 2000,[7–30] which represents more than a 10-fold increase in incidence or awareness during the past 5 years. Outside of the published medical literature, there is additional evidence that the GHB withdrawal syndrome is occurring with greater frequency. GHB withdrawal accounted for 8.4% of the toxicity from GHB exposures (30/356 GHB exposures) recorded by the California Poison Control System in 1999, and an Internet help site for GHB addiction recorded 184 cases of withdrawal in 33 U.S. states in 2001.[18]

A rapidly emerging disease of GHB addiction with severe and potentially life-threatening clinical consequences, the GHB withdrawal syndrome shares some clinical similarities with those of alcohol withdrawal, including occurrence of tremor, tachycardia, anxiety, restlessness, hallucinations (primarily visual and auditory), delirium, insomnia, delusions, paranoia, diaphoresis, hypertension, nausea or vomiting, and psychosis.[1–30] Two seizures have been reported during GHB withdrawal, one of which was associated with death.[18,30] While the clinical symptoms and signs of GHB withdrawal are becoming identified and well defined, the neurobiology, pathophysiology, and treatment of the GHB withdrawal syndrome are poorly understood. A significant impediment in the progress in these aspects of GHB withdrawal research is the lack of a validated animal model. We describe a series of experiments that evaluated the occurrence of GHB withdrawal in several rat lines and report success in generating audiogenic withdrawal seizures in only the selectively bred line of Sardinian alcohol-preferring (sP) rats.

MATERIALS AND METHODS

Materials

We evaluated for signs of GHB withdrawal in four different rat lines: Experiment 1—Wistar (Charles River Laboratories, Calco, LC, Italy); Experiment

2—Sprague-Dawley (Charles River Laboratories, Wilmington, MA); Experiment 3—GHB-sensitive (GHB-S); and and Experiment 4—sP rats. Rats of the GHB-S and sP lines were bred at the CNR Institute of Neuroscience, Cagliari, Italy. In all experiments, four rats were housed per cage in standard plastic cages with wood chip bedding under standard environmental conditions. Water and standard rat chow were available *ad libitum* in the home cages. GHB (sodium salt; donated by Laboratorio Farmaceutico CT, Sanremo, IM, Italy, for Experiments 1, 3, and 4; purchased from Sigma-Aldrich, St. Louis, MO, for Experiment 2), 1,4-BD (Sigma-Aldrich, Milan, Italy, for Experiment 4; Sigma-Aldrich for Experiment 2), and GBL (Sigma-Aldrich for Experiment 2) were dissolved in distilled water in a volume of 10 mL/kg. SCH 50911 [(2*S*)-5,5-dimethyl-2-morpholineacetic acid; Tocris Cookson, Bristol, UK] was dissolved in saline in a volume of 1 mL/kg. NCS-382 (sodium salt of 6,7,8,9-tetrahydro-5-hydroxy-5H-benzocyclohept-6-ylideneacetic acid; Tocris Cookson) was dissolved in saline containing 0.1 N sodium bicarbonate in a volume of 2 mL/kg.

Study Protocols

Experiment 1—Wistar Rats

GHB (15% w/v) or control vehicle (water) was administered intragastrically (i.g.), 4 times/day (06:00, 12:00, 18:00 and 24:00) for five consecutive days, to 35 male Wistar rats (n = 30 GHB-treated rats, n = 5 control rats). The intoxication procedure involved the administration of doses of GHB chosen on the basis of the level of intoxication of each single rat immediately before each GHB administration: neutrality (absence of any intoxication sign) = 2.5 g/kg; ataxia 1 (locomotion only when stimulated, modest muscle flaccidity) = 2 g/kg; ataxia 2 (immobility, marked muscle flaccidity) = 1.5 g/kg; and ataxia 3 (slow regaining of the righting reflex) = 0.75 g/kg; loss of righting reflex = 0 g/kg. This scale was conceived from the Majchrowicz scale for alcohol intoxication.[31] After 5 days of drug administration, rats were observed and scored for withdrawal signs between 9 and 21 h after the last GHB administration; the GHB receptor-selective antagonist NCS 382 (400 mg/kg, i.p.) was administered to four rats 12 h after the last GHB administration. Due to the paucity of published research on GHB withdrawal in laboratory animals, we evaluated study animals for a broad spectrum of GHB-related withdrawal signs that included the presence or absence of a number of spontaneous behaviors and responses to handling that have characterized rodent withdrawal syndromes from other drugs of abuse, including alcohol, opioids, and nicotine. Specifically, we evaluated experimental rats for locomotor hyperactivity, running episodes, treading, reverse motion, back arching, head shaking, wet dog shakes, teeth chattering, chewing, grooming, dipping, excessive sniffing, aggression, salivation, rhinorrhea, lacrimation, penile erection, penile ejaculation, diarrhea, piloerection, body tremors, head tremors, tail tremors, muscle rigidity, tail rigidity, altered posture, spontaneous and handling-stimulated vocalization, and seizures.

Experiment 2—Sprague-Dawley Rats

Twenty-four adult male Sprague-Dawley rats were divided into four groups ($n = 6$) that received a 6-day treatment regimen with control vehicle or equimolar doses of GHB (1025 mg/kg, intraperitoneal [i.p.]), GBL (700 mg/kg, i.p.), and 1,4-BD (732 mg/kg, i.p.) every 3 h. The intoxication procedure involved the administration of doses of GHB, GBL, and 1,4-BD chosen on the basis of the level of intoxication of each single rat immediately before each GHB, GBL, or 1,4-BD administration: mild sedation and ataxia or none at all = full dose of GHB, GBL, or 1,4-BD; moderate sedation and ataxia = half dose of GHB, GBL, or 1,4-BD; and coma, loss of righting reflex, or severe ataxia = no dose. At the end of the dosing regimen, rats were scored for GHB withdrawal by employing an alcohol withdrawal scoring system originally described by Lal *et al.* and modified by Colombo *et al.*[32,33] This withdrawal scoring system used a simple 4-point Likert scale (0–3, paralleling increased frequency of occurrence and/or degree of severity) to assess 11 separate neurobehavioral outcome measures. Some outcome measures (general activity, shakes, jerks, head tremors, bracing posture, and spontaneous convulsions) were rated before touching the rat, while assessment of other outcome measures required palpation (namely, general tremors, tail tremors, rigidity of muscle tone, and tail rigidity) or handling stimulation (vocalization). The sum of the 11 values was the total score assigned to each rat on each observation. In this modified alcohol withdrawal rating scale, total scores of 8–9 indicate a neutral clinical state, corresponding to a healthy and undrugged rat. Lower scores indicate intoxication, with scores ≤ 4 indicating severe intoxication. Higher scores indicate withdrawal, with scores of ≥ 18 indicating severe withdrawal. A total score was calculated for each rat at 3, 6, 9, 12, 24, 48, and 72 h after the last dose of GHB, GBL, 1,4-BD, or control vehicle.

Experiment 3—GHB-S Rats

Twenty GHB-S rats were administered control vehicle ($n = 10$) or GHB ($n = 10$) i.g. twice daily in the following escalating dosing regimen over 11 days: GHB 1.5 g/kg for day 1; GHB 2 g/kg for day 2; GHB 2.5 g/kg GHB for days 3–7; GHB 3 g/kg GHB for days 8–9; and GHB 3.5 g/kg GHB days 10–11. On day 12, rats were administered the $GABA_B$ receptor-selective antagonist, SCH 50911 (50 mg/kg, i.p.), in an attempt to precipitate a withdrawal syndrome.

Fifteen minutes later, rats were evaluated for signs of withdrawal-related motor hyperactivity and anxiety-related behaviors by observation with open field testing. The floor of the open field was divided into 25 squares, 16 in an outer circle, and 9 in an inner area; this permitted differentiation between behaviors performed in the "safe" and "comfortable" portion of the arena (outer circle), and those behaviors that occurred in the "uncomfortable" and "anxiogenic" portion (the inner area) of the arena. Specifically, the following variables were assessed in an open field test: time spent moving, number of crossings, number of rearings, number of fecal boluses, time spent grooming, and number of wet dog shakes. Rats were exposed to the open field test for 10 consecutive min.

Experiment 4—sP Rats

Experiment 4 was conducted in three phases. In Experiment 4A, sP rats ($n =$ 15) were treated with GHB i.g. twice daily (at 8:00 AM and 8:00 PM) for nine consecutive days, with increasing doses of GHB. Specifically, the following escalating schedule of GHB administration was used: 1.5 g/kg on day 1; 2 g/kg on days 2 and 3; 2.5 g/kg on days 4 and 5; 3 g/kg on days 6 and 7; and 3.5 g/kg on days 8 and 9. Control rats ($n = 10$) received an equal volume (10 mL/kg) of distilled water vehicle. The escalating dosing regimen for GHB was derived from preliminary experiments in this lab, which succeeded in maintaining the rats in a steady state of intoxication and compensated for the development of tolerance. In Experiment 4B, rats ($n = 40$) were treated with increasing doses of 1,4-BD i.g. twice daily (at 8:00 AM and 8:00 PM) for nine consecutive days. Specifically, the following escalating schedule of 1,4-BD administration was adopted: 500 mg/kg on day 1; 650 mg/kg on days 2 and 3; 850 mg/kg on days 4 and 5; and 1000 mg/kg on days 6–9. Control rats ($n = 30$) received an equal volume (10 mL/kg) of distilled water vehicle. The dosing regimen of 1,4-BD was adapted for its higher potency in comparison with that of GHB; indeed, sedation/hypnosis of comparable duration was observed in rats with 500 mg/kg 1,4-BD and 1 g/kg GHB. In Experiment 4C, SCH 50911 (50 mg/kg, i.p.) was acutely injected, 30 min before the administration of acoustic stimuli and assessment for audiogenic seizures, to 1,4-BD chronically treated rats ($n = 10$) and control rats ($n = 10$). In all experiments, rats were tested for audiogenic seizures as a sign of withdrawal syndrome at 18–24 h after the last administration of GHB or 1,4-BD. Specifically, rats were placed, one at a time, in a plastic cylindrical chamber (60 cm diameter, 100 cm high) and exposed to acoustic stimuli for 60 consecutive seconds by manually shaking a ring of 10 metal keys (sound pressure level: 102 $dB_{re20\mu Pa}$, with acoustic energy [99.99%] concentrated in the high frequency range [>2 kHz] as revealed by a spectrum analyzer [Larson Davis, Provo, UT]). The cylinder was located in a quiet, soundproof, and dimly lit room adjacent to the housing room. An operator who was blinded to group allocation administered the acoustic stimuli.

Data Analysis

Data from Experiments 1 and 2 were not subjected to any statistical analysis. Data from Experiment 3 were statistically analyzed as follows: data on total time spent moving, time spent moving in the inner area, total number of crossings, number of crossing in the inner area, number of rearings, number of fecal boluses and time spent moving were analyzed by separate unpaired, 2-tailed Mann-Whitney U tests; and data on the number of rats displaying episodes of wet dog shakes were analyzed by the Fisher's exact test for a 2 $\times$ 2 table (treatment [vehicle, GHB] $\times$ wet dog shakes [presence, absence]). In Experiment 4, occurrence of audiogenic seizures was evaluated by a Fisher's exact test for a 2 $\times$ 2 table (treatment [vehicle, GHB or 1,4-BD] $\times$ seizure [presence, absence]). In all data analyses, statistical significance was set an alpha value of 0.05.

RESULTS

Experiment 1—Wistar Rats

Thirteen of 30 rats died during the intoxication procedure, likely due to overdose. TABLE 1 illustrates the number of rats, out of the 13 undergoing the withdrawal phase, that displayed some bizarre behaviors or responses to handling. Specifically, GHB-withdrawn rats displayed some episodes of eye closing, dipping, chewing, treading, reverse motion, back arching, grooming, and yawning, which were virtually absent in control rats. NCS 382 administration did not increase the occurrence of any of the above bizarre behaviors or responses to handling.

Experiment 2—Sprague-Dawley Rats

Mortality for treated animals was high: two of six GHB rats, six of six GBL rats, and three of six 1,4-BD rats. The results, summarized in TABLE 2, suggest that there were no differences in the withdrawal scores among GHB-rat groups.

Experiment 3—GHB-S Rats

No rat died during the intoxication phase. When rats were tested in the open field arena, there were no differences for any of the withdrawal-related outcome measures between GHB-S rats chronically treated with GHB and their vehicle

TABLE 1. Occurrence of bizarre behaviors or responses in handling in GHB-withdrawn Wistar rats (Experiment 1)

Bizarre behaviors or responses to handling	Time (in h) after the last GHB administration																							
	9			10			11			12			14			16			18			21		
	C	S	T	C	S	T	C	S	T	C	S	T	C	S	T	C	S	T	C	S	T	C	S	T
Head tremors																				1				
Treading					1	1		2	1		1	2		2						1	1			
Reverse motion		2			1			2			2			1										
Arched back		2			1												1							
Head shake					1						1													
Teeth chattering					1						1													
Chewing					2			1			5	1		2	2		5	2		1	1			
Grooming				1	3	3		3	1		2	2		1						1				
Dipping		6			6	1		5			3	1		3	2		2	1		2				
Closed eyes		7	2		10	3	1	9	3		11	4		9	4		10	4		7	2		2	
Diarrhea																	1							
Penile erection																	1							
Yawning					1			3			2	2		1										
Handling-induced Vocalization											1													

NOTE: The rats were divided into three experimental groups: one group (C; n = 5) consisted of rats treated with control vehicle (water) for 5 consecutive days; one group (S; n = 13) was treated with intoxicating doses of GHB for 5 consecutive days and then underwent a withdrawal phase without any pharmacological, precipitating treatment; and one group (T; n = 4) was treated with intoxicating doses of GHB for 5 consecutive days and then underwent a withdrawal phase, which included the acute injection of NCS 382 (400 mg/kg, i.p.) 12 h after the last GHB administration.

TABLE 2. Withdrawal scores in Sprague-Dawley rats treated with control vehicle, GHB, GBL, and 1,4-BD from Experiment 2

	Withdrawal score (hour after last dose)						
Animal	3	6	9	12	24	48	72
Control 1	10	9	7	7	8	9	10
Control 2	10	8	7	7	10	10	9
Control 3	10	9	7	7	8	10	8
Control 4	10	9	7	7	9	9	10
Control 5	10	10	7	7	10	10	9
Control 6	10	9	7	7	9	9	10
GHB 1	10	9	7	7	9	9	10
GHB 2	8	6	5	4	9	4	Expired
GHB 3	10	8	8	7	5	10	9
GHB 5	11	9	9	7	10	9	9
1,4-BD 1	10	11	8	8	8	8	11
1,4-BD 4	13	8	8	7	10	9	9
1,4-BD 6	8	8	8	7	11	9	10

NOTE: Twenty-four rats were divided into 4 groups ($n = 6$) that received a 6-day treatment regimen with control vehicle or equimolar doses of GHB (1025 mg/kg, i.p.), GBL (700 mg/kg, i.p.), and 1,4-BD (732 mg/kg, i.p.) every 3 h. The intoxication procedure involved the administration of doses of GHB, GBL, and 1,4-BD chosen on the basis of the level of intoxication of each single rat immediately before each administration: mild sedation and ataxia or none at all = full dose of GHB, GBL, or 1,4-BD; moderate sedation and ataxia = half dose; and coma, loss of righting reflex, or severe ataxia = no dose. At the end of the dosing regimen, the rats were scored for GHB withdrawal by employing an alcohol withdrawal scoring system that assessed 11 separate neurobehavioral outcome measures for frequency and intensity of occurrence. There was 100% (6/6) mortality for GBL-treated rats.

controls, except for wet dog shakes that occurred in some GHB-withdrawn rats and in no control rat (TABLE 3).

Experiment 4—sP Rats

Data are illustrated in TABLE 4. In Experiment 4A, 5 of 15 GHB-treated rats died during the intoxication phase, likely due to overdose. No rats of the control group exhibited seizures after the delivery of the auditory stimulus; in contrast, audiogenic seizures occurred in 6 of 10 GHB-withdrawn rats ($P = 0.01$). In Experiment 4B, 10 of 40 1,4-BD-treated rats died during the intoxication phase, likely due to overdose. Again, no control rat displayed audiogenic seizures; in contrast, audiogenic seizures occurred in a statistically significant portion (6/22) of 1,4-BD-withdrawn rats ($P = 0.02$). In Experiment 4C, acute administration of SCH 50911 did not induce any seizure episode in control rats; in contrast, most of the rats of the 1,4-BD-withdrawn group (8/10) had audiogenic seizures ($P = 0.0007$).

TABLE 3. Measures of exploratory behavior or anxiety-related responses in GHB-S rats exposed to an open field arena after treatment with either control vehicle ($n = 10$) or GHB ($n = 10$) i.g. twice daily in the escalating dosing regimen (1.5–3.5 g/kg; see Materials and Methods for details) over 11 days (Experiment 3)

Experiment	Total time spent moving (s)	Time spent moving in inner (s)	Total number of crossings	Number of crossings in inner	Number of rearings	Number of fecal boluses	Time spent grooming (s)	Number of rats with wet dog shakes
Control rats	264.9 ± 30.2	26.1 ± 6.0	89.5 ± 15.0	12.6 ± 3.7	16.6 ± 5.1	0.7 ± 0.3	10.2 ± 3.7	0/10
GHB-withdrawn rats	228.4 ± 42.3	25.7 ± 9.8	59.3 ± 14.2	14.9 ± 2.9	12.3 ± 3.4	0.9 ± 0.4	17.0 ± 4.4	5/10*

NOTE: Exposure to the open field arena occurred on day 12, 15 min after the acute administration of the $GABA_B$ receptor-selective antagonist SCH 50911 (50 mg/kg, i.p.), and lasted for 10 consecutive min. $P < 0.05$ with respect to control rats (Fisher's exact test for a 2×2 table).

TABLE 4. Occurrence of audiogenic seizures in sP rats treated with GHB, 1,4-BD, and 1,4-BD/SCH 50911 from Experiments 4A-C, respectively

Experiment	Treated rats	Control rats	*P* value
4A- GHB treatment	6/10	0/10	0.01
4B- 1,4-BD treatment	6/22	0/20	0.02
4C- 1,4-BD treatment followed by SCH 50911 challenge	8/10	0/10	0.02

NOTE: In Experiment 4A, rats were treated twice daily, and for 9 consecutive days, with increasing doses of GHB (1.5–3.5 g/kg; see Materials and Methods for details). In Experiment 4B, rats were treated twice daily, and for 9 consecutive days, with increasing doses of 1,4-BD (500–1000 mg/kg; see Materials and Methods for details). In Experiment 4C, SCH 50911 (50 mg/kg, i.p.) was acutely injected 30 min before exposure to acoustic stimuli to 1,4-BD chronically treated rats and control rats. In all experiments, control rats received an equal volume (10 mL/kg) of distilled water vehicle. Rats were tested for audiogenic seizures as a sign of withdrawal syndrome at 18–24 h after the last administration of GHB or 1,4-BD.

DISCUSSION

Although different intoxication procedures were used, the results of the present series of experiments suggest an apparent differential sensitivity of four rat species to GHB withdrawal-related effects. Experiments 1 and 2 failed to generate withdrawal effects in Wistar and Sprague-Dawley rats following chronic treatment with either GHB, GBL, or 1,4-BD. The findings of Experiment 2 are in direct contrast to Bania *et al.*, who used a similar 6-day course of escalating GHB i.p. administration to generate withdrawal scores of 13.7–14.7, indicating what the authors characterized as "a mild withdrawal syndrome," and no seizures occurred in any rat during the withdrawal period.[34] However, it is important to note that small experimental animal samples were employed in this study (2 rats per GHB treatment group). Conversely, our data from Experiments 1 and 2 are in agreement with Cook *et al.*, who attempted, but failed, to produce GHB physical dependence and withdrawal in Long Evans rats (4 groups of rats; n = 6–8 rats/group), following escalating GHB i.p. injections over a consecutive 5-day period. Following abrupt termination of GHB administration, with and without pharmacological challenge with the putative GHB receptor-selective antagonist NCS 382, neither spontaneous nor NCS 382-precipitated signs of physical dependence and withdrawal were observed.[35]

The results from our initial experiments with Wistar and Sprague-Dawley rats, in agreement with the work reported by Cook *et al.* in Long Evan rats, led us to hypothesize that rats with a unique genetically determined sensitivity to the toxic effects of GHB may serve as better animal models to investigate GHB physical dependence and withdrawal. We have recently used selective bidirectional breeding techniques to produce GHB-S and GHB-resistant (GHB-R) rat lines, which have been shown to display opposite sensitivity to the sedative/hypnotic effect produced by the acute administration of GHB 1 g/kg i.p.[36–39] The selective breeding of GHB-S and GHB-R rats provided evidence that sensitivity to the pharmacological and toxicological effects of GHB is under genetic control. We therefore hypothesized that, unlike the Wistar and Sprague-Dawley rats we had previously studied, GHB-S rats may possess a genetic predisposition for developing withdrawal manifestations following abrupt cessation from chronic administration of GHB, GBL, and 1,4-BD. In Experiment 3, however, GHB-S rats demonstrated no withdrawal effects compared to controls following an 11-day course of escalating GHB dosing. However, only one dosing schedule was employed and only GHB was studied; higher doses or longer periods of administration of GHB, in addition to GBL and 1,4-BD, warrant additional future study in GHB-S rats, given their known unique genetic sensitivity to GHB.

Our attention next focused on sP rats that have been selectively bred in this lab for high alcohol preference/intake and represent a longstanding, well-validated genetic model of high alcohol intake.[40] Utilizing sP rats in Experiment 4, we successfully demonstrated the spontaneous occurrence of audiogenic seizures following abrupt cessation from chronic administration of GHB and 1,4-BD, as well as precipitated audiogenic seizures following the administration of the $GABA_B$ receptor-selective antagonist, SCH 50911. These findings of spontaneous and precipitated GHB withdrawal-related audiogenic seizures in sP rats suggest a genetic predisposition. Accordingly, sP rats have been shown to have greater sensitivity to some other GHB-related effects. Compared to Sardinian non-alcohol-preferring (sNP) rats, sP rats have a greater sensitivity to the sedative/hypnotic effect of GHB 0.75 and 1.0 g/kg i.p., as evidenced by a significantly shorter latency to losing the righting reflex and a significantly longer time to regain the righting reflex.[41] Thus, sensitivity to the sedative/hypnotic effect of GHB is positively correlated to alcohol preference in sP and sNP rats, an indication that it may be genetically controlled. In another study examining GHB voluntary intake in sP and sNP rats, sP rats orally consumed larger daily amounts of GHB and displayed higher preference for GHB than sNP rats.[42]

In summary, results from the series of experiments in the present study indicate that a reliable sign of GHB or 1,4-BD withdrawal syndrome, audiogenic seizures, can be elicited by repeated administration of intoxicating doses of these drugs in selectively bred sP rats. Indeed, severe audiogenic seizures occurred at a significantly higher rate in GHB- and 1,4-BD-withdrawn rats than in water-treated rats. We propose that the genetically determined high sensitivity of sP rats to different GHB-associated responses has produced the observation of a withdrawal phenomenon that had previously been undetected in other rat strains, including Wistar, Sprague-Dawley, and Long Evans. SCH 50911 appeared to precipitate or exacerbate the 1,4-BD withdrawal syndrome, as its acute administration significantly increased seizure occurrence in 1,4-BD-withdrawn rats, suggesting that $GABA_B$ receptor-selective antagonists may constitute a powerful pharmacological tool to generate or exacerbate neurobehavioral signs of the withdrawal syndrome from GHB and its precursors, and it confirms previous data suggesting that the $GABA_B$ receptor is a major component of the neural substrate mediating the pharmacological and toxicological actions of GHB and its precursors.[43–47]

ACKNOWLEDGMENTS

These studies were supported in part by the Italian National Research Council (CNR, Drs. Colombo, and Carai) and the National Institutes of Health (NIH)/National Institute on Drug Abuse (NIDA) grant 1R03 DA14951-02. (Dr. Quang).

REFERENCES

1. Galloway, G.P., S.L. Frederick & F. Staggers Jr. 1994. Physical dependence on sodium oxybate [letter]. Lancet **343:** 57.
2. Friedman, J., R. Westlake & M. Furman. 1996. 'Grievous bodily harm': gamma hydroxybutyrate abuse leading to Wernicke-Korsakoff syndrome. Neurology **46:** 469–471.
3. Dyer, J.E. & K.M. Andrews. 1997. Gamma hydroxybutyrate withdrawal. J. Toxicol. Clin. Toxicol. **92:** 89–96.
4. Galloway, G.P., S.L. Frederick & F.E. Staggers Jr., *et al.* 1997. Gamma-hydroxybutyrate: an emerging drug of abuse that causes physical dependence. Addiction **92:** 89–96.
5. Hernandez, M., C.H. McDaniel, C.D. Costanza, *et al.* 1998. GHB-induced delirium: a case report and review of the literature of gamma hydroxybutyric acid. Am. J. Drug Alcohol Abuse **24:** 179–183.
6. Addolorato, G., F. Caputo, E. Capristo, *et al.* 1999. A case of gamma-hydroxybutyric acid withdrawal syndrome during alcohol addiction treatment: utility of diazepam administration. Clin. Neuropharmacol. **22:** 60–62.
7. Craig, K., H.F. Gomez, J.L. McManus, *et al.* 2000. Severe gamma-hydroxybutyrate withdrawal: a case report and literature review. J. Emerg. Med. **18:** 64–70.
8. Hutto, B., A. Fairchild & R. Bright. 2000. γ-Hydroxybutyrate withdrawal and chloral hydrate. Am. J. Psychiatry **157:** 10.
9. Miglani, J.S., K.Y. Kim & R. Chahil. 2000. Gamma-hydroxybutyrate withdrawal delirium: a case report. Gen. Hosp. Psychiatry **22:** 213–215.
10. Price, G. 2000. In-patient detoxification after GHB dependence. Br. J. Psychiatry **177:** 181.
11. Greene, T., T. Dougherty & A. Rodi. 2000. Gamma-butyrolactone withdrawal presenting as acute psychosis. J. Tox. Clin. Tox. **37:** 651.
12. Sharma, A.N., L. Nelson & R.S. Hoffman. 2000. Severe gamma-butyrolactone withdrawal. J. Tox. Clin. Tox. **38:** 535.
13. Catalano, M.C., J.M. Glass, G. Catalano, *et al.* 2001. Gamma butyrolactone (GBL) withdrawal syndromes. Psychosomatics **42:** 83–88.

14. MULLINS, M.E. & S.C. FITZMAURICE. 2001. Lack of efficacy of benzodiazepines in treating gamma-hydroxybutyrate withdrawal. J. Emerg. Med. **20:** 418–420.
15. SHARMA, A.N. & M.H. LOMBARDI. 2001. Management of gamma-hydroxybutyrate withdrawal. Ann. Emerg. Med. **38:** 605–607.
16. SU, M., S.J. TRAUB, E. HUSSAIN, *et al.* 2001. 1,4-Butanediol withdrawal complicated by urinary retention. J. Toxicol. Clin. Toxicol. **39:** 542.
17. BOWLES, T.M., R.W. SOMMI & M. AMIRI. 2001. Successful management of prolonged γ-hydroxybutyrate and alcohol withdrawal. Pharmacotherapy **21:** 254–257.
18. DYER, J.E., B. ROTH & B.A. HYMA. 2001. Gamma-hydroxybutyrate withdrawal syndrome. Ann. Emerg. Med. **37:** 147–153.
19. MAHR, G., C.L. BISHOP & D.J. ORRINGER. 2001. Prolonged withdrawal from extreme gamma-hydroxybutyrate (GHB) abuse. Psychosomatics **42:** 439–440.
20. MCDANIEL, C.H. & K.A. MIOTTO. 2001. Gamma hydroxybutyrate (GHB) and gamma butyrolactone (GBL) withdrawal: five case studies. J. Psychoactive Drugs **33:** 143–149.
21. MIOTTO, K., J. DARAKJIAN, J. BASCH, *et al.* 2001. Gamma-hydroxybutyric acid: patterns of use, effects and withdrawal. Am. J. Addict. **10:** 232–241.
22. SCHNEIR, A.B., B.T. LY & R.F. CLARK. 2001. A case of withdrawal from the GHB precursors gamma-butyrolactone and 1,4-butanediol. J. Emerg. Med. **21:** 31–33.
23. SIVILOTTI, M.L., M.J. BURNS, C.K. AARON, *et al.* 2001. Pentobarbital for severe gamma-butyrolactone withdrawal. Ann. Emerg. Med. **38:** 660–665.
24. MYCYK, M.B., C. WILEMON & S.E. AKS. 2001. Two cases of withdrawal from 1,4-butanediol use. Ann. Emerg. Med. **38:** 345–346.
25. CHIN, R.L. 2001. A case of severe withdrawal from gamma-hydroxybutyrate. Ann. Emerg. Med. **37:** 551–552.
26. ZVOSEC, D.L., S.W. SMITH, J.D. MCCUTCHEON, *et al.* 2001. Adverse events, including death, associated with the use of 1,4-butanediol. N. Engl. J. Med. **344:** 87–94.
27. HAROLD, A.H. & K.B. SNEED. 2002. Treatment of a young adult taking gamma-butyrolactone (GBL) in a primary care clinic. J. Am. Board Family Pract. **15:** 161–163.
28. MCDONOUGH, M., N. KENNEDY, A. GLASPER, *et al.* 2004. Clinical features and management of gamma-hydroxybutyrate (GHB) withdrawal: a review. Drug Alcohol Depend. **75:** 3–9.
29. ZVOSEC, D.L. & S.W. SMITH. 2004. γ-Hydroxybutyrate addiction and withdrawal: from the γ-hydroxybutyrate addiction study. Ann. Emerg. Med. **44:** pS91.
30. CHEW, G. & A. FERNANDO III. 2004. Epileptic seizure in GHB withdrawal. Australas. Psychiatry **12:** 410–411.
31. MAJCHROWICZ, E. 1975. Induction of physical dependence upon ethanol and the associated behavioural changes in rats. Psychopharmacologia **43:** 245–254.
32. LAL, H., C.M. HARRIS, D. BENJAMIN, *et al.* 1988. Characterization of a pentylenetetrazol-like interoceptive stimulus produced by ethanol withdrawal. J. Pharmacol. Exp. Ther. **247:** 508–518.
33. COLOMBO, G., R. AGABIO M.A.M. CARAI, *et al.* 2000. Ability of baclofen in reducing alcohol intake and withdrawal severity: I—preclinical evidence. Alcohol Clin. Exp. Res. **24(1):** 58–66.
34. BANIA, T.C., T. ASHAR, G. PRESS, *et al.* 2003. Gamma-hydroxybutyric acid tolerance and withdrawal in a rat model. Acad. Emerg. Med. **10:** 697–704.

35. Cook, C.D., M.D. Aceto, A. Coop, *et al.* 2002. Effects of the putative antagonist NCS382 on the behavioral pharmacological actions of gammahydroxybutyrate in mice. Psychopharmacology **160:** 99–106.
36. Lobina, C., G. Colombo, G. Brunetti, *et al.* 2001. Procedure of bidirectional selective outbreeding for production of two rat lines differing in sensitivity to the sedative/hypnotic effect of gamma-hydroxybutyric acid. Brain Res. Brain Res. Protoc. **8:** 74–81.
37. Colombo, G., C. Lobina, R. Agabio, *et al.* 2001. Selective breeding of two rat lines differing in sensitivity to GHB and baclofen. Brain Res. **902:** 127–130.
38. Lobina, C., G. Colombo, G.L. Gessa, *et al.* 2004. Completion by the 10th Generation of the Bidirectional Selective Breeding of GHB-Sensitive and GHB-Resistant Rats. Brain Res. Brain Res. Protoc. **13:** 53–56.
39. Lobina, C., G. Colombo, G.L. Gessa, *et al.* 2005. Different sensitivity to the motor in coordinating effects of gamma-hydroxybutyric acid (GHB) and baclofen in GHB-sensitive and GHB-resistant rats. Brain Res. **1033:** 109–112.
40. Colombo, G. 1997. Ethanol drinking behaviour in Sardinian alcohol preferring rats. Alcohol Alcohol. **32:** 443–453.
41. Colombo, G., R. Agabio, C. Lobina, *et al.* 1998. High sensitivity to gamma-hydroxybutyric acid in ethanol-preferring sP rats. Alcohol Alcohol. **33:** 121–125.
42. Colombo, G., R. Agabio, G. Diaz, *et al.* 1998. Gamma-hydroxybutyric acid intake in ethanol-preferring sP and -non preferring sNP rats. Physiol. Behav. **64:** 197–202.
43. Lingenhoehl, K., R. Brom, J. Heid, *et al.* 1999. γ-Hydroxybutyrate is a weak agonist at recombinant GABAB receptors. Neuropharmacology **38:** 1667–1673.
44. Carai, M.A.M., G. Colombo, G. Brunetti, *et al.* 2001. Role of $GABA_B$ receptors in the sedative/hypnotic effect of γ-hydroxybutyric acid. Eur. J. Pharmacol. **428:** 315–321.
45. Carai, M.A.M., G. Colombo, R. Reali, *et al.* 2002. Central effects of 1,4-butanediol are mediated by $GABA_B$ receptors via its conversion into γ-hydroxybutyric acid. Eur. J. Pharmacol. **441:** 157–163.
46. Carai, M.A.M., G. Colombo & G.L. Gessa. 2005. Resuscitative effect of a $GABA_B$ receptor antagonist on γ-hydroxybutyric acid (GHB) mortality in mice. Ann. Emerg. Med. **45:** 614–619.
47. Quang, L.S., M.C. Desai, J.C. Kraner, *et al.* 2002. Enzyme and receptor antagonists for preventing toxicity from the gamma-hydroxybutyric acid precursor 1,4-butanediol in CD-1 mice. Ann. N. Y. Acad. Sci. **965:** 461–472.

γ-Hydroxybutyrate (GHB) in Humans

Pharmacodynamics and Pharmacokinetics

SERGIO ABANADES,[a,b] MAGI FARRÉ,[a,b] MIREIA SEGURA,[c] SIMONA PICHINI,[d] DIEGO BARRAL,[a] ROBERTA PACIFICI,[d] MANUELA PELLEGRINI,[d] FRANCINA FONSECA,[c,e] KLAUS LANGOHR,[a] AND RAFAEL DE LA TORRE[a,c]

[a]*Pharmacology Research Unit, Human Pharmacology and Clinical Neurosciences Research Group, Institut Municipal d'Investigació Mèdica (IMIM), 08003 Barcelona, Spain*

[b]*Universitat Autònoma de Barcelona, 08003 Barcelona, Spain*

[c]*Universitat Pompeu Fabra, Barcelona, 08003 Barcelona, Spain*

[d]*Drug Research and Evaluation Department, Istituto Superiore di Sanità, 00161 Roma, Italy*

[e]*Drug Addiction Unit, IAPS, Barcelona, 08003 Barcelona, Spain*

ABSTRACT: Despite γ-hydroxybutyrate (GHB) therapeutic uses and the increasing concern about its toxicity, few studies have addressed GHB dose-related effects under controlled administration and their relationship with its pharmacokinetics. The study design was double-blind, randomized, crossover, and controlled. As a pilot pharmacology phase I study, increasing doses of GHB were given. Single oral sodium GHB doses (40, 50, 60, and 72 mg/kg) were administered to eight volunteers. Plasma and urine were analyzed for GHB by gas chromatography–mass spectrometry. Physiological effects, psychomotor performance, and subjective effects were examined simultaneously. GHB produced dose-related changes in subjective effects as measured by questionnaires and VAS. GHB showed a mixed stimulant-sedative pattern, with initially increased scores in subjective feeling of euphoria, high, and liking followed by mild-moderate symptoms of sedation with impairment of performance and balance. Mean peak GHB plasma concentrations were 79.1, 83.1, 113.5, and 130.1 μg/L for 40, 50, 60, and 72 mg/kg, respectively. GHB-mediated physiological and subjective effects were dose dependent and related to GHB plasma concentrations. GHB urinary excretion was mainly related to administered doses. GHB-mediated

Address for correspondence: Sergio Abanades, Pharmacology Research Unit, Human Pharmacology and Clinical Neurosciences Research Group, Institut Municipal d'Investigació Mèdica (IMIM), c/ Doctor Aiguader 80, 08003 Barcelona, Spain. Voice: +34-93-2211009; fax: +34-93-2213237. e-mail: sabanades@imim.es

Ann. N.Y. Acad. Sci. 1074: 559–576 (2006). © 2006 New York Academy of Sciences. doi: 10.1196/annals.1369.065

subjective and physiological effects seem dose dependent and related to GHB plasma concentrations. Results suggest a high abuse liability of GHB in the range of dose usually consumed.

KEYWORDS: γ-hydroxybutyric acid; γ-hydroxybutyrate; GHB; subjective effects; abuse liability

INTRODUCTION

γ-hydroxybutyrate (GHB, "liquid ecstasy") is also known as γ-hydroxybutyric acid, 4-hydroxybutyiric acid, 4-hydroxybutanoic acid, and oxybate (sodium oxybate is the United States approved name). GHB is a short chain fatty acid that can be considered both an endogenous metabolite and a precursor of the neurotransmitter γ-aminobutyric acid (GABA). GHB acts in the central nervous system as a neuromodulator. GHB can be formed in human peripheral tissues from two precursors, γ-butyrolactone and 1,4-butanediol.[1] GHB is marketed in the United States with the name of Xyrem® (Jazz Pharmaceuticals, Palo Alto, CA) for the treatment of cataplexy in patients with narcolepsy,[2] and in some European countries as an anesthetic agent and for the treatment of alcohol withdrawal (e.g., Alcover®; CT Laboratorio Farmaceutico, SRL, San Remo, Italy). On the other hand, GHB is a recreational drug commonly consumed at nightclubs and "raves" in conjunction with alcohol, cannabis and drugs, such as 3,4-methylenedioxymethamphetamine (MDMA, ecstasy), or ketamine, also known as "club drugs."[3] In humans, γ-butyrolactone and 1,4-butanediol have also been abused. During the last years, GHB has become a major concern in emergency rooms of some countries due to an important increase in the number of cases of intoxications.[4–6] GHB has also been used for narcotizing victims in drug-facilitated sexual assaults because its capacity to induce short-term antegrade amnesia, increased libido, and suggestibility.[7,8] Recreational users of GHB experience euphoria, relaxation, reduction of social inhibitions, decreased motor skills, and other effects similar to those reported for a moderate alcohol intoxication.[9] These effects can explain its abuse liability in humans, but this aspect has not been yet characterized under controlled administration. After GHB ingestion, a mild intoxication may be observed with nausea, dizziness, and difficulty in focusing the eyes.[10] Acute severe intoxications have been reported, where individuals may experience vomiting, extreme dizziness, disorientation, amnesia, and unconsciousness[4–6,11] that may evolve to convulsions, deep coma, and rarely death.[12] The range between high recreational doses and overdose is narrow; and acute intoxications are quite common in humans.

GHB has been detected in blood and urine of subjects after acute intoxications and in the context of clinical trials.[13–16] Results from these reports indicate that GHB is eliminated from the body very rapidly; being detection dependent on the time elapsed between consumption and sample collection. Because GHB is an endogenous compound, there are measurable baseline concentrations in blood and urine.[17–20]

The range of GHB doses typically abused by subjects range between 2 and 6 g (25–75 mg/kg). Most reports available are focused on the pharmacokinetic of GHB in humans.[15–17,21–23] Nevertheless, little is known on the physiological and subjective effects and alterations in psychomotor performance induced by this drug in the range of doses commonly abused. In addition, despite its therapeutic uses and the increasing concern about the toxicity of GHB, few studies addressed dose-related effects under controlled administration and the correlation of drug effects and concentrations in biological fluids.

The aims of this article were as follows: (*a*) to select appropriate doses for a series of GHB clinical pharmacology studies (interval: lowest dose with noticeable effects and doses that lead to significant somnolence); (*b*) to describe time course of physiological, subjective variables, and psychomotor performance following drug administration; (*c*) to investigate the presence and the time course of GHB in plasma and urine; and (*d*) to assess the eventual correlation between GHB pharmacokinetics and drug effects in a range of doses compatible with those usually consumed by recreational users.[24]

MATERIALS AND METHODS

Human Subjects

Eight male subjects were recruited by ''word of mouth'' and included in the study. Eligibility criteria required the recreational use of GHB on at least five occasions. Exclusion criteria included daily consumption of more than 20 cigarettes and more than 30 g of ethanol (3 units per day). All subjects gave their written informed consent before inclusion and were economically compensated for inconveniences caused by their participation in the study. The study was conducted in accordance with the Declaration of Helsinki, approved by the local Ethical Committee (CEIC-IMAS), and authorized by the Spanish Ministry of Health (Agencia Española del Medicamento). Eligible subjects were interviewed by a psychiatrist (structured clinical interview for Diagnostic and Statistical Manual version N [DSM-IV-TR] in order to exclude psychiatric disorders, including schizophrenia, psychosis, and major affective disorders. Each participant underwent a general physical examination, routine laboratory tests, urinalysis, and a 12-lead electrocardiogram. The participants had a mean age of 28.1 years (range 25–32), mean weight of 71.9 kg (range 60.5–84.2), and mean height of 179.1 cm (range 167.5–194.0). Participants were non-smokers ($n = 7$) except for one, and their average consumption of alcohol was 9 units per week. All of them had previous experience with the consumption of alcohol, cannabis, sedatives, stimulants, and "club drugs," with at least five previous consumptions of GHB. None had history of abuse or drug dependence according to DSM-IV criteria (except for nicotine dependence), nor had experienced any medical or psychiatric adverse reaction following GHB consumption.

Study Design

This study is a preliminary phase of a series of clinical trials of GHB administration in humans. As a pilot pharmacology phase I study, increasing doses of GHB were given. The study design was double-blind, randomized, crossover, and controlled. Subjects participated as outpatients in two different randomly assigned 6-h study sessions with a washout period of 7 days, in which they were given single doses of 40 (33.1), 50 (41.4), 60 (49.7), and 72 (60.1) mg/kg of sodium (GHB) or placebo by the oral route. Participants and evaluators (two physicians) were blind to treatments although they were told that GHB or placebo would be given during the sessions. Thus, in a dose escalation schedule, two different doses of sodium GHB were given to every subject (40 mg/kg dose was given in four occasions, 50 mg/kg given in four occasions, 60 mg/kg given in five occasions, 72 mg/kg given in two occasions, and placebo given in one occasion). Participants were requested to abstain from consumption of any drug of abuse during the study period and urine drug testing was performed before each study session for cannabinoids, cocaine, opiates, amphetamine/methamphetamine, barbiturates, benzodiazepines, and phencyclidine. For all groups of substances, participants tested negative before each experimental session. In each session, subjects arrived at the laboratory at 8 AM after an overnight fast and had an indwelling intravenous catheter inserted into a subcutaneous vein in the forearm of the non-dominant arm. Thereafter, they remained seated in a quiet room throughout the session. GHB (Alcover OS® sodium GHB, 17.5% syrup, CT Laboratorio Farmaceutico) or matched placebo (syrup, CT Laboratorio Farmaceutico) were orally administered around 9:00 AM in a fasting state. The different doses corresponding to appropriate volumes of syrup and placebo were diluted to 250 mL of a soda orange-based drink. Participants were told to drink the beverage as soon as possible (mean of 10.2 s; range: 5–20 s). Placebo consisted of syrup diluted to the same 250 mL of a soda orange-based drink.

Collection of Blood and Urine Samples

Blood was collected at 0, 0.25, 0.5, 0.75, 1, 1.5, 2, 3, 4, 5, and 6 h after GHB administration in heparinized tubes and immediately centrifuged. Urine samples were collected before, and at 0–3 and 3–6 h after drug administration. All biological specimens were frozen at −20°C until analysis. No preservatives were added to the specimens.

Determination of GHB Concentrations in Biological Fluids

Frozen, plasma, and urine samples were allowed to thaw at room temperature. Aliquots of 100 μL plasma and urine were added with 5 μg (5 μL of the 1 mg/mL methanolic solution) of GHB hexadeuterated analoge, GHB-d_6 as internal standard, and 200 μL of acetonitrile. After 30-s vortex and 5-min centrifugation at 1400 rpm, 150 μL of the organic phase were transferred to a clean extraction tube and evaporated to dryness. The dried extracts were derivatized with 50 μL of BSTFA-1% TMCS for 30 min at 70°C.

A 1-μL aliquot of derivatized samples was injected onto a Hewlett-Packard (HP) 6890 gas chromatograph coupled to a HP5973 quadrupole mass spectrometer (Agilent, Palo Alto, CA, USA). The capillary column was a cross-linked 5% phenyl-methylsilicone (12 m × 0.2 mm i.d. and 0.33-μm film thickness, Ultra-2, Agilent). The samples were injected in split-less mode and helium gas was used as carrier at a flow rate of 1.2 mL/min (measured at 180°C). The injector and detector temperatures were both maintained at 280°C, respectively. The temperature program was initially set at 60°C for 2 min and increased to 180°C at 20°C/min, then 35°C to 250°C, and then held for 4 min, being the total run time 14 min. The mass spectrometer was operated in the electron impact ionization and selected ion monitoring (SIM) acquisition mode and the following ions were monitored (underlined ions used for quantification): GHB-bis-TMS: m/z 233, <u>204</u>, 117; GHB-d_6-bis-TMS: m/z <u>239</u>. Under these analytical conditions, the limit of quantification (LOQ) was 0.5 μg/mL and the intra-day precision and accuracy were always better than 4.2% and 13.4%. Similarly, inter-day precision and accuracy were lower than 13.4% and 12.1% at the GHB LOQ.

PHARMACOLOGICAL EFFECTS

Physiological Measures

Non-invasive systolic blood pressure (SBP), diastolic blood pressure (DBP), heart rate, oral temperature, and pupil diameter were recorded at −15 min and immediately before drug administration (time 0, baseline) and at 0.25, 0.50, 0.75, 1, 1.50, 2, 3, 4, 5, and 6 h after GHB administration using a DinamapTM 8100-T vital signs monitor (Critikon, Tampa, FL). Pupil diameter was recorded with a Haab pupil gauge.[25]

Psychomotor Performance Measures

The psychomotor performance battery included the digit symbol substitution test (DSST), the Maddox-wing device, and the balance task. This battery has been used previously in the evaluation of psychostimulants and sedatives.[26,27] The DSST is a subtest of the Wechsler Adult Intelligence Scale-Revised.[28] A computerized version was used and scores were based on the number of correct patterns keyed in 90 s (correct responses). The Maddox-wing device measures the balance of extraocular muscles and quantifies exophoria, as an indicator of extraocular musculature relaxes, and esophoria. Results were expressed in diopters along the horizontal scale of the device.[29] The Balance Task assessed the participant's ability to stand upright for a maximum of 30 s on each foot.[30] The score was the total number of seconds the participant was able to balance (maximum of 60 s). The DSST and balance task were performed at −15 min and immediately before drug administration (time 0, baseline) and at 0.50, 1, 1.50, 2, 3, 4, and 6 h after drug administration. Measurements with the Maddox-wing device were performed at −15 min and at 0.25, 0.50, 0.75, 1, 1.50, 2, 3, 4, 5, and 6 h after drug administration.

Subjective Effects Rating Scales

Subjective effects were measured using the Addiction Research Center Inventory (ARCI), the VESSPA (Evaluation of the Subjective Effects of Substances with Potential of Abuse) questionnaire, and a set of 13 different visual analog scales (VAS). ARCI is a true–false questionnaire with empirically derived scales that are sensitive to the effects of a variety of classes of drugs of abuse.[31] The Spanish validated version of a 49-item short form of ARCI was used.[32] The questionnaire included five scales: PCAG (pentobarbital-chlorpromazine-alcohol group, a measure of sedation); MBG (morphine-benzedrine group, a measure of euphoria); LSD (lysergic acid diethylamide group, a measure of dysphoria and somatic symptoms); BG (benzedrine group, a stimulant scale consisting mainly of items relating to intellectual efficiency and energy); and A (amphetamine, an empirically derived scale sensitive to the effects of D-amphetamine). ARCI was administered at −15 min (immediately before drug administration), and at 0.50, 1, 1.50, 2, 3, 4, 5, and 6 h after GHB administration. VESSPA (evaluation of the subjective effects of substances with potential of abuse) is an in-house developed and validated questionnaire specifically created to measure changes in subjective variables caused by MDMA.[33] It contains six scales: sedation (SED), psychosomatic anxiety (ANX), changes in perception (PER), pleasure and sociability (SOC), activity and energy (ACT), and psychotic symptoms (PSY). Each scale consists of six questions with a five-point Likert response (0 to 4 depending on the intensity of the effect). VESSPA scales were administered at −15 min (before drug administration), and at 1, 2, 3, 4, and 6 h after GHB administration.

A total of 13 VAS (100 mm) labeled with different adjectives marked at opposite ends with "not at all" and "extremely" were used. Subjects were asked to rate effects of "stimulated," "high", "any effect," "good effects," "bad effects," "liking," "content," "drunkenness," "drowsiness," "dizziness," "confusion," "depression or sadness," and "relax." Scales were administered at −15 min (immediately before drug administration), 0.25, 0.50, 0.75, 1, 1.50, 2, 3, 4, 5, and 6 h after GHB administration.

Pharmacodynamic and Pharmacokinetics Parameters

The following parameters were determined from GHB plasma concentrations over time: peak concentration (C_{max}), time to reach peak concentrations (t_{max}), area under the concentration-time curve from 0 to 6 h (AUC_{0-6}), elimination half-life ($t_{1/2}$), and elimination constant (Ke). Taking into account the duration of GHB physiological and subjective effects, area under the effects-time curve from 0 to 2 h (AUC_{0-2}), and maximal effect (E_{max}) were also determined. AUCs were calculated by the linear trapezoidal rule.

Pharmacokinetic parameters were obtained with use of specific functions of computer program (PK Functions for Microsoft Excel, Microsoft Corporation, USA).

Data Analysis: Statistical Methods

Data are represented as mean ± standard deviation (SD) or median. The nonparametric Kruskal–Wallis test was applied to compare the distributions of AUC_{0-6} and C_{max} values (pharmacokinetics) and AUC_{0-2} and E_{max} values (pharmacodynamics) between the different sodium GHB doses assayed without assuming any parametric form of these distributions. The Kruskal–Wallis test was applied to test the null hypothesis, which assumes equal distribution functions versus the alternative that, at least, two distributions differ with respect to the median. Since the power of the test was low because of only two observations in the GHB dose group of 72 mg/kg, posterior comparisons of GHB doses groups of 40 and 60 mg/kg were also carried out. In this latter case, the Wilcoxon Mann-Whitney test was applied. Given the small sample sizes, tests were carried out using the add-on module SPSS Exact of the statistical software package SPSS, version 12.0 (SPSS Inc., Chicago, IL).

RESULTS

A summary of results for pharmacological effects and pharmacokinetics showing statistical significant differences between treatments is presented in TABLE 1.

Pharmacological Effects

Time course of several GHB pharmacological dose-related effects in humans are presented in FIGURES 1 (physiological effects and Maddox wing),

TABLE 1. Variables showing statistically significant differences between treatments. Mean, minimum, maximum values for the four doses tested and comparisons performed

		40 mg/kg ($n = 4$)		50 mg/kg ($n = 5$)		60 mg/kg ($n = 4$)		72 mg/kg ($n = 2$)		
	Criteria	Mean	Median	Mean	Median	Mean	Median	Mean	All	40 and 60
GHB Plasma concentrations	AUC_{0-6h}	106.5	108.5	143.7	133.9	183.9	185.8	301.1	0.004	0.029
Pupil diameter	AUC_{0-2h}	1.2	1.2	.65	.69	.22	.13	1.4	0.014	
VAS any effect	AUC_{0-2h}	14.2	12.2	46.1	40.9	61.8	57.1	67.2		0.029
VAS drunkenness	AUC_{0-2h}	3.7	3.6	33.6	21.9	49.7	38.8	33.1		0.029
VAS good effects	AUC_{0-2h}	13.4	11.7	45.6	48.6	60.2	58.1	64.8		0.029
VAS high	AUC_{0-2h}	15.3	14.4	47.5	49.1	59.4	55.4	65.2		0.029
VAS content	AUC_{0-2h}	13.9	11.8	39.5	13.4	53.3	53.5	23.1		0.029
VAS stimulated	AUC_{0-2h}	7.2	6.4	34.3	16.6	53.3	57.4	68.1	0.040	0.029
	E_{max}	10.2	10.5	30.4	33.0	43.2	46.5	61.5	0.020	0.029
VAS liking	AUC_{0-2h}	14.1	12.6	44.6	47.1	54.2	54.2	58.9		0.029
VAS bad effects	AUC_{0-2h}	0.7	0.6	15.1	0.0	30.2	27.9	16.9		0.029
	E_{max}	1.7	1.5	15.4	0.0	33.2	29.0	20.0		0.029
VAS dizziness	AUC_{0-2h}	7.8	5.4	34.4	19.9	67.3	68.2	56.6		0.029
	E_{max}	10.0	9.5	32.6	32.0	63.0	67.0	62.0	0.049	0.029
VAS relax	AUC_{0-2h}	7.3	3.4	29.8	9.1	59.3	57.1	19.4		0.029
	E_{max}	7.7	5.5	25.6	15.0	49.2	48.0	9.7		0.029
ARCI A	E_{max}	1.7	2.0	3.6	4.0	4.0	3.5	2.0	0.048	0.029

[a] P values < 0.05.

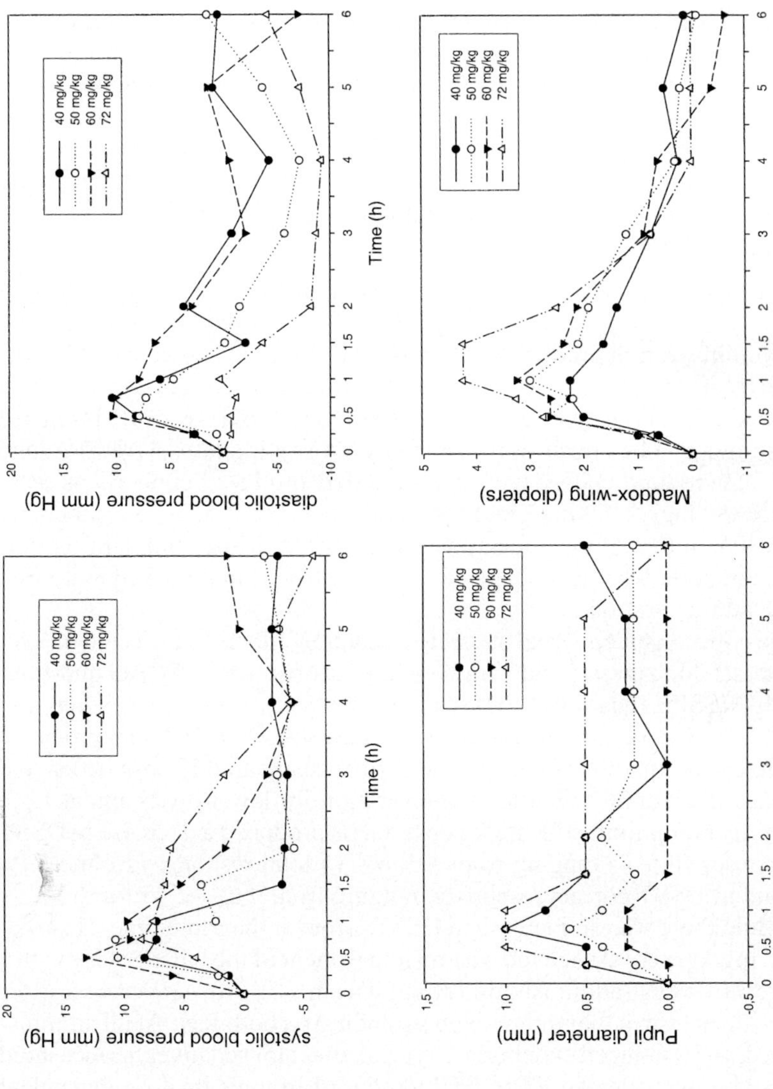

FIGURE 1. Time course of GHB dose-related physiological effects (mean values) in humans (SBP, DBP, pupil diameter, and Maddox wing).

2 (subjective effects: VAS), and 3 (subjective effects: ARCI and VESSPA and DSST performance).

Physiological Effects

GHB produced a slight increase in systolic and diastolic blood pressure for all doses tested, with a peak effect between 30 and 45 min and a return to previous values at 3 h after GHB administration, without reaching statistical significance between different doses (FIG. 1). No apparent changes in heart rate or oral temperature were observed. GHB produced a significant (AUC 0–2 h comparison) dose-related pupil diameter increase from 0.5 mm to 1 mm between 30 min and 1-h post-administration.

Subjective Effects and Psychomotor Performance

GHB administration produced dose-related changes in subjective effects as measured by questionnaires and VAS. GHB showed a mixed sedative-stimulant pattern mediating both types of effects (see FIGS. 2 and 3). GHB produced marked stimulant-like effects as measured by VAS "stimulated," ARCI A, and VESSPA activity and energy (ACT) scale. GHB produced euphoria as measured by VAS "high," "liking," and "good effects," ARCI MBG questionnaire and VESSPA pleasure and sociability (SOC) scale. Most stimulant-like effects and euphoria were dose dependent (see TABLE 1) and peaked at 45 min post-drug administration.

GHB produced objective and subjective sedation effects as reflected in VAS "drowsiness," "dizziness," and "drunkenness" scores, ARCI PCAG questionnaire and VESSPA sedation (SED) scale. Peak effects were achieved between 1 and 1.5 h after drug administration and lasted for 3 h. GHB also produced a slight deterioration of psychomotor performance apparently dose dependent with a peak effect at 30 min after administration for lower doses and at 1.5 h post-administration for the 72 mg/kg dose. GHB produced a decrease in DSST total responses (FIG. 3) ranging from −5 to −11 total responses for the E_{max} values, and in DSST correct responses, ranging from 0 to −2.75 for the E_{max} values, while there was an increase in DSST errors at the same time. Doses of 60 and 72 mg/kg were associated with an impairment of the balance task with a peak effect at 1 h post-administration ranging from −15 s to −19 s decrease for the E_{max} values from a maximum of 60 s standing on both feet. At all administered doses, GHB induced exophoria, a typical effect for sedatives, as measured by the Maddox-wing device. Thus, GHB produced an apparent dose-dependent increase in diopters with a peak effect at 1 h post-administration (E_{max} 2.25 40 mg/kg, 2.7 50 mg/kg, and 3.25 60 mg/kg), that lasted 4 h post-administration (see FIG. 1).

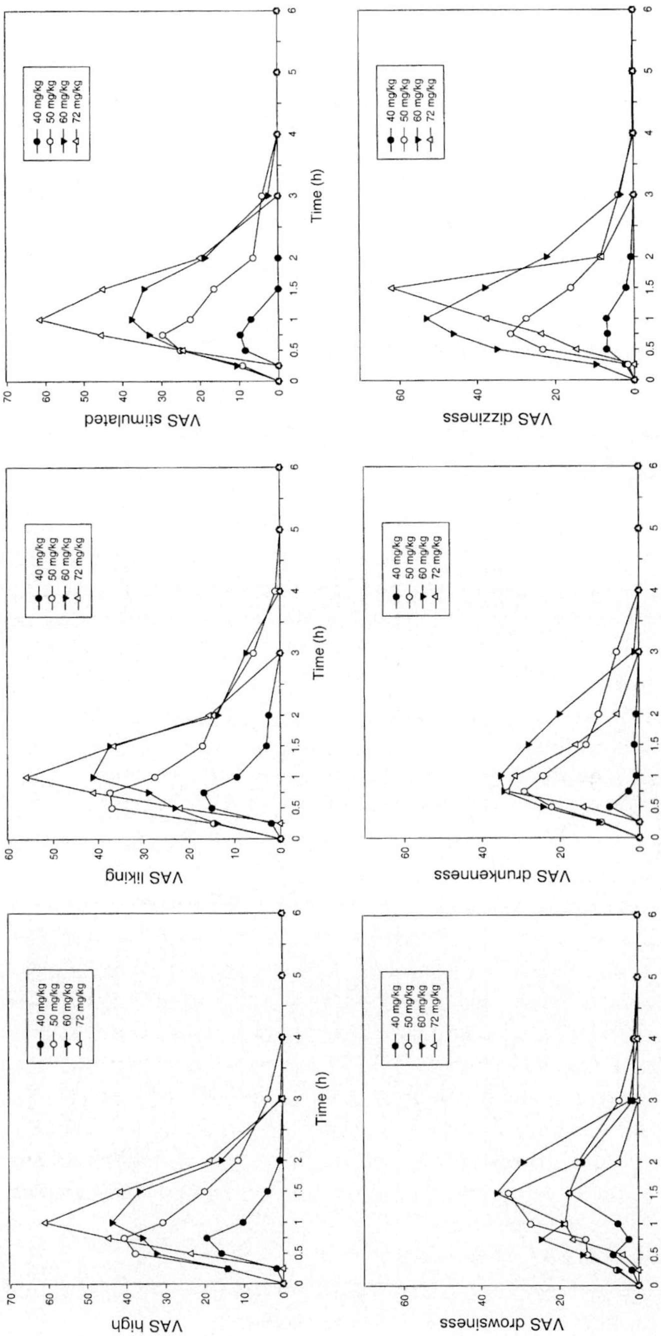

FIGURE 2. Time course of GHB dose-related subjective effects (VAS).

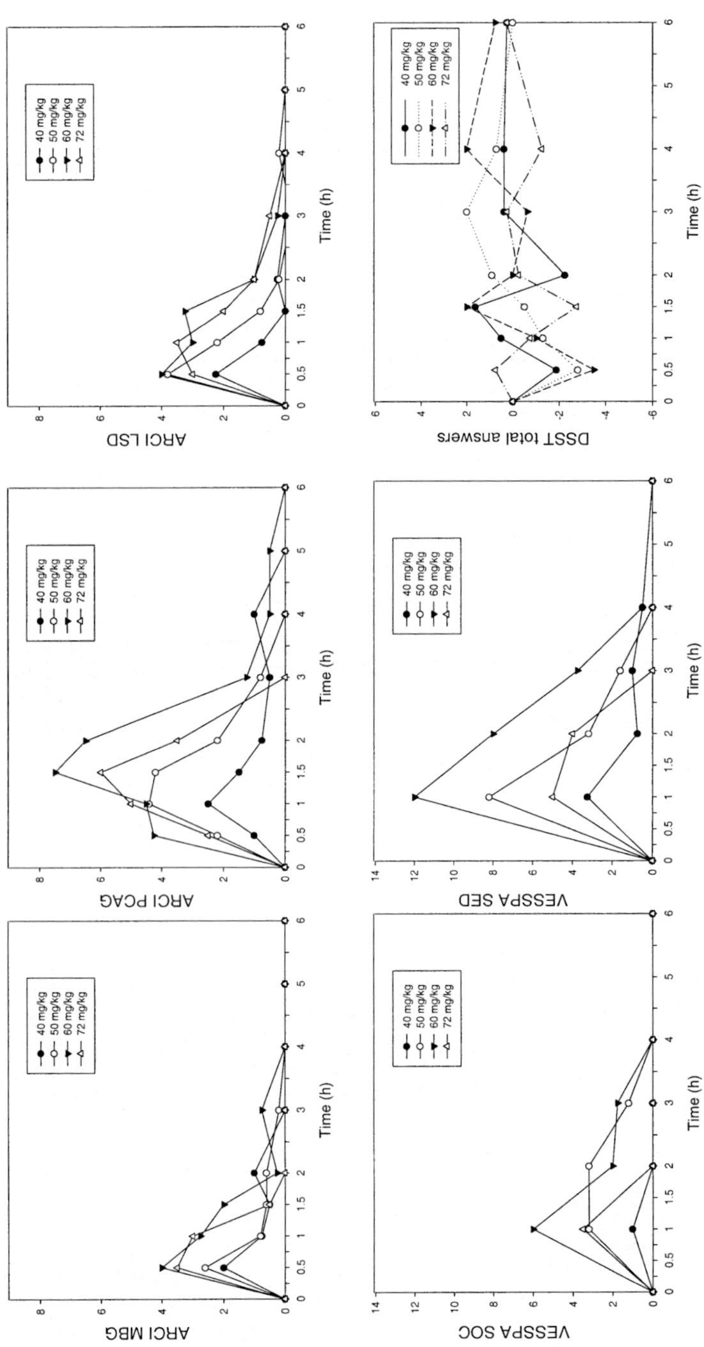

FIGURE 3. Time course of GHB dose-related subjective effects (ARCI and VESSPA questionnaires) and psychomotor performance (DSST total responses).

TABLE 2. Pharmacokinetic parameters of GHB in plasma (mean ± SD values given)

Parameter	40 mg/kg[a]	50 mg/kg[a]	60 mg/kg[a]	72 mg/kg[a]
C_{max} (μg/mL)	79.1 ± 26.4	83.1 ± 28.8	113.5 ± 20.1	130.1 ± 10.7
t_{max} (h)	0.7 ± 0.2	0.6 ± 0.1	0.6 ± 0.14	0.9 ± 0.2
$AUC_{0–6}$ (μg/mL h)	106.5 ± 6.7	143.7 ± 36.4	183.9 ± 47.0	301.1 ± 11.4
K_e (h^{-1})	0.98 ± 0.21	1.01 ± 0.18	1.06 ± 0.18	1.23 ± 0.11
$t_{1/2}$ (h)	0.73 ± 0.17	0.71 ± 0.15	0.67 ± 0.12	0.57 ± 0.05

[a]Sodium GHB doses.

None of the participants required specific therapy or special care during the study. Serious adverse events were not observed, although one subject vomited 1 h after the administration of the 60 mg/kg dose. No hallucinations, psychotic episodes, or any other psychiatric symptoms were observed during the experimental sessions.

Concentration-Time Profiles of GHB in Plasma

Pharmacokinetic parameters of GHB in plasma after oral doses of 40, 50, 60, and 72 mg/kg of sodium GHB are presented in TABLE 2.

GHB was detected in all baseline plasma samples, with mean concentrations of 0.04 ± 0.01 μg/mL. After drug administration, concentrations peaked between 30 and 60 min after drug administration (C_{max} range: 45.8–109.3 μg/mL for 40 mg/kg; 51.0 – 123.5 μg/mL for 50 mg/kg, 90.3 – 134.7 for 60 mg/kg, and 122.5 – 137.6 for 72 mg/kg) (TABLE 2). Following the absorption phase, concentrations declined to a mean values at 6 h that ranged from 0.5 to 0.9 mg/mL for all doses tested.[13,34] GHB was readily absorbed after oral administration and rapidly eliminated (t_{max} and $t_{1/2} < 1$ h). $AUC_{0–6h}$ derived from plasma GHB concentrations were significantly different upon comparing the four different doses ($P < 0.05$) (TABLE 1). No significant differences were observed for C_{max}, t_{max}, Ke, and $t_{1/2}$ between different drug doses. Normalized (1 mg/kg) values for AUC were similar for 40, 50, and 60 mg/kg doses (2.7, 2.9, and 3.1). For the 72 mg/kg dose, this value was higher (4.2). Normalized C_{max}, values were similar for all doses tested.

Excretion of GHB in Urine

A summary of GHB urinary excretion is shown in TABLE 3. GHB was detected in urine at baseline samples, with mean concentrations of 0.21 ± 0.14 μg/mL. The highest GHB recovery was found in the 0–3 h urine samples. Less than 2% of doses tested were recovered in urine for the 0–6 h collection period.

TABLE 3. Urinary excretion of GHB following different oral doses

		Urinary collection period		
Dose[a] mg/kg	Mean dose given (g)	0–3 h	3–6 h	0–6 h
40	2.9 ± 0.4	305.8 ± 121.4[b]	125.3 ± 214.4[b]	431.2 ± 202.4 (1.60%)[c]
50	3.7 ± 0.3	593.1 ± 297.9[b]	113.2 ± 155.0[b]	706.3 ± 433.8 (1.98%)[c]
60	3.9 ± 0.4	440.1 ± 114.1[b]	104.9 ± 118.6[b]	545.0 ± 106.8 (1.50%)[c]
72	5.2 ± 1.2	821.8 ± 149.8[b]	96.9 ± 33.3[b]	918.7 ± 116.5 (1.90%)[c]

[a]As sodium GHB.
[b]Mean ± SD, values given in micromoles.
[c]Recoveries (0–6 h) as a percentage of the administered dose.

DISCUSSION

Results of the study provide new insights on GHB pharmacodynamics and pharmacokinetics in humans. To our knowledge, there are no previous reports of the evaluation of GHB physiological and subjective effects after controlled administration of doses compatible with those consumed by recreational users. The main finding of the study is that GHB-mediated physiological and subjective effects are dose dependent and related to GHB plasma concentrations.

Our study, although somehow limited by both a dose escalation schedule design and the number of volunteers tested, provides new knowledge about its induced subjective effects and alterations of psychomotor performance. GHB produced dose-related changes in subjective effects as measured by specific questionnaires and VAS. GHB showed a mixed stimulant-sedative pattern with a biphasic time profile as described for other sedatives (alcohol or cannabis).[35,36] Psychostimulant effects were predominant in the first hour while sedative effects initiate more slowly and predominate in the second hour after drug administration. In reference to its abuse liability, GHB induced euphoria, well being, pleasurable effects, and liking effects that are on the basis of its misuse as recreational drug and similar to those reported by GHB abusers.[9,37] In the case of the sedative effects, they were similar to those elicited by low doses of benzodiazepines and alcohol[26,27] and included subjective feelings of sedation, a decrease in psychomotor performance, ataxia, and exophoria.

Regarding physiological effects, GHB administration produced a constant slight increment in SBP and DBP for all doses tested, lasting for 1–2 h post-administration that did not reached statistical significance when comparing doses assayed. Interestingly, this effect was not reported in none of the therapeutic studies previously performed. Furthermore, following GHB intoxication hypotension is frequently reported.[10] However, recent results suggest that GHB has also sympathomimetic cardiovascular effects that could induce increases in blood pressure following its acute administratrion.[38] Further studies with a larger population of subjects are needed to confirm these findings.

GHB given by the oral route is rapidly absorbed and eliminated. Drug consumption can be differentiated from GHB endogenous concentrations both in plasma and urine in a time-window of 6 h post-ingestion. Our results are in agreement with those obtained in healthy subjects administered with 4.5 g of oxybate[13] (equivalent to 50–60 mg/kg of GHB) and lower to those observed in severe acute intoxications.[39] GHB elimination follows a nonlinear process as suggested by comparison of normalized AUCs. In the dose range of 40–60 mg/kg, elimination is linear in agreement with previous reports,[13,17] although nonlinearity can be observed at the 72 mg/kg dose. GHB elimination appears to be capacity-limited at higher doses as it has been observed in some narcoleptic patients administered at a fixed dose of 3 g twice nightly at a 4-h interval.[23] The accumulation of GHB in the body as a result of a nonlinear disposition of GHB might have some implications in the susceptibility of some subjects to develop acute intoxications.

GHB urinary excretion was mainly related to administered doses and in accordance with previous reports.[13,16,40] However, there was a slightly higher recovery of GHB for the 50 mg/kg dose than for 60 mg/kg dose. Higher mean weights of the subjects (resulting in similar total mean dose given), and an increased percentage of the administered dose recovery in the 50 mg/kg dose group, account for these results. In line with early reports, less than 2% of doses administered were recovered in the collection period.

Plasma concentrations reached in the range of doses administered are lower than that observed in acute intoxications and therefore is not surprising that, in our study, strong sedation or coma were not observed.[39] GHB plasma concentrations correlated better with psychostimulant-like effects rather than with sedative ones. At higher doses, sedative effects would predominate leading to the observed effects in acute intoxications. Our results suggest a high abuse liability of GHB in the range of doses usually abused. Further studies are needed to confirm these results.

ACKNOWLEDGMENTS

The work was supported in part by grants from Fondo de Investigación Sanitaria FIS (02/0824, Red de Trastornos Adictivos G03/005, Red CIEN, C03/06), Generalitat de Catalunya (CIRIT 2001SGR00407), and Istituto Superiore di Sanità, Rome, Italy (funded by the Dipartimento Nazionale per le politiche antidroga della Presidenza del Consiglio dei Ministri). Sergio Abanades is the recipient of a fellowship from the Spanish Health Authorities [Ayudas para contratar profesionales sanitarios que hayan finalizado el período de Formación Sanitaria Especializada,. Instituto Carlos III (CM04/00216)]. We are indebted to research nurses Esther Menoyo, Olga Sanchez, and Marta Perez for their valuable assistances throughout the clinical trial. We are also grateful to the work made by Pere Roset MD, Ph.D.

REFERENCES

1. NICHOLSON, K.L. & R.L. BALSTER. 2001. GHB: a new and novel drug of abuse. Drug Alcohol Depend. **63:** 1–22.
2. U.S. XYREM® MULTICENTER STUDY GROUP. 2003. A 12-month, open-label, multicenter extension trial of orally administered sodium oxybate for the treatment of narcolepsy. Sleep **26:** 31–35.
3. ABANADES, S., A.M. PEIRO & M. FARRE. 2004. Club drugs: old medicines as new party drugs. Med. Clin. (Barc.) **123:** 305–311.
4. MIRO, O., S. NOGUE, G. ESPINOSA, J. TO-FIGUERAS & M. SANCHEZ. 2002. Trends in illicit drug emergencies: the emerging role of gamma-hydroxybutyrate. J. Toxicol. Clin. Toxicol. **40:** 129–135.
5. CHIN, R.L., K.A. SPORER, B. CULLISON, *et al.* 1998. Clinical course of gamma-hydroxybutyrate overdose. Ann. Emerg. Med. **31:** 716–722.
6. LIECHTI, M.E. & H. KUPFERSCHMIDT. 2004. Gamma-hydroxybutyrate (GHB) and gamma-butyrolactone (GBL): analysis of overdose cases reported to the Swiss Toxicological Information Centre. Swiss. Med. Wkly. **134:** 534–537.
7. ELSOHLY, M.A. & S.J. SALAMONE. 1999. Prevalence of drugs used in cases of alleged sexual assault. J. Anal. Toxicol. **23:** 141–146.
8. VARELA, M., S. NOGUE, M. OROS, *et al.* 2004. Gamma hydroxybutirate use for sexual assault. Emerg. Med. J. **21:** 255–256.
9. DEGENHARDT, L., S. DARKE & P. DILLON. 2002. GHB use among Australians: characteristics, use patterns and associated harm. Drug Alcohol Depend. **67:** 89–94.
10. MASON, P.E. & W.P. KERNS 2nd. 2002. Gamma hydroxybutyric acid (GHB) intoxication. Acad. Emerg. Med. **9:** 730–739.
11. ABANADES, S., M.L. IGLESIAS, J.L. ECHARTE, *et al.* 2001. Gammahydroxibutyrate: a novel toxicological emergency. Meth. Find. Clin. Exp. Pharmacol **23:** 326.
12. FERRARA, S.D., L. TEDESCHI, G. FRISON, *et al.* 1995. Fatality due to GHB and heroin intoxication. J. Forensic Sci. **40:** 501–504.
13. PALATINI, P., L. TEDESCHI, G. FRISON, *et al.* 1993. Dose-dependent absorption and elimination of gamma-hydroxybutyric acid in healthy volunteers. Eur. J. Clin. Pharmacol. **45:** 353–356.
14. MCCUSKER, R.R., H. PAGET-WILKES, C.W. CHRONISTER, *et al.* 1999. Analysis of gamma-hydroxybutyrate (GHB) in urine by gas chromatography-mass spectrometry. J. Anal. Toxicol. **23:** 301–305.
15. FERRARA, S.D., S. ZOTTI, L. TEDESCHI, *et al.* 1992. Pharmacokinetics of gamma-hydroxybutyric acid in alcohol dependent patients after single and repeated oral doses. Br. J. Clin. Pharmacol. **34:** 231–235.
16. BRENNEISEN, R., M.A. ELSOHLY, T.P. MURPHY, *et al.* 2004. Pharmacokinetics and excretion of gamma-hydroxybutyrate (GHB) in healthy subjects. J. Anal. Toxicol. **28:** 625–630.
17. BORGEN, L.A., R.A. OKERHOLM, A. LAI, *et al.* 2004. The pharmacokinetics of sodium oxybate oral solution following acute and chronic administration to narcoleptic patients. J. Clin. Pharmacol. **44:** 253–257.

18. LeBeau, M.A., R.H. Christenson, B. Levine, *et al.* 2002. Intra- and interindividual variations in urinary concentrations of endogenous gamma-hydroxybutyrate. J. Anal. Toxicol. **26:** 340–346.
19. Elliott, S.P. 2003. Gamma hydroxybutyric acid (GHB) concentrations in humans and factors affecting endogenous production. Forensic Sci. Int. **133:** 9–16.
20. Yeatman, D.T. & K. Reid. 2003. A study of urinary endogenous gamma-hydroxybutyrate (GHB) levels. J. Anal. Toxicol. **27:** 40–42.
21. Caputo, F., G. Addolorato, F. Lorenzini, *et al.* 2003. Gamma-hydroxybutyric acid versus naltrexone in maintaining alcohol abstinence: an open randomized comparative study. Drug Alcohol Depend. **70:** 85–91.
22. Borgen, L.A., R. Okerholm, D. Morrison, *et al.* 2003. The influence of gender and food on the pharmacokinetics of sodium oxybate oral solution in healthy subjects. J. Clin. Pharmacol. **43:** 59–65.
23. Scharf, M.B., A.A. Lai, B. Branigan, *et al.* 1998. Pharmacokinetics of gammahydroxybutyrate (GHB) in narcoleptic patients. Sleep **21:** 507–514.
24. Gonzalez, A. & D.J. Nutt. 2005. Gamma hydroxy butyrate abuse and dependency. J. Psychopharmacol. **19:** 195–204.
25. Pickworth, W.B., R.V. Fant & E.B. Bunker. 1998. Effects of abused drugs on papillary size and the light reflex. *In* Drug Abuse Handbook. S.B. Karch, Eds.: 266–275. CRC Press. Boca Raton, FL.
26. Farre, M., M.T. Teran & J. Cami. 1996. A comparison of the acute behavioral effects of flunitrazepam and triazolam in healthy volunteers. Psychopharmacology (Berl.) **125:** 1–12.
27. Hernandez-Lopez, C., M. Farre, P.N. Roset, *et al.* 2002. 3,4-Methylenedioxymethamphetamine (ecstasy) and alcohol interactions in humans: psychomotor performance, subjective effects, and pharmacokinetics. J. Pharmacol. Exp. Ther. **300:** 236–244.
28. Wechsler, D. 1958. The Measurement and Appraisal of Adult Intelligence. Williams & Wilkins. Baltimore.
29. Hannington-Kiff, J.G. 1970. Measurement of recovery from out patient general anesthesia with a simple ocular test. Br. Med. J. **3:** 132–135.
30. Evans, S.M., J.R. Troisi II & R.R. Griffiths. 1994. Tandospirone and alprazolam: comparison of behavioral effects and abuse liability in humans. J. Pharmacol. Exp. Ther. **271:** 683–694.
31. Haertzen, C.A. 1974. An overview of the Addiction Center Research Inventory: an appendix and manual of scales DHEW Pub. no. (ADM) 79. Department of Health, Education and Welfare, Washington.
32. Lamas, X., M. Farré, M. Llorente, *et al.* 1994. Spanish version of the 49-item short version of the Addiction Research Center Inventory (ARCI). Drug Alcohol Depend. **35:** 203–209.
33. Poudevida, S., M. Farré, P.N. Roset, *et al.* 2003. Construcción de un cuestionario para la Valoración de los Efectos Subjetivos de Sustancias con Potencial de Abuso (VESSPA): Evaluación del éxtasis. Adicciones **15:** 115–126.
34. Elian, A.A. 2001. GC-MS determination of gamma-hydroxybutyric acid (GHB) in blood. Forensic Sci. Int. **122:** 43–47.
35. Davidson, D., K. Hutchison, C. Dagon, *et al.* 2002. Assessing the stimulant effects of alcohol in humans. Pharmacol. Biochem. Behav. **72:** 151–156.
36. Heishman, S.J., K. Arasteh & M.L. Stitzer. 1997. Comparative effects of alcohol and marijuana on mood, memory, and performance. Pharmacol. Biochem. Behav. **58:** 93–101.

37. Miotto, K., J. Darakjian, J. Basch, *et al.* 2001. Gamma-hydroxybutyric acid: patterns of use, effects and withdrawal. Am. J. Addict. **10:** 232–241.
38. Hicks, A.R., D.R. Kapusta & K.J. Varner. 2004. Mechanisms underlying the sympathomimetic cardiovascular responses elicited by [gamma]-hydroxybutyrate. J. Cardiovas. Pharmacol. **44:** 631–638.
39. Sporer, K.A., R.L. Chin, J.E. Dyer, *et al.* 2003. Gamma-hydroxybutyrate serum levels and clinical syndrome after severe overdose. Ann. Emerg Med. **42:** 3–8.
40. Kavanagh, P.V., P. Kenny, J. Feely. 2001. The urinary excretion of gamma-hydroxybutyric acid in man. J. Pharm. Pharmacol. **53:** 399–402.

CNS Aspects of Prenatal Drug Exposure

Drugs of Abuse, Toxins, and Corticosteroids

LIBOR VELÍŠEK

The Saul R. Korey Department of Neurology and the Dominick P. Purpura Department of Neuroscience, Albert Einstein College of Medicine, Einstein/Montefiore Comprehensive Epilepsy Management Center, Bronx, New York 10461, USA

ABSTRACT: Studies of the effects of prenatal exposure (to drugs or environmental factors) on postnatal brain morphology and function have an important role in assessing adverse effects of prenatal administration of corticosteroids in obstetrics, in studying the impairment of the offspring due to maternal drug abuse, as well as in studies of the influence of other environmental factors (such as toxins or stress). Timing, duration, and dose of the prenatal exposure play a significant role in the postnatal expression of the impact. However, data interpretation may be complicated by additional factors. As mixed litters of prenatally exposed subjects are evaluated, significant differences between males and females may occur. Additionally in females, cyclical changes in ovarian steroids may interfere with the effects of prenatal impact. Developmental differences may be also present, and data from infant, juvenile, prepubertal, and adult individuals cannot be simply compared. Finally, prenatal treatment is a stressful event and may present itself as prenatal stress, misguiding the interpretation. Postnatal environmental factors in raising the offspring, such as housing, maternal care, light–dark cycle, and weaning age can also change the data in such a way, which makes comparisons between different research laboratories impossible.

KEYWORDS: morphine; betamethasone; methotrexate; methylazoxymethanol; sex; development; gonadal hormones; stress; environmental factors

INTRODUCTION

Understanding the effects of prenatal exposure (to drugs or other environmental factors) on postnatal brain morphology and function is an important issue in developmental studies. There are many types of prenatal exposures

Address for correspondence: Dr. Libor Velíšek, AECOM, K314, 1300 Morris Park Ave, Bronx, NY 10461. Voice: 718-430-2490; fax: 718-430-8899.
e-mail: velisek@aecom.yu.edu

**Ann. N.Y. Acad. Sci. 1074: 577–589 (2006). © 2006 New York Academy of Sciences.
doi: 10.1196/annals.1369.057**

(events), which may affect the developing individual throughout postnatal life. Some of these prenatal impacts are naturally occurring and unavoidable, such as maternal stress, other events may be associated with therapeutic interventions, such as antenatal administration of corticosteroids (invariably life-saving for the fetus endangered by premature delivery), some of these exposures may be the result of maternal drug abuse, and finally, environmental toxins may exert their harmful effects during prenatal period. Each of these events may leave a significant imprint for further development.

In humans, maternal drug abuse during gestation may induce permanent neurological and behavioral abnormalities.[1] Offspring exposed to exogenous opiates (e.g., morphine, heroin, or methadone), as a result of maternal drug abuse, may exhibit deleterious, long-term functional alterations expressed as psychological and behavioral impairments.[2–4] These effects can persist till adulthood as demonstrated in numerous animal studies.[5–10] The scale of this problem is enormous. During 1970s and 1980s only in the United States alone, more than 300,000 people were exposed to opiates early in life.[11] Since prospective human studies are very prolonged and costly,[12,13] studies in animals with a relatively short life span are essential to identify potential neurochemical and behavioral consequences of prenatal drug exposure for the development of human nervous system and possibly, behavior.

Methodological Aspects of the Exposure

The *timing* of the exposure is critical. Significant impact during first two trimesters of pregnancy may be abortive, resulting in the interruption of pregnancy or in teratogenicity, with gross organ impairments.[14,15] However, events occurring at the end of the second trimester and especially during the third trimester of pregnancy may cause more subtle changes, yet similarly important for growth, development and general health of the offspring.[16–18]

The *duration and dosage* of the exposure is also significant. Brief periods of exposure usually leave a lesser footprint than a long-term exposure. However, some events even in a brief exposure and in a low dose may affect the offspring for the rest of the life, if the exposure coincides with a critical developmental period for a particular brain structure or function.[19] If a human condition is modeled, the duration and dosage of exposure should mimic human situation.

The *mechanism of action* of the treatment (or prenatal event) is also important for the consequences of the impact. Therefore, toxic chemicals, e.g., directly impairing DNA synthesis during critical growth periods, may provide significant morphological and functional alterations postnatally.[20–22] On the other hand, events with more generalized effects, such as prenatal stress,[23] may result in no overt morphological changes and only functional outcome may appear postnatally,[24] yet still significant for the health outcome of the offspring.[25] Yet, advanced techniques may eventually discover that even subtle alterations in behavioral outcome may be associated with changes in morphology.[26]

Although these methodological issues are important for developing the models of prenatal exposure, they are not subject of this text. In this article, the focus is on the other, less obvious factors, which may affect outcome of prenatal exposure studies and appropriate data interpretation. These factors should be always controlled for or at least considered. Several models of prenatal drug exposure will be appraised with a special emphasis on effects of prenatal exposure to the drugs of abuse, particularly morphine on nervous system development and function.

Examples of Models of Prenatal Drug Exposure

This laboratory is interested in the effects of different prenatal exposures on the development of the offspring with special emphasis on seizure susceptibility. We tested the effects of prenatal morphine exposure as an example of maternal drug abuse. Other models (methylazoxymethanol and methotrexate) were developed to study the effects of some toxins, which lead to neuronal migration disorders in the offspring, as many (developmental) types of epilepsy develop in the terrain of preexisting brain damage.[27] Finally, as an example of iatrogenic interventions, betamethasone administration, which is commonly used as a life-saving treatment for improved lung development in those pregnant women where there is a high risk of premature delivery, was studied. Yet, interpretational outcomes in all these models often overlap and, are subjected to similar errors especially if comparisons are attempted across different scientific groups.

Morphine was used to simulate prenatal opiate abuse. A treatment paradigm of two daily doses of 5–10 mg/kg administered between E11 and E18 produced very complex changes in the offspring.[10,28] Alterations in the offspring were clearly sex-specific as well as dependent on the postnatal developmental stage and involved changes in behavior, in endogenous opioid systems, reactivity of the hypothalamus-pituitary-adrenal (HPA) axis, synaptic plasticity, and seizure susceptibility.[29–37]

Methylazoxymethanol (MAM), a cycas toxin, is a DNA alkylating agent, which attacks DNA during the G_0 phase.[38–41] If administered during critical period of development of hippocampal pyramidal cells, it causes disruptions of neuronal migration resulting in occurrence of clustered neocortical neurons in the hippocampus.[20,22,42] Timing is critical in the case of MAM: the largest neuronal dysplasias can be induced by a single 25 mg/kg dose of MAM on day 15 (E15) of fetal development in the rat.[43,44] The offspring of MAM-treated rats dams were repeatedly tested for seizure susceptibility in various *in vivo* and *in vitro* models. The effects of prenatal MAM exposure were invariably proconvulsant without any obvious sex-specific features.[21,22,44–46]

Methotrexate (MTX, amethopterin), a folic acid antimetabolite, disrupts DNA synthesis during the S phase.[47–49] If a single dose of 5 mg/kg was

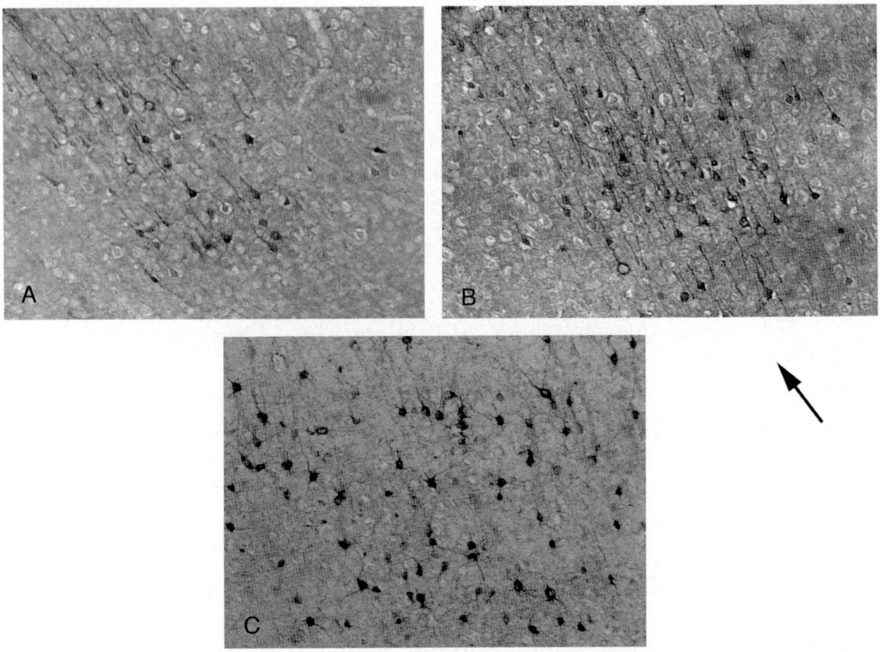

FIGURE 1. Sagittal sections through neocortex in two prenatally MTX-exposed rats (**A**, **B**) and a prenatally saline-exposed rat (**C**). In both sections from MTX-exposed rats (5 mg/kg on gestational day 15), there are clusters of GAD67-immunopositive (GABAergic) cells with processes perpendicular to the surface of the neocortex (direction indicated by an arrow). In contrast, GAD67-immunopositive cells in prenatally saline-exposed rat are randomly dispersed in the neocortex without clustering. GAD67-immunopositivity was more intense in the saline-exposed rat (**C**).

administered on E15, the offspring invariably demonstrated increased resistance to evoked seizures, i.e., this exposure had anticonvulsant features.[50] Similarly, there was an increased resistance to low Mg^{2+}-induced epileptiform activity in slices from prenatally MTX-exposed rats.[51] There was no sex difference in these effects of prenatal MTX. Morphologically, we observed increased cellularity in parts of the cortex[51] as well as clusters of GABAergic cells in the neocortex (FIG. 1).

Betamethasone is commonly used in pregnant women in the third trimester of pregnancy as a life-saving treatment to improve lung development of the fetus during periods of imminent premature delivery.[52] Our model of two administrations of 0.4 mg/kg betamethasone on E15 was developed to mimic human situation and make possible long-term follow-up in the offspring.[53,54] This treatment paradigm resulted in distinct sex-specific behavioral changes (decreased anxiety) and with sex-specific changes in seizure susceptibility. Morphologically, we found increased expression of neuropeptide Y (NPY) in the hippocampus, but not in the amygdala, consistent with findings of decreased anxiety.

Sex-Specific Outcomes

Effects of prenatal drug exposure are sometimes extremely complex. We studied effects of prenatal morphine exposure on seizure susceptibility in various models of primarily generalized seizures (such as flurothyl and bicuculline)[31,55–59] as well as secondarily generalized seizures (such as kainic acid).[60] We found that effects of prenatal morphine exposure in one model cannot be predicted from the effects in another model and that the effects on seizure susceptibility are significantly modified by gonadal steroids, i.e., are dependent not only on the sex of the animals, but also on the stage of estrous cycle in females.[55] For review of the effects of sex and estrous cycle stage on seizure susceptibility in adult rats (postnatal day 60 and older; >PN 60), see TABLE 1.

Similar differences were recorded in the *in vitro* model of epileptiform activity. Removal of Mg^{2+} from the perfusing medium results in occurrence of

TABLE 1. Effects prenatal morphine exposure on seizure susceptibility in adult (>PN 60) rats *in vivo:* modification by sex and female gonadal steroids

		Females			
Models	Males	OVX	OVX+ E	OVX+ P	OVX+E+P
Flurothyl	Anticonvulsant	0	Anticonvulsant	0	Proconvulsant
Bicuculline	0	Anticonvulsant	Anticonvulsant	N/T	0
Kainic acid (KA)	0	Anticonvulsant	Anticonvulsant	N/T	N/T
N-methyl-D-aspartic acid (NMDA)	0	0	0	N/T	N/T

NOTE: In this overview, only unambiguous behavioral seizures are considered. OVX females were used either injected with oil (OVX) or supplemented with E (3 μg s.c. 48 h prior to testing) or P (500 μg s.c 4 h prior to testing) or with a combination of E + P. In the flurothyl test, rats were subjected to inhalant convulsant drug flurothyl delivered to an air-tight, 9.38 L chamber at the rate of 20 μL/s). KA-treated male rats received 15 or 20 mg/kg dose, female rats 10–15 mg/kg dose i.p. NMDA-treated rats received 150–250 mg/kg doses, female rats received 200 mg/kg dose i.p. Although flurothyl produces two seizure types, clonic and tonic–clonic, the effects on these two seizure types were never the opposite. Both KA and NMDA elicit automatisms and seizures. Here, only the effects on seizures are shown.

OVX: ovariectomy.

E: estradiol replacement.

P: progesterone replacement.

Anticonvulsant: seizures occurred later compared to prenatally saline-exposed controls under the same seizure test conditions.

0: no difference in seizure onset compared to prenatally saline-exposed controls.

Proconvulsant: seizures occurred earlier compared to prenatally saline-exposed controls.

N/T: not tested.

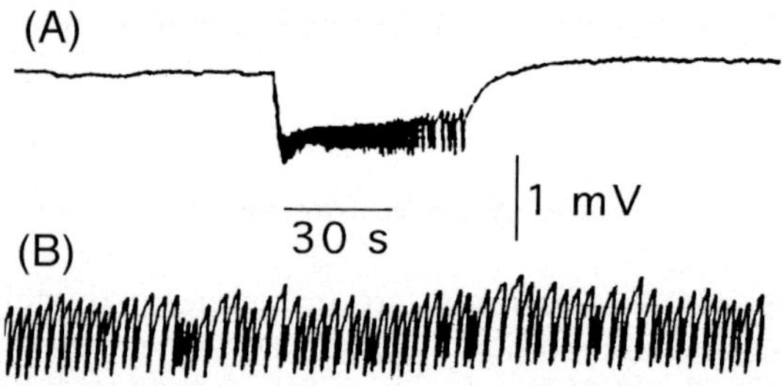

FIGURE 2. Examples of discharges induced in the medial entorhinal cortex by low extracellular Mg^{2+} *in vitro*. (**A**) Long-lasting SLE is the first sign of epileptiform activity in the medial entorhinal cortex. (**B**) Eventually, SLEs develop into status of short recurrent discharges continuing as long as the Mg^{2+} in the extracellular environment stays low.

epileptiform discharges in combined hippocampus–entorhinal cortex slices.[61] In the medial entorhinal cortex, initially long ictal discharges are recoded, lasting 1–7 min associated with a significant negative DC shift (seizure-like events [SLE]; FIG. 2A). These discharges eventually develop into a status of recurrent discharges (FIG. 2B) and last as long the perfusing solution stays Mg^{2+}-free. Latency to onset of SLEs and status of recurrent discharges in slices from prenatally morphine-exposed rats was significantly modified by sex and ovarian steroids (TABLE 2).[36,62]

Additionally, we determined synaptic plasticity in the hippocampal CA1 region in hippocampal slices *in vitro*.[37,63] After high-frequency stimulation of Schaffer collaterals, synaptic responses were recorded in the stratum radiatum of CA1. Indeed, we found sex-specific alterations of the short-term plasticity

TABLE 2. Effects prenatal morphine exposure on low Mg^{2+}-induced epileptiform activity in adult (>PN 60) rats *in vivo*: modification by sex and female gonadal steroids

		Females			
Feature	Males	OVX	OVX+ E	OVX+ P	OVX+E+P
SLE	Proconvulsant	0	Anticonvulsant	0	0
Status of recurrent discharges	Proconvulsant	0	Anticonvulsant	0	0

NOTE: Combined horizontal hippocampus–entorhinal cortex slices were prepared. Slices from both morphine- and saline-exposed rat were placed side by side in one recording in vitro chamber for similar conditions. Order of preparing slices was alternated. Extracellular recordings were performed in the layers IV–V of the medial entorhinal cortex.

OVX: ovariectomy.

E: estradiol replacement.

P: progesterone replacement.

Proconvulsant: epileptiform events occurred earlier compared to prenatally saline-exposed controls.

0: no difference in seizure onset compared to prenatally saline-exposed controls.

Anticonvulsant: epileptiform events occurred later compared to prenatally saline-exposed controls under same seizure test conditions.

TABLE 3. Effects prenatal morphine exposure on CA1 hippocampal synaptic plasticity in adult (>PN 60) rats *in vitro*: modification by sex and female estrous cycle stages

		Females	
Parameter	Males	Diestrus	Proestrus
Short-term plasticity	0	Enhanced	Suppressed
LTP	Suppressed	0	Suppressed

NOTE: Short-term plasticity was evaluated 5 min after the high-frequency stimulation. LTP was assessed at 30 min after high-frequency stimulation. Extracellular excitatory postsynaptic potential (EPSP) slopes were determined.

0: no difference from saline-exposed controls.

Enhanced: increase compared to saline-exposed controls.

Suppressed: decrease compared to saline-exposed controls.

and long-term potentiation (LTP) as well as a significant role of female gonadal steroids (TABLE 3).

These data illustrate that the prenatal exposure studies represent an extreme interpretational challenge. As the outcome of pregnancy is usually a mix of males and females, the results of postnatal tests in both sexes are not equal and cannot be considered equal unless statistically proven. Further, if adult females are used, their estrous cycle stage may additionally modify the outcome of the studies, unless properly determined and controlled for.

Age-Specific Outcomes

In our studies, we also performed developmental evaluation of seizure susceptibility in prenatally morphine-exposed rats. Postnatal susceptibility to seizures was further affected by developmental stages, though still with the influence of sex.[31,59,64] For review of age-specific modification of prenatal morphine exposure effects on seizure susceptibility, see TABLE 4.

As the prenatally exposed offspring develops, one is presented with further challenge in the interpretation of prenatal drug exposure data. Results can be compared only at the corresponding ages. As shown in TABLE 4, results obtained in PN 25 rats cannot be compared to PN 38 rats and on top of this developmental difference, there is still a sex difference.

Masking Effects of Stress

Every prenatal drug administration is a stressful event. In the evaluation of postnatal effects of drug exposure stress effects can completely overlap the effects of prenatal treatment. This can be seen in examples of behavioral testing of three groups of subjects: prenatally saline- and morphine-exposed rats in addition to the offspring of noninjected dams. In fact, it has been demonstrated that in Porsolt forced swim test and in the open field test, there was no difference

TABLE 4. Effects prenatal morphine exposure on seizure susceptibility in immature (PN 15–38) rats *in vivo*: modification by developmental stage and sex

	Flurothyl		Bicuculline	
Postnatal age	Males	Females	Males	Females
PN 15	0	Proconvulsant	N/T	N/T
PN 25	Proconvulsant	Anticonvulsant	Proconvulsant	0
PN 38	Anticonvulsant	0	Anticonvulsant	0

NOTE: In this overview, only unambiguous behavioral seizures are considered. In the flurothyl test, rats were subjected to inhalant convulsant drug flurothyl delivered to an air-tight, 9.38 L chamber at the rate of 20 μL/s. In the bicuculline test, PN 25 rats received 5 mg/kg, while PN 38 rats received 7.5 mg/kg i.p. Although both flurothyl and bicuculline produce two seizure types, clonic and tonic–clonic, the effects on these two seizure types were never the opposite.

0: no difference in seizure onset compared to prenatally saline-exposed controls.

Proconvulsant: seizures occurred earlier compared to prenatally saline-exposed controls.

Anticonvulsant: seizures occurred later compared to prenatally saline-exposed controls under the same seizure test conditions.

N/T: not tested.

between prenatally saline- and morphine-exposed groups of adult male rats. However, results in both groups differed from the offspring of noninjected mothers.[65] Similar differences were found in female rats. However, finding differences in females was further dependent on the presence of estradiol. So, again both prenatally exposed groups of adult female rats were similar in parameters measured in the Porsolt swim test and in the open field, but differed from the female offspring of noninjected mothers only in presence of estradiol.[65]

The data indicate that the effects of prenatal stress can pose as the effects of injected drug (if any) as prenatal stress has been shown to significantly affect postnatal behaviors as well as seizure susceptibility.[53,66–69]

Other Postnatal Variables

There are many additional factors, which may significantly sway the outcome of prenatal drug exposure. *Housing* can be critical for experiments in rodents. Rodents are social animals and their performance can be significantly altered if housed individually. Although individual housing does not affect HPA reactivity,[34,70] the effect of housing on performance can be indirectly verified in experiments using animals raised in enriched environment,[71,72] which usually includes larger (6–10) than normal group of animals (3–4). Discordance in *lighting* may affect outcome of the experiments as well, because of exploiting different phases of the circadian rhythm.[73,74] Usually, rats are housed on a regular light–dark cycle and the experiments are performed during the light period. This can be dramatically changed if the rats are housed on reversed light–dark cycle and as a result, all experiments are performed during the dark period. Also *maternal care* is important, as maternal behavior may be altered by the exposure during pregnancy and simulate effects of prenatal exposure in the offspring. Therefore, if possible, cross-fostering between exposed and control dams should be done. Finally, *weaning* is similarly critical. Behavioral characteristics can significantly differ based on the weaning age.[75] Weaning differences after prenatal exposure thus can skew interpretations and comparisons with other research groups.

CONCLUSIONS

Studies on the brain effects of prenatal exposure to drugs, especially illicit drugs, are very important since during pregnancy, many women continue their drug abuse. However, these studies bring many challenges. These challenges may be the result of the methodological aspects of prenatal treatment, such as timing within the pregnancy, dose, and duration. Treatment itself may be stressful and postnatally expressed similarly or identically to prenatal stress. Other interpretational challenges arise from different standards in different laboratories and include sex and hormonal status of the subjects as well as their age. Postnatal environmental challenges include breeding condition such as light–dark cycle, individual versus group housing, maternal care, and age of weaning. All these factors need to be considered for interpretation of the data and for comparisons between laboratories.

ACKNOWLEDGMENTS

Based on the presentation "Stress or Drug Abuse? Mechanisms of Long-Term Impact of Prenatal Morphine Exposure" at the ISN/ESN Satellite Meeting "Cellular and Molecular Mechanisms of Drugs of Abuse and Neurotoxicity: Cocaine, GHB and Substituted Amphetamines", Isola di San Servolo, Venice, Italy, August 16–19, 2005. This work was supported by the NIH grants NS-41366, NS-20253, and NS-36238 and by the CURE Foundation. The author wishes to thank Dr. Jana Velíšková for very critical reading of the manuscript.

REFERENCES

1. CHASNOFF, J. 1985. Effects of maternal narcotic vs non narcotic addiction on neonatal neurobehavior and infant development. *In* Consequences of Maternal Drug Abuse, National Institute of Drug Abuse. T.M. Pinkert, Ed.: 84–95. National Institute of Drug Abuse. Washington, D.C.
2. WILSON, G.S. 1989. Clinical studies of infants and children exposed prenatally to heroin. Ann. N. Y. Acad. Sci. **562:** 183–194.
3. WOODS, J.R. Jr. 1996. Adverse consequences of prenatal illicit drug exposure. Curr. Opin. Obstet. Gynecol. **8:** 403–411.

4. ZUCKERMAN, B., D. FRANK & E. BROWN. 1995. Overview of the effects of abuse and drugs on pregnancy and offspring. NIDA Res. Monogr. **149:** 16–38.
5. ZAGON, I.S., P.J. MCLAUGHLIN & C.I. THOMPSON. 1979. Learning ability in adult female rats perinatally exposed to methadone. Pharmacol. Biochem. Behav. **10:** 889–894.
6. KOYUNCUOGLU, H. & F. ARICIOGLU. 1993. Prenatal exposure to morphine or naloxone intensifies morphine dependence at maturity. Pharmacol. Biochem. Behav. **44:** 939–941.
7. CASTELLANO, C. & M. AMMASSARI-TEULE. 1984. Prenatal exposure to morphine in mice: enhanced responsiveness to morphine and stress. Pharmacol. Biochem. Behav. **21:** 103–108.
8. GAGIN, R., E. COHEN & Y. SHAVIT. 1997. Prenatal exposure to morphine feminizes male sexual behavior in the adult rat. Pharmacol. Biochem. Behav. **58:** 345–348.
9. GAGIN, R. *et al.* 1997. Prenatal morphine enhances morphine-conditioned place preference in adult rats. Pharmacol. Biochem. Behav. **58:** 525–528.
10. LESAGE, J. *et al.* 1998. Consequences of prenatal morphine exposure on the hypothalamo-pituitary-adrenal axis in the newborn rat: effect of maternal adrenalectomy. J. Neuroendocrinol. **10:** 331–342.
11. ZAGON, T.S. & P.J. MCLAUGHLIN. 1992. Maternal exposure to opioids and the developing nervous system; laboratory findings. *In* Maternal Substance Abuse and the Developing Nervous System. I.S. Zagon & T.A. Slotkin, Eds.: 241–282. Academic Press. San Diego.
12. BEHNKE, M. & F.D. EYLER. 1993. The consequences of prenatal substance use for the developing fetus, newborn and young child. Int. J. Addict. **28:** 1341–1391.
13. VAN BAAR, A. & B.M.T. de GRAAFF. 1994. Cognitive development at preschool-age of infants of drug-dependent mothers. Dev. Med. Child Neurol. **36:** 1063–1075.
14. JORDAN, R.L., J.G. WILSON & H.J. SCHUMACHER. 1977. Embryotoxicity of the folate antagonist methotrexate in rats and rabbits. Teratology **15:** 73–80.
15. TSHIBANGU, K., F. LEROY & M. DOUMONT-MEYVIS. 1975. Effects of amethopterin (methotrexate) on the evolution of pregnancy in rats. Toxicology **4:** 65–73.
16. SECKL, J.R. 2000. Antenatal glucocorticoid therapy: a caveat to the applause. Clin. Sci. (Colch.) **98:** 127–128.
17. WELBERG, L.A.M. & J.R. SECKL. 2001. Prenatal stress, glucocorticoids and the programming of the brain. J. Neuroendocr. **13:** 113–128.
18. VATHY, I. *et al.* 1994. Modulation of catecholamine turnover rate in brain regions of rats exposed prenatally to morphine. Brain Res. **662:** 209–215.
19. AVISHAI-ELINER, S. *et al.* 2002. Stressed-out, or in (utero)? Trends Neurosci. **25:** 518–524.
20. GERMANO, I.M. & E.F. SPERBER. 1998. Transplacentally induced neuronal migration disorders: an animal model for the study of the epilepsies. J. Neurosci. Res. **51:** 473–488.
21. BARABAN, S.C. & P.A. SCHWARTZKROIN. 1995. Electrophysiology of CA1 pyramidal neurons in an animal model of neuronal migration disorders: prenatal methylazoxymethanol treatment. Epilepsy Res. **22:** 145–156.
22. CHEVASSUS-AU-LOUIS, N. *et al.* 1998. Neocortex in the hippocampus: an anatomical and functional study of CA1 heterotopias after prenatal treatment with methylazoxymethanol in rats. J. Comp. Neurol. **394:** 520–536.
23. VALLEE, M. *et al.* 1999. Long-term effects of prenatal stress and postnatal handling on age- related glucocorticoid secretion and cognitive performance: a longitudinal study in the rat. Eur. J. Neurosci. **11:** 2906–2916.

24. FRIDE, E. *et al.* 1986. Effects of prenatal stress on vulnerability to stress in prepubertal and adult rats. Physiol. Behav. **37:** 681–687.
25. STOTT, D.H. 1973. Follow-up study from birth of the effects of prenatal stresses. Dev. Med. Child Neurol. **15:** 770–787.
26. LEMAIRE, V. *et al.* 2000. Prenatal stress produces learning deficits associated with an inhibition of neurogenesis in the hippocampus. Proc. Natl. Acad. Sci. U.S.A. **97:** 11032–11037.
27. HOLMES, G.L. 1997. Epilepsy in the developing brain: lessons from the laboratory and clinic. Epilepsia **38:** 12–30.
28. VATHY, I., A.M. ETGEN & R.J. BARFIELD. 1985. Effects of prenatal exposure to morphine on the development of sexual behavior in rats. Pharmacol. Biochem. Behav. **22:** 227–232.
29. RIMANÓCZY, A. & I. VATHY. 1995. Prenatal exposure to morphine alters brain μ opioid receptor characteristics in rats. Brain Res. **690:** 245–248.
30. VATHY, I. & L. KÁTAY. 1992. Effects of prenatal morphine on adult sexual behavior and brain catecholamines in rats. Dev. Brain Res. **73:** 115–122.
31. VATHY, I., J. VELÍŠKOVÁ & S.L. MOSHÉ. 1998. Prenatal morphine exposure induces age-related changes in seizure susceptibility in male rats. Pharmacol. Biochem. Behav. **60:** 635–638.
32. VATHY, I. *et al.* 1995. Sex dimorphic alterations in postnatal brain catecholamines after gestational morphine. Brain Res. Bull. **36:** 185–193.
33. VATHY, I. *et al.* 2002. Prenatal morphine exposure differentially alters plasma CORT and ACTH levels in response to restraint stress of adult male rats. Society for Neuroscience 2002 Abstract Viewer/Itinerary Planner. **No. 274.6.**
34. ŠLAMBEROVÁ, R. *et al.* 2004. Hypothalamo-pituitary-adrenal axis-regulated stress response and negative feedback sensitivity is altered by prenatal morphine exposure in adult female rats. Neuroendocrinology **80:** 192–200.
35. DUTRIEZ-CASTELOOT, I. *et al.* 1999. Hypothalamic-pituitary-adrenocortical and gonadal axes and sympathoadrenal activity of adult male rats prenatally exposed to morphine. Neurosci Lett. **263:** 1–4.
36. VELÍŠEK, L. *et al.* 2000. Prenatal morphine exposure enhances seizure susceptibility but suppresses long-term potentiation in the limbic system of adult male rats. Brain Res. **869:** 186–193.
37. VELÍŠEK, L., R. ŠLAMBEROVÁ & I. VATHY. 2003. Prenatal morphine exposure suppresses mineralocorticoid receptor-dependent basal synaptic transmission and synaptic plasticity in the lateral perforant path in adult male rats. Brain Res. Bull. **61:** 571–576.
38. NAGATA, Y. & H. MATSUMOTO. 1969. Studies on methylazoxymethanol; methylation of nucleic acids in fetal rat brain. Proc. Soc. Exp. Biol. Med. **132:** 383–385.
39. ZEDECK, M.S. *et al.* 1974. Early changes induced in rat liver by methylazoxymethanol acetate: mitotic abnormalities and polyploidy. J. Nation. Cancer. Instit. **53:** 719–723.
40. MATSUMOTO, H. & H.H. HIGA. 1966. Studies on methylazoxymethanol, the aglycone of cycasin: methylation of nucleic acids *in vitro*. Biochem. J. **98:** 20c–22c.
41. HADDAD, R.K., A. RABE & R. DUMAS. 1972. Comparison of effects of methylazoxymethanol acetate on brain development in different species. Fed. Proc. **31:** 1520–1523.
42. CHEVASSUS-AU-LOUIS, N. *et al.* 1999. Cortical malformations and epilepsy: new insights from animal models. Epilepsia **40:** 811–821.

43. BARABAN, S.C. & P.A. SCHWARTZKROIN. 1996. Flurothyl seizure susceptibility in rats following prenatal methylazoxymethanol treatment. Epilepsy Res. **23:** 189–194.
44. GERMANO, I.M. *et al.* 1996. Neuronal migration disorders increase susceptibility to hyperthermia-induced seizures in developing rats. Epilepsia **37:** 902–910.
45. GERMANO, I.M. & E.F. SPERBER. 1997. Increased seizure susceptibility in adult rats with neuronal migration disorders. Brain Res. **777:** 219–222.
46. DE FEO, M.R., O. MECARELLI & G.F. RICCI. 1995. Seizure susceptibility in immature rats with microencephaly induced by prenatal exposure to methylazoxymethanol acetate. Pharmacol. Res. **31:** 109–114.
47. SCHMID, B.P. 1984. Monitoring of organ formation in rat embryos after in vitro exposure to azathioprine, mercaptopurine, methotrexate or cyclosporine A. Toxicology **31:** 9–21.
48. KAMEN, B.A. 1986. Methotrexate, folate and the brain. Neurotoxicology **2:** 209–216.
49. LAVELLE, F.W. & A. LAVELLE. 1967. Resistance of differentiating neurons to the antimetabolite, amethopterin. Exp. Neurol. **17:** 140–158.
50. KÁBOVÁ, R., J. VELÍSKOVÁ & L. VELÍSEK. 2000. Prenatal methotrexate exposure decreases seizure susceptibility in young rats of two strains. Exp. Neurol. **161:** 167–173.
51. KÁBOVÁ, R. & L. VELÍSEK. 2000. Prenatal methotrexate exposure delays onset of low Mg^{2+}-induced epileptiform discharges in the entorhinal cortex. Dev. Brain. Res. **123:** 91–94.
52. GUINN, D.A. *et al.* 2001. Single vs weekly courses of antenatal corticosteroids for women at risk of preterm delivery: a randomized controlled trial. JAMA **286:** 1581–1587.
53. VELÍŠEK, L. 2005. Prenatal corticosteroid impact on hippocampus: implications for postnatal outcomes. Epilepsy Behav. **7:** 57–67.
54. VELÍŠEK, L. 2005. Prenatal betamethasone exposure suppresses kindling epileptogenesis in immature rats. *In* Kindling 6. M.E. Corcoran & S.L. Moshé, Eds.: 11–17. Springer. New York.
55. VATHY, I. 2001. Prenatal morphine exposure induces age- and sex-dependent changes in seizure susceptibility. Prog. Neuropsychopharmacol. Biol. Psychiatry **25:** 1203–1226.
56. ŠLAMBEROVÁ, R. & I. VATHY. 2000. Estrogen differentially alters NMDA- and kainate-induced seizures in prenatally morphine- and saline-exposed adult female rats. Pharmacol. Biochem. Behav. **67:** 501–505.
57. SCHINDLER, C.J., R. SLAMBEROVA & I. VATHY. 2003. Bicuculline seizure susceptibility and nigral GABAA alpha1 receptor mRNA is altered in adult prenatally morphine-exposed females. Psychoneuroendocrinology **28:** 348–363.
58. SCHINDLER, C.J., R. SLAMBEROVA & I. VATHY. 2001. Prenatal morphine exposure decreases susceptibility of adult male rat offspring to bicuculline seizures. Brain Res. **922:** 305–309.
59. SCHINDLER, C.J. *et al.* 2000. Prenatal morphine exposure alters susceptibility to bicuculline seizures in a sex- and age-specific manner. Brain Res. Dev. Brain Res. **121:** 119–122.
60. ŠLAMBEROVÁ, R., L. VELÍŠEK & I. VATHY. 2000. Prenatal morphine exposure alters *N*-methyl-D-aspartate- and kainate-induced seizures in adult male rats. Pharmacol. Biochem. Behav. **65:** 39–42.

61. WALTHER, H. *et al.* 1986. Epileptiform activity in combined slices of the hippocampus, subiculum and entorhinal cortex during perfusion with low magnesium. Neurosci. Lett. **69:** 156–161.
62. VELÍŠEK, L. *et al.* 1998. Prenatal morphine exposure alters ovarian steroid hormonal regulation of seizure susceptibility. Brain Res. **796:** 247–256.
63. VELÍŠEK, L. & I. VATHY. 2005. Mifepristone (RU486) inhibits lateral perforant path long-term potentiation in hippocampal slices from prenatally morphine-exposed female rats. Int. J. Dev. Neurosci. **23:** 559–565.
64. VELÍŠKOVÁ, J., S.L. MOSHÉ & I. VATHY. 1999. Prenatal morphine exposure differentially alters seizure susceptibility in developing female rats. Brain Res. Dev. Brain Res. **116:** 119–121.
65. ŠLAMBEROVÁ, R., C.J. SCHINDLER & I. VATHY. 2002. Impact of maternal morphine and saline injections on behavioral responses to a cold water stressor in adult male and female progeny. Physiol. Behav. **75:** 723–732.
66. EDWARDS, H.E. *et al.* 2002. Prenatal stress alters seizure thresholds and the development of kindled seizures in infant and adult rats. Horm. Behav. **42:** 437–447.
67. EDWARDS, H.E., S. VIMAL & W.M. BURNHAM. 2002. Dose-, time-, age-, and sex-response profiles for the anticonvulsant effects of deoxycorticosterone in 15-day-old rats. Exp. Neurol. **176:** 364–370.
68. KAPOOR, A. & S.G. MATTHEWS. 2005. Short periods of prenatal stress affect growth, behaviour and hypothalamo-pituitary-adrenal axis activity in male guinea pig offspring. J. Physiol. **566:** 967–977.
69. KOENIG, J.I. *et al.* 2005. Prenatal exposure to a repeated variable stress paradigm elicits behavioral and neuroendocrinological changes in the adult offspring: potential relevance to schizophrenia. Behav. Brain Res. **156:** 251–261.
70. RIMANÓCZY, A. *et al.* 2003. Adrenocorticotropin stress response but not glucocorticoid-negative feedback is altered by prenatal morphine exposure in adult male rats. Neuroendocrinology **78:** 312–320.
71. YOUNG, D. *et al.* 1999. Environmental enrichment inhibits spontaneous apoptosis, prevents seizures and is neuroprotective. Nat. Med. **5:** 448–453.
72. NILSSON, M. *et al.* 1999. Enriched environment increases neurogenesis in the adult rat dentate gyrus and improves spatial memory. J. Neurobiol. **39:** 569–578.
73. KOEHL, M. *et al.* 1999. Prenatal stress alters circadian activity of hypothalamo-pituitary-adrenal axis and hippocampal corticosteroid receptors in adult rats of both gender. J. Neurobiol. **40:** 302–315.
74. ATKINSON, H.C. & B.J. WADDELL. 1997. Circadian variation in basal plasma corticosterone and adrenocorticotropin in the rat: sexual dimorphism and changes across the estrous cycle. Endocrinology **138:** 3842–3848.
75. NOVAKOVA, V. 1966. Weaning of young rats: effect of time on behavior. Science **151:** 475–476.

Effects of Prenatal Exposure to Methamphetamine on the Development of the Rat Retina

PEDRO MELO,[a,b] LORENA G. RODRIGUES,[a,c] M. CAROLINA SILVA,[c] AND MARIA AMÉLIA TAVARES[a,b]

[a]*Unit of Neurobehaviour, Institute for Molecular and Cell Biology;* [b]*Institute of Anatomy, Faculty of Medicine of the University of Porto;* [c]*Institute for Biomedical Sciences Abel Salazar, University of Porto, 4150-180 Porto, Portugal*

ABSTRACT: In recent years there has been growing use of methamphetamine (METH) by pregnant women, resulting in an increasing number of children exposed prenatally to this drug of abuse. METH is known to be potentially neurotoxic to human adults, but there is minimal information with respect to the consequences of such exposure to the fetus. The purpose of this study was to ascertain external parameters of animal development, as well as neurochemical and immunohistochemical alterations at three key points of retinal development (postnatal day [PND] 7, 14, and 30). Rats of the Wistar strain were used in this experimental model. Pregnant females received a dose of 5 mg/kg body weight per day of METH-HCl in 0.9% saline, from gestational day (GD) 8 to 22. The control group to be used was pair fed and saline injected. Litters were randomly culled at PND 1 to 8 pups. Analysis of maternal body weight gain during pregnancy showed that females treated with METH had lower body weights than control-treated females. The body weight on PND 1, showed that animals treated with METH prenatally had smaller body weights than the control-treated animals and also that females weighed less than males. Prenatal exposure to METH did not alter the retinal levels of 3,4-dihydroxyphenylacetic acid (DOPAC) in the male group and the level of dopamine (DA) in both female and male groups when compared with their respective pair fed control groups during the first month of life. Correlating with the neurochemical data, no obvious changes on the localization of TH immunoreactivity in the rat retina at PND 7, 14, and 30 could be detected between control and METH-treated animals. Thus, exposure to METH disrupted this pattern in a gender-dependent manner. These data confirm previous observation that developing rats are protected against the adult type of METH-induced neurotoxicity. Therefore, conventional markers used for adult animals appear to be unsatisfactory to demarcate boundaries of the PND 1 to 30 critical periods.

Address for correspondence: P. Melo, Unit of Neurobehaviour, Institute for Molecular and Cell Biology, Rua do Campo Alegre, 823, 4150-180 Porto, Portugal. Voice: +351 22 6074700; fax: +351 22 6099157.

e-mail: pmelo@ibmc.up.pt

Ann. N.Y. Acad. Sci. 1074: 590–603 (2006). © 2006 New York Academy of Sciences.
doi: 10.1196/annals.1369.058

Keywords: methamphetamine; retina; development; Wistar rat; dopamine; tyrosine hydroxylase

INTRODUCTION

It is well known that exposure to some substances, such as environmental contaminants, industrial toxics, food preservatives, pharmacological substances, drugs of abuse, and alcohol,[1] during gestation can have profound effects on the morphological, physiological, and/or behavioral development of the offspring. The severity of these effects is dependent upon many factors, but of particular importance is the time during development when the exposure occurs.[2,3]

The effects of substituted amphetamines during pregnancy have not been well characterized in humans even though the use of some of these drugs, for example, methamphetamine (METH), increased dramatically during the 1990s.[4,5] It has been suggested that in humans long-term cognitive deficits may result following exposure to amphetamine *in utero*,[6] although no retrospective studies exist for METH. In humans there have been several reports of short-term effects of METH *in utero*: decreased body weights at birth, smaller head circumferences, increased morbidity, and reduced performance in a visual recognition test during the first year of life.[7,8] It has also been shown that women who use METH throughout all of gestation have smaller babies than those who use during only the first trimester or the first and second trimesters.[9] Magnetic resonance imaging spectroscopy performed on children exposed to METH during gestation identified an increase in creatine and glutamate/glutamine concentrations in the striatum, suggesting increased cellular metabolic activity that continued years after the *in utero* exposure.[10] The volume of neurons and glia in the METH-exposed children did not appear to be altered in that study. Therefore, in humans, *in utero* METH exposure alters cellular function, while leaving the volume of cells relatively intact. Taken together, these data suggest that METH causes prolonged central nervous system changes.

A major concern among research groups that study drugs of abuse is the selection of a suitable experimental design when working with animal models. The effects of prenatal exposure to METH have been widely studied throughout the last decades. In animal models, the pharmacological effects of METH depend greatly upon the dose and pattern of administration. In rat models, for example, different effects are seen with administration of a single dose, with repeated administration of a low dose at long intervals, or with high-dose runs superimposed on chronic low administrations.[11]

Experimental studies examining the effect of prenatal exposure to METH are limited and have produced variable results. When METH is administered throughout gestation, elevations in dopamine (DA), serotonin (5-HT), s-hydroxyindoleacetic acid (5-HIAA), and norepinephrine (NE) are observed in several forebrain regions of 9-month-old rat offspring following drug treatment.[12,13] Others, however, have reported a reduction in rat cortical DA concentration as well as 5-HT receptor binding in 5-week postnatal offspring.[14] To increase this complexity, studies of other neurochemical markers have indicated that low doses (2–5 mg/kg) of METH, administered throughout pregnancy, result in a reduction in DA and 5-HT uptake sites in young adult progeny, while higher doses (10 mg/kg) of the drug, in contrast, produce an increase in DA and 5-HT uptake sites.[15] When pregnant dams are treated with METH for a more limited period, from gestational day (GD) 13 to 20, their adult offspring exhibit an attenuated elevation in plasma renin following exposure to parachloroamphetamine despite having normal levels of brain 5-HT uptake sites and 5-HT receptors.[16] The differences observed in these studies may well be related to the use of different dosage regimens, periods of gestational exposure to this psychomotor stimulant, strain of rats used or postnatal ages at which offspring are assessed.

The present study was undertaken to test whether METH impairs the normal development of the retina at different time points of its development. In order to achieve this aim a prenatal rat model was used.

MATERIALS AND METHODS

Animal Model

Handling and care of animals were according to the Association for Research into Vision and Ophthalmology (ARVO) Statement for the Use of Animals in Ophthalmic and Vision Research and the Portuguese law (Portaria n° 1005/92). Rats of the Wistar strain were used in this experimental model. At the beginning of the experimental period, 2-month-old nulliparous females, weighing an average of 250–300 g, were mated with one male, at 8:00 PM The following morning, vaginal cytology was performed. If either sperm or a vaginal plug was detected (GD 1) the female was weighed and placed in a separate cage. At GD 8, pregnant females were assigned to each experimental group.

Prenatal Administration of Methamphetamine

Pregnant females received a dose of 5 mg/kg body weight per day of METH-HCl in 0.9% saline, from GD 8 to GD 22. Each daily dose was split in two and administered between 9:00 and 9:30 AM and between 5:00 and 5:30 PM, respectively. Injections were delivered subcutaneously, in the dorsum, in a volume of 3 mL/kg per injection, with injection sites rotated to minimize damage to the dermis. No necrotic lesions in the dermis were produced using this method. Daily food consumption (weight difference to a known value) was registered during the drug exposure period (beginning on GD 8 and ending on GD 22). The control group to be used was pair fed and saline injected. Both the schedule and volume for injecting saline in the pair-fed control group were the same as for the METH dams. Each female in this group received the average amount of food daily that the METH-injected female in the same group ate the same GD. Beginning on GD 22, pregnant females were checked twice daily for the presence of a litter. Females were allowed to deliver and litters were reared by their biological mother. The day of birth was designated postnatal day (PND) 0. Litters were left undisturbed until PND 1 when the litter was sexed, weighed, and randomly culled to eight pups (four males and four females). Animals were identified by painting their paws, head, or trunk with unwashable ink according to a coding system. The pups were weighed everyday at 8:30 a.m. to avoid variances. At PND 21, litters were weaned from their mothers.

Neurochemical Studies

At the end of each experimental period (PND 7, 14, and 30) following METH or vehicle treatment, at least two females and two males per litter, were randomly selected from the litters for neurochemical studies. The animals were decapitated, eyes were enucleated, and the retinas quickly dissected. The retinas were frozen and stored at $-70°C$, until neurochemical determination. Retinas were ultrasonicated (Branson sonifier W-150, Branson Ultrasonics, Danbury, CT) in 500 μL of ice-cold 0.2 M perchloric acid containing 10 ng/mL of the internal standard 3,4-dihydrobenzylamine (DHBA). The homogenate was centrifuged (13,000 g, 15 min) and the supernatant was filtered through a 0.2-μm Nylon-66 microfilter. Aliquots of 50 μL were then analyzed for DA and 3,4-dihydroxyphenylacetic acid (DOPAC) by high-performance liquid chromatography (HPLC) with electrochemical detection (ECD) by a method modified from Ali and colleagues.[17] The Gilson Medical Electronics HPLC system (Middleton, WI) was composed of a LC234 auto-injector, LC307 delivery pump, LC142 electro-chemical detector, and 712 HPLC system controller data version 1.30 management software. The mobile phase consisted of 70 mM potassium phosphate monobasic buffer (pH was adjusted to 3.0 by adding phosphoric acid), 1 mM *l*-heptanosulfonic acid, 107.5-μM sodium EDTA, and 10% (v/v) methanol. The flow rate was maintained at 1 mL/min. Biogenic amines were separated by a Supelcosil LC (7.5 cm × 4.6 cm, 3 μm) reversed phase column. Quantification was achieved via an electro-chemical detector equipped with a glassy carbon working electrode set at + 0.75 V.

Immunohistochemical Studies

On PND 7, 14, and 30 rats used for immunohistochemistry for the prenatal and postnatal models were deeply anaesthetized using a combination of ketamine (300 mg/kg) and acepromazine (7.5 mg/kg).[18] The animals were then perfused intracardially with 0.9% saline followed by 4% paraformaldehyde in 0.1 M sodium phosphate buffer pH 7.4. The retinas were dissected and postfixed with the same fixative for 30 min at room temperature. The retinas were immersed in a 30% sucrose solution at 4°C for at least 16 h. Frozen 10-μm sections of the fixed tissues were produced on gelatinized slides and kept at –20°C until use. The sections were then incubated, overnight, in a humidity chamber at 4°C, with sheep antityrosine hydroxylase polyclonal antibody (1:500) diluted in PBST and bovine serum albumin (1% w/v). After rinsing in phosphate buffer-containing Triton X-100 (0.25% v/v) the retinal sections were incubated at room temperature for 1 h in biotinilated anti-sheep followed by two rinses in phosphate buffer. The coverslips or slides were then incubated for 30 min in avidin biotin complex (1:250) followed by a 10-min rinse first in phosphate buffer and then in 0.1 M Tris-HCl buffer (pH 7.2). Immunoreactive sites were visualized by incubating the sections with 3,3′-diaminobenzidine tetrahydrochloride (0.05% w/v) and H_2O_2 (0.025% v/v) in 0.1-M Tris-HCl (pH 7.2) for 5 min at room temperature. After a phosphate buffer rinse, the coverslips or slides were dehydrated by a series of alcohols, cleared with xylene, and mounted with DPX. Negative control sections were treated in the same way as described above except for the omission of the primary or secondary antibody, which was replaced with phosphate buffer-containing Triton X-100 (0.25 % v/v).

STATISTICS

Model for Body Growth and Comparison of Growth Patterns

Logistic curves were fitted to the measurements of body weight of the rats in the pre- and postnatal models, from PND1 to PND30. Curves were fitted using SPSS for Windows software (SPSS Statistical Software Programs version 11.5). Growth patterns, defined by measures of parameters in different times, were compared using a fixed-effect factorial analysis of variance (ANOVA) using the general linear modeling procedure. Main effects were treatment group, sex, and day and these were all treated as within-subjects factors. The experimental unit was the litter ($n = 24$, 12 litters per treatment). Nonorthogonal-planned comparisons were applied to the growth data, so that each METH-treated group was separately compared to the control group. Analysis was performed on log-transformed data to reduce differences in variance among samples. For growth evolution, only litters with a sex ratio of four males and four females were used.

Neurochemical Studies

Neurochemical determinations, defined by measures of parameters in different times were compared using a fixed-effect factorial ANOVA using the general linear modeling procedure. Main effects were treatment group, sex, and day and these were all treated as within-subjects factors. The experimental unit was the litter. Nonorthogonal-planned comparisons were applied to the growth data, so that each METH-treated group was separately compared to the control group. The statistical level of significance was considered at $P < 0.05$ with Bonferroni correction.

RESULTS

Animal Model

The effects of METH on maternal, litter, and offspring variables are shown in TABLE 1. There were no effects on maternal mortality, maternal weight, or gestational length. Maternal weight gain was determined by calculating the difference between body weight at GD 1 and GD 22. Analysis of maternal body weight gain during pregnancy showed that females treated with METH had lower body weights than control-treated females. There were no significant differences in the total number of offspring per litter among treatment groups. Analysis of body weight on PND 1 showed that animals treated prenatally with METH had smaller body weights than the control-treated animals.

The mean body weight evolution of pups did not show any significant difference between groups at any studied age (PND 7, PND 14, or PND 30) as shown in TABLE 2.

Neurochemical Studies

The effect of METH on the DA level in the rat retina of prenatally exposed females and males on PND 7, 14, and 30, and the respective control is shown

TABLE 1. Effects of METH on maternal and litter variables

	Control	Methamphetamine
Number of pregnant females	19	21
Maternal weight (G1)	288.59 ± 44.01	289.48 ± 40.19
Maternal weight gain (g)	109.42 ± 24.35^{a}	83.14 ± 30.04^{a}
Gestational Length (days)	21.88 ± 0.33	21.86 ± 0.37
Number of litters	19	21
Litter size	12.47 ± 0.72	12.76 ± 0.69
Mean birth weight of the litter (g)	6.60 ± 0.66	6.13 ± 0.78
Total number of pups	234	266
Number of postnatal deaths	0	0
Total number of male pups	107	153
Mean weight of males at PND 1 (g)	$6.82 \pm 0.56^{a,c}$	$6.30 \pm 0.72^{a,d}$
Total number of female pups	127	113
Mean weight of females at PND 1 (g)	$6.42 \pm 0.68^{b,c}$	$6.13 \pm 0.78^{b,d}$

The results represent the mean ± SD. For dams, ^{a} $P < 0.05$; For pups ^{a,b,c,d} $P < 0.001$.

TABLE 2. Mean body weight (g) of prenatally exposed females and males to METH on PND 1, 7, 14, and 30, and respective controls

	Female		Male	
PND	Control	METH (5 mg/kg/day)	Control	METH (5 mg/kg/day)
1 ($n = 44$)	6.68 ± 0.51	6.39 ± 0.36	6.95 ± 0.47	6.92 ± 0.75
7 ($n = 16$)	15.94 ± 1.94	16.04 ± 1.62	16.99 ± 1.50	16.99 ± 1.94
14 ($n = 16$)	36.18 ± 5.99	33.73 ± 3.40	37.37 ± 6.38	34.78 ± 3.62
30 ($n = 12$)	100.11 ± 3.36	96.46 ± 5.83	111.14 ± 4.97	106.35 ± 5.38

n = number of litters.

Data represent body weight and are expressed as mean ± SD for n = 4 litters per group (each litter comprising four males and four females).

in FIGURE 1. Animals treated prenatally with METH had a similar DA level to the control-treated animals. For the DA level, a main effect of age was shown and also between litters (treatment × age).

Planned comparisons revealed that, within the control group, the level of DA, in both females and males, was higher on PND 14 than on PND 7 ($P < 0.001$ and $P < 0.001$, respectively) and lower on PND 30 than on PND 14 ($P < 0.001$ and $P < 0.001$, respectively). Within the METH-exposed group, the level of DA, for females and males, was higher on PND 14 than on PND 7 ($P < 0.001$ and $P < 0.001$, respectively) and lower on PND 30 than on PND 14 ($P < 0.001$ and $P < 0.001$, respectively).

The effect of METH on the DOPAC level in the rat retina of prenatally exposed females and males on PND 7, 14, and 30, and the respective controls is shown in FIGURE 2. Animals treated prenatally with METH had a similar DOPAC level to the control-treated animals. Also, there was no main effect of age or sex. For the DOPAC level, a main effect between litters (treatment × age) was found.

Planned comparisons revealed that METH-treated females on PND 30 group had a higher DOPAC level when compared to the control-treated group ($P < 0.001$) and a higher level of DOPAC on PND 14 than on PND 7, for both females and males ($P < 0.001$ and $P < 0.001$, respectively). Within the control group, significant differences were found in the level of DOPAC in both females and males, which were higher on PND 14 than on PND 7 ($P < 0.001$ and $P < 0.001$, respectively).

Immunohistochemical Studies

The effect of prenatal exposure to METH on the localization of tyrosine hydroxylase immunoreactivity in the rat retina at PND 7, 14, and 30 is shown in FIGURE 3.

At PND 7, the cells and their projections toward inter plexiform layer (IPL) became more distinct (FIG. 3 A). At this stage, it is well established that

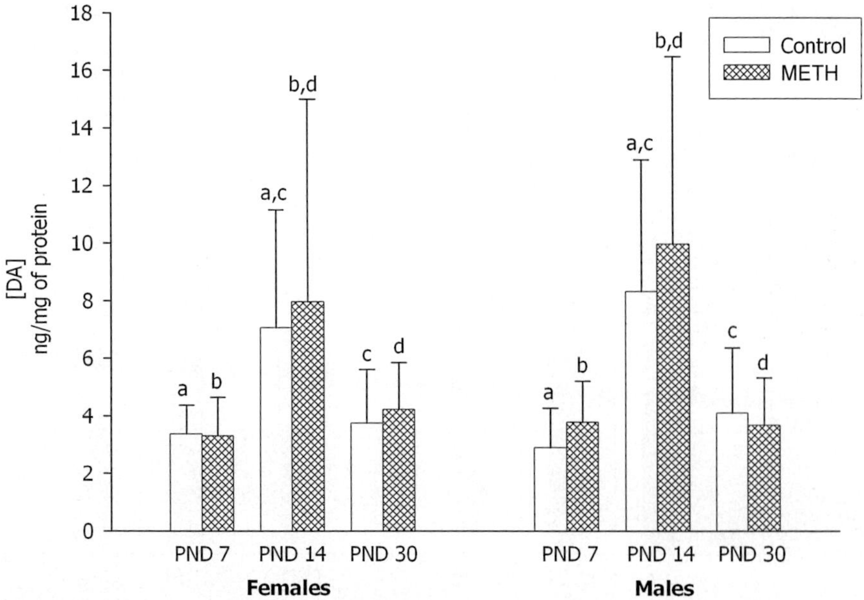

FIGURE 1. Retinal level of DA at PND 7, PND 14, and PND 30 in female and male rats exposed prenatally to METH. Also shown are the respective controls. Data are expressed as mean ± SD (from 9 to 19 animals per group). Columns with the same letter are significantly different from each other. For females: a-d $P < 0.001$. For males: a–d $P < 0.001$.

immunoreactive cells are also present in relatively more peripheral parts of the retina. At PND 14, two sublaminations of the immunoreactive plexus in IPL, and a faint immunoreactivity in outer plexiform layer (OPL) could be identified (FIG. 3 C). In this, and the later stages, it was observed that the distal sublamina in the immunoreactive plexus in the IPL was thicker than the proximal one (FIG. 3 C, E). At PND 30, the immunoreactivity reached the adult level (FIG. 3 C) such that the pattern of immunoreactivity remained unchanged throughout adulthood. No obvious changes in this antigen could be detected between control-treated (FIG. 3 A, C, E) and METH prenatally exposed (FIG. 3B, D, F) animals for any of the ages chosen for this study.

DISCUSSION

The animal model developed for this study comprised a prenatal exposure from GD 8 to 22, this stage being considered the major period for organogenesis and CNS development in the rat.[19,20] The 5 mg/kg/day dose was chosen on the basis of the findings of Weissman and Caldecott–Hazard[15] that this dose alters locomotor and exploratory behaviors. Further, other studies have shown that METH in doses of 5 or 10 mg/kg administered to pregnant females results in

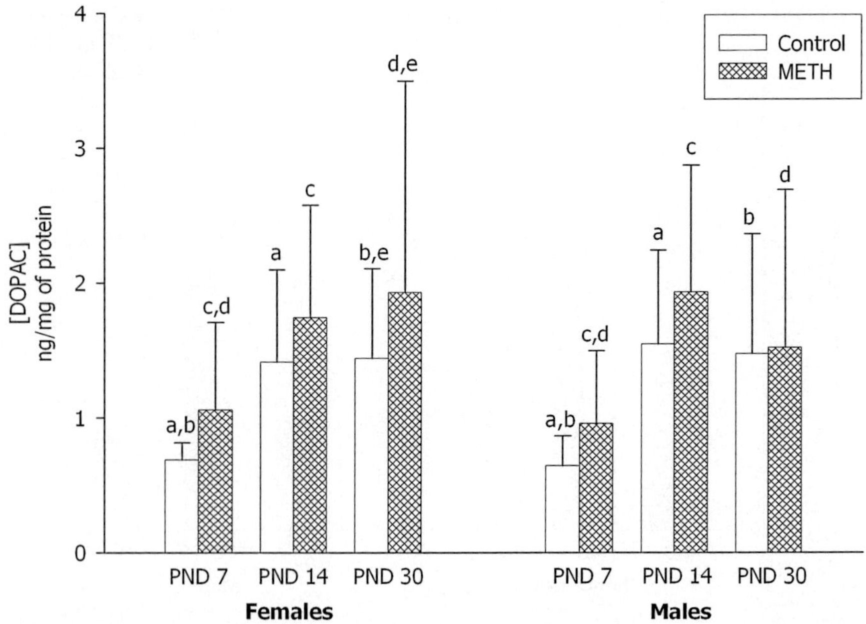

FIGURE 2. Retinal level of DOPAC at PND 7, PND 14, and PND 30 in female and male rats exposed prenatally to METH. Also shown are the respective controls. Data are expressed as mean ± SD (from 9 to 19 animals per group). Columns with the same letter are significantly different from each other. For females: a–d: $P < 0.001$; e: $P < 0.05$. For males: A–D $P < 0.001$.

fetal brain drug concentrations, which approximate those reported in human infants whose mothers abused METH.[21–23] Several previous prenatal studies used extremely high doses of METH (up to 50 mg/kg as free base) leading, for instance, to eye defects (i.e., anophthalmia, microphthalmia, and folded retina) and a high incidence of delivery failure and maternal deaths relative to controls[22,24,25]; these effects were unwanted in this study.

At birth, the rat retina consists of a ganglion cell layer, an inner plexiform layer, and a large neuroblastic layer[26–28]; within the inner plexiform layer many amacrine cells are observed.[26] At the first point chosen, 7 days after birth (PND 7) the outer plexiform layer is almost formed. The second time point selected is the 14th postnatal day (PND 14). By PND 14, all retina layers are present.[26] In addition, this age corresponds to the day of eye opening.[29] The third time point chosen is the end of the first month of life (PND 30) where the maturation of retinal neurons, for example, ganglion cells,[30] is complete.

In this model, each female in the pair-fed group received the daily average amount of food that the METH-injected female in the same group ate on the same GD. This procedure allowed the number of dams involved throughout the study to be kept to the minimum, on account of the occurrence of miscarriages

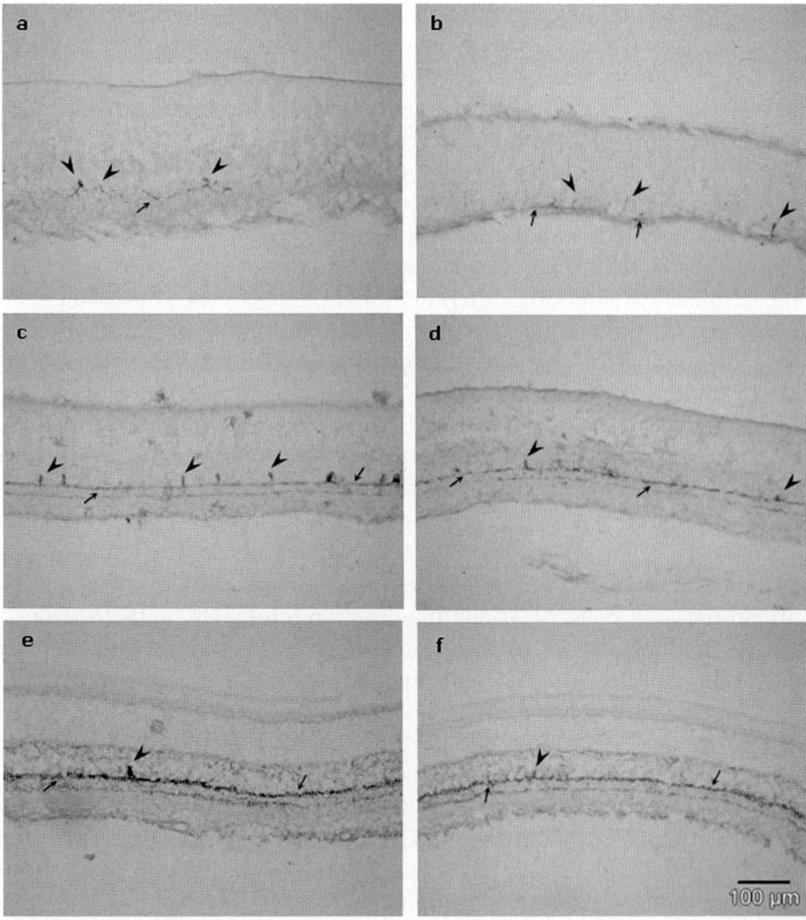

FIGURE 3. Localization of tyrosine hydroxylase immunoreactivity in the normal rat retina at PND 7 (A), PND 14 (C), and PND 30 (E), and after prenatal exposure to METH at PND 7(B), PND 14 (D), and PND 30 (F). Normal tyrosine hydroxylase immunoreactivity is associated with a set of terminals located as a single stratum of labeling in the inner plexiform layer (small arrows) and a few cell bodies in the inner nuclear layer (arrow heads). It can be seen that METH causes no obvious change in the localization of tyrosine hydroxylase immunoreactivity. Figures are representative of four litters per age (with two females and two males). Scale bars = 100 μm.

and mortality in METH-treated females, as well as differences in evolution in control and METH-treated females.[31,32] In contrast to the work of Martin and colleagues showing shorter gestation period in METH-treated mothers,[21] in our study there was no difference between METH-treated mothers and their respective controls. Although the food intake of pregnant females of the control group was controlled (i.e., animals were pair fed with the correspondent METH group), a small decrease in weight gain during pregnancy in the METH-treated group was apparent; however, the difference was not significant on any of the days and the pair fed is a valid control used by other authors.[16,31–33] Further, we did not see the decreasing effect of maternal METH injection on litter size found by Martin.[34] The possible explanation as to why we did not observe the negative effects of METH on the length of gestation and litter size might be on account of different doses used in both studies.

The finding that METH administered during pregnancy decreases birth weight is in agreement with clinical evidence showing decreased body weight, length, and head circumference in neonates born to mothers who abused METH during pregnancy.[35] Similarly, others demonstrated decreased birth weight after prenatal METH administration.[21,31,32,36] Although offspring were not cross-fostered to noninjected dams, the administration of METH daily to the pregnant female (5 mg/kg/day) from GD 8 to 22 had no apparent effect on nutritional status of the pups as estimated by body weight measured at PND 7, 14, and 30 when compared to the control-treated groups and thus correlate with studies of others.[16,24,33]

The dopaminergic neurons are among the first neurochemical systems to appear in the developing retina (for review see Djamgoz *et al.*[37]). DA is involved in neurotransmission and neuromodulation in various parts of the central and peripheral nervous systems. In the mammalian retina, DA is the neurotransmitter of a small number of amacrine and interplexiform cell types, stratifying mainly in the outermost part of the inner plexiform layer but also extending processes into the inner plexiform layer, the inner nuclear layer, and outer plexiform layer.[38,39]

Prenatal exposure to METH did not alter the retinal level of DOPAC in the male group and the level of DA in both female and male groups when compared with their respective pair-fed control groups during the first month of life. These last results can be supported by the TH immunoreactivity studies.

These results show that prenatal exposure to METH has a mild effect on the neurotransmitter system, only depicted on DOPAC level for females at PND 30. At PND 30 the level of DOPAC in females was significantly higher when compared with its respective control group. This higher content on DOPAC can imply a higher DA turnover that can be related to the neurotoxicity of METH.

The results obtained in this study support the view that, during the critical periods in which the catecholamines can influence the development of neurons, prenatal exposure to METH subtly affects the pattern of the dopaminergic system in the developing retina.

ACKNOWLEDGMENTS

The research presented in this article was supported by Fundação para a Ciência e Tecnologia (FCT) by awarding a grant to Pedro Melo (PRAXIS

XXI/BD/3395/2000) and Lorena G. Rodrigues (PRAXIS XXI/BD/18508/98), by the project PRAXIS/P/SAU/12287/1998 approved by FCT and supported by FEDER and Plurianual funds from IBMC.

REFERENCES

1. Aust, S.D. *et al.* 1993. Free radicals in toxicology. Toxicol. Appl. Pharmacol. **120:** 168–178.
2. Bowen, S.E. *et al.* 2005. Abuse pattern of gestational toluene exposure and early postnatal development in rats. Neurotoxicol. Teratol. **27:** 105–116.
3. Aziz, M.H. *et al.* 2001. Neurodevelopmental consequences of gestational exposure (GD14–GD20) to low dose deltamethrin in rats. Neurosci. Lett. **300:** 161–165.
4. Johnston, L.D. *et al.* 2004. Monitoring the Future National Survey Results on Drug Use, 1975–2003. Volume I: Secondary school students (NIH Publication No. 04–5507). National Institute on Drug Abuse: Bethesda, MD.
5. Johnston, L.D. *et al.* 2004. Monitoring the future national results on adolescent drug use: Overview of key findings, 2003 (NIH Publication No. 04–5506). Bethesda, MD: National Institute on Drug Abuse.
6. Cernerud, L. *et al.* 1996. Amphetamine addiction during pregnancy: 14-year follow-up of growth and school performance. Acta. Paediatr. **85:** 204–208.
7. Oro, A.S. & S.D. Dixon. 1987. Perinatal cocaine and methamphetamine exposure: maternal and neonatal correlates. J. Pediatr. **111:** 571–578.
8. Dixon, S.D. & R. Bejar. 1989. Echoencephalographic findings in neonates associated with maternal cocaine and methamphetamine use: incidence and clinical correlates. J. Pediatr. **115:** 770–778.
9. Smith, L. *et al.* 2003. Effects of prenatal methamphetamine exposure on fetal growth and drug withdrawal symptoms in infants born at term. J. Dev. Behav. Pediatr. **24:** 17–23.
10. Smith, L.M. *et al.* 2001. Brain proton magnetic resonance spectroscopy in children exposed to methamphetamine in utero. Neurology **57:** 255–260.
11. Segal, D.S. & R. Kuczenski. 1997. Repeated binge exposures to amphetamine and methamphetamine: behavioral and neurochemical characterization. J. Pharmacol. Exp. Ther. **282:** 561–573.
12. Tonge, S. 1973. Permanent alterations in 5-hydroxyindole concentrations in discrete areas of rat brain produced by the pre- and neonatal administration of methylamphetamine and chlorpromazine. J. Neurochem. **20:** 625–627.
13. Tonge, S.R. 1973. Permanent alterations in catecholamine concentrations in discrete areas of brain in the offspring of rats treated with methylamphetamine and chlorpromazine. Br. J. Pharmacol. **47:** 425–427.
14. Sato, M. & Y. Fujiwara. 1986. Behavioral and neurochemical changes in pups prenatally exposed to methamphetamine. Brain Dev. **8:** 390–396.
15. Weissman, A.D. & S. Caldecott-Hazard. 1993. In utero methamphetamine effects: I. Behavior and monoamine uptake sites in adult offspring. Synapse **13:** 241–250.
16. Cabrera, T.M. *et al.* 1993. Prenatal methamphetamine attenuates serotonin mediated renin secretion in male and female rat progeny: evidence for selective long-term dysfunction of serotonin pathways in brain. Synapse **15:** 198–208.

17. ALI, S.F. *et al.* 1994. MPTP-induced oxidative stress and neurotoxicity are age-dependent: evidence from measures of reactive oxygen species and striatal dopamine levels. Synapse **18:** 27–34.
18. WOLFENSOHN, S. & M. LLOYD. 1998. Handbook of Laboratory Animal Management and Welfare. Blackwell Science. Oxford.
19. CHURCH, M.W., G.W. OVERBECK & A.L. ANDRZEJCZAK. 1990. Prenatal cocaine exposure in the Long-Evans rat: I. Dose-dependent effects on gestation, mortality, and postnatal maturation. Neurotoxicol. Teratol. **12:** 327–334.
20. HENCK, J.W. 2002. Developmental neurotoxicology: testing and interpretation. *In* Handbook of Neurotoxicology, Vol. II. E.J. Massaro Ed.: 3–56. Humana Press. Totowa, NJ.
21. MARTIN, J.C. & D.C. MARTIN. 1981. Voluntary activity in the aging rat as a function of maternal drug exposure. Neurobehav. Toxicol. Teratol. **3:** 261–264.
22. ACUFF-SMITH, K.D. *et al.* 1996. Stage-specific effects of prenatal d-methamphetamine exposure on behavioral and eye development in rats. Neurotoxicol. Teratol. **18:** 199–215.
23. CHO, D.H. *et al.* 1991. Behavioral teratogenicity of methamphetamine. J. Toxicol. Sci. **16**(Suppl 1)**:** 37–49.
24. ACUFF-SMITH, K.D. *et al.* 1992. Preliminary evidence for methamphetamine-induced behavioral and ocular effects in rat offspring following exposure during early organogenesis. Psychopharmacology (Berl.) **109:** 255–263.
25. ACUFF-SMITH, K.D. 1993. Neurobehavioral, neurochemical, and ocular effects of prenatal methamphetamine exposure in rats as a function of dose and gestational stage. PhD, University of Cincinnati.
26. FLETCHER, E.L. & M. KALLONIATIS. 1997. Localisation of amino acid neurotransmitters during postnatal development of the rat retina. J. Comp. Neurol. **380:** 449–471.
27. WEIDMAN, T.A. & T. KUWABARA. 1968. Postnatal development of the rat retina. An electron microscopic study. Arch. Ophthalmol. **79:** 470–484.
28. WEIDMAN, T.A. & T. KUWABARA. 1969. Development of the rat retina. Invest. Ophthalmol. **8:** 60–69.
29. KATO, S., T. NAKAMURA & K. NEGISHI. 1980. Postnatal development of dopaminergic cells in the rat retina. J. Comp. Neurol. **191:** 27–36.
30. PERRY, V.H. & M. WALKER. 1980. Morphology of cells in the ganglion cell layer during development of the rat retina. Proc. R. Soc. Lond. B. Biol. Sci. **208:** 433–445.
31. GOMES-DA-SILVA, J. 2002. Efeito da metanfetamina na ontogenia das vias dopaminérgicas do sistema nervoso do rato. PhD, University of Porto, Porto.
32. GOMES-DA-SILVA, J. *et al.* 2002. Prenatal exposure to methamphetamine in the rat: ontogeny of tyrosine hydroxylase mRNA expression in mesencephalic dopaminergic neurons. Ann. N. Y. Acad. Sci. **965:** 68–77.
33. MELO, P. *et al.* 2005. Methamphetamine and lipid peroxidation in the rat retina. Birth Defects Res. A Clin. Mol. Teratol. **73:** 455–460.
34. MARTIN, J.C. 1975. Effects on offspring of chronic maternal methamphetamine exposure. Dev. Psychobiol. **8:** 397–404.
35. PLESSINGER, M.A. 1998. Prenatal exposure to amphetamines. Risks and adverse outcomes in pregnancy. Obstet. Gynecol. Clin. North Am. **25:** 119–138.
36. MARTIN, J.C. *et al.* 1976. Growth, development and activity in rat offspring following maternal drug exposure. Exp. Aging Res. **2:** 235–251.

37. DJAMGOZ, M.B. *et al.* 1997. Neurobiology of retinal dopamine in relation to degenerative states of the tissue. Vision Res. **37:** 3509–3529.
38. POURCHO, R.G. 1996. Neurotransmitters in the retina. Curr. Eye Res. **15:** 797–803.
39. NGUYEN LEGROS, J. *et al.* 1981. Tyrosine hydroxylase-like immunoreactive interplexiform cells in the rat retina. Neurosci. Lett. **27:** 255–259.

Effects of Postnatal Exposure to Methamphetamine on the Development of the Rat Retina

LORENA G. RODRIGUES,[a,b] PEDRO MELO,[a,c] M. CAROLINA SILVA,[b] AND MARIA AMÉLIA TAVARES[a,c]

[a]*Unit of Neurobehaviour, Institute for Molecular and Cell Biology, University of Porto, 4150-180 Porto, Portugal*

[b]*Institute for Biomedical Sciences Abel Salazar, University of Porto, 4150-180 Porto, Portugal*

[c]*Institute of Anatomy, Faculty of Medicine of the University of Porto, 4150-180 Porto, Portugal*

ABSTRACT: Since the development of different cell types in the retina occurs at different rates, it is possible that exposure to an exogenous substance may produce effects during one time period, but not during another. This study aims to analyze the effects of methamphetamine (METH) in the growth pattern of an experimental model as well as neurochemical and immunohistochemical parameters of the dopaminergic system of the rat retina. The three development stages chosen in this study are key markers in rat eye development. Rats were given 15 mg/kg body weight per day of METH as subcutaneous injections in 0.9% saline (3 mL/kg weight/day) from the day after birth PND 1 to PND 6, PND 13, and PND 29. Each daily dose was split into two. The control group was injected subcutaneously with saline. Both the schedule and volume for injecting saline in the control group were the same as for the METH-treated group. There were no significant differences in the total number of offspring per litter among treatment groups. All offspring had similar body weight at birth. Analysis of body weight on PND 1, showed that animals treated with METH had similar body weights to control-treated animals and females had smaller weights than males. For growth evolution, only litters with a sex ratio of four males and four females were used. Animals treated with METH had smaller body weights than the control-treated animals for all ages studied (PND 7, 14, and 30). Within the control group at PND 30, a significant difference was found in the body weight of females, which was lower when compared with males. For the postnatal model, 7 deaths occurred for the METH-exposed group. No deaths occurred in the control group in a total of 16 saline-injected litters comprising 186 pups. Although the levels of dopamine (DA) was

Address for correspondence: Lorena G. Rodrigues, UniLiPe, Institute for Molecular and Cell Biology, Rua do Campo Alegre, 823, 4150-180 Porto, Portugal. Voice: +351 226074900; fax: +351 226099157. e-mail: lorena@ibmc.up.pt

Ann. N.Y. Acad. Sci. 1074: 604–619 (2006).
doi: 10.1196/annals.1369.059

within normal values for the postnatally exposed METH group when compared with its respective control group at PND 7 and 30, at PND 14 this was not the case: in this experimental group, the level of DA was lower than in the control group for both females and males. Support for this result was not evident from the TH immunoreactivity studies, probably because the methodology lacks the sensitivity to distinguish any mild effects, such as that observed in the postnatal model at PND 14. The level of the DA metabolite 3, 4-dihydroxyphenylacetic acid (DOPAC) remained unaffected at all ages studied, for both females and males. The results obtained in this study support the view that, during the critical periods in which the catecholamines can influence the development of neurones, METH transiently affects the pattern of the dopaminergic system in the developing retina.

KEYWORDS: methamphetamine; Wistar rat; retina development; postnatal model; dopamine

INTRODUCTION

Methamphetamine (METH) abuse increased significantly in the early 1990s and continued to gain popularity until 1998, plateauing thereafter.[1,2] In recent years there has been growing use of this drug by pregnant women,[3] resulting in a fairly large number of children born to METH-abusing mothers. Women, especially during pregnancy, take METH because it reduces appetite, and consequently helps to control weight, and it also increases energy. METH is known to be potentially neurotoxic to human,[4,5] but there is minimal information with respect to the consequences of such exposure to the fetus. Nevertheless, METH use during pregnancy has been associated with adverse physical defects for the human fetus or neonate, including low birth weight, cleft palate, reduced head circumference, and cerebral hemorrhage (for review see Plessinger[6]). Children who have been exposed prenatally to amphetamines may also be predisposed to increased risk for altered neurobehavioral function.[7,8] It is well established that METH is neurotoxic to central dopaminergic and serotonergic projections of adult animals.[9–12] It is also known that METH can exacerbate the effect of other toxic substances, for example, it enhances kainic acid-induced toxicity in the adult rat retina.[13] Yet, despite this knowledge, there are a relatively limited number of experimental studies indicating that gestational exposure to METH can also have long-term consequences on monoaminergic neurons development as well as on behavior. Conversely, neurochemical and functional alterations in dopaminergic and serotonergic neurons in adolescent and adult offspring following prenatal METH exposure have been reported.[14–17] In addition, METH-exposed progeny are less active than offspring from control-treated mothers.[14,17] Studies on the effects of prenatal exposure to psychomotor stimulants on developing neurons are complicated by a number of experimental variables, including dosage, exposure regimens, gestational age, duration of exposure, and postnatal age at which the offspring are examined.

The first three weeks of postnatal life in rats are comparable to middle and late prenatal periods in humans; the rat brain is approaching the appearance of the adult within approximately 6 weeks after fertilization, while the human brain takes nearly seven times longer to reach the same maturational state.[18,19] Throughout this study animals were exposed to METH postnatally all through the first 29 days of postnatal life, covering a period of development where events of general development like functional maturation occur; as well, events involving the central nervous system (CNS) development, like neurogenesis and cell migration, dendritic growth and differentiation, gliogenesis, synaptogenesis, and myelination processes are still occurring, and as a result an insult during this period can produce adverse effects. Development processes in the CNS are most vulnerable to insults during the time of their rapid growth, that is, during "brain growth spurt" that occur in the rat from birth to weaning (peaking at approximately postnatal day [PND] 10),[20] although some important events (like gliogenesis and synaptogenesis) continue beyond this stage (for review, see Henck[21] and Insel[22]).

The three development stages chosen in this study are key markers in rat eye development. At birth, the rat retina consists of a ganglion cell layer, an inner plexiform layer, and a large neuroblastic layer [23–25]; within the inner plexiform layer many amacrine cells are present.[23] At the first point chosen, 7 days after birth (at PND 7) the outer plexiform layer is almost formed. The second time point selected is the 14th postnatal day (PND 14). By PND 14, all retina layers are present.[23] In addition, this stage corresponds to the day of eye opening.[26] The third time point chosen is the end of the first month of life (PND 30) where retinal neurons, for example, ganglion cells,[27] are fully developed.

The present study was undertaken to test whether METH impairs the normal development of the retina at different time points of its development. In order to achieve this goal, a postnatal rat model was used where METH 15 mg/kg/day was injected from PND 1 to PND 6, 13, and 29.

MATERIALS AND METHODS

Animal Model

Handling and care of animals were according to the Association for Research into Vision and Ophthalmology (ARVO) Statement for the Use of Animals in Ophthalmic and Vision Research and the Portuguese law (Portaria n° 1005/92). Rats of the Wistar strain were used in this experimental model. At the beginning of the experimental period, 2-month-old nulliparous females, weighing an average of 250–300 g were used. Beginning on GD 21, pregnant females were checked twice daily for the presence of a litter. Females were allowed to deliver and litters were reared by their biological mother. Litters were left undisturbed until PND 1 when the litter was sexed, weighed, and randomly culled to eight pups (four males and four females). Animals were identified by painting their paws, head, or trunk with unwashable ink according to a coding system. At PND 21, litters were weaned from their mothers.

Postnatal Administration of Methamphetamine

Rats were given 15 mg/kg body weight/day of *d*-N,α-dimethylphenethylamine hydrochloride (METH-HCl; Sigma-Aldrich, St. Louis, MO), as subcutaneous injections in 0.9% saline (3 mL/kg weight/day) from the day after birth PND 1 to PND 6, and to PND 13 and to PND 29. Each daily dose was split into two and administered between 9:00 and 9:30 AM and between 5:00 and 5:30 PM, respectively. The control group was injected subcutaneously with saline. Both the schedule and volume for injecting saline in the control group were the same as for the METH-treated group.

Neurochemical Studies

At the end of each experimental period (PND 7, 14, and 30) following METH or vehicle treatment, at least two females and two males per litter, were randomly selected from the litters for neurochemical studies. The animals were decapitated, the eyes were enucleated, and the retinas quickly dissected. The retinas were frozen and stored at –70°C, until neurochemical determination. Retinas were ultrasonicated (Branson sonifier W-150, Branson Ultrasonics, Danbury, CT) in 500 μL of ice-cold 0.2 M perchloric acid containing 10 ng/mL of the internal standard 3,4-dihydrobenzylamine (DHBA). The homogenate was centrifuged (13,000 *g*, 15 min) and the supernatant was filtered through a 0.2-μm Nylon-66 microfilter. Aliquots of 50 μL were then analyzed for dopamine (DA) and 3,4-dihydroxyphenylacetic acid (DOPAC) by high-performance liquid chromatography (HPLC) with electrochemical detection (ECD) by a method modified from Ali and colleagues.[28] The Gilson Medical Electronics HPLC system (Middleton, WI) was composed of a LC234 auto-injector, LC307 delivery pump, LC142 electro-chemical detector, and 712 HPLC system controller data version 1.30 management software. The mobile phase consisted of 70 mM potassium phosphate monobasic buffer (pH was adjusted to 3.0 by adding phosphoric acid), 1 mM *l*-heptanosulfonic acid, 107.5-μM sodium EDTA, and 10% (v/v) methanol. The flow rate was maintained at 1 mL/min. Biogenic amines were separated by a Supelcosil LC (7.5 cm × 4.6 cm, 3 μm) reversed phase column. Quantification was achieved via an electro-chemical detector equipped with a glassy carbon working electrode set at + 0.75 V.

Immunohistochemical Studies

On PND 7, 14, and 30, rats used for immunohistochemistry for the postnatal models were deeply anaesthetized using a combination of ketamine (300 mg/kg) and acepromazine (7.5 mg/kg).[29] The animals were then perfused intracardially with 0.9% saline followed by 4% paraformaldehyde in 0.1-M sodium phosphate buffer pH 7.4. The retinas were dissected and post-fixed with the same fixative for 30 min at room temperature. The retinas were immersed in a 30% sucrose solution at 4°C for at least 16 h. Frozen 10-μm sections of the fixed tissues were produced on gelatinized slides and kept at –20°C until use. The sections were then incubated overnight, in a humidity chamber at 4°C, with sheep antityrosine hydroxylase polyclonal antibody (1:500) diluted in PBST and bovine serum albumin (1% w/v). After rinsing in phosphate buffer-containing Triton X-100 (0.25% v/v) the retinal sections were incubated at room temperature for 1 h in biotinilated anti-sheep followed by two rinses in phosphate buffer. The slides were then incubated for 30 min in avidin biotin complex (1:250) followed by a 10-min rinse first in phosphate buffer and then in 0.1 M Tris-HCl buffer (pH 7.2). Immunoreactive sites were visualized by incubating the sections with 3,3′-diaminobenzidine tetrahydrochloride (0.05 % w/v) and H_2O_2 (0.025% v/v) in 0.1-M Tris-HCl (pH 7.2) for 5 min at room temperature. After a phosphate buffer rinse, the slides were dehydrated by a series of alcohols, cleared with xylene, and mounted with DPX. Negative control sections were treated in the same way as described above except for the omission of the primary or secondary antibody, which was replaced with phosphate –buffer-containing Triton X-100 (0.25 % v/v).

STATISTICS

Model for Body Growth and Comparison of Growth Patterns

Logistic curves were fitted to the measurements of body weight of the rats in the postnatal models, from PND 1 to PND 30. Curves were fitted using SPSS for Windows software (SPSS Statistical Software Programs version 11.5). Growth patterns, defined by measures of parameters in different times, were compared using a fixed-effect factorial analysis of variance (ANOVA) using the general linear modeling procedure. Main effects were treatment group, sex, and day and these were all treated as within-subjects factors. The experimental unit was the litter ($n = 24$, 12 litters per treatment). Nonorthogonal-planned comparisons were applied to the growth data, so that each METH-treated group was separately compared to the control group. Analysis was performed on log-transformed data to reduce differences in variance among samples. For growth evolution, only litters with a sex ratio of four males and four females were used.

Neurochemical Studies

Neurochemical determinations, defined by measures of parameters in different times were compared using a fixed-effect factorial ANOVA using the general linear modeling procedure. Main effects were treatment group, sex, and day and these were all treated as within-subjects factors. The experimental unit was the litter. Nonorthogonal-planned comparisons were applied to the growth data, so that each METH-treated group was separately compared to the control group. The statistical level of significance was considered at $P < 0.05$ with Bonferroni correction.

RESULTS

Animal Model

As indicated in TABLE 1, there were no significant differences in the total number of offspring per litter among treatment groups ($F[1, 34] = 0.99$, $P > 0.3$). All offspring had similar birth body weight. Analysis of the male versus female ratio on PND 1, showed no difference when litters were distributed randomly for different treatments ($F[1, 34] = 2.56$, $P > 0.1$). Analysis of body weight on PND 1, showed that animals treated with METH had similar body weights to control-treated animals ($F[1, 36] = 0.42$, $P > 0.5$) and females had smaller weights than males ($F[1, 39] = 27.18$, $P < 0.001$).

For the postnatal model, seven deaths occurred for the METH-exposed group (one male on PND 3 and PND 8, one female on PND 5, PND 8, and PND 11, and two females on PND 12) in a total of 20 exposed litters comprising 269 pups. No deaths occurred in the control group in a total of 16 saline-injected litters comprising 186 pups. Consequently, there was a 2.6% mortality rate for the

TABLE 1. Litter variables in the postnatal model

	Control	METH
Number of litters	16	20
Litter size	12.06 ± 2.84	13.10 ± 3.31
Litters with less than 8 pups	0	0
Litters with 8 to 16 pups	16	18
Litters with more than 16 pups	0	2
Male: female ratio	0.99 ± 0.55	1.99 ± 2.51
Mean birth weight of the litter (g)	6.68 ± 0.55	6.69 ± 0.64
Total number of pups	186	269
Total number of male pups	96	135
Mean weight of males at PND 1 (g)	6.85 ± 0.55	6.82 ± 0.61
Total number of female pups	90	134
Mean weight of females at PND 1 (g)	6.52 ± 0.50	6.55 ± 0.63
Number of postnatal deaths	0	7

The results represent mean ± SD.

TABLE 2. Mean body weight (g) of female and male rats exposed postnatally to METH

	Female		Male	
PND	Control	METH (15 mg/ kg/day)	Control	METH (15 mg/ kg/day)
1 ($n = 48$)	6.76 ± 0.42	6.70 ± 0.35	7.07 ± 0.375	7.07 ± 0.54
7 ($n = 16$)	16.71 ± 0.62^{a}	14.69 ± 1.11^{a}	17.35 ± 0.79^{b}	15.16 ± 0.88^{b}
14 ($n = 16$)	30.67 ± 2.67^{c}	27.78 ± 3.01^{c}	32.21 ± 2.09^{d}	28.51 ± 3.80^{d}
30 ($n = 16$)	$97.86 \pm 5.75^{e,g}$	70.12 ± 5.72^{e}	$105.98 \pm 7.68^{f,g}$	73.40 ± 7.23^{f}

Significant differences due to treatment $^{a-f}$ $P < 0.001$, and sex ^{g} $P < 0.01$. Values represent mean $\pm$ SD. n = number of litters.

Rats were injected with METH (7.5 mg/kg) twice daily from day 1 until the day before the analysis was performed (PND 7, 14, and 30). Also shown are the respective controls. Data are expressed as mean $\pm$ SD of $n = 4$ litters per group (each litter comprising 4 males and 4 females).

METH-treated group. These numbers included all the litters used throughout this study (TABLE 1).

For growth evolution, only litters with a sex ratio of four males and four females were used. Mean body weight values (and respective SD) on PND 1, 7, 14, and 30, for both groups are represented in TABLE 2. Prior to the first daily dose, animals were weighed. The animals treated with METH had smaller body weights than the control-treated animals ($F[1, 18] = 52.08$, $P < 0.001$) and females had smaller weights than males ($F[1, 18] = 29.82$, $P < 0.001$) (TABLE 2). Animals gained weight over days as shown by a significant main effect of age ($F[2, 18] = 1245.63$, $P < 0.001$). The highest order significant interaction with treatment was treatment $\times$ age ($F[2, 18] = 7.54$, $P < 0.004$). Analysis of the following interactions: treatment $\times$ sex ($F[1, 18] = 1.93$, $P > 0.1$), treatment $\times$ age $\times$ sex ($F[2, 18] = 0.31$, $P > 0.7$) and age $\times$ sex ($F[2, 18] = 1.09$, $P > 0.3$) showed no differences. Planned comparisons revealed that the animals treated with METH had smaller body weights than the control-treated animals for all ages studied (PND 7, 14, and 30). Within the control group at PND 30, a significant difference was found in the body weight of females, which was lower when compared with males.

Neurochemical Studies

The effect of postnatal exposure to METH on the levels of DA and DOPAC in the rat retina at PND 7, 14, and 30, and the respective controls is shown in FIGURES 1 and 2.

The effect of METH on the level of DA in the rat retina of postnatally exposed females and males on PND 7, PND 14, and PND 30, and respective controls is shown in FIGURE 1. Animals treated with METH had a similar DA level to control-treated animals ($F\ [1, 20] = 2.58$, $P > 0.1$) and also there were no main effects of age ($F\ [2, 20] = 2.97$, $P > 0.06$) or sex ($F\ [1, 23] = 0.98$,

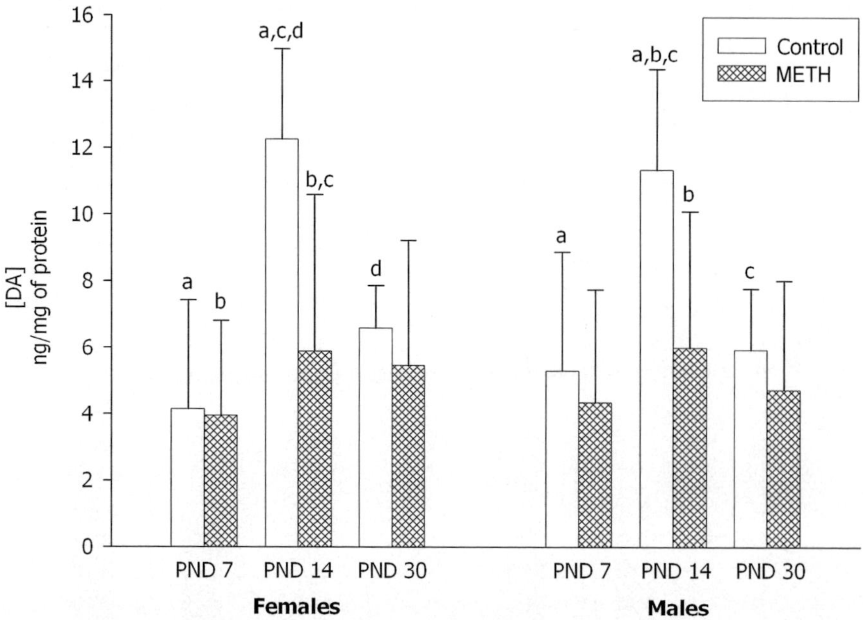

FIGURE 1. DA level in the retinas of female and male rats exposed postnatally to METH. Rats were injected with METH (7.5 mg/kg) twice daily from day 1 until the day before the analysis was performed (PND 7, 14, and 30). Also shown are the respective controls. Data are expressed as mean ± SD (from 9–23 animals per group). For females: a,c,d $P < 0.001$; [b] $P < 0.05$. For males: a–c $P < 0.001$.

$P > 0.3$). For the DA level, a main effect between litters (treatment × age) was shown ($F[20, 20] = 32.24$, $P < 0.001$) and also of age × sex ($F\ [2, 22] = 3.61$, $P < 0.05$). Analysis of the following interactions: treatment × age ($F[2, 20] = 0.99$, $P > 0.3$), treatment × sex ($F[1, 22] = 0.87$, $P > 0.3$) and treatment × age × sex ($F[2, 22] = 1.0$, $P > 0.3$) showed no differences.

Planned comparisons revealed that within the METH group, significant differences were found in the DA level for both females and males, which were lower on PND 14 when compared to their control-treated group ($P < 0.001$). For females, also, the DA level was higher on PND 14 than on PND 7 ($P < 0.05$). Within the control group, significant differences were found in the DA level for both females and males, which were higher on PND 14 than on PND 7 ($P < 0.001$ and $P < 0.001$, respectively) and lower on PND 30 than on PND 14 (see FIG. 1 for results).

The effect of METH on the level of DOPAC in the rat retina of postnatally exposed females and males on PND 7 and PND 30 and respective controls, is shown in FIGURE 2. The animals treated with METH had a similar DOPAC level to the control-treated animals ($F\ [1, 14] = 0.51$, $P > 0.8$) and also there were no main effects of age ($F\ [2, 14] = 2.43$, $P > 0.1$) and sex ($F\ [1, 12] =$

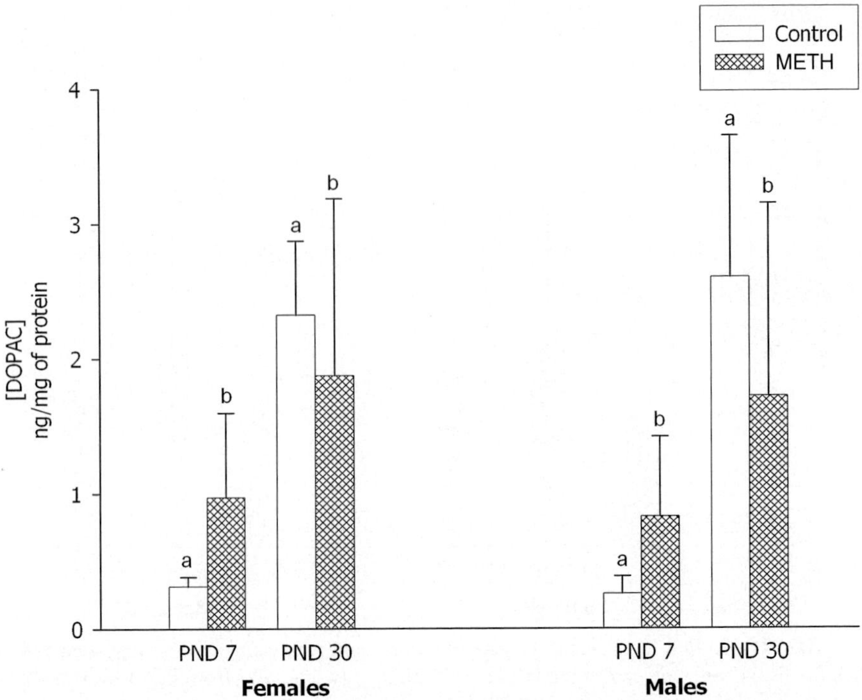

FIGURE 2. DOPAC level in the retinas of female and male rats exposed postnatally to METH. Rats were injected with METH (dose) twice daily from day 1 until the day before the analysis was performed (PND 7 and PND 30). Also shown are the respective controls. Data are expressed as mean ± SD (from 13–18 animals per group). For females: a, b $P < 0.001$. For males: a, b $P < 0.001$.

0.001, $P > 0.9$). The highest order of significant interaction with was the litters (treatment × age) ($F[14,14] = 34,9$, $P < 0.001$). Analysis of the following interactions: age × sex ($F[2,11] = 0.243$, $P > 0.7$), treatment × age ($F[1,14] = 0.99$, $P > 0.3$), treatment × sex ($F[1,11] = 0.2$, $P > 0.6$) , and treatment × age × sex ($F[2,11] = 0.5$ $P > 0.5$), showed no differences.

Planned comparisons revealed that within the control group, the level of DOPAC in both females and males was lower on PND 7 than on PND 30 ($P < 0.001$ and $P < 0.001$, respectively). Within the METH-exposed group, a lower level of DOPAC was found on PND 7 than on PND 30 for both females and males ($P < 0.001$ and $P < 0.001$, respectively) (see FIG. 2 for results).

Immunohistochemical Studies

The effect of postnatal exposure to METH on the localization of tyrosine hydroxylase immunoreactivity in the rat retina at PND 7, 14, and 30 is shown in FIGURE 3.

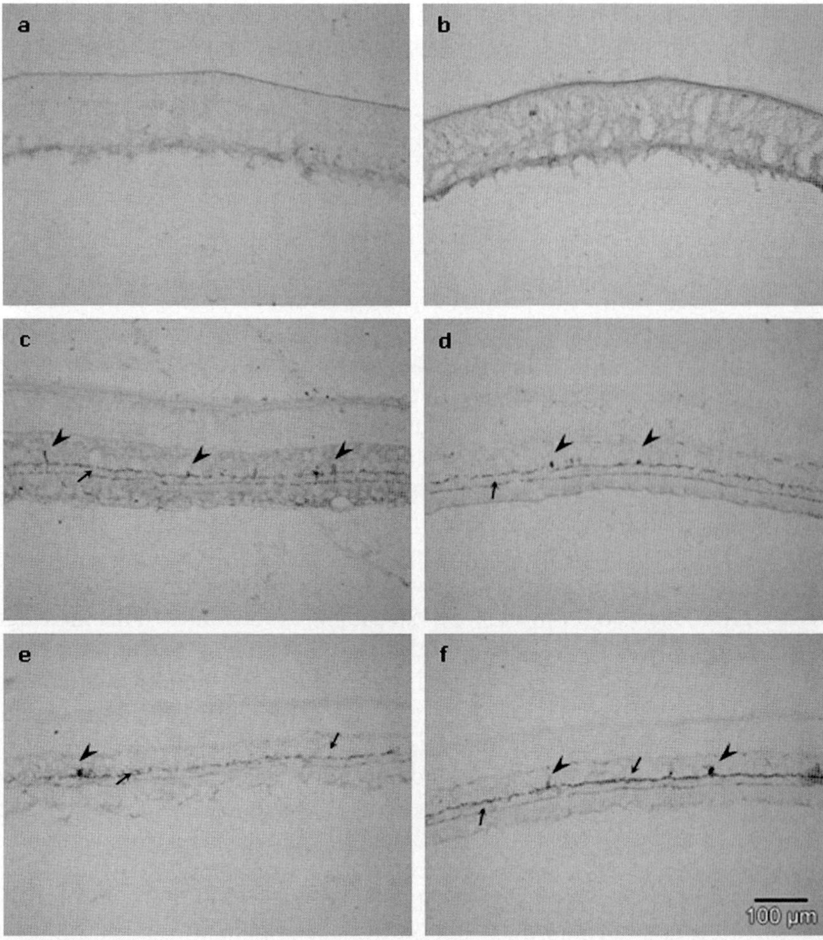

FIGURE 3. The localization of tyrosine hydroxylase immunoreactivity in the normal rat retina at PND 7(A), PND 14 (C) and PND 30 (E), and after postnatal exposure to METH at PND 7(B), PND 14 (D), and PND 30 (F). Normal tyrosine hydroxylase immunoreactivity is associated with a set of terminals located as a single stratum of labeling in the inner plexiform layer (small arrows) and a few cell bodies in the inner nuclear layer (arrow heads). It can be seen that MA causes no obvious change in the localization of tyrosine hydroxylase immunoreactivity. Figures are representative of four litters per age (with two females and two males) of separate experiments. Scale bars = 100 μm.

At PND 7, these cells and their projections toward interplexiform layer (IPL) became more distinct (FIG. 3 A). At PND 14, two sublaminations of the immunoreactive plexus in IPL, and a faint immunoreactivity in outer plexiform layer (OPL) could be identified (FIG. 3 C). In this, and the later stages, it was noted that the distal sublamina in the immunoreactive plexus in the IPL was thicker than the proximal one (FIG. 3 C, E). At PND 30, the immunoreactivity reached the adult level (FIG. 3 C) such that the pattern of immunoreactivity remained unchanged throughout adulthood. No obvious changes in this antigen could be detected between control-treated (FIG. 3 A, C, E) and METH postnatally exposed (FIG. 3 B, D, F) animals for any of the ages chosen for this study.

DISCUSSION

We have been using the postnatal period of development in the rat as a model of exposure for the human third trimester, since analogous development occurs between the rat and human during these respective time points.[19] The dose was selected to produce selective effects on a vulnerable CNS region, the retina, without leading to more deleterious effects. Moreover, this dose has formerly been used in similar studies in our laboratory, not only with METH but also with different psychostimulants, and were shown to effectively disrupt the standard development of the CNS.[30–35]

It is well known that physiological growth is considered an indicator of health status, and is usually evaluated as body weight gain.[21] Therefore, the decrease in body weights observed for METH-exposed females and males of the three ages studied, that is, PND 7, 14, and 30, for the postnatal model, indicates that, even though a low dose of METH was used in this study, physiological alterations have occurred. As showed in TABLE 2, on PND 7, 14, and 30, the body weights of both males and females exposed to METH were smaller relative to the control groups. Accordingly, similar body weight differences have been noted in humans following prenatal exposure.[36–38] We have demonstrated that even a relative low dose of METH (15 mg/kg/day) administered during a period of brain development that is analogous to third trimester human development[19] can produce a reduction in body weight. These results are in agreement with those found by other groups that used substituted amphetamines, and similarly found anorectic effects in adult animals.[16,30,34,39–44]

Postnatal mortality is a parameter that should be evaluated as a rule in all pre- and postnatal developmental toxicity studies.[21] In our postnatal model, 7 deaths occurred although statistically this effect cannot be attributed to the treatment. Thus, this observation supports the evidence that the METH doses tested here are not excessively harmful. Elevated body temperatures in adult animals are known to play a role in the neurotoxic effect of substituted amphetamines,[45,46] although it has been established that in pups this is not the case. Even at 20 days of age, rats do not demonstrate hyperthermia when they are administered METH at normal room temperature.[45] Rats begin to thermoregulate on approximately PND 12 and this response continues to mature until PND 21.[47] Therefore, it is unlikely that body temperature plays a significant role in the long-term effects of METH after early exposure. It is obvious that many different changes are taking place in the rat during the PND 1 to PND

29 exposure period and some of the systems undergoing rapid development require further investigation, but it seems that body temperature does not play an important role during the time of exposure chosen for this study.

The dopaminergic neurons are among the first neurochemical systems to appear in the developing retina (for review see Djamgoz *et al.*).[48] DA is involved in neurotransmission and neuromodulation in different regions of the central and peripheral nervous systems. In the mammalian retina, DA is the neurotransmitter of a small number of amacrine and interplexiform cell types, stratifying mainly in the outermost part of the inner plexiform layer but also extending processes into the inner plexiform layer, the inner nuclear layer, and outer plexiform layer.[49–51]

Postnatal exposure to METH had no influence on the level of DA when compared with the control group at PND 7 and 30, for both females and males. Although the levels of DA was within normal values for the postnatally exposed METH group when compared with its respective control group at PND 7 and 30, at PND 14 this was not the case: in this experimental group, the level of DA was lower than in the control group for both females and males. Support for this result was not evident from the tyrosine hydroxylase immunoreactivity studies, probably because the methodology lacks the sensitivity to distinguish any mild effects, such as that observed in the postnatal model at PND 14. The level of the DA metabolite DOPAC remained unaffected at all of the age studied, for both females and males. As well, both female and male control animals presented the same pattern of variation of neurotransmitters level in the retina. The results obtained in this study support the view that, during the critical periods in which the catecholamines can influence the development of neurons, METH transiently affects the pattern of the dopaminergic system in the developing retina. It is important to detect even transient alterations in the levels of catecholamines because of their suggested role as regulatory or trophic factors in developing neurons circuits. The dopaminergic system, as well as other neurotransmitter systems, of the immature retina may play an important role in the steady-state sensitivity of retinal cells to programmed cell death during normal development.[52] Protection against glutamate excitotoxicity has also been conferred by DA.[53] Also, growth cone motility is modulated by DA in developing chick retinal cells.[54] Since a normal increase in the levels of catecholamines, especially DA, it is observed during the second week of postnatal development (also shown in this study since DA levels were also higher at PND 14 than PND 7 and 30, for both females and males), and since this is the period during which most amacrine cells differentiate and form synaptic contacts in the inner plexiform layer, any disruption of this normal pattern of development will be critical for the above events to occur.

In summary, these results demonstrate, for the first time, that the dopaminergic system in the retina of the rat is transiently affected by postnatal exposure to METH. Additional work is required to determine whether these changes are due to vasoconstrictive effects and ischemia, as it was previously demonstrated that ischemia in the retina leads to alterations in DA,[55] or to the direct effects of METH on the development of dopaminergic neurons, or if both mechanisms contribute for the alterations found in the retina under these experimental conditions.

ACKNOWLEDGMENTS

The research presented in this article was supported by Fundação para a Ciência e Tecnologia (FCT) by awarding a grant to Lorena G. Rodrigues (PRAXIS XXI/BD/18508/98) and Pedro Melo (PRAXIS XXI/BD/3395/2000), by the project PRAXIS/P/SAU/12287/1998 approved by FCT and supported by FEDER and Plurianual funds from IBMC.

REFERENCES

1. Johnston, L.D. *et al.* 2004. Monitoring the future national survey results on drug use, 1975–2003. Volume I: Secondary school students (NIH Publication No. 04–5507). Bethesda, MD: National Institute on Drug Abuse.
2. Johnston, L.D. *et al.* 2004. Monitoring the future national results on adolescent drug use: overview of key findings, 2003 (NIH Publication No. 04–5506). Bethesda, MD: National Institute on Drug Abuse.
3. Vega, W.A. *et al.* 1993. Prevalence and magnitude of perinatal substance exposures in California. N. Engl. J. Med. **329**: 850–854.
4. Volkow, N.D. *et al.* 2001. Association of dopamine transporter reduction with psychomotor impairment in methamphetamine abusers. Am. J. Psychiatry **158:** 377–382.
5. McCann, U.D. *et al.* 1998. Reduced striatal dopamine transporter density in abstinent methamphetamine and methcathinone users: evidence from positron emission tomography studies with [11C]WIN-35,428. J. Neurosci. **18**: 8417–8422.
6. Plessinger, M.A. 1998. Prenatal exposure to amphetamines. Risks and adverse outcomes in pregnancy. Obstet. Gynecol. Clin. North Am. **25**: 119–138.
7. Cernerud, L. *et al.* 1996. Amphetamine addiction during pregnancy: 14-year follow-up of growth and school performance. Acta. Paediatr. **85**: 204–208.
8. Eriksson, M. & R. Zetterstrom. 1994. Amphetamine addiction during pregnancy: 10-year follow-up. Acta. Paediatr. Suppl. **404**: 27–31.
9. Bakhit, C. & J.W. Gibb. 1981. Methamphetamine-induced depression of tryptophan hydroxylase: recovery following acute treatment. Eur. J. Pharmacol. **76**: 229–233.
10. Hotchkiss, A.J. & J.W. Gibb. 1980. Long-term effects of multiple doses of methamphetamine on tryptophan hydroxylase and tyrosine hydroxylase activity in rat brain. J. Pharmacol. Exp. Ther. **214**: 257–262.
11. Hotchkiss, A.J., M.E. Morgan & J.W. Gibb. 1979. The long-term effects of multiple doses of methamphetamine on neostriatal tryptophan hydroxylase, tyrosine hydroxylase, choline acetyltransferase and glutamate decarboxylase activities. Life Sci. **25**: 1373–1378.

12. SEIDEN, L.S. & K.E. SABOL. 1996. Methamphetamine and methylenedioxymethamphetamine neurotoxicity: possible mechanisms of cell destruction. NIDA Res. Monogr. **163**: 251–276.
13. RODRIGUES, L.G. *et al.* 2004. Methamphetamine exacerbates the toxic effect of kainic acid in the adult rat retina. Neurochem. Int. **45**: 1133–1141.
14. WEISSMAN, A.D. & S. CALDECOTT HAZARD. 1993. In utero methamphetamine effects: I. Behavior and monoamine uptake sites in adult offspring. Synapse **13**: 241–250.
15. ACUFF-SMITH, K.D. 1993. Neurobehavioral, neurochemical, and ocular effects of prenatal methamphetamine exposure in rats as a function of dose and gestational stage. PhD, University of Cincinnati.
16. CABRERA, T.M. *et al.* 1993. Prenatal methamphetamine attenuates serotonin mediated renin secretion in male and female rat progeny: evidence for selective long-term dysfunction of serotonin pathways in brain. Synapse **15**: 198–208.
17. SATO, M. & Y. FUJIWARA. 1986. Behavioral and neurochemical changes in pups prenatally exposed to methamphetamine. Brain Dev. **8**: 390–396.
18. RICE, D. & S. BARONE, JR. 2000. Critical periods of vulnerability for the developing nervous system: evidence from humans and animal models. Environ. Health Perspect. **108**(Suppl 3): 511–533.
19. BAYER, S.A. *et al.* 1993. Timetables of neurogenesis in the human brain based on experimentally determined patterns in the rat. Neurotoxicology **14**: 83–144.
20. DOBBING, J. & J. SANDS. 1979. Comparative aspects of the brain growth spurt. Early Hum. Dev. **3**: 79–83.
21. HENCK, J.W. 2002. Developmental neurotoxicology: testing and interpretation. *In* Handbook of Neurotoxicology, Vol. II. E.J. Massaro Ed.: 3–56. Humana Press. Totowa, NJ.
22. INSEL, T.R. 1995. The development of brain and behavior. *In* Psychopharmacology: the Fourth Generation of Progress. F.E. Bloom & D.J. Kupfer, Eds.: 683–694. Raven Press. New York.
23. FLETCHER, E.L. & M. KALLONIATIS. 1997. Localisation of amino acid neurotransmitters during postnatal development of the rat retina. J. Comp. Neurol. **380**: 449–471.
24. WEIDMAN, T.A. & T. KUWABARA. 1968. Postnatal development of the rat retina. An electron microscopic study. Arch. Ophthalmol. **79**: 470–484.
25. WEIDMAN, T.A. & T. KUWABARA. 1969. Development of the rat retina. Invest. Ophthalmol. **8**: 60–69.
26. KATO, S., T. NAKAMURA & K. NEGISHI. 1980. Postnatal development of dopaminergic cells in the rat retina. J. Comp. Neurol. **191**: 27–36.
27. PERRY, V.H. & M. WALKER. 1980. Morphology of cells in the ganglion cell layer during development of the rat retina. Proc. R. Soc. Lond. B. Biol. Sci. **208**: 433–445.
28. ALI, S.F. *et al.* 1994. MPTP-induced oxidative stress and neurotoxicity are age-dependent: evidence from measures of reactive oxygen species and striatal dopamine levels. Synapse **18**: 27–34.
29. WOLFENSOHN, S. & M. LLOYD. 1998. Handbook of Laboratory Animal Management and Welfare. Blackwell Science. Oxford.
30. GOMES-DA-SILVA, J. 2002. Efeito da metanfetamina na ontogenia das vias dopaminérgicas do sistema nervoso do rato. PhD, University of Porto, Porto.

31. SILVA-ARAUJO, A. *et al.* 1995. Effects of prenatal cocaine exposure in the retinal ganglion cell layer of the rat. A morphometric analysis. Mol. Neurobiol. **11**: 87–97.
32. SILVA-ARAUJO, A. *et al.* 1996. The effects of prenatal exposure to cocaine on the dopaminergic cells in the rat retina. An immunocytochemical and neurochemical study. Exp. Eye Res. **62**: 697–708.
33. SILVA-ARAUJO, A. & M.A. TAVARES. 1996. Development of the eye after gestational exposure to cocaine. Vascular disruption in the retina of rats and humans. Ann. N. Y. Acad. Sci. **801**: 274–288.
34. TAVARES, M.A. & M.C. SILVA. 1993. Body weight gain and hippocampal volumes of rats exposed neonatally to psychostimulants. Brain Res. **619**: 137–145.
35. MELO, P. *et al.* 2005. Methamphetamine and lipid peroxidation in the rat retina. Birth Defects Res. A Clin. Mol. Teratol. **73:** 455–460.
36. DIXON, S.D. & R. BEJAR. 1989. Echoencephalographic findings in neonates associated with maternal cocaine and methamphetamine use: incidence and clinical correlates. J. Pediatr. **115**: 770–778.
37. ORO, A.S. & S.D. DIXON. 1987. Perinatal cocaine and methamphetamine exposure: maternal and neonatal correlates. J. Pediatr. **111**: 571–578.
38. SMITH, L. *et al.* 2003. Effects of prenatal methamphetamine exposure on fetal growth and drug withdrawal symptoms in infants born at term. J. Dev. Behav. Pediatr. **24**: 17–23.
39. ACUFF-SMITH, K.D. *et al.* 1996. Stage-specific effects of prenatal d-methamphetamine exposure on behavioral and eye development in rats. Neurotoxicol. Teratol. **18**: 199–215.
40. CHO, D.H. *et al.* 1991. Behavioral teratogenicity of methamphetamine. J. Toxicol. Sci. **16**(Suppl 1): 37–49.
41. TAVARES, M.A. & M.C. SILVA. 1996. Differential effects of prenatal exposure to cocaine and amphetamine on growth parameters and morphometry of the prefrontal cortex in the rat. Ann. N. Y. Acad. Sci. **801**: 256–273.
42. TAVARES, M.A. *et al.* 1996. Effects of prenatal exposure to amphetamine in the medial prefrontal cortex of the rat. Int. J. Dev. Neurosci. **14**: 585–596.
43. WILLIAMS, M.T., M.S. MORAN & C.V. VORHEES. 2003. Refining the critical period for methamphetamine-induced spatial deficits in the Morris water maze. Psychopharmacology (Berl.) **168**: 329–338.
44. WILLIAMS, M.T. *et al.* 2003. Developmental D-methamphetamine treatment selectively induces spatial navigation impairments in reference memory in the Morris water maze while sparing working memory. Synapse **48**: 138–148.
45. CAPPON, G.D., L.L. MORFORD & C.V. VORHEES. 1997. Ontogeny of methamphetamine-induced neurotoxicity and associated hyperthermic response. Brain Res. Dev. Brain Res. **103**: 155–162.
46. FARFEL, G.M. & L.S. SEIDEN. 1995. Role of hypothermia in the mechanism of protection against serotonergic toxicity. II. Experiments with methamphetamine, p-chloroamphetamine, fenfluramine, dizocilpine and dextromethorphan. J. Pharmacol. Exp. Ther. **272**: 868–875.
47. CONKLIN, P. & F.W. HEGGENESS. 1971. Maturation of temperature homeostasis in the rat. Am. J. Physiol. **220**: 333–336.
48. DJAMGOZ, M.B. *et al.* 1997. Neurobiology of retinal dopamine in relation to degenerative states of the tissue. Vision Res. **37**: 3509–3529.
49. NGUYEN LEGROS, J. *et al.* 1981. Tyrosine hydroxylase-like immunoreactive interplexiform cells in the rat retina. Neurosci. Lett. **27**: 255–259.

50. VERSAUX-BOTTERI, C. *et al.* 1986. Regional specialization of the rat retina: catecholamine-containing amacrine cell characterization and distribution. J. Comp. Neurol. **243**: 422–433.
51. WITKOVSKY, P. & M. SCHUTTE. 1991. The organization of dopaminergic neurons in vertebrate retinas. Vis. Neurosci. **7**: 113–124.
52. VARELLA, M.H., F.G. DE MELLO & R. LINDEN. 1999. Evidence for an antiapoptotic role of dopamine in developing retinal tissue. J. Neurochem. **73**: 485–492.
53. KASHII, S. *et al.* 1994. Protective action of dopamine against glutamate neurotoxicity in the retina. Invest. Ophthalmol. Vis. Sci. **35**: 685–695.
54. LANKFORD, K.L., F.G. DEMELLO & W.L. KLEIN. 1988. D1-type dopamine receptors inhibit growth cone motility in cultured retina neurons: evidence that neurotransmitters act as morphogenic growth regulators in the developing central nervous system. Proc. Natl. Acad. Sci. USA. **85**: 4567–4571.
55. CAO, W. *et al.* 1993. Effects of experimentally induced ischemia on dopamine metabolism in rabbit retina. Invest. Ophthalmol. Vis. Sci. **34**: 3140–3146.

Prenatal Exposure to Cocaine and Enriched Environment

Effects on Social Interactions

ANA MAGALHÃES,[a,b] TERESA SUMMAVIELLE,[a,c] PEDRO MELO,[a,d] RUI ROSA,[a] MARIA AMÉLIA TAVARES,[a,d] AND LILIANA DE SOUSA[a,b]

[a]*Institute for Molecular and Cellular Biology, University of Porto, 4150-180 Porto, Portugal*

[b]*Institute for Biomedical Sciences Abel Salazar, University of Porto, 4099-003 Porto, Portugal*

[c]*ESTSP, Instituto Politécnico do Porto, 4000-294 Porto, Portugal*

[d]*Institute of Anatomy, Medical School of Porto, University of Porto, 4200-319 Porto, Portugal*

ABSTRACT: Exposure to cocaine throughout gestation may produce several deleterious outcomes in the offspring that include effects on neurotransmitter systems and structure of the central nervous system. Such changes are most likely correlated with behavioral alterations. Environmental enrichment (EE) in early stages is a factor that affects structural and behavioral development. This article examines the effects, upon social interactions, of EE during the first month of life in rats prenatally exposed to cocaine. Wistar dams were subcutaneously exposed to 60 mg/kg of cocaine divided in two daily doses from gestational day (GD)8 to GD22. Pair-fed controls were given saline vehicle in the same protocol. Offspring were distributed to the different environments in four experimental groups. Group 1: offspring from dams prenatally exposed to cocaine as previously described and reared in EE from postnatal day (PND)1 to PND28; Group 2: pups from cocaine-exposed dams and reared in a standard environment (SE); Group 3: pups from pair-fed saline-exposed dams and reared in EE; Group 4: offspring from saline-exposed dams and reared in SE. On PND21, 24, and 28, rats were examined in several social behavioral categories (play fighting, social investigation, comfort behaviors, and solicitation to play) for 10 min. Animals reared in SE do not display any differences due to treatment in the behavioral categories analyzed. Control offspring reared in EE presented decreased play fighting, decreased solicitation to play, and decreased social investi-

Address for correspondence: Ana Magalhães, Neurobehavior Unit, Institute for Molecular and Cellular Biology, University of Porto, Rua do Campo Alegre 823, 4150-180 Porto, Portugal. Voice: +351-22-6074945; fax: +351-22-6099157.
e-mail: anam@ibmc.up.pt

Ann. N.Y. Acad. Sci. 1074: 620–631 (2006).
doi: 10.1196/annals.1369.060

gation compared to the control SE group, while cocaine-exposed animals reared in EE did not present these variations. These results suggest that EE rearing may unmask hidden effects of prenatal cocaine exposure.

Keywords: cocaine; development; enriched environment; social interactions

INTRODUCTION

Rats exhibit a complex and well-organized repertoire of social behavior. In juvenile rats, social activities are different from social play, which suggests that within the social repertoire of juvenile rats, it is possible to formulate a distinction between social behaviors related to play (pinning, boxing/wrestling, following/chasing) or unrelated to play (social exploration, contact behavior).[1–3] Social behaviors related to play occur mainly before sexual maturation, peaking at a midpoint of the periadolescent period, while other forms of social repertoire occur during the entire life span, such as social investigation and social contact behavior.[2,4,5] Play behavior seems to be an affiliate form of behavior, functioning to facilitate different aspects of social development, such as establishment of social organization in a group[6] and development of the ability to express and understand intraspecific-communicating signals,[4,7] which may serve to inhibit aggression[6,8] and increase group stability. Social play may be seen as facilitating the ability to cope with social conflicts.[9]

Behavioral studies have indicated that social play is a separate and relevant category of behavior and have reported that play and social investigation are influenced differentially by drugs' treatments.[10–12] Former studies suggest that behaviors related to play may be regulated through neuronal systems different from those that regulate social behaviors unrelated to play.[8,13] It was found that opioid systems have an important role in regulation and expression of social play. The motivational and rewarding aspects of play behavior are thought to be regulated by the endogenous opioid system.[13] The implication of the reward system in the regulation of social play suggested that long-term changes in this system probably would alter the expression of social play.

Cocaine reinforcing proprieties also utilize, in part, the same circuit implicated in the reinforcing properties of opiates.[14] Cocaine exposure throughout gestation results in an altered dopaminergic system[15,16] and this alteration produces some deficits in social behaviors.[17–21] Studies linking cocaine and social interaction showed that prenatal cocaine exposure results in diminished social play,[17,22] increased aggression,[19–21,23] and potentiation of responsiveness to acute or chronic stress.[24–27] Other groups reported that animals postnatally exposed to cocaine decreased aggression (acute treatment),[28] elicited less play solicitation from conspecifics, or did not differ from controls in their own play behavior.[22] These discrepancies in published data may be associated to the variety of test paradigms, animal models, and dosing regimens that have been utilized. However, there is some convergence in basic research which suggests that exposure to drugs throughout development may lead to persistent abnormalities of in-brain systems and behavior. These permanent changes in the development of the brain circuits that process reward or reinforcement may result in a greater vulnerability to additive behaviors in adulthood.[29]

There are indications that both formal training on complex spatial tasks and living in spatially complex environments (environmental enrichment [EE]) alter neurochemistry, brain weight, and behavior in rats.[30] An environment that supplies a great variety of incentives provides a learning space to the animal, with increased possibilities of interaction, manipulation, and exploration of the environment.[31] Exploration presupposes the occurrence of learning, which probably alters the behavioral sequences (for review see Ref. 32). A complex environment increases the opportunity not only of social play but also of object interaction. Several studies found evidence of neurogenesis in response to EE (for review see Ref. 33), which might explain its beneficial effects on the course of neurodegeneratives diseases,[34] aging,[35] and recovery from brain damage.[36] The stimulation provided via EE, applied early in life, alters both brain and behavior and may be beneficial for the behavior development.[32]

The main objective of the present article was to analyze the effects of prenatal exposure to cocaine on development social behavior and to verify if a postnatal environmental condition (EE/standard) would affect the expression of social behaviors in rats exposed to cocaine during prenatal life.

MATERIAL AND METHODS

Subjects and Protocol of Drug Exposure

Rats used in this study were offspring born from Wistar females purchased from the Colony of the Gulbenkian Institute of Science, Oeiras, Portugal. They were bred at the Institute of Molecular and Cell Biology, University of Porto, Portugal. Animals were housed in a temperature- and humidity-controlled colony room, maintained on a 12/12-h light/dark cycle, with free access to food and water. At the onset of breeding, adult nulliparous females, weighing an average of 250–300 g, were mated with one male of the same strain. The morning a copulatory plug or sperm-positive vaginal cytology was observed was considered as gestational day 1 (GD1). Pregnant females were weighed, housed individually in standard cages containing wood bedding, and assigned to one of the following prenatal groups: a cocaine-exposed group (COC) and a control group, pair-fed to the COC group (PF). Dams in the COC group received subcutaneous injections (s.c.) of cocaine hydrochloride (Sigma Chemical Co., St. Louis, MO) at 60 mg/kg of body weight/day from GD8 to 22 and were given *ad libitum* food and water. The period of exposure comprises the major periods of organogenesis and of neurogenesis, migration and gliogenesis, covering also the onset of synaptogenesis.[37,38] Each daily dose was divided into two equal parts, administered between 8:30–9:00 AM and 5:00–6:00 PM. Dams in the PF group received daily s.c. injections of vehicle (saline 0.9%), isovolumetric to cocaine and were submitted to food restriction (pair-fed to the cocaine females).

On the day after birth, postnatal day (PND)1, each litter was culled to eight pups, gender balanced, and pups weighed, marked with a felt-tip pen for identification, and housed in standard polycarbonate cages, living directly on wooden bedding. Pups were weaned on PND21. All procedures used were approved by the Portuguese Agency for Animal Welfare (General Board of Veterinary Medicine).

Housed Conditions

EE: large acrylic cage (100 × 70 × 70 cm) with wooden bedding and equipped with various objects (polyvinyl chloride [PVC] tubes, ping-pong and paper balls, wood objects, ladders, toys) that were replaced every 3 days. Standard environment (SE) standard acrylic cage type III, living directly on wooden bedding without objects.

Experimental Groups

Offspring were distributed into these two different environments completing 4 experimental groups: Group1 COC/EE: offspring from dams prenatally exposed to COC as previously described and reared in EE from PND 1 to PND28; Group 2 COC/SE: pups from COC exposed dam and reared in SE; Group 3 SAL/EE: pups from PF and saline (SAL)-exposed dam and reared in EE; Group 4 SAL/SE: offspring from SAL-exposed dams and reared in SE.

Behavioral Testing: Social Interactions

Social interactions were assessed in three periods of development: PND21—weaning and beginning of play-fighting behaviors,[39] PND24 and 28—prepubescent period. The social interaction test was performed in a sound-attenuated room, during the dark phase of the light cycle. The testing arena consisted in a (PVC) cage measuring 60 × 53 × 40 cm with wood shaving covered floor, containing the following objects: three ladders, a block and a siring, illuminated by an infrared light mounted 1 m above. The test was carried out between 4 PM and 5 PM, 6.5 h after the daily drug treatment. This period of time was chosen, to allow enough time to eliminate the influence of acute cocaine, considering a 2-h half-life after subcutaneous administration of cocaine (reviewed in Ref. 40). Behavior sessions were recorded by a video camera (SONY DCR-TRV9E; Sony Corp., Tokyo, Japan), for 10 min, after allowing a 5-min period for habituation to the test arena. Test was performed in groups of four rats from the same experimental group but only one rat was observed by focal–animal method. The following behavioral categories were analyzed using the software Observer 4.1 (Noldus Information Technology, Wageningen Netherlands): frequency of play-fighting behaviors, divided into play-dominant (wrestling, boxing, pouncing, aggressive grooming, on-top-posture, chase, attack) and play-submissive (pining, escape, evade) behaviors; comfort behaviors (social grooming and pile-up behavior); play solicitation (crawl over/under, nosing); social investigation (sniffing the conspecific's body including the anogenital area); and total frequency social interaction.

Data Analyses

Behavioral data were analyzed by a Mann-Whitney U test. Since this Mann-Whitney U test did not indicate a significant effect of the gender factor, data were collapsed across gender and reanalyzed. Results were analyzed at a significance level of 5%, using the software Statistica version 5.5 (Statsoft Inc., 1999; Tulsa, OK).

RESULTS

Effects of Postnatal Exposure to Cocaine in SE

Prenatal exposure to cocaine had no significant effect on social behavior of developing rat pups reared in SE when compared to SAL/SE animals. No significant differences were found on frequency of play solicitation (see FIG. 1 A), play-fighting behaviors (dominant or submissive) (see FIG. 1 B,C), or social investigation (FIG. 1 D) comfort behaviors (FIG. 1 E) in rats COC/SE when compared to SAL/SE.

Effects of EE

For data concerning effects of EE, Mann-Whitney U test revealed a significant effect of housing conditions in several behavioral categories. Animals of SAL/EE group decreased play-dominant behaviors on PND21 ($Z = -2.92$; two-tailed $P < 0.01$) and on PND24 ($Z = -2.323$; two-tailed $P < 0.05$) (see FIG. 1 B), play-submissive behaviors on PND21 ($Z = -2.542$; two-tailed $P < 0.05$) and on PND24 ($Z = -3.192$; two-tailed $P < 0.001$) (see FIG. 1 C), social investigation on PND28 ($Z = -2{,}226$; two-tailed $P < 0.05$) (FIG. 1 D) and also decreased play solicitation on PND21 ($Z = -3.241$; two-tailed $P < 0.001$); and PND24 ($Z = -2.427$; two-tailed $P < 0.05$) (FIG. 1 A) when compared to SAL/SE rats.

Man-Whitney test showed a significant alteration in behavior of rats prenatally exposed to cocaine when they were reared in EE during the first month of life in three behavioral categories. COC/EE rats showed a decreased play-dominant behavior on PND21 ($Z = -2.353$; two-tailed $P < 0.05$) (see FIG. 1 B), of play-submissive behavior on PND21 ($Z = -2.672$; two-tailed $P < 0.01$) (see FIG. 1 C), and decreased social investigation on PND21 ($Z = -2.4$; $P < 0.05$) (FIG. 1 D). No other behavioral categories presented a significant effect for EE.

DISCUSSION

In the present study, effects of EE on prenatal cocaine-exposed rats were examined in several categories of social behavior. In the rat, the first month of postnatal life is a particularly sensitive developmental period in which environmental influences can have a significant effect on subsequent behavioral development.[11]

In an attempt to identify the effects of prenatal cocaine exposure on rat social behavior, we have examined the effects of chronic cocaine exposure on several behavioral categories of social interaction at three different points during the prepubescent period. However, control and prenatal cocaine-exposed rats reared in SE do not display any differences in the behavioral categories analyzed. Some studies report that prenatal cocaine exposure results in diminished social behavior,[17,22,41] decreased solicitation to play,[17,20,22] and increased aggression[18,20,21] in the offspring. These positive effects may be explained, in part, by methodological differences such as subject age at testing, dose of drug administered, and other differences in the protocol used.

Control animals reared in an EE (SAL/EE) displayed decreased play fight when compared to SE-reared rats (SAL/SE). This result is consistent with other studies, where a significant reduction of play-related behaviors on animals reared in EE was shown.[39,42] The reduction of social play in SAL/EE rats may reflect the fact that, in this study, rats were tested in an arena with novel objects. The novelty of objects' arrangements may have facilitated the exploration of environment.[42,43] Also, there is evidence that social interactions may increase object interaction.[43] Animals reared in an EE are more exploratory and seem to prefer to explore the novel environment instead of being engaged in social play,[42] which would reduce attention to the surroundings. The EE also decreased social investigation in SAL/EE when compared to SAL/SE-reared rats. This social behavior, unrelated to play, has the immediate goal of exploring cospecifics.[3] Social memory, the ability to form and retain information related to conspecifics,[44] seems to be improved in EE-housed animals. This result suggests that EE facilitated the retention of specific information, which is in accordance with the increased plasticity in the hippocampus described to be caused by EE.[33]

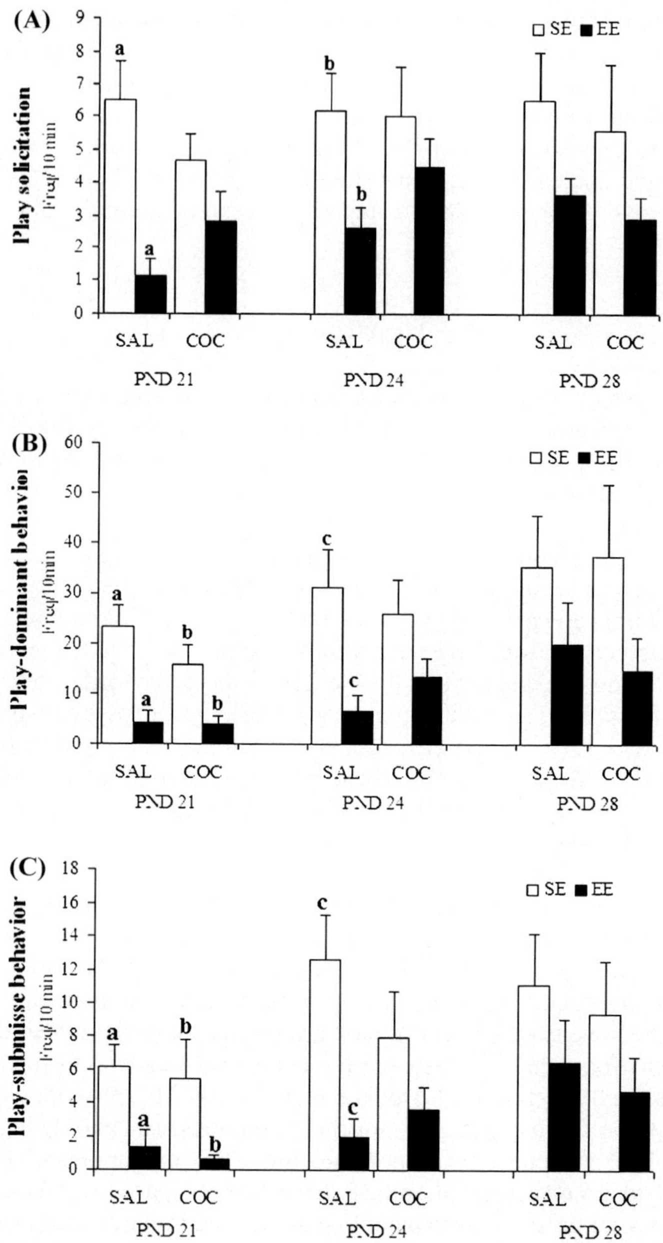

FIGURE 1. Effect of prenatal cocaine exposure and environmental enrichment on frequencies per 10 min of the follows behavioral categories: (**A**) play solicitation: (**a**) $P < 0.001$, (**b**) $P < 0.05$; (**B**) play-dominant behaviors: (**a**) $P < 0.01$, (**b, c**) $P < 0.05$; (**C**) play-submissive behaviors: (**a**) $P < 0.05$, (**b**) $P < 0.001$, (**c**) $P < 0.01$; (**D**) social investigation: (**a, b**) $P < 0.05$; and (**E**) comfort behaviors. Data are presented as means + SEM.

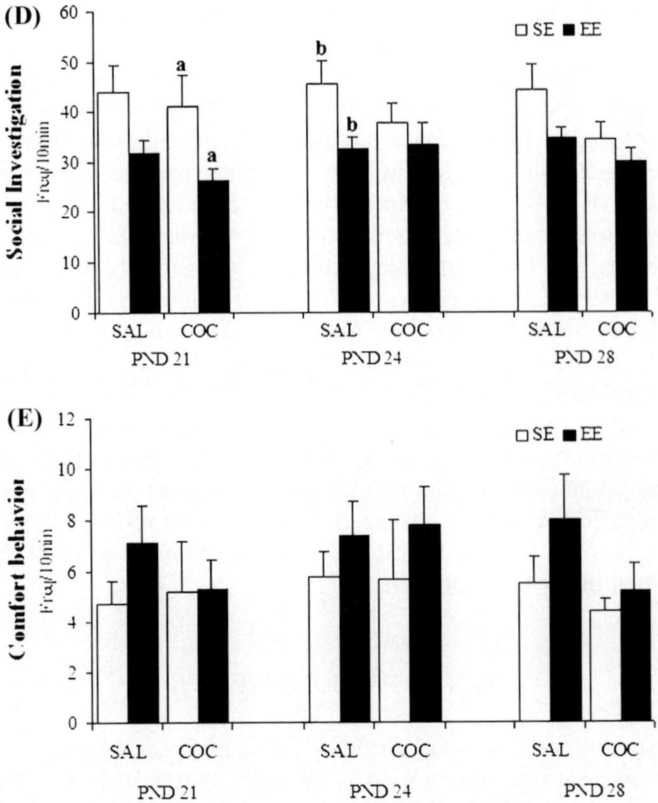

FIGURE 1. *Continued*

Play solicitation is less frequent in rats of SAL/EE group when compared to rats reared in SE. In the juvenile rat, specific behaviors classified as play solicitation include pounce, tail pulling, crawl over/under and darting, and precede bouts or sequences of play fighting.[4] Play solicitation has been described as a set of behaviors functionally inciting social play.[45] So, this decrease in solicitation to play can be related with the decreased play-fighting behavior.

Rats prenatally exposed to cocaine, when reared in EE, display decreased play-fighting behaviors (play-dominant and play-submissive behaviors) compared to COC/SE group. As already mentioned, reduction of play in animals reared in EE may be related with their preference to explore the novel environment instead of being engaged in social play.[42] Animals in EE present reduced levels of offensive and submissive behaviors such chasing, attacking, pining and fighting, suggesting that a complex environment most markedly affects play fighting. In fact, EE environment enhances the opportunities to spread out and to stay away, expanding the exploration of the behavioral repertoire.

Rats prenatally exposed to cocaine and reared in EE also decreased social investigation when compared to COC/SE animals. These results suggest that EE improves social memory in rats postnatally exposed to cocaine. Rats who were engaged in playful behavior with conspecifics in EE present increased dendritic arboration, have heavier cerebral cortices, and show improved learning abilities when compared to play-deprived rats in impoverished environment (for review see Ref. 46). Social exploration is not associated with play behavior. This social category, unrelated to play, seems to be regulated through different neural systems.[13] While social play seems to be primarily regulated through the opioid system,[47] cocaine is known to affect mainly the dopaminergic and serotonergic systems.[48,49] However, although these circuitries are not fully understood, there are strong evidences of direct and indirect (via GABAergic inhibition) influence of one system onto the other (for review see Ref. 10).

In the present work, no differences between cocaine-exposed and control rats could be determined when both groups were reared in a SE, nevertheless, when rats were given an extra developmental stimuli, such as those promoted by an EE, several differences were observed. Therefore, we propose that rearing in an EE may unmask hidden deficits of prenatal cocaine exposure that would not be evident under SE conditions.

ACKNOWLEDGMENTS

The present research was supported by Fundação para a Ciência e Tecnologia (FCT) by awarding grants to Ana Magalhães (PRAXISXXI/BD/20075/99), Pedro Melo (PRAXIS XXI/BD/3395/2000) and Teresa Summavielle (SFRH/BPD/20997/2004), and also through the Project POCTI/PSI/39491/2001 approved by FCT and supported by FEDER and by Plurianual funds from IBMC.

REFERENCES

1. NIESINK, R., L. VANDERSCHUREN & J.M. VAN REE. 1996. Social play in juvenile rats after in utero exposure to morphine. Neurotoxicology **17:** 905–912.
2. HOLE, G. 1991. Proximity measures of social play in laboratory rat. Dev. Psychobiol. **24:** 117–133.
3. VANDERSCHUREN, L. *et al.* 1995. Influence of environmental factors on social play behavior of juvenile rats. Physiol. Behav. **58:** 119–123.
4. MEANEY, M.J. & J. STEWART. 1981. A descriptive study of social development in the rat (*Rattus norvegicus*). Anim. Behav. **29:** 34–45.
5. POOLE, T.B. & J. FISH. 1975. An investigation of playful behavior in *Rattus norvegicus* and *Mus musculus* (Mammalia). J. Zool. Lond. **175:** 61–71.
6. VANDERSCHUREN, L., R. NIESINK & J.M. VAN REE. 1997. The neurobiology of social play behavior in rats. Neurosci. Behav. Rev. **21:** 309–326.

7. TAKAHASHI, L. 1986. Postweaning environmental and social factors influencing the onset and expression of agonistic behavior in Norway rats. Behav. Proc. **12:** 237–260.
8. VARLINSKAYA, E., L. SPEAR & N. SPEAR. 1999. Social behavior and social motivation in adolescent rats: role of housing conditions and partner's activity. Physiol. Behav. **67:** 475–482.
9. AKBARI, H. *et al.* 1992. Prenatal cocaine exposure disrupts the development of the serotonergic system. Brain Res. **572:** 57–63.
10. BEATTY, W. *et al.* 1982. Psychomotor stimulants, social deprivation and play in juvenile rats. Pharmacol. Biochem. Behav. **16:** 417–422.
11. HARRISON, R. *et al.* 2000. Chronic low-dose cocaine treatment during adolescence facilitates aggression in hamsters. Physiol. Behav. **69:** 555–562.
12. HOL, T. *et al.* 1996. Prenatal exposure to morphine affects juvenile play behavior and adult social behavior in rats. Pharmacol. Biochem. Behav. **55:** 615–618.
13. VANDERSCHUREN, L. *et al.* 1996. Sequential analysis of social play behavior in juvenile rats: effects of morphine. Behav. Brain Res. **72:** 89–95.
14. KOOB, G., P. SANNA & F. BLOOM. 1998. Neuroscience of addiction. Neuron **21:** 467–476.
15. SPEAR, L., C. KIRSTEIN & N. FRAMBES. 1989. Cocaine effects on developing central nervous system: behavioral, psychopharmacological, and neurochemical studies. Ann. N. Y. Acad. Sci. **562:** 290–307.
16. SPEAR, L. *et al.* 1989. Effects of prenatal cocaine exposure on behavior during the early postnatal period. Neurotoxicol. Teratol. **11:** 57–63.
17. WOOD, R.D., M.D. BANNOURA & I.B. JOHANSON. 1994. Prenatal cocaine exposure: effects on play behavior in juvenile rat. Neurotoxicol. Teratol. **16:** 139–144.
18. WOOD, R.D. & L.P. SPEAR. 1998. Prenatal cocaine alters social competition of infant, adolescent, and adult rats. Behav. Neurosci. **112:** 419–431.
19. JOHNS, J.M. *et al.* 1994. Prenatal exposure to cocaine effects on aggression in Sprague-Dawley rats. Dev. Psycholobiol. **27:** 227–239.
20. JOHNS, J.M. & L.R. NOONAN. 1995. Prenatal cocaine exposure affects social behavior in Sprague-Dawley rats. Neurotoxicol. Teratol. **17:** 569–576.
21. ESTELLES, J. *et al.* 2005. Prenatal cocaine exposure alters spontaneous and cocaine-induced motor and social behaviors. Neurotoxicol. Teratol. **27:** 449–457.
22. WOOD, R. *et al.* 1995. Play behavior and stress responsivity in periadolescent offspring exposed prenatally to cocaine. Pharmacol. Biochem. Behav. **52:** 367–374.
23. WOOD, R. & L. SPEAR. 1998. Prenatal cocaine alters social competition of infant, adolescent, and adult rats. Behav. Neurosci. **112:** 419–431.
24. BILITZKE, P.J. & M.W. CHURCH. 1992. Prenatal cocaine and alcohol exposure affect rat behavior in a stress test (the Porsolt swim test). Neurotoxicol. Teratol. **14:** 359–364.
25. CAMPBELL, J. *et al.* 2000. Effects of prenatal cocaine on behavioral adaptation to chronic stress in adult rats. Neurotoxicol. Teratol. **22:** 845–850.
26. GOODWIN, G.A. *et al.* 1997. Immediate early gene expression to examine neural activity following acute and chronic stressors in rat pups: examination of neurophysiological alterations underlying behavioral consequences of prenatal cocaine exposure. Physiol. Behav. **61:** 895–902.
27. MOLINA, V.A., J.M. WAGNER & L.P. SPEAR. 1994. The behavioral response to stress is altered in adult rats exposed prenatally to cocaine. Physiol. Behav. **55:** 941–945.

28. RADEMACHER, D. *et al.* 2002. Effects of cocaine and putative atypical antipsychotics on rat social behavior: an ethopharmacological study. Pharmacol. Biochem. Behav. **73:** 769–778.
29. MALANGA, C. & B. KOSOFSKY. 2003. Does drug abuse beget drug abuse? Behavioral analysis of addiction liability in animal models of prenatal drug exposure. Brain Res. Dev. Brain Res. **147:** 47–57.
30. ROSENZWEIG, M. & E. BENNETT. 1996. Psychobiology of plasticity: effects of training and experience on brain and behavior. Behav. Brain Res. **78:** 57–65.
31. JURASKA, J.M., C. HENDERSON & M. JUTTA. 1983. Difference rearing experience, gender, radial maze performance. Dev. Psychol. **17:** 209–215.
32. RENNER, M. & M. ROSENZWEIG. 1987. Enriched and Impoverished Environments: Effects on Brain and Behavior. Spring-Verlag. New York.
33. VAN PRAAG, H., G. KEMPERMANN & F. GAGE. 2000. Neural consequences of environmental enrichment. Nat. Rev. Neurosci. **1:** 191–198.
34. VAN DELLEN, A. *et al.* 2000. Delaying the onset of Huntington's in mice. Nature **404:** 721–722.
35. WINOCUR, G. 1998. Environmental influences on cognitive decline in aged rats. Neurobiol. Aging **19:** 589–597.
36. HORNER, P. & F. GAGE. 2000. Regenerating the damaged central nervous system. Nature **407:** 963–970.
37. HENCK, J.W. 2002. Developmental neurotoxicology: testing and interpretation. *In* Handbook of Neurotoxicology, Vol. II. E.J. Massaro, Ed.: 3–56. Humana Press. Totowa.
38. INSEL, T. 1995. Development of brain and behavior. *In* Psychopharmacology—The Fourth Generation of Progress. F.E. Bloom & D.J. Kupfer, Eds.: 683–693. Raven Press, Ltd. New York.
39. PANKSEPP, J. 1981. The ontogeny of play in rats. Dev. Psychobiol. **14:** 327–332.
40. VORHEES, C. 1996. Long-term effects of developemental exposure to cocaine on learned and unlearned behaviors. *In* Behavioral Studies of Drug-Exposure Offspring: Methological Issues in Human and Animal Research, Vol. NIDA Research Monograph 164. C.L. Wetherington, V.L. Smeriglio & L.P. Finnegan, Eds.: 3–52. U.S Department of Health and Human Services—National Institute of Health.
41. WANG, H., J. YEUNG & E. FRIEDMAN. 1995. Prenatal cocaine exposure selectively reduces mesocortical dopamine release. J. Pharmacol. Exp. Ther. **273:** 1211–1215.
42. RENNER, M.J. & M.R. ROSENZWEIG. 1986. Social interactions among rats housed in grouped and enriched conditions. Dev. Psychobiol. **19:** 303–313.
43. JURASKA, J.M. & M. MEYER. 1986. Behavioral interactions of postweaning male and female rats with a complex environment. Dev. Psychobiol. **19:** 493–500.
44. BURMAN, O. & M. MENDL. 1999. The effects of environmental context on laboratory rat social recognition. Anim. Behav. **58:** 629–634.
45. FAGEN, R. 1981. Animal Play Behavior. Oxford: Oxford University Press.
46. FERCHMIN, P.A. & V.A. ETEROVIC. 1982. Play stimulated by environmental complexity alters the brain and improves learning abilities in rodents, primates, and possibly humans. Behav. Brain Sci. **5:** 164.
47. VANDERSCHUREN, L. *et al.* 1995. Sequential analysis of social play behavior in juvenile rats: effects of morphine. Behav. Brain Res. **72:** 89–95.

48. Carelli, R.M., S.G. Ijames & A.J. Crumling. 2000. Evidence that separate neural circuits in the nucleus accumbens encode cocaine versus "natural" (water and food) reward. J. Neurosci. **20:** 4255–4266.
49. Broderick, P.A., D.N. Rahni & Y. Zhou. 2003. Acute and subacute effects of risperidone and cocaine on accumbens dopamine and serotonin release using in vivo microvoltammetry on line with open-field behavior. Prog. Neuropsychopharmacol. Biol. Psychiatry **27:** 1037–1054.

Nitric Oxide and Oxidative Stress in the Brain of Rats Exposed *In Utero* to Cocaine

VALENTINA BASHKATOVA,[a] JOHANN MEUNIER,[b] ANATOLY VANIN,[c] AND TANGUI MAURICE[b]

[a]*Department of Neurochemical Pharmacology, Institute of Pharmacology, Russian Academy of Medical Sciences, 125315 Moscow, Russia*

[b]*INSERM U. 710, EPHE, University of Montpellier II, 34095 Montpellier cedex 5, France*

[c]*Department of Physical Chemistry of Biopolimeres, Semenov Institute of Chemical Physics, Russian Academy of Sciences, 119113 Moscow, Russia*

ABSTRACT: The role of nitric oxide (NO) and lipid peroxidation (LPO) processes in the physiological deficits induced by *in utero* cocaine exposure was examined in rats. NO generation in the hippocampus and cortex was detected using the electron paramagnetic resonance and LPO products were measured as thiobarbituric acid reactive species (TBARS). Pregnant Sprague-Dawley rats received a daily intraperitoneal injection of 20 mg/kg cocaine (IUC) or saline solution for control dams (IUV) between E17–E20. NO level was lower in the brain of IUC rats at postnatal day 1 and 2, but not 4, as compared with IUV rats. TBARS content was increased at day 1–4. Animals were used for behavioral testing at 25 days of age. Both NO and TBARS were elevated in the hippocampus of IUC rats as compared with IUV rats. Juvenile IUC rats developed significant learning impairments in the water-maze, as revealed by probe test retrieval deficits. Behavioral sessions resulted in a significant increase of TBARS levels only in IUV animals. Therefore, IUC rats showed a significant oxidative stress in basal conditions that may be related to their impaired learning ability. We did not find direct correlation between the changes in NO generation and intensity of LPO processes. It may probably mean that changes in intensity of LPO processes observed during prenatal cocaine exposure are not directly linked to NO pathway activation.

KEYWORDS: cocaine; *in utero*; exposure; lipid peroxidation; NO; oxidate stress; postnatal development

Address for correspondence: V. Bashkatova, Institute of Pharmacology, Russian Academy of Medical Sciences, 8 Baltiyskaya Street, 125315, Moscow, Russia. Voice: 007-095-1554753; fax: 007-095-1511261.
e-mail: bashkatovav@yahoo.com

**Ann. N.Y. Acad. Sci. 1074: 632–642 (2006). © 2006 New York Academy of Sciences.
doi: 10.1196/annals.1369.061**

INTRODUCTION

It is well known that popular drugs of abuse, such as methamphetamine, amphetamine, 3,4-methylenedioxymethamphetamine ("Ecstasy"), or cocaine might produce selective toxic effects on striatal monoamine-containing neurons in a variety of experimental animal models. This process is believed to be mediated by the production of free radicals. Meanwhile, results of our group[1] and other studies[2,3] have led to the proposal that neuron-damaging effects of psychostimulant drugs are mediated by nitric oxide (NO). It has been recently shown using the pharmacological and genetic manipulations with the neuronal-type of NO synthase (NOS) that NO is also involved in the rewarding properties of cocaine.[2,4]

Cocaine abuse among pregnant women continues at an alarming frequency. In utero cocaine exposure leads to pre-term birth, developmental delays, and behavioral abnormalities.[5] Exposed children often show selective impairments of attention, arousal, and information processing, that appear early in lifetime and develop to major cognitive and emotional disorders.[6,7] In particular, they exhibit marked learning and memory problems, as observed in reasoning and verbal tasks.[7,8] The mechanisms by which cocaine perturbates the brain development are rather unclear still now. It was shown recently that the neurochemical and behavioral alterations in offspring rats provoked by in utero cocaine exposure probably include generation of a sustained oxidative stress related to fetal vasoconstriction and may be involved in the memory impairments observed in offspring rats. Indeed, in utero cocaine-exposed rats showed significant learning impairments.[9,10]

The task of this article was to elicidate the role of NO and lipid peroxidation (LPO) processes in the pathophysiological mechanisms elicited by in utero exposure to cocaine. In this article, we examined whether a long-lasting oxidative stress is induced in rats after in utero cocaine exposure, which could be coherent with the learning deficits observed in these animals. We therefore measured the NO generation and LPO products in the hippocampus and cortex of juvenile rats exposed in utero to cocaine (IUC rats) or from dams receiving vehicle solution (IUV rats). Analyses were performed at days 1, 2, 4, and 25 after birth and in animals that performed a behavioral task, place learning in the water-maze.

MATERIALS AND METHODS

Experiments were carried out on male Sprague-Dawley rats (250–320 g). Protocols of experiments were approved by and in adherence of European Union Directive of 24 November 1986 (86-609).

Drugs and Drug Administration

Male Sprague-Dawley rats, originating from pregnant female rats (Depré, St-Doulchard, France) were used. Between E17 and E20, pregnant dams received a daily intraperitoneal injection of 20 mg/kg cocaine or saline solution for control dams. Delivery, weaning, and male offspring rats selection and breeding was conducted as previously detailed.[10] Rats were maintained on a constant 12h/12h light/dark cycle (lights on at 7:00 AM), at constant room temperature (21°C) and humidity (50%) with food and water *ad libitum*. Litters were divided into two groups and half of the animals were used for behavioral testing at 25 days of age. Cocaine hydrochloride was from Cooper (Melun, France). Other chemicals were from Sigma-Aldrich (St-Quentin-Fallavier, France).

Measurement of NO Generation

Diethyldithiocarbamate (DETC, 500 mg/kg) was administered intraperitoneally simultaneously with a mixture of $FeSO_4$ (37.5 mg/kg) and sodium citrate (165 mg/kg), injected subcutaneously.[11] Animals were sacrificed by decapitation 30 min after the injections and the frontal cortex and whole hippocampus were quickly dissected out and immediately frozen in liquid nitrogen. The EPR spectra were recorded at 77 K on a Brucker ESR 300E spectrometer at a frequency of 9.33 kHz.[11]

Measurement of LPO Secondary Products

Determination of LPO processes in the frontal cortex and hippocampus was performed in different animals by measuring as thiobarbituric acid reactive species (TBARS).[12]

Place Learning in the Water-Maze

The maze was a circular pool (160 cm diameter, 40 cm height) that the videotracking systems could arbitrarily divide into four quadrants. The water temperature (24° ± 2°C), light intensity, external cues in the room, and water opacity, obtained by suspension of lime carbonate, were rigorously reproduced. A transparent Plexiglas platform, 10 cm in diameter, could be immersed 2 cm under the water surface at the center of each quadrant during training sessions. This quadrant was termed the training (T) quadrant and the others opposite (O), adjacent right (AR), and adjacent left (AL) quadrants, during the subsequent retention session. Swimming was recorded using a CCD camera connected to a computer, trajectories being analyzed in terms of latencies and distances, and thus swim speed, using the Videotrack® (version NT) software (Viewpoint, Champagne-au-Mont-d'Or, France).

Animals were trained to learn a fixed platform location during 5 days. Training consisted of 3 swims per day with a 20-min inter-trial time interval. Start positions, set at each limit between quadrants, were randomly selected. Each animal was allowed a 90-s swim to find the platform and was left for a further 30 s on the platform. Animals failing to find the platform were placed on it manually. On day 5, 1 h after the last swim, a probe test was carried out. The platform was removed and each animal was allowed a free 60-s swim. The percentage of time spent in each quadrant was determined.

Statistical Analyses

Levels of NO and TBARS were expressed as mean ± SEM and analyzed using a two-way ANOVA using prenatal treatment and postnatal day (PND) or behavior as independent factors. The median swim duration was calculated per day and expressed as mean ± SEM for each group. Latencies were analyzed over trials using the nonparametric Friedman repeated measures test (Fr values), comparisons between groups being made using Dunn's test. The level of statistical significance was $P < 0.05$.

RESULTS

The in utero exposure to cocaine provoked in the offspring pup cortex marked changes in TBARS and NO contents (FIG. 1). For TBARS measures, the two-way ANOVA showed a significant effect for the in utero treatment ($F_{(1,32)} = 20.53, P < 0.0001$), but not for the PND ($F_{(2,32)} = 0.99, P > 0.05$) or the day × in utero treatment interaction ($F_{(2,32)} = 1.16, P > 0.05$). Indeed, TBARS levels were found significantly elevated in IUC rats on day 1 and day 4 after birth (FIG. 1 A). On the contrary, NO levels were found decreased after in utero exposure to cocaine. The two-way ANOVA showed significant effects for the in utero treatment ($F_{(1,33)} = 11.53, P < 0.01$), for the PND ($F_{(2,33)} = 5.52, P < 0.01$) and for the day × in utero treatment interaction ($F_{(2,32)} = 3.58, P < 0.05$). Indeed, on days 1 and 2, the NO levels were significantly lower in IUC rats as compared with IUV controls (FIG. 1 B). In juvenile rats, at PND 30, concentrations of TBARS and NO in the hippocampus and cortex were higher than the levels measured immediately after birth (FIG. 2). Both TBARS and NO were elevated in the hippocampus of IUC rats as compared with IUV rats. Animals were used for behavioral testing at 25 days of age. Behavioral sessions resulted in a significant increase of TBARS levels only in CTL animals at 30 days of age.

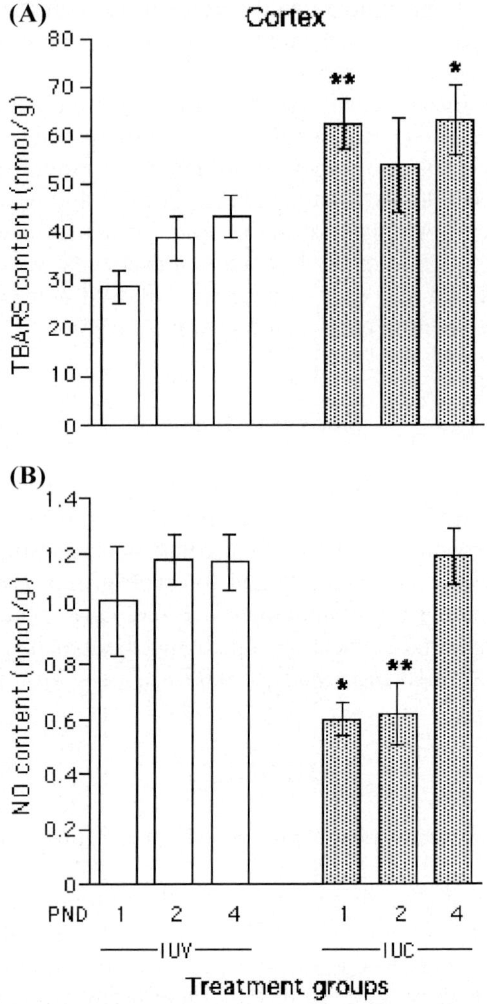

FIGURE 1. Effect of in utero cocaine exposure on LPO products (**A**) and NO production (**B**) in the cortex of rats. The cortex of pups exposed in utero to vehicle (IUV) or cocaine (IUC) was dissected out at PND 1, 2, or 4 and the TBARS and NO contents analyzed. The number of animals was $n = 6$–7 per group. $^*P < 0.05$, $^{**}P < 0.01$ versus IUV data on the same day; Newman–Kuel's test.

Two-way analysis of hippocampal TBARS contents showed the main effect of prenatal treatment ($F_{(1,20)} = 11.7, P < 0.01$) and behavior ($F_{(1,20)} = 5.3, P < 0.05$), but not of the prenatal treatment × behavior interaction ($F_{(1,20)} = 0.85, P > 0.05$). Indeed, basal levels of TBARS were highly significantly augmented in IUC rats as compared with IUV animals, and that spatial learning resulted

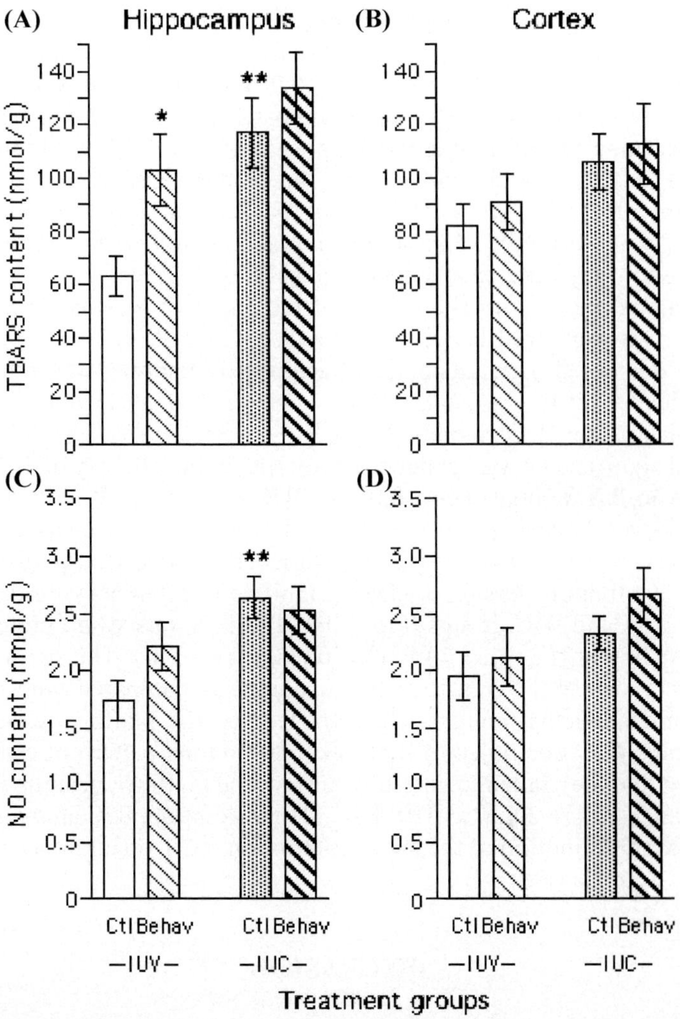

FIGURE 2. Effect of in utero cocaine exposure and place learning on TBARS products (**A, B**) and NO generation (**C, D**) in the hippocampus (**A, C**) and cortex (**B, D**) of rats. IUV and IUC rats, submitted to place learning (Behav) or not (Ctl), were dissected out and the TBARS and NO contents analyzed. $n = 6$ per group. $^{*}P < 0.05$, $^{**}P < 0.01$ versus IUV control group data; Newman–Keul's test.

in a significant induction of TBARS formation in IUV, but not IUC, animals (FIG. 2 A). In the cortex, only the prenatal treatment resulted in a significant effect ($F_{(1,19)} = 4.4$, $P < 0.05$; $F_{(1,19)} = 0.52$, $P > 0.05$ for behavior and $F_{(1,19)} = 0.01$, $P > 0.05$ for the interaction). However, no difference was measured between groups (FIG. 2 B). Two-way analysis of hippocampal NO contents showed only a significant effect for prenatal treatment ($F_{(1,20)} = 9.91$, $P < 0.01$), but not for behavior ($F_{(1,20)} = 0.90$, $P > 0.05$) or prenatal treatment × behavior interaction ($F_{(1,20)} = 2.29$, $P > 0.05$). Indeed, basal NO levels were significantly augmented in IUC rats as compared with IUV animals (FIG. 2 C). Spatial learning tended to increase hippocampal NO content, but nonsignificantly (FIG. 2 C). In the cortex, only the prenatal treatment resulted in a significant effect ($F_{(1,20)} = 4.59$, $P < 0.05$; $F_{(1,20)} = 1.32$, $P > 0.05$ for behavior and $F_{(1,19)} = 0.17$, $P > 0.05$ for the interaction), but *post hoc* comparisons failed to show any difference among groups (FIG. 2 D).

No major difference in acquisition of the platform location in the water-maze test was observed between IUV and IUC rats (FIG. 3 A). Swimming latencies decreased over the course of acquisition training, with a high level of significance for IUV animals ($F_{(4,29)} = 18.9$, $P < 0.0001$) and a lower level of significance for IUC animals ($F_{(4,29)} = 12.7$, $P < 0.05$). The difference in statistical significance was related to a lower matching efficacy of the repeated measures in IUC animals ($P > 0.05$ for IUC rats versus $P < 0.05$ for IUV rats). However, latencies measured for each training day decreased similarly among IUV and IUC rats (FIG. 3 A). During the probe test, performed 1 h after the last training session on day 5, significant differences were observed between IUV and IUC groups (FIG. 3 B). The IUV rats swam preferentially in the T quadrant ($F_{(3,23)} = 14.9$, $P < 0.0001$, FIG. 3 B). The swim duration appeared significantly greater in this quadrant as compared with the three others, indicating that animals correctly learned the platform location. On the contrary, IUC rats failed to show such differential pattern of exploration, indicating that they failed to correctly retrieve the platform position in testing conditions ($F_{(3,23)} = 2.6$, $P > 0.05$, FIG. 3 B). In addition, IUC animals showed a significant diminution of the swim duration in the T quadrant as compared with IUV animals (FIG. 3 B).

DISCUSSION

The findings indicate that NO level was lower in the brain of IUC rats immediately after birth (at days 1 and 2) in comparison with IUV rats. On the contrary, TBARS content was increased at PND 1–4 after birth. Also both NO and TBARS were increased in the hippocampus of IUC rats as compared with IUV rats. In addition to the biochemical alterations, juvenile IUC rats developed significant learning impairments in the water-maze, as revealed by probe test retrieval deficits. Moreover, impairments in place learning correlated, within the hippocampus, with diminution of the task-induced TBARS formation, suggesting a physiological substratum to the cognitive deficits observed in IUC rats.

There is a growing number of recent studies concerning the role of NO, a molecule which is regarded as universal neuronal messenger in the central

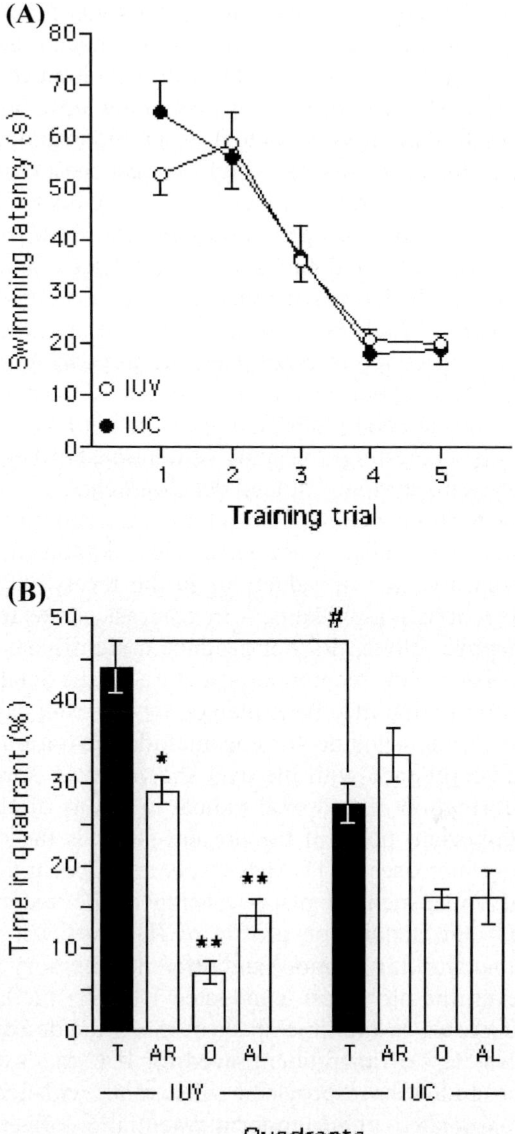

FIGURE 3. Acquisition profiles (**A**) and probe test performances (**B**) of control rats exposed in utero to vehicle injection (IUV, open circles) or cocaine (IUC, closed circles) for place learning in the water-maze. Rats were submitted during 5 days to 3 swims per day, with an inter-trial time interval of 10 min. One hour after the last swim trial, the platform was removed and animals were submitted to a 60-s swim. The presence in each quadrant was measured. Quadrants: T, training; AL, adjacent left; O, opposite; AR, adjacent right. $n = 6$ per group. $^{*}P < 0.05$, $^{**}P < 0.01$ versus time spent in the T quadrant for the same group; # $P < 0.05$ versus time spent in the T quadrant for the IUV group; Dunn's test.

nervous system, in the pathophysiology of neurotoxicity produced by psychostimulant drugs including cocaine.[1,3,13] It was established that reduced brain NOS activity blunts the processes that underlie the development of sensitization to cocaine.[4] A single administration of cocaine at low dose failed to affect coproduct of NO synthesis citrulline content in the hippocampus. By contrast, repeated administration of cocaine or its high dose caused a significant increase in the citrulline formation and this effect has been abolished by nonselective NOS inhibitor.[14] NO and the neuropeptide C-type natriuretic peptide (CNP) are now considered as potential regulators of cocaine-related effects on behavior.[15] We found that NO levels decreased in the brain of rat pups at PND 1–4 in comparison with that of adult rats. These results are in agreement with data demonstrating that expression of NOS rises in brain during the first week of postnatal life in rat pups.[16] Our results showed that NO generation was lower in the brain of IUC rats at PND 1 and 2 as compared with IUV. Our observation supports hypothesis suggesting a very close relationship between serotomin (5-HT) and NO systems during postnatal development.[17]

Although NO acts independently, it also may cause neuronal damage in cooperation with other free radicals. Recently, it was demonstrated that chronic exposure to cocaine resulted in reductions in the levels of glutathione, one of the main endogenous antioxidants.[18] In contrast, acute fetal cocaine exposure, unlike hypoxia alone, did not produce a significant increase in the LPO products in brain cell membrane structure in the fetal guinea pigs.[19] This apparent contradiction may be explained by different experimental conditions (the doses, time schedule for cocaine administration, etc.). Our observations are in accordance with the data showing that small doses of cocaine increased formation of hydroxyl radical in brains of chicken embryos on E18.[20] One important point of the present study is the observation that behavioral training increases in TBARS levels in hippocampus of IUV rats. IUC rats showed impairment of place-learning in the water-maze. As previously reported,[10] the acquisition profile of IUC rats was similar to IUV rats, suggesting that working memory and reference memory components are preserved. However, the probe test, conducted 1 h after the last training session, showed a decrease in the time spent in the T quadrant. Therefore, the mnesic engram was less efficiently engraved for IUC rats as compared with IUV rats. Recent studies have provided substantial evidence that oxidative stress is closely associated with long-term potentiation, a persistent increase in synaptic activity implicated in certain forms of learning and memory.[21] Moreover, blockade of NOS activity in the brain with NOS inhibitors has been shown to impair learning and memory in adult[22] and neonatal rats.[23] Therefore, LPO products and NO levels may be differentially in physiological processes. Indeed, we did not observe any significant increase of NO generation after learning experiments. In turn, changes in intensity of LPO processes observed during prenatal cocaine exposure are not directly linked to NO pathway activation.

In conclusion, our results may contribute to the understanding of neurochemical and behavior mechanisms of neurotoxicity produced by cocaine admitted in utero. Findings of our study might open ways to new strategies for neuroprotection against toxic effects of cocaine, which is widely used drug of abuse.

ACKNOWLEDGMENTS

This work was supported by the CNRS project #16350 PECO-NEI Russian-French cooperation program and by RFBR 03-04-49050 and RFH 03-06-00085 to V. Bashkatova.

REFERENCES

1. BASHKATOVA, V., M. KRAUS, A. VANIN, *et al.* 2004. Comparative effects of NO-synthase inhibitor and NMDA antagonist on generation of nitric oxide and release of amino acids and acetylcholine in the rat brain elicited by amphetamine neurotoxicity. Ann. N. Y. Acad. Sci. **1025:** 221–230.
2. ITZHAK, Y., J.L. MARTIN, M.D. BLACK & P.L. HUANG. 1998. The role of neuronal nitric oxide synthase in cocaine-induced conditioned place preference. Neuroreport **9:** 2485–2488.
3. ITZHAK, Y. & S.F. ALI. 2006. Role of nitrergic system in behavioral and neurotoxic effects of amphetamine analogs. Pharmacol. Ther. **109:** 246–262.
4. ITZHAK, Y., S.F. ALI, J.L. MARTIN, *et al.* 1998. Resistance of neuronal nitric oxide synthase-deficient mice to cocaine-induced locomotor sensitization. Psychopharmacology **140:** 378–386.
5. SOBRIAN, S.K., S.F. ALI, W. SLIKKER. JR. & R.R. HOLSON. 1995. Interactive effects of prenatal cocaine and nicotine exposure on maternal toxicity, postnatal development and behavior in the rat. Mol. Neurobiol. **11:** 121–143.
6. MAYES, L.C. 2002. A behavioral teratogenic model of the impact of prenatal cocaine exposure on arousal regulatory systems. Neurotox. Teratol. **24:** 385–395.
7. SINGER, L.T., S. MINNES, E. SHORT, *et al.* 2004. Cognitive outcomes of preschool children with prenatal cocaine exposure. J. Am. Med. Assoc. **291:** 2448–2456.
8. NULMAN, I., J. ROVET, D. ALTMANN, *et al.* 1994. Neurodevelopment of adopted children exposed in utero to cocaine. Can. Med. Assoc. J. **151:** 1591–1597.
9. INMAN-WOOD, S.L. M.T. WILLIAMS, L.L. MORFORD & C.V. VORHEES. 2000. Effects of prenatal cocaine on Morris and Barnes maze tests of spatial learning and memory in the offspring of C57BL/6 mice. Neurotox. Teratol. **22:** 547–557.
10. MEUNIER, J. & T. MAURICE. 2004. Beneficial effects of the $sigma_1$ receptor agonists igmesine and dehydroepiandrosterone against learning impairments in rats prenatally exposed to cocaine. Neurotoxicol. Teratol. **26:** 783–797.
11. MIKOYAN, V.D., N.V. VOEVODSKAYA, L.N. KUBRINA, *et al.* 1995. The influence of antioxidants and cycloheximide on the level of nitric oxide in the livers of mice in vivo. Biochim. Biophys. Acta. **1269:** 19–24.
12. OHKAWA, H., N. OHISHI & K. YAGI. 1979. Assay for lipid peroxides in animal tissues by thiobarbituric acid reaction. Anal. Biochem. **95:** 351–358.

13. IMAM, S.Z., F. ISLAM, Y. ITZHAK, *et al.* 2000. Prevention of dopaminergic neurotoxicity by targeting nitric oxide and peroxynitrite: implications for the prevention of methamphetamine-induced neurotoxic damage. Ann. N. Y. Acad. Sci. **914:** 157–171.
14. BAGETTA, G., S. PICCIRILLI, C. DEL DUCA, *et al.* 1999. Systemic administration of cocaine, given alone or in combination with sensory stimuli, differentially affects L-arginine-nitric oxide metabolism in discrete regions of the brain of rat. Neurosci. Lett. **356:** 183–186.
15. JOUVERT, P., M.O. REVEL, A. LAZARIS, *et al.* 2004. Activation of the cGMP pathway in dopaminergic structures reduces cocaine-induced EGR-1 expression and locomotor activity. J. Neurosci. **24:** 10716–10725.
16. LABUDA, C., B. LITWINOWICZ, P. KOWIANSKI, *et al.* 2003. Developmental changes in nitric oxide synthase protein expression in the rat striatum and cerebral cortex. Folia Morphol. (Warsz.) **62:** 171–174.
17. TAGLIAFERRO, P., A.J. RAMOS, J.J. LOPEZ-COSTA, *et al.* 2003. Changes in the postnatal development on nitric oxide system induced by serotonin depletion. Brain Res. Dev. Brain Res. **146:** 39–49.
18. LIPTON, J.W., S.E.D. GYAWALI, *et al.* 2003. Prenatal cocaine administration increases glutathione and alpha-tocopherol oxidation in fetal rat brain. Dev. Brain Res. **147:** 77–84.
19. LIEN, R., O.P. MISHRA, E. GRAHAM, *et al.* 1994. Alteration of brain cell membrane function following cocaine exposure in the fetal guinea pig. Brain Res. **637:** 249–254.
20. CASTELLI, M.C., L. VENTURINI & S.B. SPARBER. 2001. Cocaine and salicylate: documentation of hydroxyl radical formation in hearts and brains of 18-day-old chick embryos and unexpected interactive toxicity. Psychopharmacology **156:** 23–31.
21. SERRANO, F. & E. KLANN. 2004. Reactive oxygen species and synaptic plasticity in the aging hippocampus. Ageing Res. Rev. **3:** 431–443.
22. MEYER, R.C., E.L. SPANGLER, H. KAMETANI & D.K. INGRAM. 1998. Age-associated memory impairment. Assessing the role of nitric oxide. Ann. N. Y. Acad. Sci. **854:** 307–317.
23. CAI, Z., F. XIAO, B. LEE, I.A. PAUL & P.G. RHODES. 1999. Prenatal hypoxia-ischemia alters expression and activity of nitric oxide synthase in the young rat brain and causes learning deficits. Brain Res. Bull. **49:** 359–365.

MDMA in Adolescent Male Rats

Decreased Serotonin in the Amygdala and Behavioral Effects in the Elevated Plus-Maze Test

RAQUEL FARIA,[a] ANA MAGALHÃES,[a] PEDRO R.R. MONTEIRO,[a,b]
JOANA GOMES-DA-SILVA,[a,c] MARIA AMÉLIA TAVARES,[a,d]
AND TERESA SUMMAVIELLE[a,b]

[a]*Neurobehavior Unit, Institute for Molecular and Cellular Biology, University of Porto, 4150-180 Porto, Portugal*

[b]*Department of Biomedical Sciences, ESTSP, Polytechnic Institute of Porto,4000-294 Porto, Portugal*

[c]*ESSUA, University of Aveiro, 3810-193 Aveiro, Portugal*

[d]*Institute of Anatomy, Medical School of Porto, University of Porto, 4200-319 Porto, Portugal*

ABSTRACT: Long-term behavioral consequences of the neurotoxicity produced by 3,4-methylenedioxymethamphetamine (MDMA) in the adolescent rat are still mostly unknown. Here, adolescent male rats (postnatal day 45 PND [45]) were exposed to 10 mg/kg of MDMA, intraperitoneally, every 2 h for 6 h. Controls were given 0.9% saline in the same protocol. Ten days after exposure, the behavioral effects of MDMA were assessed in the elevated plus-maze ($n = 6$ per group). After behavioral testing, animals were sacrificed and the amygdalae were dissected and processed for HPLC determination of dopamine (DA), serotonin (5-HT), and metabolites. Results showed a significant decrease in the 5-HT content ($P <$ 0.05), but no significant alterations in DA or its metabolites. Behavioral observation in the elevated plus-maze showed a decreased number of entries in the unprotected arms ($P < 0.05$), which were correlated to the number of entries and time spent in the central platform. Rearing was also decreased ($P < 0.05$). No differences were observed in head dips, grooming, or number of entries in the protected arms of the apparatus. Therefore, we conclude that, as in the adult rat, exposure to MDMA in the adolescent rat is associated to long-term depletion of the 5-HT content and increased anxiety-like behavior.

KEYWORDS: MDMA; ecstasy; serotonin; dopamine; amygdala; anxiety

Address for correspondence: Teresa Summavielle, IBMC - Neurobehavior Unit, Rua do Campo Alegre, 823, 4150-180 Porto, Portugal. Voice: +351-22-6074945; fax: +351-22-6099157.
e-mail: tsummavi@ibmc.up.pt

**Ann. N.Y. Acad. Sci. 1074: 643–649 (2006). © 2006 New York Academy of Sciences.
doi: 10.1196/annals.1369.062**

INTRODUCTION

Exposure to MDMA (3,4-methylenedioxymethamphetamine) in the adult rat is known to produce short- and long-term neurotoxicity mainly affecting the serotonergic system (for revision see Ref. 1). Although short- and long-term cellular, molecular, and behavioral neurotoxic effects of MDMA abuse were extensively studied in the adult, its consequences in the adolescent rat are still mostly unknown.

The amygdala is a limbic structure that integrates positive and aversive emotional information mediating behavioral reactions, and there is a relevant number of studies pointing to its essential role in the acquisition of both emotional and motor-conditioned responses.[2,3] This brain structure has an active role in the conditioning of autonomic fear responses through its projections to the hypothalamus, that in turn project to brain stem areas and spinal premotor neurons.[4,5] The involvement of amygdala in the addictive behavior seems to be fairly specific,[6] comprehending conditioned associations, stress responses, and anxiety behaviors, which are usually related to altered dopamine (DA) and serotonin (5-HT) levels.[7] The elevated plus-maze is a standard test of fear and anxiety, useful in testing the effects of anxiolytic and anxiogenic drugs. Therefore, this article aimed to evaluate the effects of exposure to MDMA in the levels of neurotransmitters, mainly DA and 5-HT, in the amygdala of adolescent rats and to relate these levels with behavioral observations in the elevated plus-maze.

MATERIALS AND METHODS

Wistar rat litters were culled to eight pups each, with equivalent sex representation, on postnatal day 1 (PND 1). On PND 45, male animals were given 10 mg/kg of MDMA, intraperitoneally, every 2 h for a period of 6 h,[8] or an isovolumetric dose of saline vehicle to control subjects. All procedures used were approved by the Portuguese Agency for Animal Welfare (General Board of Veterinary Medicine).

Ten days later, behavioral effects of MDMA were assessed in the elevated plus-maze ($n = 6$ per group) in sessions of 5 min, which were recorded and analyzed using the software Observer 4.1 (Noldus Information Technology, Wageningen, Netherlands). After behavioral testing, animals were sacrificed by decapitation, the brains were rapidly removed and dissection of the amygdalae were performed on ice. Tissue samples were frozen by immersion in 4-methylbutane cooled over dry ice and stored at $-70°C$ until used for neurochemical determinations. Levels of 5-HT and its metabolite 5-hydroxyindoleacetic acid (5-HIAA) and dopamine (DA) and its metabolites, dihydroxyphenylacetic acid (DOPAC) and homovanillic acid (HVA), were quantified by a modified method[9] of high performance liquid chromatography combined with electrochemical detection (HPLC/EC) in a system from Gilson Inc. (Middleton, WI). The analytic column was a Supelco Inc. (Bellefonte, PA) Supelcosil LC-18 3 μM (7.5 cm × 4.6 mm). Concentrations of neurotransmitters were calculated using standard curves. Standards were purchased from Sigma (St. Louis, MO). Final results were expressed in terms of monoamine content per amount of protein. The total content of protein was assayed in duplicate using a colorimetric microassay from Bio-Rad (Munchen, Germany) based on the Bradford assay.[10]

Neurochemical determinations and elevated plus-maze data were analyzed using one-way ANOVA (treatment). Significant main effects and interactions were further explored using *post hoc* tests. The statistical level of significance was considered at $P < 0.05$. All tests were performed using the software Statistica 5.5A (Statsof Inc., 2000; Tulsa, OK).

RESULTS

Analysis of data obtained in the elevated plus-maze, by one-way ANOVA (treatment), followed by *post hoc* analysis using Tukey Honest Significant Difference (HSD), revealed a significantly increased number of entries in the protected arms ($P < 0.05$) and a decreased number of entries and time spent in the central platform ($P < 0.05$). Behavioral analysis showed also a decrease in rearing ($P < 0.05$). No differences were observed in head dips, grooming, or number of entries in the protected arms of the apparatus. Also, there were no differences in the latency of any of the assessed behavioral categories (see FIG. 1).

Analysis of neurochemical data showed a significant decrease in the levels of both 5-HT and 5-HIAA ($P < 0.05$) and no differences in the levels of DA and its metabolites (see FIG. 2) or DA turnover.

DISCUSSION

MDMA in the adult rat is known to be selectively neurotoxic to the serotonergic system causing almost no deleterious effects on the dopaminergic system.[1] Nevertheless, there is evidence for a possible interaction between these two systems concerning the behavioral effects of MDMA,[11,12] which is likely to be expected, since these two systems are intimately connected.[11,13] As previously described for the adult rat in the amygadala[14] and other brain areas,[15,16] also in the adolescent rat, we have found that the amygdalar 5-HT content is markedly decreased 10 days after exposure and therefore, behavioral alterations are likely to appear at this stage. Regardless of the possible relation between 5-HT and DA, in the present work we could not determine any significant differences in the dopaminergic system.

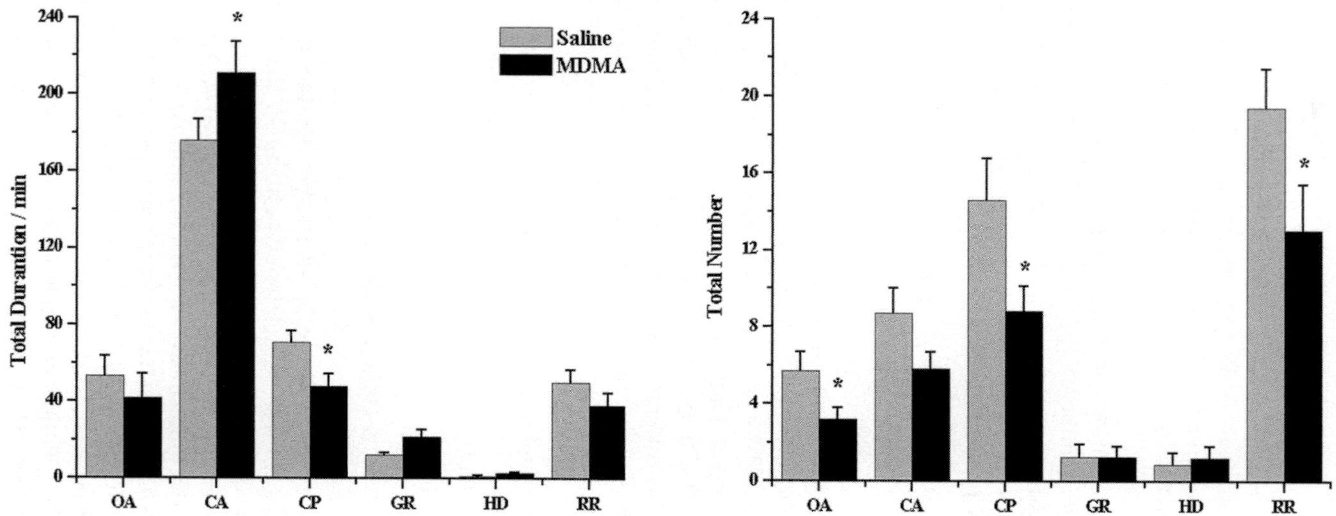

FIGURE 1. Behavioral effects of MDMA in the elevated plus-maze, tested 10 days after exposure to MDMA (4 × 10 mg/kg i.p. every 2 h for 6 h), representing the total number of times that each behavior was repeated and the total time spent in each category. Data expressed as mean values + SEM ($n = 6$ per group). OA = open arms, CA = closed arms, CP = central platform, GR = grooming, HD = head dips, RR = rearing. *Significantly different from control ($P < 0.05$).

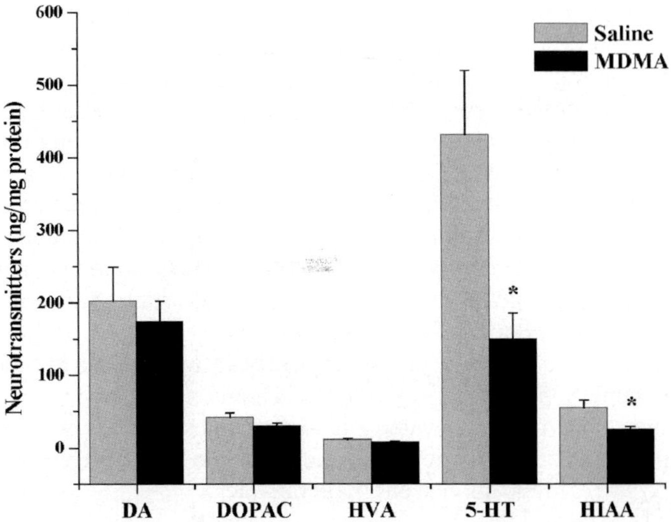

FIGURE 2. Effects of MDMA exposure in the amygdalar levels of monoamines, determined by HPLC/EC. Each column represents mean + SEM for six animals per group. *Significantly different from control ($P < 0.05$).

Acutely, MDMA is known to be anxiogenic in the elaveted plus-maze, reducing the percentage of entries and the time spent in the open arms, as well as all other exploratory behaviors.[8] Albeit, when testing social interaction, acute MDMA causes a marked increase in the displayed interaction,[17] which probably results from the interaction of different neurotransmitter systems. In a previous study, no differences in the time spent in the open arms of the elevated plus-maze were seen in adult rats MDMA pretreated (12.5 mg/kg, i.p.) and tested 8 days after exposure.[18] Likewise, another study, using the same protocol of exposure to MDMA as the present work, also failed to identify long-term (14 days later) behavioral effects in the elevated plus-maze.[8] However, using a similar pretreatment dose, other authors were able to observe increased anxiety in the plus-maze in adult rats tested 9 weeks after exposure to MDMA, which was also associated to 5-HT depletion in the amygdala, hippocampus, and caudate–putamen.[14]

Here, we describe that adolescent rats pretreated with MDMA and tested in the elevated plus-maze 10 days after treatment, presented anxiety-related behavior, spending more time in the closed arms of the apparatus and making a reduced number of entries in the open arms and central platform, evidencing reduced exploration and increased fear. Likewise, these rats also presented reduced rearing behavior, which is considered to reflect emotional behavior components and that may be associated with increased fear. Therefore, it seems that in the adolescent rat the behavioral neurotoxic effects of MDMA are evidenced earlier than in the adult. On PND 45 gliogenesis, synaptogenesis, and myelination processes are still occurring at a high rate, which increases the risk of suffering a neurotoxic insult.[19]

Although traditionally amygdala-related behavioral alterations are associated to changes in the DA content,[20,21] we did not observe any changes in either DA or its metabolites. Our findings are in agreement with previous results describing increased anxiety in adult rats pretreated with MDMA, which was also associated to serotonin depletion but not to DA changes.[14] However, it is important to remember that MDMA induced sustained hyperthermia (data not shown) through all the period of exposure, which is known to have a significant role in producing 5-HT depletion.[22,23]

In conclusion, we report here that exposure to MDMA in the adolescent rat induced depletion of the amygdalar 5-HT content, increasing anxiety-like behavior measured in the elevated plus-maze; these effects were observed 10 days after exposure and evidence the presence of long-term neurotoxic effects of MDMA in the adolescent male rat.

ACKNOWLEDGMENTS

This work was supported by project Fundação Calouste Gulbenkian ref. 65710 and Programa de Financiamento Plurianual do IBMC. Teresa Summavielle was partially granted by Fundação para a Ciência e Tecnologia (FCT) SFRH/BPD/20997/2004.

REFERENCES

1. LYLES, J. & J.L. CADET. 2003. Methylenedioxymethamphetamine (MDMA, Ecstasy) neurotoxicity: cellular and molecular mechanisms. Brain Res. Brain Res. Rev. **42:** 155–168.
2. MINTZ, M. & Y. WANG-NINIO. 2001. Two-stage theory of conditioning: involvement of the cerebellum and the amygdala. Brain Res. **897:** 150–156.
3. LEDOUX, J. 2000. The amygdala and emotion a view through fear. *In* The Amygdala. J.P. Aggleton, Ed.: 289–310. Oxford University Press. Oxford.
4. ANTONIADIS, E.A. & R.J. MCDONALD. 2001. Amygdala, hippocampus, and unconditioned fear. Exp. Brain Res. **138:** 200–209.
5. PACKARD, M.G., L. CAHILL & J.L. MCGAUGH. 1994. Amygdala modulation of hippocampal-dependent and caudate nucleus-dependent memory processes. Proc. Natl. Acad. Sci. USA. **91:** 8477–8481.
6. EVERITT, B.J., R.N. CARDINAL, J. HALL, *et al*. 2000. Differential involvement of amygdala subsystems in appetitive conditioning and drug addiction. *In* The Amygdala. J.P. Aggleton, Ed. 353–390. Oxford University Press. Oxford.
7. GREBA, Q., A. GIFKINS & L. KOKKINIDIS. 2001. Inhibition of amygdaloid dopamine D(2) receptors impairs emotional learning measured with fear-potentiated startle. Brain Res. **899:** 218–226.

8. SUMNALL, H.R. *et al.* 2004. The effects of MDMA pretreatment on the behavioural effects of other drugs of abuse in the rat elevated plus-maze test. Pharmacol. Biochem. Behav. **77:** 805–814.
9. ALI, S.F., S.N. DAVID & G.D. NEWPORT. 1993. Age-related susceptibility of MPTP-induced neurotoxicity in mice. Neurotoxicology **14:** 29–34.
10. BRADFORD, M.M. 1976. A rapid and sensitive method for the quantitation of microgram quantities of protein utilizing the principle of protein-dye binding. Ann. Biochem. **72:** 248–254.
11. BANKSON, M.G. & K.A. CUNNINGHAM. 2001. 3,4-Methylenedioxymethamphetamine (MDMA) as a unique model of serotonin receptor function and serotonin-dopamine interactions. J. Pharmacol. Exp. Ther. **297:** 846–852.
12. MCCREARY, A.C., M.G. BANKSON & K.A. CUNNINGHAM. 1999. Pharmacological studies of the acute and chronic effects of (+)-3,4-methylenedioxymethamphetamine on locomotor activity: role of 5-hydroxytryptamine(1A) and 5-hydroxytryptamine(1B/1D) receptors. J. Pharmacol. Exp. Ther. **290:** 965–973.
13. BRODERICK, P.A. & C.F. PHELIX. 1997. I. Serotonin (5-HT) within dopamine reward circuits signals open-field behavior. II. Basis for 5-HT-DA interaction in cocaine dysfunctional behavior. Neurosci. Biobehav. Rev. **21:** 227–260.
14. GURTMAN, C.G. *et al.* 2002. Increased anxiety in rats after 3,4-methylenedioxymethamphetamine: association with serotonin depletion. Eur. J. Pharmacol. **446:** 89–96.
15. COLADO, M.I., J.L. WILLIAMS & A.R. GREEN. 1995. The hyperthermic and neurotoxic effects of 'Ecstasy' (MDMA) and 3,4 methylenedioxyamphetamine (MDA) in the Dark Agouti (DA) rat, a model of the CYP2D6 poor metabolizer phenotype. Br. J. Pharmacol. **115:** 1281–1289.
16. O'SHEA, E. *et al.* 1998. The relationship between the degree of neurodegeneration of rat brain 5-HT nerve terminals and the dose and frequency of administration of MDMA ('ecstasy'). Neuropharmacology **37:** 919–926.
17. MORLEY, K.C. & I.S. MCGREGOR. 2000. (±)-3,4-methylenedioxymethamphetamine (MDMA, 'Ecstasy') increases social interaction in rats. Eur. J. Pharmacol. **408:** 41–49.
18. MECHAN, A.O. *et al.* 2002. A study of the effect of a single neurotoxic dose of 3,4-methylenedioxymethamphetamine (MDMA; "ecstasy") on the subsequent long-term behaviour of rats in the plus maze and open field. Psychopharmacology (Berl.) **159:** 167–175.
19. INSEL, T.R. 1995. The development of brain and behavior. *In* Psychopharmacology: the Fourth Generation of Progress. D.J. Kupfer, Ed.: 683–694. Raven Press. New York.
20. GREBA, Q., A. GIFKINS & L. KOKKINIDIS. 2001. Inhibition of amygdaloid dopamine D2 receptors impairs emotional learning measured with fear-potentiated startle. Brain Res. **899:** 218–226.
21. ANTONIADIS, E.A. & R.J. MCDONALD. 2001. Amygdala, hippocampus, and unconditioned fear. Exp. Brain Res. **138:** 200–209.
22. O'LOINSIGH, E.D. *et al.* 2001. Behavioural, hyperthermic and neurotoxic effects of 3,4-methylenedioxymethamphetamine analogues in the Wistar rat. Prog. Neuropsychopharmacol. Biol. Psychiatry **25:** 621–638.
23. GREEN, A.R., E. O'SHEA & M.I. COLADO. 2004. A review of the mechanisms involved in the acute MDMA (ecstasy)-induced hyperthermic response. Eur. J. Pharmacol. **500:** 3–13.

Morphological Evidence that Xenon Neuroprotects against *N*-Methyl-DL-Aspartic Acid-Induced Damage in the Rat Arcuate Nucleus

A Time-Dependent Study

GIANFRANCO NATALE,[a] DAVIDE CATTANO,[b] ANTONIO ABRAMO,[b] FRANCESCO FORFORI,[b] FEDERICA FULCERI,[a] FRANCESCO FORNAI,[a] ANTONIO PAPARELLI,[a] AND FRANCESCO GIUNTA[b]

[a]*Department of Human Morphology and Applied Biology, University of Pisa, I-56126 Pisa, Italy*

[b]*Department of Surgery, University of Pisa, Pisa, Italy*

ABSTRACT: The hyperactivation of glutamate receptors, especially those of the *N*-methyl-D-aspartate subtype (NMDA), can induce excess calcium entry into cells, leading to neuronal death. Since the anesthetic gas xenon behaves as an NMDA antagonist, the present article investigated, by distinct morphological approaches and after different times, the possible neuroprotectant effects of this gas in a model of neuronal damage induced by *N*-methyl-DL-aspartic acid (NMA) on rat arcuate nucleus. Rats were assigned to the following groups: controls; xenon exposure; NMA treatment; or xenon exposure + NMA treatment. Animals were placed in an experimental cage and after 10 min a mixture of xenon (or nitrogen) 70% and oxygen 30% was delivered. After 3 h, 1, 2, 5, or 7 days from gas exposure, rats were euthanized and the whole brain was removed and processed for either transmission electron microscopy or light microscopy. In the arcuate nucleus from NMA-treated animals only 40–60% of cell population survived in all times with several degenerating neurons giving the typical appearance of a "bull's eye." At ultrastructural level, chromatin margination, nuclear shrinkage, mitochondria with matrix dilution, dilated endoplasmic cisternae, and electrondense cytoplasm were detected. Xenon alone did not induce changes, but reduced of about 50% NMA-induced cell loss as well as degenerating neurons, with the maximal neuroprotection at 7 days. These results confirm that in the rat arcuate nucleus NMA can induce a severe neuronal damage that is

Address for correspondence: Gianfranco Natale, M.D., Department of Human Morphology and Applied Biology, University of Pisa, Via Roma 55, I-56126 Pisa, Italy. Voice: +39-50-2218610; fax: +39-50-2218606.

e-mail: gianfranco.natale@anist.med.unipi.it

Ann. N.Y. Acad. Sci. 1074: 650–658 (2006). © 2006 New York Academy of Sciences. doi: 10.1196/annals.1369.063

already marked after 3 h. Xenon significantly reduced the neuronal damage at all times and can be then regarded as a promising neuroprotectant agent.

Keywords: arcuate nucleus; neuroprotection; NMDA receptor; *N*-methyl-DL-aspartic acid; xenon

INTRODUCTION

Xenon is a chemical element belonging to the group 0 of the periodic table, together with other noble gases. Since 1940 noble gases have been studied as possible anesthetics and only xenon resulted as a promising agent.[1,2] In fact, xenon has many of the properties of the ideal anesthetic and it is the only noble gas which exhibits anesthetic effects under normobaric conditions.[3] Since the 1950s xenon has been used in humans.[4] Clinical trials demonstrated that it offers rapid induction and recovery from anesthesia. Subjective sensations from the anesthesia were pleasant and significant alterations of the hemodynamic and cardiovascular patterns were not observed.[5] In comparative clinical trials, xenon was shown to be superior in comparison with other anesthetics.[6–8]

From a morphological point of view, Bracken *et al.*[1] did not find significant alterations in major organs of rabbits exposed to xenon. We showed that the subchronic exposure to a mixture of xenon 70% and oxygen 30% did not induce significant morphological alterations in lung, liver, kidney, and adrenal gland of the rat and also it did not affect corticosterone plasma levels.[9,10]

In contrast to most general anesthetics, xenon produces little or no potentiation at GABAergic synapses.[11,12] Unlike other volatile anesthetics, it is a potent noncompetitive inhibitor of the glutamatergic NMDA (*N*-methyl-D-aspartate) receptor.[11] Although excitatory amino acids are essential for normal brain function, the presence of excessive synaptic release of this amino acid (i.e., in ischemic–ipoxic stress conditions) or the administration of NMDA receptor agonists can be responsible of neurodegeneration. This neurotoxic effect has been well-documented in the past years, leading Olney to formulate the concept of "excitotoxicity" to indicate the damaging effects depending on the excitatory amino acid receptor hyperactivation.[13] A large body of evidence has shown that NMDA receptor antagonists can be neuroprotectant in both *in vitro* and *in vivo* models of neuronal injury.[14,15] However, the development of several NMDA receptor antagonists has had to be abandoned, because clinical trials revealed that they possessed their own inherent neurotoxicity.[16] Previous studies showed that xenon does not exhibit neurotoxicity and protects against the injury induced by ketamine or other agents.[17,18]

Since it can be easily administered and rapidly enters the brain, xenon may be regarded as a good candidate for neuroprotectant agent. The hypothalamic region, including the arcuate nucleus–median eminence complex, has been frequently used in studies dealing with glutamate neurotoxicity.[19–23] Indeed, this area appears the most glutamatesensitive among the circumventricular organs where the fenestrated endothelium allows free access to amino acids present in circulating blood.

The present article investigated, by distinct morphological approaches and after different times, the possible neuroprotectant effects of this gas in a model of neuronal damage induced by *N*-methyl-DL-aspartic acid (NMA) on the rat arcuate nucleus. Samples of arcuate nucleus were examined under light microscopy(LM) for the quantitative analysis of the damage. Ultrastructural investigations were also performed under transmission electron microscopy (TEM) to evaluate subcellular alterations.

MATERIALS AND METHODS

Female Sprague-Dawley rats (180–200 g body weight) were used throughout the study. Each animal was placed in an experimental cage, sealed with material impervious to xenon and subjected to a denitrogenation process by allowing them to breathe pure oxygen delivered at high flow rate. After 10 min, a gas mixture of xenon 70% and oxygen 30% (or nitrogen 70% and oxygen 30%) was delivered into the cage for the experimental period of 3 h. Gas concentrations were monitored by capnography (carbon dioxide) and gas chromatography (xenon). The bottom of the cage was provided by a layer of sodalime to keep the carbon dioxide levels below 0.6% and silica gel to keep the humidity between 40–60%. At the end of the experiment, animals were euthanized by an intraperitoneal overdose of sodium pentobarbital (100 mg/kg).

Animals were randomly assigned to four major experimental groups:

Control group ($n = 5$ for each subgroup): rats were injected with 1 mL of phosphate buffered saline (PBS), then maintained in the experimental cage breathing a gas mixture of nitrogen 70% and oxygen 30% for 3 h. The animals were then euthanized and processed for LM or TEM.

Xenon-exposed group ($n = 5$ for each subgroup): rats were injected with 1 mL of PBS and exposed in the experimental cage to xenon 70% and oxygen 30% for 3 h. After this experimental time, some animals were euthanized and processed for LM or TEM, while other animals were brought back to their home cages and euthanized 7 days after xenon exposure and processed for LM or TEM in order to assess possible late morphological changes attributable to xenon.

NMA-treated group ($n = 5$ for each subgroup): rats were injected with NMA (100 mg/kg) and immediately placed into the experimental cage, breathing a gas mixture of nitrogen 70% and oxygen 30% for 3 h. Then, some animals were euthanized and processed for LM or TEM, while other animals, were brought back to their home cages and euthanized 1, 2, 5, or 7 days after the treatment with NMA and processed for LM or TEM (only 1- and 7-day subgroups).

NMA plus xenon-exposed group (n = 5 for each subgroup): rats were injected with NMA (100 mg/kg) and immediately placed into the experimental cage breathing a gas mixture of xenon 70% and oxygen 30% for 3 h. Then, some animals were euthanized and processed for LM or TEM, while other animals, were brought back to their home cages and euthanized 1, 2, 5, or 7 days after the treatment with NMA and processed for LM or TEM (only 1- and 7-day subgroups).

For LM, the brain was removed by opening the skull and frozen in isopenthane at −80°C. Ten-micrometer thick coronal cryocut sections were taken at the level of arcuate nucleus and processed thereafter for hematoxylin–eosin (H/E) staining. A quantitative evaluation was performed and the extent of the damage was estimated as the number of altered cells over the total number of cells, and expressed as percentage values.

For TEM the perfusion was performed after thoracotomy. After a quick wash with saline, perfusion solution (0.1 M PBS followed by 300 mL per animal of 4% paraformaldehyde in 0.1 M PBS) was injected by a 16-gauge cannula through the left ventricle into ascending aorta with a peristaltic pump. The brain was then carefully removed and definitively fixed overnight in a 4% paraformaldehyde solution. A 2-mm thick slice was obtained through coronal plane rostrally to cerebellum. Under stereomicroscope, samples of the arcuate nucleus were bilaterally taken from the paraventricular area and processed for TEM. After 24 h of fixation, specimens were postfixed in buffered 1% osmium tetroxide for 2 h, dehydrated in series of ethanol, and embedded in Epon-araldite. Thin sections of each specimen were cut with an LKB ultramicrotome, stained with uranyl acetate and lead citrate, and finally examined under a TEM (Jeol JEM 100 SX; Jeol Ltd., Tokyo, Japan).

The following drugs were used: NMA (Sigma Chemicals Co., St. Louis, MO); xenon (SIAD S.p.A., Bergamo, Italy); sodium penthobarbital (Abbot S.p.A., Campoverde di Aprilia, Latina, Italy). NMA was dissolved in PBS (0.1 M PBS) and administered subcutaneously using a 25-gauge needle in a volume of 1 mL subdivided into two injections of 0.5 mL on the back of the animal.

RESULTS

In the arcuate nucleus from control and xenon-exposed animals, the cell population conformed to standard descriptions (FIG. 1A).

After all times examined, NMA administration induced a marked cell loss: degenerated cells were identified by their pyknotic nuclei and edematous swelling of the surrounding cytoplasmic compartment giving the typical appearance of a "bull's eye" (FIG. 1B). In NMA 3 h, 2- and 7-day groups a marked cell depletion ranging between −40% and −50% was observed. In contrast,

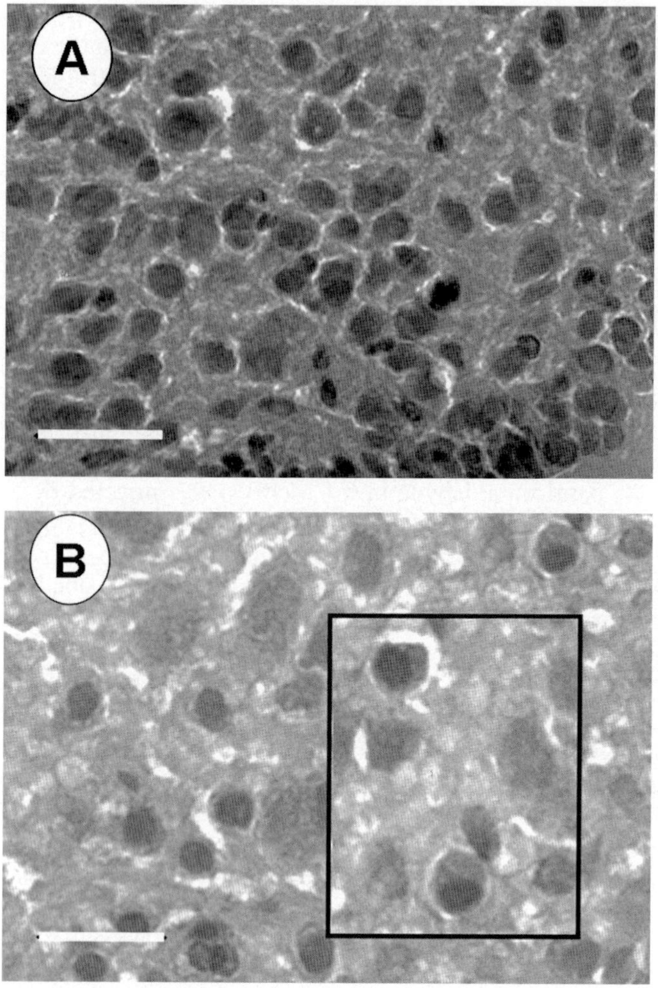

FIGURE 1. H/E staining of rat arcuate nucleus. (**A**) Control rat. (**B**) NMA-treated rat. Cell population is markedly reduced and degenerated cells are identified by their pyknotic nuclei and edematous swelling of the surrounding cytoplasmic compartment giving the typical appearance of a "bull's eye" (insert). *Scale bars* = 100 μm.

1 day after NMA injection cell depletion appeared attenuated. Pyknotic cell count was higher in 2- and 7-day groups.

Xenon induced a significant reduction of cell loss after all times examined, with a peak effect in the 7-day group, where the NMA-induced cell loss was reduced by about 50%. Cellular alterations like pyknosis and swelling of cytoplasm were also noticeably reduced.

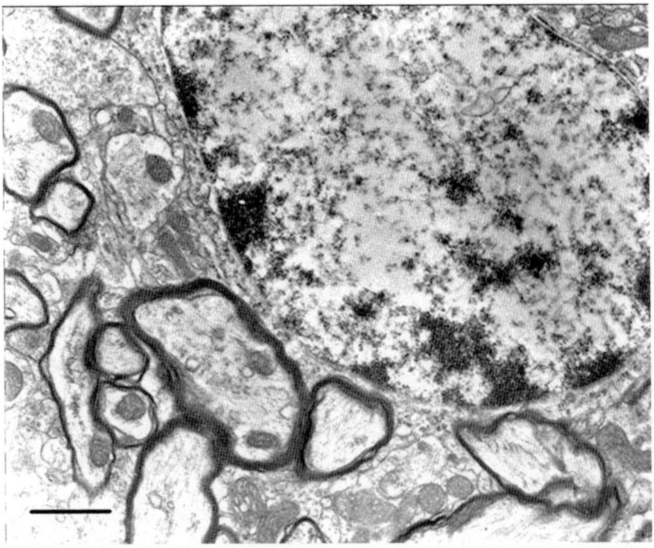

FIGURE 2. TEM of arcuate nucleus from an NMA-treated rat: a neuron exhibits morphological signs of apoptosis with chromatin margination. *Scale bar* = 5 μm.

TEM of arcuate nucleus from control and xenon-exposed animals showed neuronal and glial cells exhibiting an ultrastructural pattern superimposable to standard descriptions.

NMA treatment induced several ultrastructural alterations in neurons and glia, including chromatin margination, nuclear shrinkage, mitochondria with matrix dilution, dilated endoplasmic cisternae, and electrondense cytoplasm (FIG. 2). These pathologic pictures were typical of degeneration and cell death, with aspects resembling both necrosis, mainly in the 3-h group, and apoptosis, mainly in the 7-day group.

All ultrastructural alterations were less marked in the NMA plus xenon-exposed group, in particular in the 3-h group where the ultrastructural pattern is superimposable to controls.

DISCUSSION

The excitatory amino acid glutamate is probably the most important and abundant neurotransmitter in the mammalian nervous system and it is essential for normal brain functions. Indeed, it is involved in many functional aspects, including long-term potentiation and depression at central synapses, formation of synapses and neuronal circuitry, learning, neuroendocrine regulation, and addictive behavior.[24,25] However, the presence of excessive amounts of glutamate can be responsible of excitotoxicity. Indeed, the hyperactivation of glutamate receptors, especially those of NMDA, can lead to excess calcium entry into cells which in turn results in neuronal death.[13]

The present data showed that in the arcuate nucleus from control animals both neuronal and glial cells conformed to standard descriptions.[19,20,26] By contrast, in NMA-treated rats, LM showed a typical marked cell depletion; furthermore, degenerated cells were identified by their pyknotic nuclei and edematous swelling of the surrounding cytoplasmic compartment giving the typical appearance of a "bull's eye." These findings are in agreement with previous studies that reported cell loss and the appearance of degenerated neurons in the arcuate nucleus of rats and mice after NMDA receptor agonist administration.[18–21] At ultrastructural level, NMA induced several alterations including chromatin margination, nuclear shrinkage, mitochondria with matrix dilution, dilated endoplasmic cisternae, and electron dense cytoplasm. Interestingly, the ultrastructure of both cell damage and death are represented in a continuum. Correctly, with the actual knowledge of general pathology, the distinction between apoptosis and necrosis slowly fades away.[27] In fact, we can notice how the "dying" neurons present a morphological profile typical of the apoptosis and another profile typical of the necrosis. The tendency toward one or the other form of cell death is based principally in the environmental microconditions specific for each cell and in the theory of dose–response to the neurotoxin.[28] The present damaging effects induced by NMA can be explained taking into account that the rat arcuate nucleus was found to contain the highest levels of NMDA subunit mRNAs.[29] We noticed different morphological pictures in accordance with the different time intervals. They might be attributable to the changes induced in the tissue by the excitotoxic damage and to the non-neuronal response to neuronal death. The damage reached the highest severity after 3 h from NMA administration, with a marked neuronal cell loss, while it appeared as inflammatory cell engorgement after 1 day and became quite stable but not definite after 7 days.

Xenon was found not to affect the morphology of the rat arcuate nucleus, but it significantly prevented the neuronal injury evoked by NMA administration. Ma *et al.*[30] also found a neuroprotectant effect of xenon after 3 h in the rat arcuate nucleus against NMA injection, but the present data showed for the first time, under both light and electron microscopy, that this gas is able to neuroprotect after 7 days, as well. Neuroprotection by xenon was also reported when neuronal damage was induced after transient middle cerebral artery occlusion[31] or by application of NMDA or glutamate or by oxygen deprivation in mouse neuronal-glial cell co-colture.[18]

In conclusion, the present results confirm that NMA is able to induce a severe neuronal damage in the rat arcuate nucleus and that the injury is already marked 3 h after drug administration. However, the neuronal loss appears to be time dependent and after 7 days from the injury it is still possible to find degenerating neurons and a marked cell depletion. Ultrastructural examinations confirm that NMA can induce a severe damage at both nuclear and cytoplasmic level in neuronal and in glial cells as well. Xenon was shown to provide a significant reduction of neuronal damage at all times and can be then regarded as a promising neuroprotectant agent, in particular against ischemic–ipoxic stress conditions.

REFERENCES

1. BRACKEN, A. *et al.* 1956. A trial of xenon as a non-explosive anesthetic. Anaesthesia **11:** 40–49.
2. BAUMERT, J.H. *et al.* 2005. Hemodynamic effects of hemorrhage during xenon anesthesia in pigs. Br. J. Anaesth. **94:** 727–732.
3. GIUNTA, F. *et al.* 1996. Xenon: a review of its anesthetic and pharmacological properties. Appl. Cardiopulm. Pathophysiol. **6:** 95–103.
4. BEDI, A. *et al.* 2002. The effects of subanesthetic concentrations of xenon in volunteers. Anaesthesia **57:** 233–241.
5. LUTTROPP, H.H. *et al.* 1994. Clinical experience with minimal flow xenon anesthesia. Acta Anaesthesiol. Scand. **38:** 121–125.
6. YAGI, M. *et al.* 1995. Analgesic and hypnotic effects of subanesthetic concentrations of xenon in human volunteers: comparison with nitrous oxide. Br. J. Anaesth. **74:** 670–673.
7. BAUMERT, J.H. *et al.* 2005. Xenon anesthesia may preserve cardiovascular function in patients with heart failure. Acta Anaesthesiol. Scand. **49:** 743–749.
8. SANDERS, R.D. *et al.* 2005. Xenon: elemental anesthesia in clinical practice. Br. Med. Bull. **22:** 115–135.
9. NATALE, G. *et al.* 1998. Main organ morphology and blood analysis after subchronic exposure to xenon in rats. Appl. Cardiopulm. Pathophysiol. **7:** 227–233.
10. NATALE, G. *et al.* 2002. Effects of repeated exposures to xenon on rat adrenal cortex ultrastructure. J. Submicrosc. Cytol. Pathol. **34:** 329–334.
11. FRANKS, N.P. *et al.* 1998. How does xenon produce anesthesia? Nature **396:** 324.
12. DE SOUSA, S.L. *et al.* 2000. Contrasting synaptic actions of the inhalational general anesthetics isoflurane and xenon. Anesthesiology **92:** 1055–1066.
13. OLNEY, J.W. 1969. Brain lesions, obesity, and other disturbances in mice treated with monosodium glutamate. Science **164:** 719–721.
14. HARADA, H. *et al.* 1999. Isoflurane reduces N-methyl-D-aspartate toxicity in vivo in the rat cerebral cortex. Anesth. Analg. **89:** 1442–1447.
15. KUDO, M. *et al.* 2001. Effects of volatile anesthetics on N-methyl-D-aspartate excitotoxicity in primary rat neuronal-glial cultures. Anesthesiology **95:** 756–765.
16. ARROWSMITH, J.E. *et al.* 1998. Neuroprotection of the brain during cardiopulmonary bypass: a randomized trial of remacemide during coronary artery bypass in 171 patients. Stroke **29:** 2357–2362.
17. NAGATA, A. *et al.* 2001. Xenon inhibits but N_2O enhances ketamine-induced c-Fos expression in the rat posterior cingulate and retrosplenial cortices. Anesth. Analg. **92:** 362–368.
18. WILHELM, S. *et al.* 2002. Effects of xenon on in vitro and in vivo models of neuronal injury. Anesthesiology **96:** 1485–1491.

19. HOLZWARTH-MCBRIDE, M.A. *et al.* 1976. Monosodium glutamate induced lesions of the arcuate nucleus. I. Endocrine deficiency and ultrastructure of the median eminence. Anat. Rec. **186:** 185–196.
20. HOLZWARTH-MCBRIDE, M.A. *et al.* 1976. Monosodium glutamate induced lesions of the arcuate nucleus. II. Fluorescence histochemistry of catecholamines. Anat. Rec. **186:** 197–206.
21. XUE, Y.-D. *et al.* 1997. Nitric oxide synthase-, N-methyl-D-aspartate receptor-, glutamate- and aspartate-immunoreactive neurons in the mouse arcuate nucleus: effects of neonatal treatment with monosodium glutamate. Acta Neuropathol. **94:** 572–582.
22. HU, L. *et al.* 1998. Exogenous glutamate enhances glutamate receptor subunit expression during selective neuronal injury in the ventral arcuate nucleus of postnatal mice. Neuroendocrinology **68:** 77–88.
23. GOLDSMITH, P.C. 2000. Neuroglial responses to elevated glutamate in the medial basal hypothalamus of the infant mouse. J. Nutr. **130:** 1032S–1038S.
24. NAKANISHI, N. 1992. Molecular diversity of glutamate receptors and implications for brain functions. Science **258:** 597–603.
25. BRANN, D.W. 1995. Glutamate: a major excitatory transmitter in neuroendocrine regulation. Neuroendocrinology **61:** 213–225.
26. ETCHEVERRY, G.J. & A.P. DE IRALDI. 1968. Ultrastructure of neurons in the arcuate nucleus of the rat. Anat. Rec. **160:** 239–254.
27. MARTIN, L.J. *et al.* 1998. Neurodegeneration in excitotoxicity, global cerebral ischemia, and target deprivation: a perspective on the contributions of apoptosis and necrosis. Brain Res. Bull. **46:** 281–309.
28. SATTLER, R. & M. TYMIANSKI. 2001. Molecular mechanisms of glutamate receptor-mediated excitotoxic neuronal cell death. Mol. Neurobiol. **24:** 107–129.
29. EYIGOR, O. *et al.* 2001. Distribution of ionotropic glutamate receptor subunit mRNAs in the rat hypothalamus. J. Comp. Neurol. **434:** 101–124.
30. MA, D. *et al.* 2002. Neuroprotective and neurotoxic properties of the "inert" gas, xenon. Br. J. Anaesth. **89:** 739–746.
31. ABRAINI, J.H. *et al.* 2005. Potentially neuroprotective and therapeutic properties of nitrous oxide and xenon. Ann. N. Y. Acad. Sci. **1053:** 289–300.

Mechanism-Based Approaches for the Reversal of Drug Neurobehavioral Teratogenicity

JOSEPH YANAI,[a,b] TAMAR L. BEN-SHAANAN,[a] HANA HAIMOVITCH,[a] SOPHIA KATZ,[a] AND MEITAL KAZMA[a]

[a]*The Ross Laboratory for Studies in Neural Birth Defects, Department of Anatomy and Cell Biology, The Hebrew University-Hadassah Medical School, 91010 Jerusalem, Israel*

[b]*Department of Pharmacology and Cancer Biology, Duke University Medical Center, Durham, North Carolina 27710, USA*

ABSTRACT: Understanding the mechanism of neurobehavioral teratogenicity is the primary prerequisite for reversal of the defect. Progress in such studies can be best achieved if the investigation focuses on behaviors related to a specific brain region and innervation. Our model focused on teratogen-induced deficits in hippocampus-related eight-arm and Morris maze behaviors. Different "cholinergic" teratogens, mainly heroin, induced both pre- and postsynaptic hyperactivity in the hippocampal cholinergic innervation that terminated in desensitization of Protein Kinase C (PKC) isoforms to cholinergic receptor stimulation. Understanding this mechanism enabled its reversal with a pharmacological therapy—nicotine infusion. Studies by others provided similar findings by targeting the deficits respective to the model investigated. Consistently, destruction of the A10-septal dopaminergic pathways that downregulate the septohippocampal cholinergic innervation ameliorated maze performance. Grafting of embryonic differentiated cholinergic cells or neural progenitors similarly reversed the biochemical/molecular alterations and the resulting deficits. Reversal therapies offer a model for the understanding of neurobehavioral teratogenicity and, clinically, offer a model for potential treatment of these deficits. Whereas neural progenitor grafting appears to be the most effective treatment, pharmacological reversal with nicotine infusion seems to possess the most feasible and immediate therapy for neurobehavioral birth defects produced by various teratogens, including drugs. This is true even though the effect of pharmacological therapies is diffuse, affecting multiple areas of the brain.

Address for correspondence: Dr. Joseph Yanai, The Ross Laboratory for Studies in Neural Birth Defects, Department of Anatomy and Cell Biology, The Hebrew University-Hadassah Medical School, Box 12272, 91010 Jerusalem, Israel. Voice: 972-2-675-8439; fax: 972-2-675-8443.
e-mail: yanai@md.huji.ac.il

Ann. N.Y. Acad. Sci. 1074: 659–671 (2006). © 2006 New York Academy of Sciences.
doi: 10.1196/annals.1369.066

KEYWORDS: A10; heroin; hippocampal cholinergic innervation; hippocampal behavior; grafting of neural progenitors; neurobehavioral teratogenicity; nicotine therapy; PKC isoforms; reversal therapies

"Everybody is talking about the weather but nobody does anything about it."
(Mark Twain)

INTRODUCTION

Neurobehavioral teratology research was initiated as a science that identifies behavioral and neural birth defects, many of them related to prenatal drug exposure.[1,2] Most early studies of behavioral teratology were only descriptive, fulfilling the necessary first requirement in a new field. Following the normal course of scientific development, studies were published which tied the neural and behavioral events into a causal relationship, that is, ascertaining of the mechanisms of the behavioral birth defects. As was predicted more than 20 years ago,[3] these developments made the reversal of neurobehavioral birth defects more likely. The current neurobehavioral teratology research is characterized by an increasing number of studies that establish a model for the reversal of defined prenatally induced neurobehavioral deficits.

Reversal of deficits inflicted experimentally on the adult or of genetic defects, usually those which have a well-described mechanism, is often performed using methods similar to the ones that will be described below. The situation is more complex with prenatal insults as most neuroteratogens act diffusely in the brain, thereby affecting multiple regions, neural pathways and transmitter systems, and, consequently, causing multiple behavioral deficits. The purpose of the present article is to argue that, despite this, understanding of the mechanism of prenatally induced deficits in a specific process, while keeping in mind that other structures and innervations were affected simultaneously, already enables restoration of normalcy by different therapies, all targeting the teratogen-impaired process.

The uniqueness of our approach is, first, that although effective therapies developed by other groups (to be discussed below) as well as our nicotine therapy model[4] most often target the particular relevant innervation, they also act throughout the entire brain, or even throughout the entire organism, beyond the region related to the deficit. In contrast, our grafting and manipulating of the regulating pathways target the pertinent innervation in the locus related to the impaired behavior. Second, most pharmacological therapies represent a treatment that has to be administered regularly on a permanent basis. Our grafting and manipulating of the regulating pathways, however, represent a permanent reversal of the deficits to facilitate a cure. It is hoped that these reversal models in animals will provide the groundwork for future clinical applications.

In our lab, we established a model for ascertaining the mechanisms of behavioral deficits related to hippocampal cholinergic innervation induced by prenatal exposure to drugs of use and abuse, as well as other substances. Fine scrutiny of this mechanism enabled the reversal of behavioral deficits by several therapies, to be described in the present paper.

METHODS

Our models for the reversal of neurobehavioral birth defects used mainly heroin or phenobarbital as teratogens, since both drugs act on the cholinergic innervation: barbiturates act directly,[5,6] whereas heroin action appears to be via opioidergic regulation of the cholinergic function.[7,8]

In our model[9] pregnant heterogeneous stock (HS/Ibg) mice received single daily heroin injections (10 mg/kg, s.c.) on gestation days (GD) 9–18. Phenobarbital was given in the milled food (0.3%) on GD 9–18. At various postnatal ages, the offspring and their respective controls underwent various treatments for the reversal of the teratogens' effects. At adulthood they were tested for hippocampus-related behaviors, followed by molecular/neurochemical evaluations of hippocampal cholinergic function. When a chick model was employed for the evaluation of heroin neurobehavioral teratogenicity, eggs were injected with 20 mg/kg eggs of heroin on incubation days 0 and 5. Soon after hatching they were tested for imprinting and the brains were studied immediately afterward.[10]

RESULTS AND DISCUSSION

Hippocampal acetylcholinesterase and choline acetyltransferase activities were not affected by prenatal drug exposure.[11,12] Whereas these enzymes are not rate limiting, it is important that the number of choline transporter sites ([^{3}H]hemicholinium-3 binding) increased in drug-exposed offspring,[13] since the transporter activity represents a rate-limiting step and is responsive to the rate of neural firing.[14,15] Acetylcholine release, assessed indirectly by measuring inositol phosphate (IP) formation in the presence of K^+, was also increased after prenatal exposure to heroin,[16] which further supports the suggestion of presynaptic hyperactivity. In the adulthood exposure models, this kind of presynaptic hyperactivity was usually offset by adaptive postsynaptic hypoactivity. Unexpectedly however, mice exposed to heroin prenatally had an increase in the postsynaptic components—muscarinic receptors number (B_{max}),[17] most pertinent, the M1 subtype, G protein (GP) activation, and muscarinic receptor induced (carbachol-induced) IP formation.[9,13,16,18] Consistently, there was a global elevation of basal membrane-bound PKC activity,[9,13] but the postsynaptic hyperactivity terminated in the total abolishment of cholinergic receptor-induced translocation/activation of PKC.[9,18] This occurred, among the conventional isoforms, in PKC-γ and-β but not PKC-α, which is not relevant to the behavioral deficits and was neither induced by cholinergic stimulation, nor affected by prenatal teratogen exposure.[4,19,20] The biochemical/molecular alterations paralleled deficits in the hippocampus-related behavior in the eight-arm and Morris mazes.[4,9,18] It is interesting that whereas the cellular function (translocation/activation of PKC) was totally abolished, the behavior deficit was only relative; that is, the animal functioned in a maze, however, with a reduced level of performance.

These findings were confirmed with prehatch exposure to heroin and other cholinergic teratogens—nicotine and chlorpyrifos—in a chick model, where the behavior studied was filial imprinting as related to function of PKC in the intermedial part of the hyperstriatum ventrale (IMHV).[10]

Reversal of Neurobehavioral Teratogenicity by Diverse, yet Related Therapies

Ascertaining the mechanism of neurobehavioral teratogenicity is a prerequisite for its reversal. In the adult, the most successful models of the reversal of brain defects are those where the mechanism was established. A prime example is Parkinson's disease, where the ascertainment of the nigrostriatal defects enabled restoration of normalcy in an animal model by grafting, either of differentiated embryonic cells[21,22] or of neural progenitors.[23,24] In turn, the therapy provided further understanding of the mechanisms of the teratogen action. In our model, abolishment of translocation/activation of PKC-γ was established as a major component in the mechanism of cholinergic teratogen action, which paved the way for attempting to reverse the defects with different therapies, all targeting the cholinergic innervation.

Reversal of Neurobehavioral Teratogenicity with Nicotine Therapy[4]

This model employed mice that were exposed prenatally to phenobarbital and were expected to show deficiencies in hippocampus-related Morris maze behavior and a concomitant PKC-γ desensitization. On postnatal day (PN) 44 they were implanted with osmotic minipumps containing nicotine bitartrate set to deliver 10 mg/kg of nicotine/day for 14 days.[4] Nicotine reversed the behavioral deficits and restored the normal response of hippocampal PKC-γ to cholinergic receptor stimulation. Although nicotine acts diffusely in the brain, its effects were, to a large extent regionally specific as PKC-γ in the cerebellum was unaffected by either phenobarbital or nicotine; furthermore, in the hippocampus, the PKC-α isoform unrelated to the behavioral deficits showed no changes. Unlike reversal by manipulating the A10 and similar to neural grafting (see below) the restoration of normalcy was not learning dependent, as grafted animals showed normal performance level from the beginning of testing.

Thus, it is evident that understanding the mechanism enabled reversal of the deficits. This is confirmed by studies published recently that also used pharmacological therapies. Although some of these studies used models of neonatal exposure to insult[25–28] and therefore are less relevant to the present discussion, it should still be remembered that the neonatal period in mice and rats is equivalent to late pregnancy in humans. When early ethanol exposure in rats was applied, there was an induction of NMDA (*N*-methyl-D-aspartate) receptor-mediated excitotoxicity. Identifying this damage enabled its reversal with the NMDA receptor antagonists MK-801[26] or eliprodil.[27] Similarly, deficits in LTP in rats, and thereby in their memory, could be reversed by physical exercises, which lead to enhanced long-term potentiation (LTP) and brain-derived neurotrophic factor (BDNF) in the hippocampus.[29] Phencyclidine (PCP) is known to induce neuro-degeneration, associated with neuro-dysfunction, in the limbic and cortical structures in the rat. Chronic treatment with D-serine, an agonist of the glycine site of the NMDA receptor, normalized cognitive dysfunction in rats by the reactivation of the NMDA receptor.[25] Another example, the dopaminergic (D2) antagonist, haloperidol, is often employed as a model for altering the characteristics of the dopaminergic receptors, which thereby cause alteration in motor function. Exposure to haloperidol during the lactation period normalized the changes induced by prenatal exposure to haloperidol.[30]

Further studies are still required to ascertain whether the effect of nicotine infusion is long-lasting, as were our models of manipulating of the regulating pathways and grafting (see below), or that this model represents a therapy that has to be administered continually without which there is no long-term restoration of normalcy. These studies are necessary, since, in addition to the short-term effect that is typical in the studies cited above, some of the pharmacological therapies did have a long-term effect.[26,27,30]

The length of the pharmacological treatment is another issue that deserves further attention. Whereas our treatment was carried out over an extended period of time, acute nicotine therapy also appeared to be effective in a model of early exposure to lead in rats.[28] Lead exposure, in our opinion, represents a less than adequate model for neurobehavioral teratogenicity, as it remains in the brain and continues to affect it long after its administration has ceased. Moreover, in the study discussed, lead was administered both pre- and postnatally. Despite all of this, acute nicotine therapy reversed cholinergic alteration and their related behavioral deficits induced by early exposure to lead.

Long-lasting reversal therapy could, in some cases, be implemented concomitantly to the developmental insult or to the immediate alteration that follows the exposure.[26,27] This led to the prevention of the ensuing defects. Although, in those studies, the insult was exacted neonatally, this approach appears to have clinically significant potential since it represents an element of prevention, and not merely therapy.

Regardless of the question of duration of the effect of our nicotine therapy, it is significant that this therapy is clinically feasible and can be implemented with an already available tool such as a nicotine patch.[31–33]

Reversal of Neurobehavioral Teratogenicity by Manipulating Regulating Pathways[34–36]

The activity of the septohippocampal cholinergic innervation is regulated, in part, by inhibitory input from the A10 (ventral tegmental area)-septal dopaminergic projection. The innervation with the cholinergic cell bodies in the septum and the diagonal band nuclei is mostly mediated via GABAergic interneurons.[37–39] Destruction of these dopaminergic pathways enhanced the activity of the septohippocampal cholinergic innervation and their related behaviors, including performance in the eight-arm maze.[40] Consistently, in our studies, destruction of the A10-septal dopaminergic projection with 6-hydroxydopamine (6-OHDA) in mice, which reduced septal dopaminergic levels by 70%, induced, presynaptically, an increase in hippocampal choline acetyltransferase (ChAT) and in K^+ stimulated IP formation, the latter suggesting an increase in acetylcholine release. Postsynaptically, there was an increase in muscarinic receptors B_{max}; nevertheless, cholinergic receptor-induced (carbachol stimulated) IP formation was unaffected.[36]

In our model, mice were exposed prenatally to phenobarbital, as described above, resulting in multiple alterations in the hippocampal cholinergic innervation and in the related behavioral deficits. Some of the offspring were injected bilaterally in the septum with 6-OHDA, which reduced their septal dopamine level by 54%. The treatment increased hippocampal ChAT activity, but this affect was unspecific, as it occurred in both prenatally exposed and control groups. Destruction of the regulating A10-septal dopaminergic pathways with 6-OHDA restored normal maze performance in the phenobarbital exposed offspring, which was most marked with increased experience. In the controls the respective behavioral changes were small and did not reach statistical significance, possibly due to the ceiling effect of this behavior.[34] It is suggested that destruction of the A10-septal dopaminergic pathways, which downregulate the septohippocampal cholinergic innervation, enhances the activity of this innervation, which in turn, induces a nonspecific augmentation of the related behavior. The unique features of this therapy are: (*a*) the effects are nonspecific in that the performance of both treated and control offspring was ameliorated, but the effect was more marked in the exposed group where more improvement was possible (ceiling effect); and (*b*) the amelioration was not of restoration of normalcy per se but in the ability to restore normal behavior with experience. Whereas this therapy does not appear to be clinically feasible, it provides a probe for the understanding of the mechanisms of the neurobehavioral teratogenicity.

Reversal of Neurobehavioral Teratogenicity with Grafting of Embryonic, Differentiated, Cholinergic Cells

Mice were exposed prenatally to phenobarbital or heroin, as described above, resulting in multiple alterations in the hippocampal cholinergic innervation and in the related behavioral deficits. At age 35 days, they received a graft of septal, embryonic, cholinergic cells into the teratogen-impaired hippocampus; behavioral and neurochemical evaluation took place 60 days later. The neural grafting restored normal performance in the eight-arm and Morris mazes among the phenobarbital and heroin-exposed offspring.[9,18,41,42] Biochemically, the prenatally induced hyperactivity in the presynaptic component of the hippocampal cholinergic innervation—the choline transporter—was partially reversed by neural grafting.[9] Postsynaptically, the teratogen-induced increase in the number (B_{max}) of cholinergic receptors was reversed by neural grafting; again partially.[42] Downstream from the receptor, neural grafting *completely* restored carbachol-induced IP formation[18] and both basal level and carbachol-induced translocation/activation of PKC.[9] Grafting studies suggest that the more downstream postsynaptic alterations, IP formation and PKC, are more relevant mechanistically to the behavioral deficits than the presynaptic alterations and this notion is supported by correlation studies, which demonstrated higher correlation scores between the behavioral deficits and PKC than for the number of choline transporter sites.[9,18]

Reversal of Neurobehavioral Teratogenicity with Grafting of Neural Progenitors[43]

Grafting of embryonic differentiated nerve cells failed to provide, to date, findings of clinical significance.[44] Stem cells seem to offer great potential for restoration of normalcy in various organ systems, and clinical application appears more feasible than that of grafted differentiated embryonic cells. It has been long assumed that the impaired tissue releases trophic factors, which direct the differentiation of the stem cells to replace or enhance the function of the impaired cells, as was more recently confirmed.[45–49] That is, they will "search and replace" damaged neurons.[50] Based on this assumption, more than a decade ago we grafted totipotent stem cells into the hippocampus in an attempt to establish a model for the reversal of neurobehavioral teratogenicity in mice. However, instead of repairing the damaged hippocampus, the stem cells rapidly developed into a huge teratoma, even larger than the brain itself—as a result of which the mice died.[51]

Recent developments, including the addition of appropriate growth factors into the medium, the choice of the specific origin of the cells, and multiple *in vitro* passages,[52] enabled the production of neural progenitors, which differentiated into nerve cells, this time devoid of the risk of tumor development.[43,45,53] Restoration of normal function by transplantation of neural progenitors was successfully demonstrated in models where the etiology of the defects was previously established, such as animal models for Parkinson's disease[24] or reversal of behavioral deficits related to the hippocampal function.[54] We attempted a similar reversal, but in a model of neurobehavioral birth defects where the reversal was of a specific known damaged process, despite the likely presence of multiple other deficits.

In our model, pregnant female mice were exposed to heroin as described above. The offspring showed deficits in the Morris maze, along with the loss of the PKC-γ and PKC-βII responses to cholinergic stimulation. Mice that were exposed prenatally to heroin and vehicle control mice were then grafted on PN35 with neural progenitors.[43] Importantly, most grafted cells differentiated to astrocytes. Neural progenitors reversed the behavioral deficits and restored the normal response of hippocampal PKC-γ and PKC-βII to cholinergic receptor stimulation. The effects were specific since the PKC-α isoform, which is unrelated to the behavioral deficits, showed almost no changes.

The mechanism by which transplanted neural progenitors restored molecular/biochemical and behavioral function is a subject of the central enigma of stem cell research. It is tempting to claim that the neural progenitors searched and replaced the neurons damaged by the teratogen and restored damaged circuitries, which we believe is at least part of the actuality.[55,56] However, there is an increasing number of studies that, despite having great success in reversing the neurobehavioral deficits, show a low survival rate of the grafted cells.[57] More so, of those which did in fact survive, a high proportion of cells differentiated into glial cell types.[58] Indeed, in our studies, we identified mainly astrocytes in the population of the grafted cells at the time of the neurobehavioral restoration. This apparent paradox can be explained by the fact that grafted neural progenitors can affect behavior via alternative routes than differentiation to neurons. Glial cell culture is known to restore normal behaviors when grafted to the brain,[59] possibly due to the known role of astrocytes in neural function, including the expression of PKC isoforms.[60] Furthermore, grafted neural progenitors possess the ability to create a host environment sufficiently rich in trophic and/or neuroprotective support to enable the rescuing of damaged host cells.[61] An intriguing possibility is that one of the routes by which grafted neural progenitors restore normalcy is the induction of the brain production of endogenous neural progenitors. Indeed, in our recent study, the grafting of neural progenitors increased the production of endogenous neural precursors that migrated to the dentate gyrus of the heroin-exposed offspring by 78% as compared to the heroin sham-grafted group.[62]

CONCLUSION

In conclusion, our studies, as well as studies published by others, show that understanding the mechanism by which the neuroteratogen exerts its effect already enables us to reverse the deficit, at least in an animal model. In turn, the reversal therapies provide a model for elucidating these mechanisms.

Despite acting diffusely in the brain and affecting regions unrelated to the deficits, and despite the fact that their effect is mostly short term, therefore requiring continuous administration, pharmacological therapies will be the most feasible for the near future. This is particularly true of nicotine therapy, which is being shown to be effective in cases such as Alzheimer's disease or in aging.[31–33] Another point in favor of pharmacological therapies is the fact that some of them seem, like grafting, to have a long-lasting effect. Furthermore, in some cases, they even appear to have a preventative effect. Since, of all pharmacological therapies, nicotine therapy is currently the one with the best clinical potential, further studies in that direction will probably prove useful.

At the same time, therapies that involve the grafting of normal cells or the surgical manipulation of regulating pathways seem to be the ultimate therapies of choice since they target the exact defective locus and have long-lasting effect. In this they represent a therapy where the patient is "cured" and does not require any further medical attention. From a clinical point of view, manipulation of the regulating pathways[34] appears to be the least feasible, since it is likely to produce extensive side effects. Grafting of embryonic differentiated cells raised great hopes in the previous decades and worked very well in almost every experimental model, yet failed to produce any clinical benefit.[44] Grafting of stem cells, in our case, neural progenitors, is emerging as promising and works extremely well in a large range of experimental models.[24,54] Its effectiveness in clinical situation is yet to be assessed.

REFERENCES

1. WERBOFF, J. & J.S. GOTTLIER. 1963. Drug in pregnancy: behavioral teratology. Obstet. Gynecol. Surv. **18:** 420–423.
2. HUTCHINGS, D.E. 1978. Behavioral teratology: embryopathic and behavioral effects of drugs during pregancy. *In* Studies on the Development of Behavior and the Nervous System. Vol. 4, Early Influences. G. Gottlieb, Ed.: 7–34. Academic Press. New York.
3. YANAI, J. 1984. Preface. *In* Neurobehavioral Terarology. J. Yanai, Ed.: V–IX. Elsevier. Amsterdam.
4. BEER, A. *et al.* 2005. Nicotine therapy in adulthood reverses the synaptic and behavioral deficits elicited by prenatal exposure to phenobarbital. Neuropsychopharmacology **30:** 156–165.
5. NORDBERG, A. & G. WAHLSTROM. 1980. Acute and chronic effects of barbiturates on regional turnover of acetylcholine in brain. Adv. Exp. Med. Biol. **126:** 165–179.

6. NORDBERG, A. & G. WAHLSTROM. 1992. Cholinergic mechanisms in physical dependence on barbiturates, ethanol and benzodiazepines. J. Neural. Transm. Gen. Sect. **88:** 199–221.
7. KEARNS, I.R. *et al.* 2001. Opioid receptor regulation of muscarinic acetylcholine receptor-mediated synaptic responses in the hippocampus. Neuropharmacology **41:** 565–573.
8. LAPCHAK, P.A., D.M. ARAUJO & B. COLLIER. 1989. Regulation of endogenous acetylcholine release from mammalian brain slices by opiate receptors: hippocampus, striatum and cerebral cortex of guinea-pig and rat. Neuroscience **31:** 313–325.
9. STEINGART, R.A. *et al.* 2000. Neural grafting reverses prenatal drug-induced alterations in hippocampal PKC and related behavioral deficits. Brain Res. Dev. Brain Res. **125:** 9–19.
10. IZRAEL, M. *et al.* 2004. Cholinergic synaptic signaling mechanisms underlying behavioral teratogenicity: effects of nicotine, chlorpyrifos, and heroin converge on protein kinase C translocation in the intermedial part of the hyperstriatum ventrale and on imprinting behavior in an avian model. J. Neurosci. Res. 499–507.
11. KLEINBERGER, N. & J. YANAI. 1985. Early phenobarbital-induced alterations in hippocampal acetylcholinesterase activity and behavior. Brain Res. **354:** 113–123.
12. ROGEL-FUCHS, Y. *et al.* 1992. Hippocampal cholinergic alterations and related behavioral deficits after early exposure to phenobarbital. Brain Res. Bull. **29:** 1–6.
13. STEINGART, R.A. *et al.* 1998. Pre- and postsynaptic alterations in the septohippocampal cholinergic innervations after prenatal exposure to drugs. Brain Res. Bull. **46:** 203–209.
14. KRISTOFIKOVA, Z. *et al.* 1995. (3H)hemicholinium-3 binding sites in postmortem brains of human patients with Alzheimer's disease and multi-infarct dementia. Exp. Gerontol. **30:** 125–136.
15. SIMON, J.R., S. ATWEH & M.J. KUHAR. 1976. Sodium-dependent high affinity choline uptake: a regulatory step in the synthesis of acetylcholine. J. Neurochem. **26:** 909–922.
16. ABU-ROUMI, M., M.E. NEWMAN & J. YANAI. 1996. Inositol phosphate formation in mice prenatally exposed to drugs: relation to muscarinic receptors and postreceptor effects. Brain Res. Bull. **40:** 183–186.
17. YANAI, J. *et al.* 1992. Alterations in septohippocampal cholinergic innervations and related behaviors after early exposure to heroin and phencyclidine. Brain Res. Dev. Brain Res. **69:** 207–214.
18. STEINGART, R.A. *et al.* 2000. Neurobehavioral damage to cholinergic systems caused by prenatal exposure to heroin or phenobarbital: cellular mechanisms and the reversal of deficits by neural grafts. Brain Res. Dev. Brain Res. **122:** 125–133.
19. SHAHAK, H., T.A. SLOTKIN & J. YANAI. 2003. Alterations in PKCγ in the mouse hippocampus after prenatal exposure to heroin: a link from cell signaling to behavioral outcome. Brain Res. Dev. Brain Res. **140:** 117–125.
20. YANIV, S.P., Z. NAOR & J. YANAI. 2004. Prenatal heroin exposure alters cholinergic receptor stimulated translocation and basal levels of the PKCβII and PKCγ isoforms. Brain Res. Bull. **63:** 339–349.

21. Bjorklund, A. & U. Stenevi. 1979. Reconstruction of the nigrostriatal dopamine pathway by intracerebral nigral transplants. Brain Res. **177:** 555–560.
22. Perlow, M.J. *et al.* 1979. Brain grafts reduce motor abnormalities produced by destruction of nigrostriatal dopamine system. Science **204:** 643–647.
23. Wang, X. *et al.* 2004. Distinct efficacy of pre-differentiated versus intact fetal mesencephalon-derived human neural progenitor cells in alleviating rat model of Parkinson's disease. Int. J. Dev. Neurosci. **22:** 175–183.
24. Bjorklund, L.M. *et al.* 2002. Embryonic stem cells develop into functional dopaminergic neurons after transplantation in a Parkinson rat model. Proc. Natl. Acad. Sci. USA **99:** 2344–2349.
25. Andersen, J.D. & B. Pouzet. 2004. Spatial memory deficits induced by perinatal treatment of rats with PCP and reversal effect of D-serine. Neuropsychopharmacology **29:** 1080–1090.
26. Thomas, J.D., S.L. Fleming & E.P. Riley. 2002. Administration of low doses of MK-801 during ethanol withdrawal in the developing rat pup attenuates alcohol's teratogenic effects. Alcohol Clin. Exp. Res. **26:** 1307–1313.
27. Thomas, J.D. *et al.* 2004. Administration of eliprodil during ethanol withdrawal in the neonatal rat attenuates ethanol-induced learning deficits. Psychopharmacology (Berl.) **175:** 189–195.
28. Zhou, M. & J.B. Suszkiw. 2004. Nicotine attenuates spatial learning deficits induced in the rat by perinatal lead exposure. Brain Res. **999:** 142–147.
29. Christie, B.R. *et al.* 2005. Voluntary exercise rescues deficits in spatial memory and long-term potentiation in prenatal ethanol-exposed male rats. Eur. J. Neurosci. **21:** 1719–1726.
30. Wolansky, M.J. *et al.* 2004. Postnatal haloperidol eliminates the deficit in circling behavior produced by prenatal exposure to the same drug. Neurotoxicol. Teratol. **26:** 561–569.
31. White, H.K. & E.D. Levin. 1999. Four-week nicotine skin patch treatment effects on cognitive performance in Alzheimer's disease. Psychopharmacology (Berl.) **143:** 158–165.
32. White, H.K. & E.D. Levin. 2004. Chronic transdermal nicotine patch treatment effects on cognitive performance in age-associated memory impairment. Psychopharmacology (Berl.) **171:** 465–471.
33. Wilson, A.L. *et al.* 1995. Nicotine patches in Alzheimer's disease: pilot study on learning, memory, and safety. Pharmacol. Biochem. Behav. **51:** 509–514.
34. Yanai, J. *et al.* 1989. Dopaminergic denervation reverses behavioral deficits induced by prenatal exposure to phenobarbital. Brain Res. Dev. Brain Res. **48:** 255–261.
35. Yanai, J. *et al.* 1987. CNS changes after early barbiturate exposure: mechanisms and reversal. *In* Functional Teratogenesis. T. Fujii & P. Adams, Eds.: 121–130. Tokyo-University Press. Tokyo.
36. Yanai, J. *et al.* 1993. Septohippocampal cholinergic changes after destruction of the A10-septal dopaminergic pathways. Neuropharmacology **32:** 113–117.
37. Robinson, S.E. *et al.* 1979. Dopaminergic control of the septal-hippocampal cholinergic pathway. J. Pharmacol. Exp. Ther. **208:** 476–479.
38. Costa, E. *et al.* 1983. The transsynaptic regulation of the septal-hippocampal cholinergic neurons. Life Sci. **32:** 165–179.
39. Jaffard, R. *et al.* 1985. The cholinergic septohippocampal pathway, learning and memory. *In* Brain Plasticity Learning and Memory. P. Schmitt & J. Dalrymple-Alford, Eds.: 167–181. Plenum. New York.

40. GALEY, D. *et al.* 1984. Improvement in spontaneous and acquired spatial behaviors following lesions of septal dopaminergic afferents in mice: possible relations with hippocampal cholinergic activity. C. R. Acad. Sci. III. **299:** 681–686.
41. YANAI, J. & C.G. PICK. 1988. Neuron transplantation reverses phenobarbital-induced behavioral birth defects in mice. Int. J. Dev. Neurosci. **6:** 409–416.
42. ROGEL-FUCHS, Y., E.A. ZAHALKA & J. YANAI. 1994. Reversal of early phenobarbital-induced cholinergic and related behavioral deficits by neuronal grafting. Brain Res. Bull. **33:** 273–279.
43. YANAI, J. *et al.* 2005. Neural progenitors for the reversal of heroin neurobehavioral teratogenicity. Proceedings of the 3rd Annual Meeting of the International Society for Stem Cell Research 259.
44. HAGELL, P. *et al.* 2002. Dyskinesias following neural transplantation in Parkinson's disease. Nat. Neurosci. **5:** 627–628.
45. BEN-HUR, T. *et al.* 2003. Transplanted multipotential neural precursor cells migrate into the inflamed white matter in response to experimental autoimmune encephalomyelitis. Glia **41:** 73–80.
46. BRUSTLE, O., U. MASKOS & R.D. MCKAY. 1995. Host-guided migration allows targeted introduction of neurons into the embryonic brain. Neuron **15:** 1275–1285.
47. BEN-HUR, T. *et al.* 2003. Effects of proinflammatory cytokines on the growth, fate, and motility of multipotential neural precursor cells. Mol. Cell Neurosci. **24:** 623–631.
48. STUMM, R.K. *et al.* 2003. CXCR4 regulates interneuron migration in the developing neocortex. J. Neurosci. **23:** 5123–5130.
49. BAGRI, A. *et al.* 2002. The chemokine SDF1 regulates migration of dentate granule cells. Development **129:** 4249–4260.
50. BULTE, J.W. *et al.* 2003. MR microscopy of magnetically labeled neurospheres transplanted into the Lewis EAE rat brain. Magn. Reson. Med. **50:** 201–205.
51. YANAI, J. *et al.* 1995. Embryonic cultures but not embryos transplanted to the mouse's brain grow rapidly without immunosuppression. Int. J. Neurosci. **81:** 21–26.
52. BEN-HUR, T., O. EINSTEIN & J.W. BULTE. 2005. Stem cell therapy for myelin diseases. Curr. Drug Targets **6:** 3–19.
53. REUBINOFF, B.E. *et al.* 2001. Neural progenitors from human embryonic stem cells. Nat. Biotechnol. **19:** 1134–1140.
54. JELTSCH, H. *et al.* 2003. Transplantation of neurospheres after granule cell lesions in rats: cognitive improvements despite no long-term immunodetection of grafted cells. Behav. Brain Res. **143:** 177–191.
55. ENGLUND, U. *et al.* 2002. Grafted neural stem cells develop into functional pyramidal neurons and integrate into host cortical circuitry. Proc. Natl. Acad. Sci. USA **99:** 17089–17094.
56. SNYDER, E.Y. & J.F. LORING. 2005. A role for stem cell biology in the physiological and pathological aspects of aging. J. Am. Geriatr. Soc. **53:** S287–S291.
57. TODA, H. *et al.* 2001. Grafting neural stem cells improved the impaired spatial recognition in ischemic rats. Neurosci. Lett. **316:** 9–12.
58. ZHANG, H. *et al.* 2004. Elevation of NMDAR after transplantation of neural stem cells. Neuroreport **15:** 1739–1743.
59. BRADBURY, E.J. *et al.* 1995. Astrocyte transplants alleviate lesion induced memory deficits independently of cholinergic recovery. Neuroscience **65:** 955–972.

60. Van der Zee, E.A., P.G. Luiten & J.F. Disterhoft. 1997. Learning-induced alterations in hippocampal PKC-immunoreactivity: a review and hypothesis of its functional significance. Prog. Neuropsychopharmacol. Biol. Psychiatry **21:** 531–572.
61. Ourednik, J. *et al.* 2002. Neural stem cells display an inherent mechanism for rescuing dysfunctional neurons. Nat. Biotechnol. **20:** 1103–1110.
62. Yanai, J., T. Ben-Hur & T. Ben-Shaanan. 2006. Transplantation of neural progenitors into the brain of mice exposed prenatally to heroin induces proliferation of endogenous neural precursors. Neurotoxicol. Teratol. In Press.

Index of Contributors